Fifteen Years of Clinical Experience
with Hydroxyapatite Coatings
in Joint Arthroplasty

[handwritten inscription]

_With my compliments
to the leaders_

[signature]

_2004_

Springer

Paris
Berlin
Heidelberg
New York
Hong Kong
London
Milan
Tokyo

Jean-Alain Epinette, MD
Michael T. Manley, PhD

Fifteen Years of Clinical Experience with Hydroxyapatite Coatings in Joint Arthroplasty

Preface by Rudolph G.T. Geesink, MD, PhD

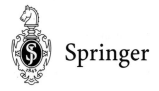 Springer

Jean-Alain Epinette, MD
Clinique Médico-Chirurgicale
200, rue d'Auvergne
62700 Bruay-Labuissière
France

Michael T. Manley, PhD
12-A Chestnut Street
Ridgewood, NJ 07450
USA

ISBN : 2-287-00508-0

SPIN: 10909850

Cover design: Nadia Ouddane

Scientific Advisory Board

BAUER Thomas W, MD, PhD
CAPELLO William N, MD
D'ANTONIO James A, MD
GEESINK Rudolph GT, MD, PhD
OONISHI Hironobu, MD, PhD
TONI Aldo, MD
TONINO Alfons J, MD, PhD
WALTER William K, MB, BS, FRCS, FRACS

Contributors

ADREY José, ARGENSON Jean-Noël, AUBANIAC Jean-Manuel, BALAY Bruno,
BARRACK Robert L, BARRERE Florence, BAUER Thomas W,
BERTEAUX Daniel, BORDINI Barbara, BRYANT Dawanna R,
CABANELA Miguel E, CAPELLO William N, CARTIER Philippe,
CHATELET Jean-Christophe, COOK Stephen D, D'ANTONIO James A,
DACULSI Gérard, DAMBREVILLE Alain, DE GROOT Klass, DELÉCRIN Joël,
DEPREZ Pascal, DHERT Wouter JA, DUMBLETON John,
DUTHOIT Etienne, EPINETTE Jean-Alain, ETTORE Pierre-Paul,
FUJIBAYASHI Shunsuke, FUJITA Hiroshi, GACON Gérard, GEESINK Rudolph GT,
GEORGE Marc, GIUNTI Armando, GOALARD Christian, GUERRA Enrico,
HABIBOVIC Pamela, HIVART Philippe, HUSSEIN Rami, JAFFE William L,
KEAST-BUTLER Oliver, LEVINE Harlan B,
LEYVRAZ Pierre-François, MANLEY Michael T., MASSIN Philippe,
MEIJERS Will, MORRIS Haydn, MUELLER Marion, NAKAMURA Takashi,
NOURISSAT Christian, OONISHI Hironobu, OOSTERBOS Kees JM,
OVERGAARD Søren, PASSUTI Norbert, PETER Bastian, PETIT Roland,
PHILIPPE Michel P, PIOLETTI Dominique P, RAHBEK Ole, RAHMY Ali,
RAKOTOMANANA Lalao R, RAY André, RUBIN Pascal, SANCHEZ-SOTELO Joaquin,
SCHAAFSMA Jelle, SEREKIAN Paul, SETIEY Louis, SHEPPERD John,
SIVERHUS Scott W, SØBALLE Kjeld, STEA Susanna, SUDANESE Alessandra,
SUTTON Kate, TAKAI Shinro, TAKIKAWA Satoshi, THÉRIN Michel, TILLIE Bruno,
TONI Aldo, TONINO Alfons J, TRAINA Francesco, TSUTSUMI Sadami,
VAN DER LINDE Mathijs, VIDALAIN Jean-Pierre,
VOGELY Charles H., WALTER William K, WITPEERD Wendy D,
YOSHINO Nobuyuki, YOUNG David

Contributors

Adrey José, MD
Clinique Saint-Roch
5 rue Gerhardt
34000 Montpellier
France

Argenson Jean-Noël, MD
Aix-Marseille University
Department of Orthopaedic Surgery
Hôpital Sainte Marguerite
13009 Marseille
France

Aubaniac Jean-Manuel, MD
Aix-Marseille University
Department of Orthopaedic Surgery
Hôpital Sainte Marguerite
13009 Marseille
France

Balay Bruno, MD
Clinique Chirurgicale du Beaujolais
Route de Longsard
69400 Arnas
France

Barrack Robert L., MD
Professor of Orthopaedic Surgery
Director, Adult Reconstructive Surgery
Department of Orthopaedic Surgery
Tulane University School of Medicine
1430 Tulane Avenue, SL-32
New Orleans, Louisiana 70112
USA

Barrère Florence, PhD
IsoTis NV
P.O. Box 98
3720 AB Bilthoven
The Netherlands

Bauer Thomas W., MD, PhD
Departments of Pathology and Orthopedic Surgery
The Cleveland Clinic Foundation
Cleveland, Ohio, 44195
USA

Berteaux Daniel, MD
Clinique de la Présentation
64 bis rue des Fossés
45400 Fleury-les-Aubrais
France

Bordini Barbara, B Sci
Laboratorio Tecnologia Medca
Istituto Codivilla Putti
Via di Barbiano 1-10
40136 Bologna
Italy

Bryant Dawanna R., CFA
The Toledo Joint Replacement & Orthopaedic
Center
2000 Regency Court
Suite 201
Toledo, Ohio 43623
USA

Cabanela Miguel E., MD
Department of Orthopedic Surgery
Mayo Clinic, 200 First St., S.W., Rochester MN 55905
USA

Capello William N., MD
Indiana University School of Medicine
542 Clinical Drive
Room 600
Indianapolis, IN 46202
USA

Cartier Philippe, MD
Clinique des Lilas
41-49 avenue du Maréchal Juin
93260 Les Lilas
France

Chatelet Jean-Christophe, MD
Polyclinique du Beaujolais
380 Route de Longsard
69400 Arnas
France

Cook Stephen D., PhD
Lee C. Schlesinger Professor
Director, Orthopaedic Research
Department of Orthopaedic Surgery
Tulane University School of Medicine
1430 Tulane Avenue, SL-32
New Orleans, Louisiana 70112
USA

D'Antonio James A., MD
Sewickley Valley Hospital
725 Cherrington Parkway, Suite 200
Moon Township, PA 15108
USA

Daculsi Gérard, PhD
Laboratoire de Recherche Biomatériaux-Tissus Calcifiés
Faculté de Chirurgie Dentaire
Université de Nantes
I, Place Alexis Ricordeau
44042 Nantes
France

Dambreville Alain, MD
21 avenue Jean Lorrain
06300 Nice
France

De Groot Klass, PhD
Biomaterials Research Group
School of Medicine
Leiden University
Rijnsburgerwerg 10
2333 AA, Leiden
The Netherlands

Delécrin Joël, PhD
Laboratoire de Recherche Biomatériaux-Tissus Calcifiés
Faculté de Chirurgie Dentaire
Université de Nantes
I, Place Alexis Ricordeau
44042 Nantes
France

Deprez Pascal, PhD
Centre d'Application des Lasers Flandres Artois (CALFA)
Université d'Artois
62400 Béthune
France

Dhert Wouter JA, PhD
Department of Orthopaedics,
University Medical Center
Utrecht
The Netherlands

Dumbleton John, DSCi, PhD
512 East Saddle River Road
Ridgewood, NJ 07450
USA

Duthoit Etienne, MD
Polyclinique de Hénin-Beaumont
Route de Courrières
B. P. 199
62256 Hénin Beaumont Cedex
France

Epinette Jean-Alain, MD
Clinique Médico-Chirurgicale
200 rue d'Auvergne
62700 Bruay-Labuissière
France

Ettore Pierre-Paul, MD
Aix-Marseille University
Department of Orthopaedic Surgery
Hôpital Sainte Marguerite
13009 Marseille
France

Fujibayashi Shunsuke, MD, PhD
Department of Orthopaedic Surgery
Kyoto University
Faculty of Medicine
54, Kawara-Machi, Shogoin
Sakyo-ku
Kyoto 606-8507
Japan

Fujita Hiroshi, MD, PhD
H. Oonishi Memorial Joint Replacement
Institute
Tominaga Hospital
4-48, 1 Chome, Minato-Machi, Naniwa-ku
Osaka-Shi, 556-0017
Japan

Gacon Gérard, MD
Centre d'Evaluation André Hermann
Fournitures Hospitalières
ZA de Mulhouse-Heimbrunn
68990 Heimsbrunn
France

Geesink Rudolph GT, MD, PhD
University Hospital Maastricht
Dept. of Orthopaedics
Peter Debyelaan 25
6202 AZ Maastricht
The Netherlands

George Marc, FRCS
Guy's Hospital
St. Thomas Street
London SE1 9RT
England

Giunti Armando, MD
Orthopaedic Department of Bologna University
Istituti Ortopedico Rizzoli
Via Pupilli 1
40136 Bologna
Italy

Goalard Christian, MD
Clinique Saint-roch
5 rue Gerhardt
34000 Montpellier
France

Guerra Enrico, MD
1st Orthopaedic Department
Istituti Ortopedici Rizzoli
Via Pupilli 1
40136 Bologna
Italy

Habibovic Pamela, B Eng
IsoTis NV
PO Box 98
3720 AB Bilthoven
The Netherlands

Hivart Philippe, PhD
Laboratoire d'Automatique et de Mécanique Industrielle et
Humaines (LAMIH)
59300 Valenciennes
France

Hussein Rami, FRCS
Department Orthopaedic Surgery
Conquest Hospital
East Sussex
England

Jaffe William L, MD
1095 Park Avenue
New York, NY 10128
USA

Keast-Butler Oliver, MRCS
Department Orthopaedic Surgery
Conquest Hospital
East Sussex
England

Kim Seok Cheol, MD, PhD
H. Oonishi Memorial Joint Replacement Institute
Tominaga Hospital
4-48, 1-Chome, Minato-Machi, Naniwa-Ku,
Osaka-Shi, 556-0017
Japan

Levine Harlan B. MD
NYU-Hospital for Joint Diseases
Resident, Department of Orthopaedic Surgery
301 E. 17th Street, 14th Floor
New York, NY 10003
USA

Leyvraz Pierre-François, MD
Hôpital Orthopédique de la Suisse Romande
Lausanne
Switzerland

Manley Michael T, PhD
12-A Chestnut Street
Ridgewood, NJ 07450
USA

Massin Philippe, MD
Service de Chirurgie Orthopédique
49100 CHU Angers
France

Meijers Will, MD
Department of Orthopaedies and Traumatology
Atrium Medisch Centrum
Postbus 4446
6401 CX Heerlen
The Netherlands

Morris Haydn, FRACS FA OrthA
Suite 80, 8th Floor
166 Gipps Street
East Melbourne 3002
Victoria
Australia

Mueller Marion. FRCS
Royal Sussex County Hospital,
Eastern Road, Brighton,
Sussex BN2 5BE
England

Nakamura Takashi, MD, PhD
Department of Orthopaedic Surgery
Kyoto University
Faculty of Medicine
54, Kawara-Machi, Shogoin
Sakyo-ku
Kyoto 606-8507
Japan

Nourissat Christian, MD
Clinique Ollier
75 rue G. Giraud
42300 Roanne
France

Oonishi Hironobu, MD, PhD
H. Oonishi Memorial Joint Replacement Institute,
Tominaga Hospital,
4-48, 1-Chome, Minato-Machi, Naniwa-Ku,
Osaka-Shi, 556-0017.
Japan

Oosterbos Kees JM, MD
Department of orthopaedics
Atrium Medisch Centrum
PO Box 4446
6401 CX Heerlen
The Netherlands

Overgaard Søren, MD, PhD
Department of Orthopaedic Surgery,
Aarhus University Hospital
Aarhus Amtssygehus
DK-8000 Aarhus C
Denmark

Passuti Norbert, MD
Laboratoire de Recherche Biomatériaux-Tissus Calcifiés
Faculté de Chirurgie Dentaire
Université de Nantes
I, Place Alexis Ricordeau
44042 Nantes
France

Peter Bastian, DSCi
Hôpital Orthopédique de la Suisse Romande
& Biomedical Engineering Laboratory
Swiss Federal Institute of Technology
1015 Lausanne
Switzerland

Petit Roland, MD
Clinique Saint-Sauveur
1 rue du Bourg
68100 Mulhouse
France

Philippe Michel P., MD
Clinique Saint Gérard
Avenue J.H. Fabre
84200 Carpentras
France

Pioletti Dominique P., PhD
Hôpital Orthopédique de la Suisse Romande
& Biomedical Engineering Laboratory
Swiss Federal Institute of Technology
1015 Lausanne
Switzerland

Rahbek Ole, MD, PhD
Department of Orthopaedic Surgery,
Aarhus University Hospital
Aarhus Amtssygehus
DK-8000 Aarhus C
Denmark

Rahmy Ali JA, MD
Department of orthopaedics
Atrium Medisch Centrum
PO Box 4446
6401 CX Heerlen
The Netherlands

Rakotomanana Lalao R., PhD
IRMAR
Université de Rennes I
35000 Rennes
France

Ray André, MD
85-87 Boulevard des Belges
69450 Lyon
France

Rubin Pascal, PhD
Hôpital Orthopédique de la Suisse Romande
Lausanne
Switzerland

Sanchez-Sotelo Joaquin, MD, PhD
Department of Orthopedic Surgery
Hospital Universitario La Paz
Madrid
Spain

Schaafsma Jelle, MD
Department of Orthopaedies and Traumatology
Atrium Medisch Centrum
Postbus 4446
6401 CX Heerlen
The Netherlands

Serekian Paul, MS
5 Aspen Court
Mahwah, New Jersey 07430
USA

Setiey Louis, MD
Polyclinique du Beaujolais
380 Route de Longsard
69400 Arnas
France

Shepperd John, FRCS
Department Orthopaedic Surgery
Conquest Hospital
The Ridge - St Leonards-on-Sea
East Sussex TN37 7RD
England

Siverhus Scott W., MD
The Toledo Joint Replacement & Orthopaedic
Center
2000 Regency Court - Suite 201
Toledo, Ohio 43623
USA

Søballe Kjeld, MD, PhD
Department of Orthopaedic Surgery,
Aarhus University Hospital
Aarhus Amtssygehus
DK-8000 Aarhus C
Denmark

Stea Susanna, B Sci
Laboratorio Tecnologia Medca
Istituto Codivilla Putti
Via di Barbiano 1-10
40136 Bologna
Italy

Sudanese Alessandra, MD
1st Orthopaedic Department
Istituti Ortopedici Rizzoli
Via Pupilli 1
40136 Bologna
Italy

Sutton Kate, MA
Advanced Technology
300 Commerce Court
Mahwah, NJ 07430
USA

Takai Shinro, MD, PhD
Department of Orthopaedic Surgery
Kyoto Prefectural University of Medicine
Kyoto
Japan

Takikawa Satoshi, MD, PhD
Departments of Pathology and Orthopedic Surgery
The Cleveland Clinic Foundation
Cleveland, Ohio, 44195
USA

Thérin Michel, MD
Cogent
69400 Villefranche sur Saône
France

Tillie Bruno, MD
Clinique Bon Secours
9, Place de la Préfecture
62000 Arras
France

Toni Aldo, MD
Orthopaedic Department
Istituti Ortopedici Rizzoli
Via Pupilli 1
40136 Bologna
Italy

Tonino Alfons J, MD, PhD
Department of orthopaedics
Atrium Medisch Centrum
PO Box 4446
6401 CX Heerlen
The Netherlands

Traina Francesco, MD
1st Orthopaedic Department
Istituti Ortopedici Rizzoli
Via Pupilli 1
40136 Bologna
Italy

Tsutsumi Sadami, PhD
Department of Medical Simulation Engineering
Institute for Frontier Medical Science
Kyoto University,
Kyoto,
Japan

Van der Linde Mathijs, MD
Department of Orthopaedies and Traumatology
Atrium Medisch Centrum
Postbus 4446
6401 CX Heerlen
The Netherlands

Vidalain Jean-Pierre, MD
Clinique du Lac
22, rue André Theuriet
74000 Annecy
France

Vogely Charles H, MD, PhD
Department of Orthopaedics
University Medical Center
Utrecht
The Netherlands

Walter William K, MB, BS, FRCS, FRACS
Level 3
100 Bay Road
Waverton
New South Wales
Australia

Witpeerd Wendy D
Department of Orthopaedics and Traumatology
Atrium Medisch Centrum
Postbus 4446
6401 CX Heerlen
The Netherlands

Yoshino Nobuyuki MD, PhD
Department of Orthopaedic Surgery
Kyoto Kujo Hospital
Kyoto
Japan

Young David, FRACS FA OrthA
Melbourne Orthopaedic Group
33, The Avenue Windsor
3181 Victoria
Australia

Foreword

Ronald J. Furlong of the United Kingdom performed the first clinical implantation of a hydroxyapatite-coated (HA) hip implant in 1985, about 18 years ago. This was followed in 1986 by other HA clinical implantations conducted by the ARTRO Group in France and Rudolf Geesink in the Netherlands. Following these pioneers, many thousands of HA-coated hip implants of various designs, from various implant manufacturers, have been implanted worldwide, by many surgeons at many institutions. The coating technology has expanded to include the revision setting in the hip, as well as unicompartmental knees, total knees, shoulders, and an assortment of minor joint implants.

In the early 1990s, we were both involved in the compilation of texts summarizing the application and function of hydroxyapatite coatings, together with the findings of favorable bone adaptation and favorable biological response to the material achieved *in vivo*. These volumes, *Hydroxyapatite Coatings in Orthopaedic Surgery, Rudolph G.T. Geesink and Michael T. Manley eds. Raven Press Ltd 1993*, together with *Hydroxyapatite Coated Hip and Knee Arthroplasty, Jean-Alain Epinette and Rudolph G.T. Geesink eds. the French Orthopaedic Society 1995*, included the early clinical results with hydroxyapatite-coated hip implants that were the results available at the time of writing. Since the publication of these volumes, many reports of clinical results with HA-coated hip implants and HA-coated knee implants have appeared in the orthopaedic literature. Clinical follow-up of about fifteen years is available now in the hip, and ten years follow-up is available in the knee. With host response data of fifteen years now available, we felt that the time was right to ask various investigators worldwide to report the current clinical results with their HA-coated implants of choice, and then to collect these manuscripts into a single volume. We trust that this compilation of results will answer the question of whether the favorable results achieved in the short term with this method of biologic fixation of total joint implants has withstood the test of time.

Our thanks are due to the authors of chapters in this volume for the effort they made to write and submit their work to us in a timely fashion. These authors, working in Europe, the United States, Japan, and Australia, do not all use English as their first language. Many made great efforts to provide us with English language documents. Where we felt the language was unclear, we made only those minor changes needed to facilitate understanding. For manuscripts submitted in a language other than English, we employed professional interpretation, and then made editorial changes if the content was unclear to us. We trust our editorial efforts have not changed the intent of the authors. In addition, each member of our Scientific Committee used their expertise to give further feedback to us. We wish to congratulate and thank each of them for this effort on our behalf. We also wish to thank Kate Sutton, MA, for her many hours of work in editing the copy of our volume. Without her help, we would never have finished this task.

Finally, we should state that results with implants manufactured by many companies are included in this volume. Our intent was simply to determine if the use of hydroxyapatite coatings for the fixation of orthopaedic implants to bone, so fascinating to us in the late 1980s, has been proven by the survivorship and satisfaction of those patients receiving hip and knee implants of the various designs described herein. We trust this monograph will be of value to researchers and to orthopaedic surgeons interested in joint replacement, and will allow them to form their own educated opinion about the utility of hydroxyapatite coatings for implant fixation.

Jean-Alain Epinette, MD

Michael T. Manley, PhD

By the authors' request, all royalties will be given to "Médecins Sans Frontières-Doctors Without Borders".

Preface

Total hip arthroplasty has been with us now for more than forty years. Since the pioneering years of Sir John Charnley, significant improvements have been achieved through better understanding of the inter-relationship between biomaterials, biomechanics, and biology. For example, structural improvements in the cement mantle were derived as cementing technique evolved from first generation to third generation methods. Modern cemented total hip arthroplasty now gives us excellent clinical results and long term implant survival, especially in elderly people. For younger patients, improvement in implant longevity was more difficult to achieve. Demands from ever younger and more active patients tended to exceed the limited mechanical properties and lifetime of acrylic bone cement. This limitation stimulated the development of alternative cementless techniques of implant fixation.

The first generation of cementless fixation included plain press-fit type implants. Without sufficient biological anchoring in bone to counteract the load-bearing forces imposed by patient activity, micro-motion between implant and bone caused bone resorbtion which contributed to complete implant loosening. However important the geometrical design of the implant may be for the initial mechanical stability of the implant in the bone, some type of stable implant-bone interface was necessary to prevent implant-bone micro-motion.

Fixation by bone ingrowth into porous-metal coatings was a development of the 1980s. Theoretical and experimental foundations were very promising. Pioneering work by Pilliar and Engh in the United States as well as Boutin, Judet and Lord in Europe contributed much to the development of cementless implants. These authors reported successful applications in many patient populations, but emphasized the need for accurate instrumentation and surgical technique. Generally, clinical results using porous-metal coatings were however rather variable and sometimes disappointing because of bead shedding, thigh-pain and unacceptable loosening rates. The causes of loosening were to be found in the inadequate biological profile of the materials involved, although this has improved considerably in the last decade. Bone ingrowth using porous-metal coatings takes a long time period for implant stabilization. Accuracy of

bone preparation and immobilization of the implant in the bone during the ingrowth period was critical to success. Improved biological surface characteristics were needed to overcome these problems.

About twenty years ago, the interesting biological profile of calcium-phosphate ceramics and its potential for implant fixation became evident, at first in dental implants, later on in orthopaedics. Through the pioneering work of Klaas de Groot of the Leiden Biomaterials Research Group, the hydroxyapatite coating technique was adapted for orthopaedic applications. Experimental studies were conducted by the author proving the excellent capability of calcium-phosphate coatings to provide a stable bony interface even under less than optimal conditions. Within the large group of calcium-phosphate materials, hydroxyapatite was and still is the most attractive choice because of its natural occurrence in bone, its well-documented biocompatibility and its reliability in establishing a stable bony interface *in vivo*. First human applications of HA-coatings in orthopaedics were reported both by Furlong and by me in 1986. Since 1987 I have enjoyed a close collaboration with Jean-Alain Epinette, one of the pioneers of HA-coatings in France. Other study teams originated in France, such as the ARTRO and ABG groups, also made significant contributions to the use of HA-coatings in orthopaedic surgery as did Michael Manley in the US. Current follow-up data suggest that HA-coatings can indeed retain reliable long term implant stability and function. The clinical results remain excellent up to current 15 year follow-up and pain rates remain very low.

Over the past two decades, numerous studies have provided an almost exponential increase in knowledge on HA-coatings in orthopaedics. This book is a welcome summary of the work so far. Some controversies still remain. Should coatings be easily resorbable or more permanent, should they be thick or thin, single phase or multiphase calcium phosphates? Today we know that HA-coatings will be transformed by osteoclastic activity and actively take part in the bone remodeling process of the bone around the implant. We know that thin (50-60 micron) HA coatings are very gradually degraded over a long period of time and the body can easily cope with the physiological material released without any tissue overload by debris and risk of osteolysis. We know that thicker coatings may suffer mechanical delamination from the implant in a short time period. We do not know if the clearance mechanisms are able to remove this debris or whether (as animal data suggests) the debris simply becomes encapsulated by bone. Some of these answers only may become apparent after many years of clinical follow-up with proper documentation of results. We know now that with the thin HA coatings, clinical results, bone adaptation and implant survivorship remain excellent at twelve to fifteen year follow-up. Only time can tell us whether this favorable trend will continue into longer term (twenty plus years) results. May this book provide a moment of contemplation on current knowledge before we continue our journey to further perfection of artificial joint reconstructions.

Rudolph GT Geesink MD, PhD

Contents

I – Introduction

II – Basic Science: Histology & Experimental Works

III – Bioactive Coatings: Clinical Works

IV – Clinical Experiences in Primary Hips at a Minimum of 10 Years

V – Hydroxyapatite in Hip Revision Surgery

VI – Clinical Experience with Hydroxyapatite Knee Implants at a minimum of 10 years

VII – Clinical Overview, Outcomes, and Perspectives in Bioactive Coatings

INTRODUCTION

1   The Early Biological History of Calcium Phosphates

John Shepperd, FRCS, MD

Calcium phosphate coatings on metal implants may seem to be avant garde innovation. However, the principal is based on events which take us back to the very dawn of life. Mineral provides the compressive strength for fundamentals such as teeth to eat with, exo or endoskeletons to walk with, and shells for protection. Small, shelly fossils exist in the lowest Cambrian series and mark the first appearance of skeletal parts (1).

The earliest life forms on our planet were monocellular algae and microbes. During the Precambrian epoch, multicellular organisms appeared in what has become known as the metazoan "explosion" (2). This "cladogenesis" is believed to have occurred up to a billion years ago, but the transition between Precambrian and Cambrian is marked by a spectacular increase in fossil records of complex animals. This remained a puzzle for Darwin that went with him to his grave. A contributing explanation for so many apparently new species was the key evolutionary development of biomineralisation, simply because it incidentally helps fossils to survive (3) (fig. 1).

The first vertebrates are found in 530 million years old fossil records from the Yunnan province in China (4). A protracted intense ice age in the late Precambrian epoch may have triggered this development, coupled with stabilisation of the atmosphere and environment (5) The epoch transition at this time saw oxygen levels on the planet increase. The continental land masses became identifiable with the present day, and a staggering array of sophisticated marine creatures appeared in the shallow seas (6). Thus, biological applications of calcium salts occur in fossil records of 500 million years ago (7).

These remarkable events evolved in a marine chemical environment. Normal physiology relies on the carbonate pool for respiratory reserve and

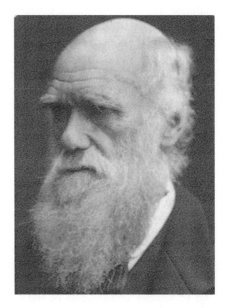

Figure 1 – Charles Darwin was mystified by Cambian explosion largely the result of biomineralisation and better fossil survival.

buffering, whereas phosphate can be committed to endoskeletal deposition. This possibly explains the fact that exoskeletons and shells are mainly calcium carbonate, and endoskeleton, enamel, dentine, and renal calculi are mainly calcium phosphates.

It is not clear whether the apatite per se has particular mechanical benefits. Carbonates are present in bone and phosphates in shells. Furthermore, normal bone has a range of phosphate forms and is by no means exclusively apatite (8). In bone, the apatite is mainly in carbonated form, with limited presence of the hydroxyl radical (9). Calcium and phosphates exist in serum at super saturation levels. In these conditions, well configured molecules bind together in close apposition, based on the physical and surface charge arrangement – a phenomenon known as epitaxy, which is responsible for all crystal formation. That calcium doesn't precipitate throughout the tissues rather than just in bone is possibly the result of the solute properties of plasma proteins (10). Solubility also rises with lowering of pH. In order to create selective precipitation of calcium phosphate at appropriate sites, specialised cell functions are required that adjust pH and possibly adjust concentrations.

The organic component of bone is mainly collagen, and provides the tensile strength of the composite material. However, it seems probable that specialised proteins within osteoid produced by osteoblasts form an epitaxial or even chemical bond with calcium apatite. All this activity is under local and systemic hormone control, which raises the question of how coatings work on metal orthopaedic implants. Local bone morphogenesis requires organisation of osteoclastic and osteoblastic cells (11). Cytokine release caused by preparation of the bone bed is a key factor. Matrix bound BMPs are generated in the surgical broaching process, which leads to recruitment of osteoblasts from marrow osteoprogenic lines, and osteoclasts from monocyte and phagiocytic cells (12). Sheets of cells are known to accumulate rapidly on a calcium apatite sprayed surface, and it is clear that several control mechanisms are involved. Included are morphology of a surface, boundary dissolution of soluble components of the calcium phosphate material, and presence of the pure apatite form. Nevertheless, regardless of the purity of the calcium apatite powder entering the reservoir on a plasma spray gun, about thirty percent is altered by the heat transport and sintering process (13).

The term apatite was coined in 1788 by the German geologist Abraham Werner (1750-1817) (14) to describe a range of Phosphate minerals that are now the major global source of phosphorous. In the same year, the French chemist Joseph-Louis Proust (1754-1826) and another German chemist Martin Klaproth (1743-1817) proposed that calcium apatite was the major inorganic component of bone. In the 19th century, several surgeons used plaster of Paris (calcium sulphate) as a bone filling substitute, notably the astonishingly innovative Themistocles Gluck (1853-1942) (fig. 2). Gluck was arguably a "Leonardo da Vinci" of orthopaedics at the time who, amongst his range of contributions, described joint replacement in a treatise in 1891 in which he reported the use of ivory

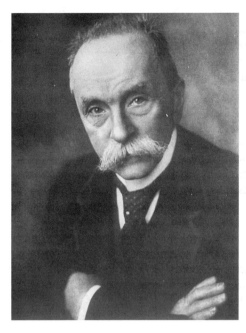

Figure 2 – Themistocles Gluck.

devices (virtually pure calcium apatite) bedded in a calcium sulphate based cement (15). This first attempt at bone cement may have been nearer the biological mark than subsequent plastic successors. Sadly though, overly ambitious surgery for the time, and probably poor patient selection, guaranteed disastrous results ; Gluck was ejected from his chair of surgery in Berlin as a discredit to German science. In 1892, Greaseman used calcium sulphate as a bone filler at the Trendelenberg clinic in Berlin, (16) and in 1922, following animal studies, Albee reported a series of forearm fractures in which he used tricalcium phosphate as a bone healing enhancer (17, 18) with allegedly good results. Hey-Groves in 1927 described pure ivory hip hemiarthroplasty for fracture the principle mineral of which is dense calcium apatite (19). Ivory devices were, and indeed still are, used quite widely, with impressive evidence of bonding. An example resides in the archive display cabinet of the British Orthopaedic Association.

During the 1950s, interest developed in the dental materials community regarding the possible application of synthetic calcium hydroxyapatite (20). With the potential benefits of exceptional biocompatibility and active bonding to osteoid, this led to accounts in 1968 of enhancement of alveolar ridges in animal experiments (21). Investigators of this component of bone metabolism increased during the 1970s, with major contributions from, Jarcho 1977 Newesley, Osborne and co-workers 1978 (22-26). Interest continued, particularly in the dental community. The ability to achieve a sintered coat of apatite on a metal substrate using the industrial process of plasma spraying offered the prospect of implant fixation.

In 1981, at St. Thomas' Hospital London, we used a plasma-sprayed, HA-coated implant for an underpinning system (fig. 3), based on information from the dental department at the London Hospital. This may have been the first orthopaedic application of the technology. During the early 1980s much laboratory work was reported, notably by Geesink in Maastricht, who undertook animal studies suggesting that fixation was transformed by coating when compared with an identical uncoated device. Several other workers confirmed these findings, including Søballe, who revealed an even more striking advantage when a prosthesis was loaded (27-32). Osborne commenced a collaboration with Furlong in 1983 (33, 34). They produced an HA-coated hip replacement, the first of which was used clinically by Furlong in 1985 (fig. 4). His femoral implant was fully coated with a 200 micron thick layer of ceramic. It had a proximal cone and distal round stem. The acetabulum had a hemispherical form with rim screw fixation. In 1986, Geesink in Maastricht, followed in 1987 by Epinette, began using a minimally modified version of the Ultrafix device intended for cemented application, namely the Omnifit. The stem was partially coated with an 60 micron thick layer of HA, and there were various acetabulum designs. In France during the same year, the Artro group developed a fully sprayed version of the Landos device. Two years later, another French group working with Howmedica produced

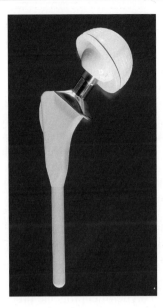

Figure 4 – The Furlong HA-coated stem.

the ABG. All of these devices included varying technologies and expertise for the spraying techniques, as well as a wide variation of implant design (35). Although each claimed the benefits of their own concepts, such claims were all anecdotal and unproven. The present volume provides an opportunity to establish the validity up to 17 years later. All these innovations of the 1980s mean that we have now accumulated a considerable range of clinical series for hip replacement devices halfway through the second decade of follow up. These include full or partial coating, thicknesses from 60 to 200 microns, sprayed in air or a vacuum, and differing claims as to the superior purity of the apatite crystals (although there is no clear evidence to suggest that this particularly matters). In addition, the implant designs vary substantially. From previous experience with cemented implants, one might expect such a spread of ideas to reveal results ranging from disastrous to excellent. In fact, it appears increasingly likely that bonding is universally superior to the best of any available cemented series.

The use of HA fixation in knee replacement has also been forging ahead. Total knee replacements have been reported from 1989, IB knees from 1990 (36), Verhaar in 1993 (37). Epinette has described extensive satisfactory experience from 1990 with both total Omnifit/Scorpio and unicompartmental Unix knees (38-40). Stability and function

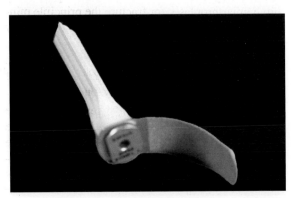

Figure 3 – HA-coated underpinning system for fractures (1981).

of a joint prosthesis at the articulating surface is of course irrelevant to the bonding issue, but it is appropriate to mention the concerns about apatite particulate possibly causing third body wear. In practice, this has not been shown to occur, although it is important that wear rates are carefully documented. When considering outcomes, it is important to focus on aspects of design related to the ability of bone to form a reliable bond with HA (41). Aseptic loosening is conspicuously absent, and debris granulomata have not appeared. If this is confirmed, it raises the question of why.

Achieving an interface with no fibrous interlayer is the ideal objective for prosthetic fixation in bone. Normal bone requires correct load transfer between varying regions and types of bone in accordance with variations in mechanical properties. The osteolytic/osteoprogenic process of bone turnover results in functional adaptation most easily seen in the trabecular patterns on X-rays. Load transfer from a prosthetic device to bone is likely to best mimic nature by transferring onto trabecular bone much in the same way stiff lamellar bone transfers to cancellous bone and then back to opposing lamellar bone in the femoral neck. The cancellous bone functions as a shock absorber.

The concept of stress protection osteopaenia is widely aired, but it of course demonstrates ignorance of Wolff's principals (42). He described functional adaptation as a normal behaviour of bone. Only when adaptation is dysfunctional is an adverse process occurring. Where fibrous tissue intervenes, bone responds with a sclerotic plate, as in a pseudarthrosis. With prostheses, a fibrous interlayer is commonplace in cemented or uncemented arthroplasties. Although this does not equal a failure of clinical outcome, it is dysfunctional and thereby a potential menace.

Avascular tissue prevents access by the reticuloendothelial system, and is thus vulnerable to bacterial colonisation. It also permits abrasion and fretting on the prosthetic interface, with consequent metallosis and or particle generation. It is possible that such a situation compromises the local immune system and allows normally non pathogenic organisms such as proprionobacter acnes and staph epidermidis to grow (43).

It seems probable that so called aseptic loosening is in most cases no such thing. Because of the nature of the bond in calcium apatite to bone as outlined earlier, less than perfect bonding with

this method is virtually never seen. This possibly explains the remarkable long term results of HA-coated implants, and evidence of its efficacy is constantly accumulating.

The chapters comprising the present volume suggest that HA has substantial benefits over cement. There is a virtual absence of negative literature and, at this stage, it is highly unlikely that adverse experience would not have been reported. Numerous reports are available comparing matching implants with and without coating. These include external fixator screws, pedicle screws, experimental blocks, revision devices. It is essential to avoid bracketing HA bonding as simply a variant of "uncemented". The consistant finding is that coating dramatically improves the reliability (fig. 5). The contrast is graphically exposed in the Swedish arthroplasty register 2000 (44). Of all options, the uncemented devices gave the worst performance; the ABG hip stem however was the only type with HA coating and the only device with 100 percent survival at 6 years including cemented. Surgeons using these devices for a decade or more are experiencing the abolition of failure due to aseptic loosening. But of the 854,000 hip replacements undertaken annually worldwide, only seven percent use hydroxyapatite coatings (45). At present the majority of orthopaedic surgeons are either not persuaded, or uninformed. The British government's "National Institute for Clinical Excellence" failed to mention HA-coated technology in its report on Hip Arthroplasty in 2000, which suggests that lack of awareness may be a significant problem. Therefore, the majority of patients undergoing hip arthroplasty may receive a suboptimal anchoring system.

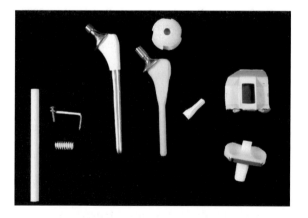

Figure 5 – Various HA-coated implants.

Perhaps this book will convey to its readership a better understanding of the highly successful and clinically proven role of HA in orthopaedics.

Use of synthetic calcium phosphates comparable to those found in the skeleton capitalise on normal biological mechanisms literally as old as the oldest hills. This is a far cry from assaulting bone cells and infrastructure with high pressure acrylic cement, which self cures by exothermic blood boiling reactions, or alien metal surfaces abrading at the interface. There remain many challenges to overcome in joint arthroplasty, but it seems logical that HA technology for fixation will be recognised as the gold standard within the coming decade.

Reference List

1. Monestersky R (1999) *Science News,* 156 (19):292.

2. Neebi C (1999) Talk Origins Archives.

3. Briggs DEG (1991) Extraordinary Fossils. *American Scientist,* 79:130-40.

4. Toewe DT, Sharnley RS. *USGS,* b2123.

5. Briggs DEG, Erwin DH, and Collier FJ (1994) The Fossils of the Burgess Shale, Smithsonian Institution Press, Washington.

6. Morris SL, Walthighe HB (1979) Animals of the Burgess Shale. *Scientific American,* :122-33.

7. Pennent Clery G, Depeachnet W (1999) Introduction to Early Palaeozoic.

8. Chemical Composition of Bone, Encyclopaedia Brittanica, 2001.

9. Betonis JD *et al.* (2001) Apatite bone is not hydroxyapatite: there must be a reason, *GSC Annual Meeting,* http: //gsc.confer.com.

10. Tiesch W *et al.* (2001) *Electron News.*

11. Stavro C (2000) Death of bone cells: basic regulatory mechanism. *Endocrine Review 21(2):113.*

12. Conference on Bone Morphogenic Proteins, June 2000, JBJS V.83 A Supplement 1-2 2001.

13. Stevenson P. of Plasma Biotal, Personal communication.

14. Deer WA *et al.* (1985) An Introduction to Rock Family Minerals. Hong Kong, Longman.

15. Gluck T (1891) *Arch. Clin. Chir.* 41, 186 & 234.

16. Dreesman H (1892) Ueber Knocknplombierung. *Beit. klin. Chir.* 9:804-10.

17. Albee FW, Morrison HF (1920) Studies in bone growth. *American Eng.* 71:31-9.

18. Albee FW. An experiemental study of bone growth and the spinal transport. *JAMA* 60, 1044:1923.

19. Hey Groves EW (1926) Some instructions on the reconstruction surgery of the hip. *Br. J.* Surg. 14:486.

20. Ray DR, Ward AA (1952) A preliminary report of studies of bone calcium phosphate in bone replacement. *Surgical Forum* 51:429.

21. Jahn TL (1968). A possible mechanism for the effects of electrical potentials on Apatite formation in bone. *Clin. Orthop. Rel. Res.* 56, 261-73.

22. Block MS, Kent JN (1984) Long term radiographic evaluation of Hydroxyapatite augmented mandibular alveolar ridges. *J. Oral. & Maxillofacial Surg.,* 42: 793-6.

23. Newesley, H, Osborrn JF (1978) Structure and textural Implications of Calcium Phosphate in ceramics. 3rd Conference on Materials for Use in Medicine and Biology. Keele University, Manchester.

24. Geesink R, De Groot K, Klein C (1987) Chemical Implant Fixation Using Hydroxyapatite. *Clin. Orth.,* 225: 147-70.

25. Jarcho M *et al.* (1977) Tissue, Cellular and Subcellular Events at a Bone-Ceramic-Hydroxyapatite Interface. *J. Bioengineer,* 1, 79-92.

26. Osborne JF and Weiss T (1978) Hydroxylapatite-ein knockenahnlicher Blowerkstoff. *Schw. Mechr. Zahnheik.* 88. 118-124.

27. Søballe K, Hansen ES, B-Rasmussen H, Pedersen CM, Bunger C (1990) Hydroxyapatite coating enhances fixation of porous coated implants. A comparison between press fit and non-interference fit. *Acta Orthopaedica Scandinavica ;* 6(4):299-306.

28. Søballe K, Hansen ES, B-Rasmussen *et al.* (1991) Gap healing enhanced by hydroxyapatite coating in dogs. *Clinical Orthopaedics* ;272:300-07.

29. Søballe K, Hansen ES, B- Rasmussen H, Pedersen CM, Bunger C (1992) Bone graft incorporation around titanium-alloy and hydroxyapatite coated implants in dogs. *Clinical Orthopaedics* ; 274:82-93.

30. Søballe K, Hansen ES, B- Rasmussen, CM, Bunger C (1992) Tissue ingrowth into titanium and hydroxyapatite coated implants during stable and unstable mechanical conditions. *Journal of Orthopaedic Research* ;10:285-99.

31. Søballe K, B- Rasmussen H, Hansen ES, Bunger C (1992) Hydroxyapatite coating modifies implant membrane formation. Controlled micromotion studied in dogs. *Acta Orthopaedica Scandinavica* ; 63(2):128-40.

32. Søballe K, Hansen ES, B-Rasmussen H, Pedersen CM, Bunger C (1993). Hydroxyapatite coating converts fibrous tissue to bone around loaded implants. *Journal of Bone and Joint Surgery* ; 75B:270.

33. Furlong R, Osborne JF (1991) The Furlong hydroxyapatite ceramic coated total hip replacement. A twenty month follow up. Presented at Osborne Memorial Symposium, Royal College of Surgeons, London, October 31.

34. Osborne JF, Histological evaluation of ceramo-osseus regeneration complexes in human bone following hydroxyapatite ceramic implantation. Implant Materials in Biofunction, edited by C. de Putter.

35. Epinette JA and Geesink RGT (1995) Hydroxyapatite Coatings: Where do we stand, where do we go ? In:

Cahiers d'Enseignement de la Sofcot, n° 51 (English Volume), "Hydroxyapatite Coated Hip and Knee Arthroplasty", pp.345-357. Paris, Expansion Scientifique Française.

36. Keast-Butler O, Shepperd J, Hinves BL Ten to twelve year results of HA coated IB knees. New York, Springer Verlag, in press.

37. Verhaar J. (1993) Early Clinical Results of Hydroxylapatite Coated Total Knee Replacements. In: Hydroxylapatite Coatings in Orthopaedic Surgery, Edited by Geesink and Manley, Raven Press.

38. Epinette JA (1995) Hydroxapatite and TKR: The HA Omnifit Knee Prosthesis; In: Cahiers d'Enseignement de la Sofcot, n° 51 (English Volume), Hydroxyapatite Coated Hip and Knee Arthroplasty, pp. 323-332. Paris, Expansion Scientifique Française.

39. Epinette JA and Edidin AA (1997) Hydroxyapatite coated unicompartmental knee replacement ; a report of five to six years' follow-up of the HA Unix Tibial Component, In: Cahiers d'Enseignement de la Sofcot, n° 61 (English Volume) Unicompartmental Knee Arthroplasty, pp. 243-259. Paris, Expansion Scientifique Française.

40. Epinette, JA (2001) HA-coated Total Knee Arthroplasty: A 9-year HA Omnifit experience – In: Arthroplasty 2000, recent advances in TJR, N. Matsui, Y. Taneda, Y. Yoshida eds., pp 189-204. Springer-Verlag Tokyo.

41. Onsten I, Nordquist A, Carlson AS, Besjarkov J., Shott S (1998) Hydroxyapatite augmentation of the porous coating improves fixation of tibial component. A randomised RSA study. JBJS (B) 80(3) : 417-25.

42. Wolff J (1892) Das Gesetz der Transformation der Knochen.

43. Tunney MM, Patrick S, Gorman SP, Nixon JR, Anderson N, Davis RI, Hanna D, Ramage G, Improved detection of infected hip replacements. A currently underestimated problem. JBJS (B) Volume 80 (4): 568-72 Jul.

44. Herberts P, Malchau H (2002), Swedish National Hip report.

45. Datamonitor: Trends & Dynamics in Global Orthopaedics: US and European Hip Implants Ref: SZME0011. 2000 April.

2 Calcium Phosphates:
A Survey of the Orthopaedic Literature

Michael T. Manley, PhD, Kate Sutton, MA and John Dumbleton, DSci, PhD

INTRODUCTION

For over two decades, calcium phosphates have been the focus of many laboratory and clinical investigations (1-8). Particular interest has surrounded calcium hydroxyapatite (HA), a naturally occurring calcium phosphate present in tooth enamel and vertebrate bone. In the early 1980's, the dental community began using HA blocks and coatings to augment bone and encourage fixation in restorative dental procedures; the chemical stability and excellent biocompatibility of HA made it an attractive material choice (1, 5, 9, 10). Subsequently, the orthopaedic community investigated and began using HA for bone defect obliteration and as an implant coating, with encouraging results (3, 11, 12). More recently, attention has been given to biphasic calcium phosphates (BCP), which combine HA and tricalcium phosphate (TCP) in different ratios. Solid, porous, and granular forms of HA and BCP materials have been employed for filling defects (13-16). Current studies involving the use of block HA as a drug delivery system and the use of HA with either bone cement or growth factors all show promise, as do HA composite materials, such as BCP (17-19).

During our review of the literature on HA and calcium phosphates, we observed inconsistencies in the way authors use the terms osteogenic, osteoconductive, and osteoinductive to describe different bone healing and forming processes. Generally, we understand osteogenic materials to contain a viable cellular component and to be derived from natural sources, such as autogenous bone-marrow grafts or autogenous bone grafts. These materials stimulate new bone formation using the cellular elements within the graft (20). Osteoconduction is a process that supports the ingrowth of sprouting capillaries, perivascular tissues, and osteoprogenitor cells from the recipient host bed into the three-dimensional structure of an implant or graft (20, 21). Osteoconductive substances cannot induce bone formation at extraskeletal sites; they must have surfaces with the necessary physical and chemical composition to support the attachment, spreading, division, and differentiation of cells and be distributed in such a way as to support the growth, vascularization, and remodeling of bone (22). Examples of osteoconductive materials are ProOsteon (Interpore International, Irvine, California) and Collagraft (Collagen Corp., Palo Alto, California). Osteoinduction is a process that supports the mitogenesis of undifferentiated mesenchymal cells, which leads to the formation of osteoprogenitor cells that have the capacity to form new bone (20, 21, 23). It promotes the differentiation of osteoblast precursors to osteoblasts (20). Unlike osteoconductive materials, osteoinductive materials can form bone at extraskeletal sites, and the osteoinductive capacity of a specific molecule (eg, a bone morphogenetic protein) may be enhanced by other factors that influence cellular responses (24). When citing various studies, we retained the authors' chosen terminology; therefore, it is important to note that the term one author uses for a particular process – osteogenesis, osteoconduction, or osteoinduction – may not always coincide with that of others.

Additionally, it should be noted that some investigators use the term "hydroxyapatite" loosely, referring to a material with a calcium-phosphorous (Ca/P) ratio ranging anywhere from 1.3 to 2.0. It can be difficult – and potentially misleading – to compare studies using various or undefined ratios to those using the generally accepted Ca/P ratio for hydroxyapatite of 1.67 (25, 26). For example, the mineral in bone (and tooth enamel) is not 100%

HA. There is substitution of sodium and fluorine for calcium, and carbonate for phosphate. It is amorphous, whereas many of the synthetic HA materials are crystalline. The Ca/P ratio of the natural mineral is typically 1.50-1.55, which deviates from the generally accepted stoichiometric value for HA. Plasma-sprayed HA coatings usually have a Ca/P ratio of 1.60 and a crystallinity of up to 95%, with the typical range being from 85% to 92%. There can be inaccuracies in the way the Ca/P ratio is determined. Therefore, it is important that the investigator detail the parameters and the method of measurement.

This chapter provides an overview of calcium phosphates with a focus on hydroxyapatite. It provides physical and biological characterizations and discusses the role of HA and biphasic calcium phosphates in established and emerging biomedical applications.

Biodegradation / Osseointegration

More research needs to be done before all the factors that govern the rate and degree of bioresorption of calcium phosphate ceramics can be clearly defined, as many factors influence the rate and degree of resorption of calcium phosphates. Some of these factors include chemical composition, grain size and crystal structure, physicochemical implant surface properties, and the overall environment at the implant site (27-31).

In the mid-1980s, Hoogendoorn *et al.* (32) reviewed studies that reached different conclusions on the degradation and resorption of HA. They concluded that this was due to the effects on dissolution properties of the different procedures used and the different HA materials employed. More contemporary investigations support these conclusions while focusing on the influence of different grain sizes and sintering temperatures on degradation and resorption rates (27, 29, 30). Generally, *in vitro* biodegradation studies of calcium phosphates have shown that tricalcium phosphates (TCP) dissolve more rapidly than HA (26, 33-36). Jarcho compared the relative dissolution rates of human dental enamel and a dense HA ceramic in buffered lactic acid and found that dental enamel appeared to dissolve ten times faster (26). However, when dissolution results were normalized for surface area, the dissolution rates were found to be the same. Klein et al conducted *in vitro* solubility tests of HA, tetracalcium phosphate, and tricalcium phosphate parti-

cles in lactate, citrate, Gomoris or Michaelis buffer with pH 6.2 or 7.2, and in distilled water (36). In general, results showed that solubility decreased in the order of tetracalcium phosphate, TCP, and HA, except for the lactate and citrate buffers, where the solubility of tetracalcium phosphate equaled that of TCP but still exceeded that of HA.

More recently, biphasic calcium phosphates (BCPs) have emerged as attractive alternatives to using HA or TCP alone. Biphasic calcium phosphates are composed of a mixture of non-resorbable HA and resorbable TCP. The goal of combining HA and TCP is to better control the process of resorption and bone substitution by adjusting the HA/TCP proportions, a concept proposed by Jarcho in the early 1980's (26).

Studies in dogs and goats have been conducted to determine the best ratio of HA to TCP (37, 38). Nery et al examined the use of BCP in periodontal osseous defects surgically created in beagle dogs (37). After six months, histological examination revealed a statistically significant higher gain in probing attachment levels in two HA/TCP treatment groups (65/35 and 85/15), outperforming the control (0/0) and three other groups (50/50, 100/0, 0/100). The higher HA ratio showed new bone formation and new attachment levels and outperformed HA alone. It was determined that the HA/TCP ratio of 85/15 provided the best results when compared to all other groups. Toth *et al.* (38) investigated the use of BP 30%, 50%, and 70% porous 50/50 HA/TCP ceramics compared to autograft in a cervical interbody fusion goat model. The porous ceramics were found to perform equally to or better than autograft. The incidence of ceramic fracture did not increase with the degree of porosity and, at three and six months, all porous ceramics had better radiographic fusion scores than the autograft.

Gao *et al.* (28) studied the bony contact of hydroxyapatite, bioactive glass, and tricalcium phosphate in a sheep diaphyseal defect model. Segmental defects were created in sheep tibiae. At four months post-implantation, with regard to bone ingrowth and bioresorption of the implants, the trabecular, web-like bone-implant contact observed with TCP appeared better than the disseminated, patchy bone-implant contact in the bioactive glass and the buttressed bone-implant contact in hydroxyapatite. The authors suggest that the differences in physicochemical properties on the surface of the three different bioceramic implants are the most probable reason for the different types of bone-implant contact.

Although chemical factors can affect bioresorbability, material structure and porosity have the potential to affect biodegradation to a greater degree than chemical factors alone. Surface area is a primary factor in determining the dissolution rate of any solid. Dissolution rates are probably best expressed as weight dissolved in relation to each unit of exposed surface area. However, porous calcium phosphate ceramics have different macro and microporosities and dissimilar pore interconnectivity and organization patterns. Therefore, comparisons of the biodegradation rates measured *in vitro* may be misleading, as it is difficult to predict specific dissolution rates for porous calcium phosphate materials. Consequently, the dissolution rate of porous calcium phosphate material is less predictable than that of the fully dense material.

Klein *et al.* (39) determined that the physiologic environment significantly affects the biodegradation of calcium phosphate ceramics and that in a given site, the chemical and crystal composition, microstructure, and porosity all affect dissolution rates. Daculsi (35) also reached similar conclusions in his work with biphasic calcium phosphate ceramics. The core issue is that dissolution is required for biological activity. Dense calcium phosphates with low dissolution rates can provide support comparable to bone, but may in some instances encourage fibrous tissue growth. Porous calcium phosphates with higher dissolution rates encourage bony ingrowth, but may not provide the structural integrity necessary to withstand physiologically compressive forces. A fundamental goal of research conducted on calcium phosphate ceramics is to develop materials with dissolution rates sufficient to encourage bone ingrowth attachment while providing adequate mechanical stability.

For mechanically stable HA implants undergoing minimal dissolution, Bauer *et al.* (40) support Jarcho's thesis of a cell-mediated resorption process by showing osteoclastic remodeling of natural and synthetic HA. Thus, for HA/bone interfaces subjected to stress, osteoclastic remodeling of bone and synthetic HA may occur followed by osteoblastic renewal of bone. However, in areas subject to stress shielding, synthetic material may be removed without being replaced by bone. Overgaard *et al.* (41) studied HA-coated porous-coated and grit-blasted surfaces in dogs. Poorer fixation and greater evidence of micromotion was found with the grit-blasted implants. The HA coating was reduced more on fibrous-anchored than bony-anchored implants, suggesting that micromotion may have accelerated the resorption of HA. Resorbed HA coating was replaced by more bone on porous-coated implants than on grit-blasted implants. Okumura *et al.* (42) examined osteoblastic phenotype expression on the surface of hydroxyapatite ceramics in rats. New bone formation was observed primarily on the HA surface with no fibrous tissue interposition. Interfacial analyses showed the appearance of osteoblastic cells on the HA surface and evidence that the cells had begun forming partially mineralized bone directly onto the surface. The existence of bone Gla protein (BGP) and mRNA in the cytoplasmic area of the cells confirmed that active osteoblast apposition generated primary bone on the HA surface, indicating the importance of the surface in supporting osteoblastic differentiation of marrow stromal stem cells (42). Removal of HA and bone by osteoclasts with replacement of bone by osteoblasts at the implant surface suggests that solid HA or HA-coated implants are involved in the remodeling process caused both by host factors and by the presence of the implant itself.

Although a thorough understanding of the factors that influence the bioresorption of calcium phosphate implant materials has yet to be achieved, it is clear that both chemistry and material structure contribute to dissolution. High-density implants of crystalline HA have a low bioresorbtion rate due to their chemical composition and small surface area. Dense tricalcium phosphate implants exhibit a measurable dissolution rate greater than that of dense HA. Porous tricalcium phosphate implants resorb at a greater rate than porous HA implants, even when the structure of both is quite similar. Macroporosity increases the degree of dissolution and, combined with the presence of microporosity, may promote the bioresorption of all calcium phosphate materials. Finally, dissolution is affected by the environment (pH), and resorption may be controlled by cellular activity.

FORMS OF CALCIUM PHOSPHATES

Blocks

Holmes *et al.* (43, 44) described the permanence, over a period of four years, of porous HA blocks as bone graft substitutes in canine mandibles and demonstrated both the osseous incorporation and long term permanence of the HA matrix. Another study on porous HA blocks with cylindrical pores found it could be a useful graft material due to its strength, osteoconductivity, and the ease with which its pore geometry could be controlled (45). Okazaki *et al.* (46) examined osseous tissue reactions around HA blocks implanted into the tibiae of rats with collagen-induced arthritis. Histological examination revealed that the amount of new bone formed around the HA block was actually greater in the arthritis group than in the control group, which suggests that bone formation around HA blocks might be enhanced even in an environment associated with highly activated bone resorption and bone formation, such as arthritis. Steffen *et al.* used a baboon model to assess the osteointegration of porous TCP blocks (15 mm plugs) into the anterior spine (47). At 6 months, complete osteointegration was observed. Using a rabbit model, Guo *et al.* investigated the efficacy of porous HA/TCP blocks as graft material for intertransverse process spinal fusion (48). Seven weeks after implantation, histomorphological observation revealed the integration of HA/TCP with the host bone.

The use of block HA as a sustained-release drug delivery system has been investigated (18, 19, 49, 50). Site-specific delivery of sustained-release drugs may be a way to reduce the side effects of some drugs, particularly those used in chemotherapy, which when delivered intravenously, exhibit strong cytotoxic and severe systemic side effects. HA blocks are attractive drug delivery systems, particularly in cases where site-specific delivery for chemotherapy or antibiotics is required. The pore structure of block HA and its excellent biocompatibility makes it especially favorable for use as a sustained-release drug delivery system.

Itokazu *et al.* (49) investigated the use of block HA as a delivery system for the chemotherapy drug adriamycin (ADR) both *in vitro* and *in vivo* (mice). The goal of the study was to suppress tumor growth and repair bone defects resulting from tumor removal. In vitro tests on the HA/ADR blocks showed acceptable sustained release capabilities. Post-implantation histological evaluations on mice with osteogenic sarcomas implanted with HA/ADR blocks were conducted at weeks one, two, three, and four. (Mice in the control group received HA blocks only.) The amount of ADR remaining in excised HA/ADR blocks decreased

during the first week and increased during the second week, after which it steadily decreased and remained at an adequate maintenance level through week four. Post-implantation tumor growth from week one to week four was shown to be significantly slower in the HA/ADR group than in the control group, and uptake of ADR into the cytoplasm and nucleus of the tumor cells was also confirmed (49). *In vivo* testing of HA as a carrier for gentamicin sulfate (GS) in goats was conducted by Rogers-Foy *et al.* (18). The authors wanted to provide a scaffold that encouraged osseous integration while eliminating infection. Cylindrical plugs of TCP, sintered HA, and sintered HA/GS were implanted in the femoral diaphysis of goats. *In vivo* data gathered six weeks post-operatively indicated that the inclusion of GS in a HA matrix had no effect on osteointegration or bone apposition. Based these results, the authors concluded that the sintered HA/GS composite had the potential to be an effective drug delivery system. A similar study on rats (50) also provided positive results for the treatment of infected osseous sites.

Although investigation into the use of HA blocks as drug delivery systems needs further evaluation, the results reflected by *in vitro* and *in vivo* studies may encourage the use of HA as a sustained-release drug delivery system in future clinical studies and applications.

Granules

In pre-clinical and clinical studies, HA and BCP have exhibited the ability to be effective as bone void fillers. The use of calcium phosphates combined with biological components such as autologous bone marrow may potentially reduce the need for allograft. Wippermann *et al.* (51) conducted a study on sheep tibia segmental defects filled with HA granules and autologous bone marrow. Animals were divided into four groups, one with HA granules and marrow, one with marrow only, one with cancellous bone graft, and one control group with no defect filler. The HA/marrow composite performed equivalently to the cancellous bone graft and better than the empty defect and the defect filled with marrow alone. Another animal study by Grundel *et al.* (52) using biphasic calcium phosphate (HA/TCP) in combination with autogenic bone marrow indicates that the mechanical properties of the delivery matrix are important in achieving a solid union. Diaphyseal defects were created in dog ulnae, and the twenty dogs were divided into four groups. The defect in the first group was filled with a graft of granular biphasic calcium phosphate (HA/TCP) and autogenic bone marrow, the second group received a graft of block BCP soaked in autogenic marrow, the third group received only bone marrow, and the fourth group (the control) received no graft. All animals were followed for 24 weeks, after which they were euthanized and the defects examined. Of the cases employing granular BCP/marrow grafts (6 dogs), five formed solid unions, and 1 progressed to a fibrous union. Of the block BCP/marrow grafts (6 dogs), three achieved solid unions, and three achieved fibrous unions. All defects filled with autogenic bone marrow united (5 dogs), and no union was seen in the ulnae of the control group (3 dogs).

A general comparison of these two animal studies seems to suggest that HA granules may have the potential to outperform BCP granules. It is possible that the tricalcium phosphate component in the BCP used in this study may not be as conducive to the formation of solid unions as HA alone. However, the HA/TCP ratio of BCPs often varies, and different ratios may yield different results. Additionally, the latter study showed a greater number of solid unions using granular BCP as opposed to block form BCP, indicating that mechanical properties and available surface area may play a significant role in determining whether a solid or fibrous union is formed.

Cement

HA cement or paste is osteoconductive, can be replaced by host bone, and avoids the potential for thermal necrosis, making it an attractive alternative to polymethylmethacrylate (PMMA) as long as it provides adequate stiffness. It is often used successfully in facial augmentation cases, where it is not subject to high compressive forces (53, 54). It differs from the ceramic form of HA used for grafting because it is produced by combining two calcium phosphates which, in the presence of water, form a paste that cures to a solid implant with a microporous structure (55).

What is occasionally referred to as HA cement is often polymethylmetacrylate (PMMA) supplemented with HA granules, which will in theory provide a way to encourage bony ingrowth at the cement/bone interfaces. An *in vivo* study investigating the response of three HA/PMMA mixtures

(0/100, 10/90, 30/70) in the distal femurs of rabbits was conducted by Kwon *et al.* (56). After six weeks, *in vivo* measurements of the interfacial shear strength showed a statistically significant increase in the 30% HA/70% PMMA specimens only. The mechanical properties of the HA/PMMA mixture resulted in linearly decreasing tensile and flexural strengths with an increasing amount of HA particles up to 30%. Dalby *et al.* (57) used human osteoblast-like cells when examining the bone/cement interface of a HA/PMMA mixture. They found a significantly higher cell proliferation and differentiation with the HA/PMMA cement compared to the PMMA cement alone. Other studies involving HA/PMMA composites have shown that cement containing HA particles adheres to bone (58, 59). Ohura *et al.* implanted two types of beta-tricalcium phosphate-monocalcium phosphate monohydrate-calcium sulfate hemihydrate (TCP-MCPM-CSH) cement into the femoral condyles of rabbits (60). One cement contained TCP granules, and the other did not. Empty femoral condyle cavities were used as the control. After 16 weeks, bone in cavities where both cements were used showed a trabecular pattern, and the control cavities remained empty and large. However, only the bone trabeculae in the cavities containing the cement with TCP granules became thick and mature.

Research involving HA and TCP as a bone void filler, in granular form or as a cement, indicates that, when used in an appropriate mixture, both offer the potential of encouraging bony ingrowth at surfaces where the particles have direct contact with bone. It also indicates that the addition of HA to PMMA may compromise the overall strength of the composite, and that further investigation with regard to this issue is merited.

Hydroxyapatite Coatings & Surface Treatments

The mechanical properties of calcium phosphates have limited their application in weight-bearing implants because they are brittle, have low impact resistance, and low tensile strength (61). In order to overcome these limitations, calcium phosphates have been applied to metallic substrates in hope of achieving the fatigue properties of metal while maintaining the biocompatibility of the ceramic (62).

In vivo studies have demonstrated the biocompatibility of calcium phosphate coatings in animals, predominantly when used with a titanium or titanium alloy substrate (63-67). Several studies have also evaluated the attachment strength between coated implants and bone (63, 64, 68). Geesink *et al.* (62) conducted a radiographic analysis using a canine model on hip implants coated with a HA/calcium oxide mixture. Proliferation of bone was seen on the implant surface from six weeks forward. Good bone integration was seen, and no radiolucent lines were observed. The uncoated controls showed no evidence of new bone formation.

Manley *et al.* (69, 70) performed histologic and quantitative analyses of HA-coated and uncoated titanium alloy intramedullary implants subjected to functional shear loading in osteotomized canine femora (61). Radiologic analysis at 10 weeks post-implantation revealed the HA-coated implants to have a slight callus formation around the osteotomy site, and evidence of cortical atrophy adjacent to the defect that was surrounded by new bone with no apparent fibrous seam. The uncoated controls exhibited large callus formation around the osteotomy site and were surrounded by a thin, fibrous seam. The authors also found that the interfacial shear strength of the HA-coated implants increased fourfold relative to the uncoated titanium implant at only five weeks post-implantation (69). These findings are similar to a later study by Chang *et al.* (27), who conducted a study to compare the *in vivo* bony response to HA coatings at different crystallinity levels in order to determine the best composition for encouraging osseointegration. The authors implanted cylindrical CP titanium implants with varying HA crystallinities into canine femora. At four weeks, greater bone contact was noted on the HA-coated implants than on the uncoated implants. Additionally, the HA-coated implants were found to have a higher interfacial attachment strength than the control from four weeks on. They concluded that HA coatings on titanium implants enhance osseointegration in the early stages of bone healing, although they noted that the uncoated titanium implants had about the same level of bone contact in the later stages of healing (27).

Another study by Manley *et al.* (71) compared grit-blasted titanium, porous titanium, and smooth titanium implants with an 80 micrometer thick HA coating. Histological examination conducted five weeks post-operatively showed bone penetrating the porous titanium coating and apposing the HA coating. The bone directly apposed to the HA coating expanded over time to the surrounding osseous structures. However, the uncoated, grit-blasted implants revealed a fibrous seam between the implant and bone. The investigators concluded that bone apposition to HA-coated implants occurs even when functional loads cause micromotion between the implant and bone (61, 71). Overgaard *et al.* (41) conducted a canine study of the effect of controlled micromotion on the porous-coated versus grit-blasted surfaces of HA-coated implants. They found that micromotion accelerates resorption of HA, and that the resorbed HA coating was replaced by more bone on porous-coated implants than on those that were grit-blasted, suggesting that the fixation of porous-coated implants would be more durable.

Some studies have shown HA-bone bridges occurring in gaps where the HA-coated implant and bone are not directly apposed (72-74). In all cases, implant stability was critical for the formation of bridges. In a canine study, Soballe compared HA-coated implants and titanium-coated implants, which were inserted into the femoral condyles of dogs (74). Gaps of 1 mm and 2 mm around the HA implants were bridged by bone. Significantly less bone filled the gap around titanium implants. A gradient of newly formed bone was found growing toward the HA coating. This may indicate that the osteoconductive effect of HA is not limited to the coated implant surface.

The ability of HA to enhance the attachment of porous-coated surfaces has been evaluated by several investigators (75, 76, 77). Overall, these studies demonstrated that HA does increase the osseous response time and volume to porous coatings, but also indicates that, ultimately, the attachment strength of the HA-coated and uncoated implant surfaces remains equivalent. In general, it can be said that all of these studies indicated a favorable biologic response to HA coatings; however, the improvements gained with HA-coated, porous-coated implants was short-term.

BIOLOGICAL CHARACTERIZATION OF HYDROXYAPATITE AND CA-P MATERIALS

Biocompatibility

The attractive biological profile of calcium phosphates is a fundamental reason why use of them in medical applications has significantly increased over the past two decades. This profile includes a lack of local or systemic toxicity, a lack of inflammatory response in solid or particulate form, and the ability of bone to bond directly without an intervening layer of fibrous tissue (53, 78-82).

HA blocks and granules have been comprehensively examined using animal models for orthopaedic and dental applications. Studies have been conducted using primates (83), dogs (84, 85), rabbits (86), and rats (85, 87), and overall results have been encouraging. Hoogendoorn *et al.* (32) investigated tissue compatibility and biodegradation of HA blocks in dog femora. Large ceramic blocks of HA were implanted for up to three and one-half years. There were no signs of inflammation or adverse tissue reactions. To gain further information on the interaction of HA particles and the bony implantation bed, Lin *et al.* (88) implanted HA particles into the tibiae of dogs. Following healing periods of 2 weeks, 1 month, and 3 months, the retrieved specimens were conventionally prepared for scanning electron microscopy (SEM) using the EDTA-KOH method. Interparticular osteogenesis progressing in a programmed sequence was observed among HA particles. Secretion of bone matrix resulted in the formation of immature bone, and this scaffold was transformed into mature lamellar bone during the subsequent bone remodeling process. The study confirmed the favorable response of HA to bone cells, and no adverse biological responses were reported.

In a study conducted by Furukawa *et al.* (89), composite rods made from ultra-high strength HA and with poly (L-lactide) (HA/PLLA) were implanted in the fascia and in the medullary cavities of rabbits. Specimens were removed at set intervals between two and fifty-two weeks. Rod surfaces were examined using a scanning electron microscope (SEM). Over time, HA particles disappeared from the rods, and the spaces left by the particles formed many pores in the composite surfaces. After four weeks, histologic analysis revealed a fibrous tissue layer around the rods in the subcutis and diaphyseal areas of the medullary canal. Bony tissue contact to the composites without fibrous tissue layers was seen in the metaphyseal area of the medullary canal. There were no inflammatory cells, and no adverse tissue reactions occurred.

Stelnicki and Ousterhout evaluated the use of synthetic HA paste (BoneSource; Leibinger Corp.,

Dallas, TX) for supraorbital and malar augmentation in rats (53). Implants were left in place for six months and subsequently examined for bone ingrowth, infection, migration, resorption, and negative effects on tissue. All implants demonstrated excellent maintenance of soft tissue contour and strong adherence to the adjacent bone. Bony ingrowth was also observed, and no evidence of gross migration or infection was found. The authors concluded that not only could the HA paste potentially be used with success to augment the supraorbital and malar regions, but its biocompatibility, excellent bony adherence, and tendency to be replaced by natural bone also made it suitable for the aesthetic patient (53).

Yoshimine *et al.* evaluated the biocompatibility of tetracalcium phosphate cement (90). No inflammation or foreign body giant cell reactions were observed in the tissue adjacent to the implanted material. Further examination showed that osteogenesis occurred directly on the surface of the material, suggesting that the tetracalcum cement is biocompatible and may possess osteoconductive properties. Liu *et al.* also found calcium phosphate cement to be highly biocompatible (91). Wu *et al.* examined the biocompatibility and systemic toxicity of magnetic porous tricalcium phosphate (MPTCP) graft in rat femurs (92). Photomicrographs, radiographs, and scanning electron photomicrographs of the rat femurs implanted with MPTCP demonstrated excellent bone association with implants and showed evidence of some new bone growth into the MPTCP.

Although the versatility and generally benign nature of calcium phosphate materials are widely reported, occasional negative reactions have been described. A few early rat studies documenting some inflammatory responses to a HA suspension were reported (93, 94). Additionally, some clinical problems were noted when HA granules used in ridge augmentation migrated due to difficulty maintaining stability at the implant site (95). Dos Santos *et al.* noted that calcium phosphate cement was somewhat cytotoxic, but that the cytotoxicity decreased the longer the calcium phosphate cement was submerged in simulated body fluid (96).

Anderson *et al.* (97) studied HA-coated and uncoated metal hip implants in 23 large dogs to determine whether or not the presence of the HA coating would increase the occurrence of synovitis in the coxofemoral joint. They found the synovial thickness of the operated side increased relative to that of the control, but that the majority of inflammatory responses among the groups were unchanged. They also concluded that, although the HA-coated components appeared to contribute somewhat to the inflammatory load within the periprosthetic environment, the effect was not marked. Furthermore, they hypothesized that the slight increase in particulate load seen in the presence of HA coatings might contribute to the development of aseptic loosening of arthroplasty components, but believed it unlikely to be a major causative factor. As with the study by Mommaerts *et al.* (98), this study also indicates that the presence of HA alone may not be completely responsible for negative immune responses.

An attractive feature of calcium phosphates, in general, is the overall lack of toxicity. Ramieres *et al.* (79) studied the behavior of human MG63 osteoblast-like cells in the presence of titanium/hydroxyapatite (TiO_2/HA) composite coatings. Biocompatibility was evaluated by means of cytotoxicity and cytocompatibility tests. Results showed the materials to have no toxic effects. Additionally, it was determined that the TiO_2/HA exhibited a positive bioactive response due to the presence of hydroxyl groups detected on the surface.

Liu *et al.* (91) examined the biocompatibility of calcium phosphate cement (CPC) in rabbit femurs. The investigation included systemic injection acute toxicity assay, cell culture cytotoxicity, gene mutation assay, chromosome aberration assay, DNA damage assay, and implant histological evaluation. The results showed that CPC had no toxicity, and all tests for mutagenicity and the resultant carcinogenicity of CPC extracts were negative.

The lack of toxicity of calcium phosphates is largely due to the fact that they contain only calcium and phosphate ions normally found in the body. De Groot (65) indicated no abnormal findings in the serum and urine analysis in different animal models of implanted resorbable and minimally resorbable calcium phosphate materials. Histologic examination of the major organs revealed no evidence of pathological reactions.

In-vivo Reactions with Bone and Bone Bonding

The physiological environment surrounding calcium phosphate implants is believed to affect the deposition of solids on their surfaces. In bone, this would generate calcium phosphate solids in the form of biologic apatite, ultimately resulting in a microscopic layer of bone mineral developing shortly after implantation (26). One study performed by Jarcho (26) involved placing dense HA implants in the femurs of dogs. Normal calcification processes were observed immediately adjacent to the implants. This was indicated by the increasing calcium and phosphate concentrations observed post-operatively (from 1.50 at one month to 1.62 at six months). At six months, mineralization within the implant sites was found to be similar to that of surrounding bone. In a clinical setting, Ayers *et al.* (13) examined porous block HA implants. Implants were placed into the lateral maxillary wall during orthognathic surgery and were harvested with patient consent after a mean implantation time of 32 months (range, 4-138 months). Histomorphometric measurements indicated that there was significant bone ingrowth in all implants, and no significant difference in microhardness values between the bone in the implant and the bone surrounding the implants was noted. This indicated that the structural integrity of the porous HA block/bone aggregate had been maintained.

Calcium phosphate implants also appear to have the desirable ability of bonding directly to bone. Early animal studies focused on using porous calcium phosphate implants to provide mechanical stabilization while encouraging bony ingrowth. In the early 1970's, Driskell *et al.* (6) performed a scanning electron microscope study of fractured samples of porous TCP at the implant site. They noted that evidence, "suggests that a chemical bond exists between the calcified tissue and the ceramic". In a later study, Chang *et al.* (27) investigated the bone-bonding properties of HA-coated titanium implants in dog femurs. The HA was defined based on its crystallinity percentage: 50% (low), 70% (medium), or 90% (high). An uncoated titanium implant was used as a control. At four weeks, a significantly higher percentage of bone contact was noted on the HA-coated implants, which were also found to have significantly higher interfacial attachment strength than the uncoated implants. All HA-coated implants provided strong bone-bonding capability, and crystallinity had no significant effect on bone forming capacity and bone bonding strength, although it should be noted that a HA coating of higher crystallinity is more desirable in maintaining osteoconductive properties.

Although the exact bonding mechanism and chemical composition of the bond between bone and HA implants have not been fully determined, optical and electron microscope observations have been conducted by several investigators. According to Cormack (99) the bone-bonding substance is very similar in character to natural bone cementing substance – initially amorphous, progressively transforming to a crystalline state, heavily mineralized, and rich in mucopolysaccharides. Jarcho (26) reported that the initial appearance of the bonding area and the first significant indication of bonding occurred with the first evidence of an acellular bone matrix from differentiating osteoblasts. In decalcified sections prepared for electron microscopy, implants were reportedly covered with a narrow (3 to 5 microns wide), amorphous, electron-dense band without distinct structural details.

Okumura *et al.* (42) analyzed the bone-bonding properties of HA ceramics in rats. Implants were harvested 3 to 4 weeks after implantation. The HA/tissue interface was analyzed by observing thin, undecalcified histological sections and fractured implant surfaces. Observations were done with a light microscope and a scanning electron microscope connected to an energy dispersive spectrometer. The interfacial analyses revealed the appearance of osteoblastic cells on the HA surface and indicated that the cells had initiated partially mineralized bone (osteoid) formation directly onto the surface. The osteoid matured into fully mineralized bone, resulting in firm bone bonding to the HA surface.

There are a variety of studies on the *in vivo* response to calcium phosphate materials at the cellular level. Calcium phosphates, used alone or mixed with autogenous bone are attractive grafting materials, particularly in spinal applications where many procedures would otherwise require harvesting bone from the iliac crest. In a goat model, Toth *et al.* (38) mixed three different HA/TCP porosities (30%, 50%, and 70%) with autograft in a 50/50 ratio to promote spinal fusion. Autograft alone was the control. All of the ceramics had better radiographic fusion scores than the autograft at 3 and 6 months. At 6 months, the union rate for autograft was 50% and 67% for each of the porous ceramics. Overall, the porous ceramics clearly outperformed autograft alone. Johnson *et al.* (100) used a canine radius model to compare the per-

formance of TCP, HA, and collagen HA, each combined with bone marrow, to cancellous bone. At 24 weeks, the TCP/bone marrow combination was found to perform most like cancellous bone. Significant degradation was shown after 24 weeks, but this occurred only after the degree of mechanical competency for weight-bearing was achieved. However, the use of collagen ceramic composite graft materials has met with mixed results. Although some studies (101, 102) have shown comparability between collagen ceramic graft materials and autogenous bone, others (103, 104) have not.

The highly biocompatible nature of calcium phosphates has encouraged investigators to evaluate the osteogenicity of calcium phosphate implants. One study using Millipore chambers (Millipore Corp., Billerica, MA) compared the osseous response to dense HA implant materials (plugs or particles) blended with hemopoietic marrow to control chambers containing marrow only. Examination at six weeks post-implantation revealed that a greater number of the control chambers contained newly formed bone (90%) compared to the chambers containing HA/marrow (35%) (26). Takaoka *et al.* (105) compared the osteogenic response of porous alumina and hydroxyapatite-coated porous alumina ceramic implants by grafting them with rat bone marrow cells and implanting them subcutaneously in syngeneic rats. They noted that osteogenesis in the HA/alumina/marrow implants began directly on the ceramic surface, but in alumina/marrow only, it began away from the surface with fibrous tissue between the new bone and implant. They concluded that a composite of marrow, HA, and alumina is a clinically useful osteogenic biomaterial. Yoshikawa *et al.* (106) examined the response of HA/marrow cells compared to HA/marrow cells/dexamethasone in a rat model. Histological analysis revealed that the dexamethasone-treated subcultured marrow cells in pore regions of HA showed a high osteogenic response immediately after transplantation. However, the HA/marrow cells not treated with dexamethasone showed no bone formation.

Calcium phosphates in some instances appear to promote the growth of bone into areas it would otherwise not occupy (26, 107). Several authors have described materials with this property as "osteoconductive" and "osteophilic". Many studies have been conducted that examined the osteoconductive properties of HA. Chang *et al.* (27) undertook a biomechanical and morphometric analysis of HA-coated implants with varying crystallinity. Sand-blasted titanium implants were compared to HA-coated implants. After histological examination at four weeks, a significantly higher percentage of bone contact was seen on the HA-coated implants than on the uncoated implants. HA-coated implants were also found to have significantly higher interfacial attachment strength than the uncoated implants at 4, 12, and 26 weeks. They concluded that HA coatings on metal implants enhanced osseointegration, and that HA coatings with higher crystallinity were more desirable in maintaining osteoconductive properties.

Initial stabilization of HA implants might also be an important component for encouraging osteoconductivity and osseous integration. In dogs, Munting (108) explored the relationship between stability and implant fixation. He noted that areas of resorption of the coating were seen on the metal implant surface in every case associated with direct bone apposition. When initial fixation was stable, osteointegration of HA-coated implants was obtained consistently, in spite of some design features known to preclude bone incorporation. He concluded that implant fixation must depend on a mechanical interlock with bone.

In summary, HA-coated implants have exhibited bone-bonding capability, particularly if initial stability is ensured. The material appears to be osteoconductive and becomes covered with bone as long as there is some bone contact at initial placement. In general, it appears calcium phosphate materials do not in themselves stimulate osteogenesis, but unlike traditional biomaterials, they appear capable of conducting bone growth into an implant surface shapes or bony defects. However, studies involving HA and bone marrow mixed with synthetic analogues of cortisol, such as dexamethasone, have shown what appear to be osteogenic properties.

HYDROXYAPATITE AND GROWTH FACTORS

With the goal of providing rapid initial implant stability and an osteoinductive alternative to autogenous bone in defect repair and reconstructive surgery, recent investigations have explored the feasibility of combining HA and BCPs with growth factors, such as bone morphogenetic proteins (BMPs). Growth factors induce the differentiation of pluripotential cells along cartilaginous and bone-forming cell lines, and bone graft substitutes containing growth factors may limit or eliminate the clinical use of autogenous bone grafting and the related donor site morbidity (109). However, growth factors need an appropriate delivery matrix in order to facilitate bone ingrowth. HA is frequently chosen as a delivery matrix because it can be preformed, has appropriate porosity, and has proven biocompatibility.

Several growth-promoting substances have been identified at the site of fractures, and these substances can be divided into two groups, the first containing the transforming growth factor-beta (TGF-ß) gene family, and the second containing immunomodulatory cytokines (23). BMP-2 through BMP-16 are part of the TGF-ß superfamily (110, 111). *In vitro* and *in vivo* research for orthopaedic applications currently appears to focus, although not exclusively, on BMP-2 and BMP-7 (also known as osteogenic protein-1, or OP-1).

Animal studies using growth factors have been encouraging. In a rabbit study, recombinant human bone morphogenetic protein-2 (rhBMP-2) was adsorbed onto porous ceramic HA to investigate the promotion of integration with host bone (112). A total of 32 HA implants were placed in unburred subperiosteal pockets, 14 HA implants saturated with saline (control), and 18 HA implants saturated with rhBMP-2. Twenty-two HA implants with saline were placed in burred pockets. After one month, histological examination revealed that one (6%) of the control implants exhibited bone growth into the implant, 10 (45%) of the implants placed in a burred pocket showed bone ingrowth, and 16 (89%) of the HA/rhBMP-2 implants showed bone ingrowth.

In a syngeneic rat model, Noshi *et al.* (113) incorporated rhBMP-2 into a composite of bone marrow mesenchymal cells (MSCs) and HA to explore the osteogenic potential of the BMP-enhanced MSCs/HA composite. Four different types of implants were used, HA alone, HA/BMP, MSCs/HA, and MSCs/HA/BMP. Composites including BMP contained 1 microgram of BMP. Post-implantation, the HA and HA/BMP composites failed to show any bone forming capability. This result is different from other studies showing osteoinductive properties in HA/BMP composites (109, 112, 114). It is possible the HA/BMP composite in this study failed to show any bone formation because of the small amount of BMP used. The MSCs/HA composite showed moderate bone formation at four weeks and extensive bone formation at eight weeks, and the MSCs/HA/BMP composite showed obvious new bone formation and active osteoblasts at two weeks, with progressive bone formation at four and eight weeks. This study provides histological and chemical evidence that MSCs/HA/BMP composites may synergistically enhance osteogenic potential (113).

Ripamonti *et al.* (115) studied the effect of surface geometry on bone induction. HA powders were sintered to form solid discs with a series of concavities on the planar surfaces. The HA discs were either treated with rhOP-1 (BMP-7) and a collagenous carrier or left untreated and implanted into heterotopic or orthotopic skullcap defects in adult baboons. After 90 days, the HA discs pretreated with rhOP-1 showed extensive bone formation ; however, the untreated HA discs also exhibited similar bone formation and healing of the skullcap defects. The authors concluded that the surface characteristics of sintered hydroxyapatites can induce intrinsic osteoinductivity in primates (115). Lind *et al.* (116) conducted a study on the stimulatory effects of allograft at different dosage levels of OP-1 in a collagen composite placed around a HA-coated implant in dogs. It was noted that higher doses of OP-1 had no effect on bone formation, and low doses had a moderate effect on bone healing around the HA-coated implants, but no effect on implant fixation.

Other studies combining BCPs and BMPs have shown encouraging results. Alam *et al.* (17) using biphasic calcium phosphate pellets (25% HA, 75% TCP) treated with rhBMP-2 and untreated (control). The pellets treated with rhBMP-2 exhibited new bone and bone marrow formation, whereas the control pellets produced fibrous connective tissues. Oda *et al.* (117) investigated ectopic bone formation by combining BCP granules (20% HA/80% TCP) and rhBMP-2 in the rat dorsum. The study contained four groups of five animals each: one control (BCP only), with the remaining three groups receiving 2/700, 10/700, and 50/700 microliters of rhBMP-2, respectively. Histological analysis was conducted three weeks post-operatively. New bone formed in all rats given the 50 microgram doses of rhBMP-2, and no bone formed in any of the rats receiving 2 micrograms of rhBMP-2 or in the control group. The results indicate that BCP/rhBMP-2 composites may induce ectopic bone formation without additional carriers, but only when the percentage of rhBMP-2 in the composite is at a high enough level.

As research involving the effect of growth factors and bone formation continues, it is important to note that adequate delivery systems for growth factors are essential to their success. The biocompatibility, mechanical structure, and chemical nature of hydroxyapatite and biphasic calcium phosphates make them reliable choices as delivery systems for growth factors.

CLINICAL RESULTS

Overall, clinical results using calcium phosphates have been encouraging. Ayers *et al.* (13) examined the ingrowth of bone into porous HA block. Twenty-five maxillary HA implants were removed from 17 patients. Implants were placed into the lateral maxillary wall and juxtapositioned to the maxillary sinus during orthognathic surgery. After voluntary consent, the implants were harvested. Microscopic examination showed normal bone morphology in all implants, and no inflammatory responses were observed. Histomorphometric measurements revealed significant ingrowth in all implants. Koshino *et al.* (12) examined the performance of porous HA wedges inserted into 10 knees (7 patients) with osteoarthritis that underwent high tibial osteotomy. At the time of hardware removal in all knees, the interface of the HA wedge and bone was histologically examined in undecalcified specimens. Total incorporation of the HA into bone was observed, with no inflammatory reaction. Many studies with HA in dental applications repeatedly show the efficacy of HA as an implant material that has no evident adverse biological effects (5, 10, 118-121).

In a study by Mommaerts *et al.* (98) involving the use HA blocks in 70 patients, 3 patients developed maxillary sinusitis. In two of the cases, the occurrence of sinusitis was directly related to fragmentation of an HA block. Overall, the authors achieved excellent results and note that complications are rare as long as the interpositional HA block is not fractured. It is possible that instability at the implantation site, not the presence of HA, may be responsible for a series of events that could potentially lead to inflammation and/or infection.

Hinz *et al.* used ultraporous TCP as a bone void filler in six patients with traumatic bone injuries (15). At a minimum of two months, radiographs showed new bone consolidating in treated sites. A biopsy was obtained 9 months postoperatively from a fractured calcaneus. Examination showed new bone growing within the ultraporous scaffold. The specimen did not indicate any significant inflammatory response or foreign body reaction. Meadows also found ultraporous TCP to be a satisfactory bone void filler in spinal arthodesis (122).

Preliminary clinical studies by Szabo *et al.* involving bilateral sinus elevations found evidence that granular TCP is a satisfactory graft material, even without autogenous bone (123). Muschik *et al.* investigated the used of granular TCP as a bone substitute for dorsal spinal fusion in adolescent idiopathic scoliosis (124). Nineteen patients received autograft bone mixed with allograft, and 9 patients received autograft bone mixed with TCP. At six months, radiographs were examined and complete fusion was noted in all cases. Preliminary results indicated that bone mineral density between the two groups was similar, and resorption of the TCP appeared to be complete at approximately 8 months. Russotti *et al.* (125) conducted a study to evaluate the efficacy of HA/TCP granules in enhancing the biologic fixation of a porous-coated femoral component without an interference fit. Neither osteoconductive nor osteoinductive properties were observed, perhaps due to the lack of initial stablilization and apposition to adjacent bone.

Oonishi *et al.* (14) used non-resorbable, sintered HA granules of varying sizes to fill massive acetabular defects in 40 revision cases. The granules were irregularly shaped and varied in size; 10% of the granules were 100-300 micrometers, 45% were from 0.9-1.2mm, and 45% were 3.0 to 5.0mm. In order to increase the mixing density and facilitate the adhesion of the granules, physiological saline was added. HA granules were placed in the defects and fixed by a layer of cement. During radiographic review, it was noted that a stable filling was attained when granules were packed densely and firmly and, in many patients, the HA layer was found to be 3 to 4 cm thick. Post-operatively, granules were stable, even in patients with massive bone loss, and hip pain was alleviated in all patients. It was determined that when HA granules are firmly packed, they become bound to bone and experience minimal absorption. Interestingly, the authors operated on one of the study patients

again two years post-operatively and found the HA granules had formed a homogeneous mass that proved difficult to cut, even with the use of a chisel. Three patients with an absent medial wall exhibited instability, but were pain free. Reinforcing the wall with allograft may have improved the stability (14).

Hydroxyapatite-coated implants have been used clinically for well over a decade. The degree of success may be influenced by the coating thickness of the HA, the location of the HA on the device, the surface preparation of the device substrate, and the overall design of the implant. Vedantam and Ruddlesdin (126) studied the clinical and radiographic results of hip stems fully coated with HA in 45 patients for an average of approximately four years. Subcortical cancellous bone formation was highest at the tip and distal portions of the stem, and radiographic evaluations suggested greater stress transfer occurring in the distal two-thirds of the stem. In 57.4% of the cases, the authors noted proximomedial femoral neck resorption. Although an excellent to good outcome was obtained with 89% of the patients, aseptic loosening in the fully coated stems was found to be higher than those of proximally HA-coated implants (126). The results of this study suggest the possibility that a stem HA-coated only proximally and not distally may distribute stresses more effectively, as reported by D'Antonio *et al.* (127).

D'Antonio *et al.* (128) reported excellent results with a proximally HA-coated stem (Omnifit-HA). At three-year follow-up with 142 cases, the authors contended that clinical and radiographic observations indicated well-fixed stems that exhibited excellent stress transfer. In a ten to thirteen year follow-up study by D'Antonio *et al.* involving 314 cases using the same proximally HA-coated hip stem design reported earlier (128), radiographic evaluation revealed progressive bone remodeling around the implants, which were 100% bone stable (129). Several histological examinations on proximally HA-coated implants retrieved at autopsy have also shown consistent evidence of new bone formation in the tissue adjacent to the HA coating (40, 130-132).

Tonino *et al.* (133) conducted a histological and histomorphometric examination of five HA-coated titanium femoral stem specimens (ABG; Howmedica, Staines, UK), and the related tissue, recovered from cadavers 3.3 to 6.2 years post-operatively. All cases showed good fixation by osseointegration. Although almost complete loss of HA was observed in one case, it did not appear to compromise fixation or osseointegration. Bone-implant contact in the proximal region of the stem did not change significantly and was similar to the other four cases.

In 23 matched pairs of patients, Thanner *et al.* investigated the clinical results of titanium-mesh porous cups plasma-sprayed with a HA/TCP coating (134). Unsprayed cups served as the control. All cups were secured with bone screws. Although clinical results did not differ between the two groups two years postoperatively, less tilting and diminished radiolucencies were found in the cups coated with HA/TCP, suggesting better bone ingrowth and sealing of the interface.

Epinette *et al.* (135) conducted a study to evaluate the clinical, radiographic, and survivorship outcomes of HA-coated titanium threaded acetabular cups (Arc2f, Osteonics, Allendale, NJ). The minimum follow-up was 10 years, with 304 cups available for analysis. Bone screws were used in all cases to provide supplementary fixation. At latest follow-up, no unstable cups were observed, all fixation interfaces were classified as "stable bone ingrown", and no cups showed any evidence of migration. Survivorship of the threaded HA cup at ten years was reported to be 99.43%

CONCLUSION

A great deal of literature on calcium phosphate materials studied *in vitro, in vivo*, and clinically exists, and a broad understanding of the chemical, physical, and biological characteristics of calcium phosphates can be obtained from it. Although block HA may have unacceptable mechanical properties as a load bearing implant, it shows promise as a site-specific, sustained-release drug delivery system, as a delivery system for growth factors, and as a filler in reconstructive surgery for areas that do not experience significant physiological loads. Several studies have shown granular forms of HA and BCP to be effective bone void fillers, and in clinical studies involving sinus reconstruction, TCP alone was found to be comparable to autogenous bone as a grafting material. Thin HA coatings applied to metallic substrates achieve the strength properties of the underlying material while providing a biocompatible environment that appears to encourage bony

attachment. Studies have shown that applying HA to an implant can eliminate the formation of the fibrous seam often seen with uncoated implants thereby enhancing the probability of long-term prosthetic stability. No adverse systemic effects have been reported with HA, which has consistently exhibited excellent biocompatibility.

Over ten-years minimum follow-up has been achieved with HA-coated implants clinically, and both pre-clinical and clinical studies have shown the ability of HA to enhance the attachment of implants to bone. The excellent biocompatibility of HA and its ability to provide a greater potential for more rapid initial implant stabilization continue to make it an attractive implant coating option. As the clinical use of HA and other calcium phosphates continues to increase, further successful use in a variety of applications is anticipated.

Reference list

1. Lacefield WR (1998) Current status of ceramic coatings for dental implants. *Implant Dent.* 7(4):315-22.

2. Spivak JM, Hasharoni A (2001) Use of hydryoxyapatite in spine surgery. *Eur. Spine J.* 10:Suppl 2: S197-S204.

3. Bucholz RW (2002) Nonallograft osteoconductive bone graft substitutes. *Clin. Orthop.* 395:44-52.

4. Geesink RGT (2002) Osteoconductive coatings for total joint arthroplasty. *Clin. Orthop.* 395:53-65.

5. Block MS, Kent JN (1984) Long term radiographic evaluation of HA-augmented mandibular alveolar ridges. *J. Oral. Maxillofac. Surg.* 42.

6. Driskell TD, Hassler CR, McCoy LR (1973) The significance of resorbable bioceramics in the repair of bone defects. Proceedings of the 26th Annual Conference on Medical Biomaterials. Vol. 15. p. 199.

7. Epinette JA, Geesink RGT (1995), eds. *Hydroxyapatite Coated Hip and Knee Arthroplasty*. Vol. 51. Cahiers d'enseignement de la SOFCOT.

8. Epinette JA (1995) HA-coated hip implants: a 10 year follow-up. *Eur. J. Orthop. Surg. Traumatol.* 9: 83-5.

9. Jarcho M (1992) Retrospective analysis of hydroxyapatite development for oral implant applications. *Dent. Clin. North. Am.* 36:19-26.

10. Kent JN, Quinn JH, Zide MF, Guerra LR, Boyne PJ (1983) Alveolar ridge augmentation using nonresorbable HA with or without autogenous cancellous bone. *J. Oral. Maxillofac. Surg.* 41:629-42.

11. Larsson S, Bauer TW (2002) Use of injectable calcium phosphate cement for fracture fixation: a review. *Clin. Orthop.* 395:23-32.

12. Koshino T, Murase T, Takagi T, Saito T (2001) New bone formation around porous hydroxyapatite wedge implanted in opening wedge high tibial osteotomy in patient with osteoarthritis. *Biomaterials.* 22:1579-82.

13. Ayers RA, Simske SJ, Nunes CR, Wolford LM (1998) Long-term bone ingrowth and residual microhardness of porous block hydroxyapatite implants in humans. *J. Oral. Maxillofac. Surg.* 56:1297-301.

14. Oonishi H, Iwaki Y, Kin N, Kushitani S, Murata N, Wakitani S, Imoto K (1997) Hydroxyapatite in revision of total hip replacements with massive acetabular defects. *J. Bone Joint Surg. Br.* 79:87-92.

15. Hinz P, Wolf E, Schwesinger G, Hartelt E, Ekkernkamp A (2002) A new resorbable bone void filler in trauma: early clinical experience and histologic evaluation. *Orthopedics.* 25:S597-S600.

16. Adenis JP, Bertin P, Lasudry JG, Boncoeur-Martel MP, Leboutet MJ, Robert PY (1999) Treatment of postnucleation socket syndrome with a new hydroxyapatite tricalcium phosphate ceramic implant. *Ophthal. Plast. Reconstr. Surg.* 15:277-83.

17. Alam I, Asahina I, Ohmamiuda K, Enomoto S (2001) Comparative study of biphasic calcium phosphate ceramics impregnated with rhBMP-2 as bone substitutes. *J. Biomed. Mater. Res.* 54:129-38.

18. Rogers-Foy JM, Powers DL, Brosnan DA, Barefoot SF, Friedman RJ, La Berge M (1999) Hydroxyapatite composites designed for antibiotic drug delivery and bone reconstruction: a caprine model. *J. Invest. Surg.* 12:263-75.

19. Itokazu M, Matsunaga T, Kumazawa S, Yang WA (1995) Novel drug delivery system for osteomyelitis using porous hydroxyapatite blocks loaded by centrifugation. *J. Appl. Biomater.* 6:167-9.

20. Greenwald AS, Boden SD, Goldberg VM, Khan Y, Laurencin CT, Rosier RN (2001) Bone-graft substitutes: facts, fictions, and applications. *J. Bone Joint Surg.* 83A(Suppl 2, Part 2):S98-S103.

21. Urist MR (1980) Bone transplants and implants, In: Fundamental and Clinical Bone Physiology, Urist, M.R., Editor. J.B. Lippincott: Philadelphia. p. 331-68.

22. Damien CJ, Parsons JR (1991) Bone graft and bone graft substitutes: a review of current technology and applications. *J. Appl. Biomater.* 2:187-208.

23. Einhorn TA (1995) Enhancement of fracture-healing. *J. Bone Joint Surg.* 77-A(6):940-56.

24. Bolander ME (1992) Regulation of fracture repair by growth factors. *Proc. Soc. Exper. Biol. and Med.* 200:165-70.

25. Black J (1988) Ceramics and composites, In: Orthopaedic Biomaterials in Research and Practice. Churchill Livingstone, Inc: New York, NY. p. 191-211.

26. Jarcho M (1981) Calcium phosphate ceramics as hard tissue prosthetics. *Clin. Orthop.* 157:259-78.

27. Chang YL, Lew D, Park JB, Keller JC (1999) Biomechanical and morphometric analysis of hydroxyapatite-coated implants with varying crystallinity. *J. Oral Maxillofac. Surg.* 57:1096-108.

28. Gao TJ, Lindholm TS, Kommonen B, Ragni P, Paronzini A, Lindholm TC (1995) Microscopic evaluation of bone-implant contact between hydroxyapatite, bioactive glass and tricalcium phosphate implanted in sheep diaphyseal defects. *Biomaterials.* 16:1175-9.

29. Malard O, Bouler JM, Guicheux J, Heymann D, Pilet P, Coquard C, Daculsi G (1999) Influence of biphasic calcium phosphate granulometry on bone ingrowth, ceramic resorption, and inflammatory reactions: preliminary *in vitro* and *in vivo* study. *J. Biomed. Mater. Res.* 46:103-11.

30. Harada Y, Wang JT, Doppalapudi VA, Willis AA, Jasty M, Harris WH, Nagase M, Goldring SR (1996) Differential effects of different forms of hydroxyapatite and hydroxyapatite/tricalcium phosphate particulates on human monocyte/macrophages *in vitro*. *J. Biomed. Mater. Res.* 31:19-26.

31. Klein CPAT, Driessen AA, de Groot K (1984) Relationship between the degradation behavior of calcium phosphate ceramics and their physical-chemical characteristics and ultrastructrual geometry. *Biomaterials.* 5:157-60.

32. Hoogendorn HA, Renooij W, Akkermans LMA, Visser W, Wittebol P (1984) Long term study of large ceramic implants (porous hydroxyapatite) in dog femora. *Clin. Orthop.* 187:281-8.

33. Lee DR, Lemmons JE, LeGeros RZ (1989) Dissolution characteristics of commercially available HA particulate. 15th Annual Meeting of the Society for Biomaterials. Vol. 161. Lake Buena Vista, FL.

34. Cleries L, Fernandez-Pradas JM, Sardin G, Morenza JL (1998) Dissolution behaviour of calcium phosphate coatings obtained by laser ablation. *Biomaterials.* 19:1483-87.

35. Daculsi G (1998) Biphasic calcium phosphate concept applied to artificial bone, implant coating and injectable bone substitute. *Biomaterials.* 19:1473-78.

36. Klein CP, de Blieck-Hogervorst JM, Wolke JG, de Groot K (1990) Studies of the solubility of different calcium phosphate ceramic particles *in vitro*. *Biomaterials.* 11:509-12.

37. Nery EB, LeGeros RZ, Lynch KL, Lee K (1992) Tissue response to biphasic calcium phosphate ceramic with different ratios of HA/beta TCP in periodontal osseous defects. *J. Periodontol.* 63:729-35.

38. Toth JM, An HS, Lim TH, Ran Y, Weiss NG, Lundberg WR, Xu RM, Lynch KL (1995) Evaluation of porous biphasic calcium phosphate ceramics for anterior cervical interbody fusion. *Spine.* 20:2203-10.

39. Klein CPAT, Driessen AA, de Groot K, van den Hooff A (1983) Biodegradation behavior of various calcium phosphate materials in bone tissue. *J. Biomed. Mater. Res.* 17:769-84.

40. Bauer TW, Geesink RGT, Zimmerman R, McMahon JT (1991) Hydroxyapatite-coated femoral stems. Histological analysis of components retrieved at autopsy. *J. Bone Joint Surg. Am.* 73:1439-52.

41. Overgaard S, Lind M, Glerup H, Bunger C, Søballe K (1998) Porous-coated versus grit-blasted surface texture of hydroxyapatite-coated implants during controlled mircomotion: mechanical and histomorphometric results. *J. Arthroplasty.* 13:449-58.

42. Okumura M, Ohgushi H, Dohi Y, Katuda T, Tamai S, Koerten HK, Tabata S (1997) Osteoblastic phenotype expression on the surface of hydroxyapatite ceramics. *J. Biomed. Mater Res.* 37:122-29.

43. Holmes RE, Hagler HK. Porous HA (1987) as a bone graft substitute in mandibular contour augmentation: a histometric study. *J. Oral Maxillofac. Surg.* 45:421-29.

44. Holmes RE, Hagler HK (1988) Porous hydroxyapatite as a bone graft substitute in maxillary augmentation. A histometric study. *J. Craniofac. Surg.* 16:199-205.

45. Chang BS, Lee CK, Hong KS, Youn HJ, Ryu HS, Chung SS, Park KW (2000) Osteoconduction at porous hydroxyapatite with various pore configurations. *Biomaterials.* 21:1291-8.

46. Okazaki A, Koshino T, Saito T, Takagi T (2000) Osseous tissue reaction around hydroxyapatite block implanted into proximal metaphysis of tibia of rat with collagen-induced arthritis. *Biomaterials.* 21:483-7.

47. Steffen T, Stoll T, Arvinate T, Schenk RK (2001) Porous tricalcium phosphate and transforming growth factor used for anterior spine surgery. *Eur. Spine J.* 10(Suppl 2):S132-S140.

48. Guo L, Guo X, Leng Y, Cheng JC, Zhang X (2001). Nanoindentation study of interfaces between calcium phosphate and bone in an animal spinal fusion model. *J. Biomed. Mater. Res.* 54:554-9.

49. Itokazu M, Kumazawa S, Wada E, Yang W (1996) Sustained release of adriamycin from implanted hydroxyapatite blocks for the treatment of experimental osteognic sarcoma in mice. *Cancer Lett.* 107:11-8.

50. Shinto Y, Uchida A, Korkusuz F, Araki N, Ono K (1992) Calcium hydroxyapatite ceramics used as a delivery system for antibiotics. *J. Bone Joint Surg. Br.* 74:600-4.

51. Wippermann B, Donow C, Schratt HE, den Boer FC, Blokhuis T, Patka P (1999) The influence of hydroxyapatite granules on the healing of a segmental defect filled with autologous bone marrow. *Ann. Chir. Gyn.* 88:194-7.

52. Grundel RE, Chapman MW, Yee T, Moore DC (1991) Autogeneic bone marrow and porous biphasic calcium phospahte ceramic for segmental bone defects in the canine ulna. *Clin. Orthop.* 266:244-58.

53. Stelnicki EJ, Ousterhout DK (1997) Hydroxyapatite paste (Bone Source) used as an onlay implant for supraorbital and malar augmentation. *J. Craniofac. Surg.* 8:367-72.

54. Petruzzelli GJ, Stankiewicz JA (2002) Frontal sinus obliteration with hydroxyapatite cement. *Laryngoscope.* 112:32-6.

55. Joosten U, Joist A, Frebel T, Walter M, Langer M (2000) The use of an in situ curing hydroxyapatite cement as an alternative to bone graft following removal of enchondroma of the hand. *J. Hand. Surg. Br.* 25:288-91.

56. Kwon SY, Kim YS, Woo YK, Kim SS, Park JB (1997) Hydroxyapatite impregnated bone cement: *in vitro* and *in vivo* studies. *Biomed. Mater. Eng.* 7:129-40.

57. Dalby MJ, Di Silvio L, Harper EJ, Bonfield W (2001) Initial interaction of osteoblasts with the surface of a hydroxyapatite-poly(methylmethacrylate) cement. *Biomaterials.* 22:1739-47.

58. Morita S, Furuya K, Kazuhiko I, Nakabayashi N (1998) Performance of adhesive bone cement containing hydroxyapatite particles. *Biomaterials.* 19:1601-6.

59. Oonishi H, Kadoya Y, Iwaki H, Kin N (2000) Hydroxyapatite granules interposed at bone-cement interface in total hip replacements: histological study of retrieved specimens. *J. Biomed. Mater. Res.* 53:174-80.

60. Ohura K, Bohner M, Hardouin P, Lemaitre J, Pasquier G, Flautre B (1996) Resorption of, and bone formation from, new beta-tricalcium phosphate-monocalcium phosphate cements: an *in vivo* study. *J. Biomed Mater Res.* 30:193-200.

61. Manley MT (1993) Calcium phosphate biomaterials: a review of the literature, In: Hydroxyapatite Coatings in Orthopaedic Surgery, Geesink, R.G.T. and Manley, M.T., Editors. Raven Press: New York. p. 1-24.

62. Geesink R, DeGroot K, Klein C (1988) Bonding of bone to apatite-coated implants. *J. Bone Joint Surg. Br.* 70:17-22.

63. Cook SD, Thomas KA, Kay JF, Jarcho M (1988) Hydroxyapatite-coated titanium for orthopedic implant applications. *Clin. Orthop.* 232:225-43.

64. DeGroot K, Geesink RGT, Klein CPAT, Serekian P (1987) Plasma sprayed coatings of HA. *J. Biomed. Mater. Res.* 21:1375-81.

65. DeGroot K (1983) Bioceramics of Calcium Phosphates, Boca Raton, FL: CRC Press, Inc.

66. Block MS, Kent JN, Kay JF (1987) HA-coated titanium dental implants in dogs. *J. Oral. Maxillofac. Surg.* 42:793-807.

67. Hayashi K, Uenoyama K, Matsuguchi N, Sugioka Y (1991) Quantitative analysis of *in vivo* tissue responses to titanium-oxide and hydroxyapatite-coated titanium alloy. *J. Biomed. Mater. Res.* 25: 515-23.

68. Boone PS, Zimmerman MC, Gutteling E, Lee CK, Parsons JR, Langrana N (1989) Bone attachment to hydroxyapatite-coated polymers. *J. Biomed. Mater. Res.* 23(A2):183-99.

69. Manley MT, Kay JF, Yoshiya S, Stern LS (1987), Stulberg BN: Accelerated fixation of weight bearing implants by HA coatings. Orthopedic Research Society 33rd Annual Meeting. Vol. 12. p. 214, San Francisco, California.

70. Manley MT, Kay JF, Uratsuji M, Stern LS, Stulberg BN (1987) Fixation of porous titanium and smooth HA interfaces in a loaded model. 13th Annual Meeting of the Society of Biomaterials. p. 210, New York, NY.

71. Manley MT, Gaisser DM, Uratsuji M, Stulberg BN, Bauer TW, Stern LS (1988) Fixation of porous titanium and smooth HA interfaces in a loaded model. 34th Annual Meeting, Orthopaedic Research Society. p. 332, Atlanta, GA.

72. Pazzaglia UE, Brossa F, Zatti G, Chiesa R, Andrini L (1998) The relevance of hydroxyapatite and spongious titanium coatings in fixation of cementless stems. An experimental comparative study in rat femur employing histological and microangiographic techniques. *Arch. Orthop. Trauma. Surg.* 117:279-85.

73. Marinoni EC, Fontana A, Castellano S (1995) Osteointegration of 96 cementless hip prostheses with hydroxyapatite coating: 5 years follow-up. *Chir. Organi Mov.* 80:147-55.

74. Soballe K (1993) Hydroxyapatite ceramic coating for bone implant fixation. Mechanical and histological studies in dogs. *Acta Orthop. Scand. Suppl.* 255:1-58.

75. Thomas KA, Cook SD, Kay JF, Jarcho M, Anderson RC, Harding AF, Reynolds MC (1986) Attachment strength and histology of HA coated implants, In: Biomedical Engineering v. Recent Developments. Proceedings of the Fifth Southern Biomedical Engineering Conference, Saha, S., Editor. Pergamon Press: New York, NY. p. 205-11.

76. Rivero DP, Fox J, Skipor AK, Urban RM, Galante JO (1988) Calcium phosphate coated porous titanium implants for enhanced skeletal fixation. *J. Biomed. Mater. Res.* 22:191-201.

77. Cook SD, Thomas KA, Dalton JE, Volkman TK, Whitecloud III TS, Kay JF (1992) HA coating of porous implants improves bone ingrowth and interface attachment strength. *J. Biomed. Mater. Res.* 26:989-1001.

78. Cook SD, Thomas KA, Kay JF, Jarcho M (1988) Hydroxyapatite-coated porous titanium for use as an orthopedic biologic attachment system. *Clin. Orthop.* 230:303-12.

79. Ramires PA, Romito A, Cosentino F, Milella E (2001) The influence of titania/hydroxyapatite composite coatings on in vitro osteoblasts behaviour. *Biomaterials.* 22:1467-74.

80. Caropreso S, Cerroni L, Marini S, Cocchia D, Martinetti R, Condo SG (1997) Necessity and validity of standard models for experimental preclinical evaluation of biomaterials. An example of biologic characterization of a hydroxyapatite-based implant material. *Minerva Stomatol.* 46:45-50.

81. Ruano R, Jaeger RG, Jaeger MM (2000) Effect of a ceramic and a non-ceramic hydroxyapatite on cell growth and procollagen synthesis of cultured human gingival fibroblasts. *J. Periodontol.* 71:540-5.

82. Sun JS, Lin FH, Hung TY, Tsuang YH, Chang WH, Liu HC (1999) The influence of hydroxyapatite particles on osteoclast cell activities. *J. Biomed. Mater. Res.* 45:311-21.

83. Gumaer KI, Salsbury RL, Sauerschell RJ, Slighter RG, Drobeck HP (1985) Evaluation of hydroxylapatite root implants in baboons. *Journal of Oral and Maxillofacial Surgery.* 44:73-9.

84. Daculsi G, LeGeros RZ, Nery E, Lynch K, Kerebel B (1989) Transformation of biphasic calcium phosphate ceramics in vivo: ultrastructural and physicochemical characterization. *Biomed. Mater. Res.* 23:883-94.

85. Drobeck HP, Rothstein SS, Gumaer KI, Sherer AD, Slighter RG (1984) Histologic observations of soft tissue responses to implanted, multifaceted particles and discs of HA. *Journal of Oral and Maxillofacial Surgery.* 42:143-9.

86. Eggli PS, Muller RW, Schenk RK (1988) Porous hydroxyapatite and tricalcium phosphate cylinders with two different pore size ranges implanted in the cancellous bone of rabbits. A comparative histomorphic and histologic study of bony ingrowth and implant substitution. *Clin. Orthop.* 232:127-38.

87. Bell R, Beirne OR (1988) Effect of HA, tricalcium phosphate, and collagen on the healing of defects in the rat mandible. *Journal of Oral and Maxillofacial Surgery.* 46:589-94.

88. Lin TC, Su CY, Chang CS (1997) Stereomorphologic observation of bone tissue response to hydroxyapatite using SEM with the EDTA-KOH method. *J. Biomed. Mater. Res.* 36:91-7.

89. Furukawa T, Matsusue Y, Yasunaga T, Shikinami Y, Okuno M, Nakamura T (2000) Biodegradation behavior of ultra-high-strength hydroxyapatite/poly (L-lactide) composite rods for internal fixation of bone fractures. *Biomaterials.* 21:889-98.

90. Yoshimine Y, Akamine A, Mukai M, Maeda K, Matsukura M, Kimura Y, Makishima T (1993) Biocompatibility of tetracalcium phosphate cement when used as a bone substitute. *Biomaterials.* 14:403-6.

91. Liu C, Wang W, Shen W, Chen T, Hu L, Chen Z (1997) Evaluation of the biocompatibility of a nonceramic hydroxyapatite. *J. Endod.* 23:490-3.

92. Wu H, Zhu TB, Du JY, Hong GX, Sun SZ, Xu XH (1992) Analysis of the biocompatibility of magnetic porous tricalcium phosphate ceramics in rat femurs. *J. Tongji Med. Univ.* 12:111-5.

93. Dieppe PA, Huskisson EC, Crocker P, Willoughby DA (1976) Apatite deposition disease. A New Arthropathy. *Lancet.* 1(7954):266-9.

94. Nagase M, Baker DG, Schumacher HR (1988) Prolonged inflammatory reactions induced by artificial ceramics in the rat air pouch model. *J. Rheumatol.* 15:1334-8.

95. Rooney T, Berman S, Indresano AT (1988) Evaluation of porous block HA for augmentation of aveolar ridges. *J. Oral. Maxillofac. Surg.* 46:15-8.

96. dos Santos LA, Carrodeguas RG, Rogero SO, Higa OZ, Boschi AO, De Arruda AC (2002) Alpha-tricalcium phosphate cement: in vitro cytotoxcity. *Biomaterials.* 23:2035-42.

97. Anderson GI, Orlando K, Waddell JP (2001) Synovitis subsequent to total-hip arthroplasty with and without hydroxyapatite coatings: a study in dogs. *Vet. Surg.* 30:311-8.

98. Mommaerts MY, Nadjmi N, Abeloos JV, Neyt LF (1999) Six years experience with zygomatic "sandwich" osteotomy for correction of malar deficiency. *J. Oral. Maxillofac. Surg.* 57:8-13.

99. Cormack DH (1987) Ham's Histology, ed. 9, Philadelphia, PA: J.B. Lippincott Co. pp. 283-87.

100. Johnson KD, Frierson KE, Keller TS, Cook C, Scheinberg R, Zerwekh J, Meyers L, Sciadini MF (1996) Porous ceramics as bone graft substitutes in long bone defects: a biomechanical, histological, and radiographic analysis. *J. Orthop. Res.* 14:351-69.

101. Zerwekh JE, Kourosh S, Scheinberg R, Kitano T, Edwards ML, Shin D, Selby DK (1992) Fibrillar collagen-biphasic calcium phosphate composite as a bone graft substitute for spinal fusion. *J. Orthop. Res.* 10:562-72.

102. Chapman MW, Bucholz R, Cornell C (1997) Treatment of acute fractures with a collagen-calcium phosphate graft material. A randomized clinical trial. *J. Bone Joint Surg. (Am).* 79:495-502.

103. Muschler GF, Negami S, Hyodo A, Gaisser D, Easley K, Kambic H (1996) Evaluation of collagen ceramic composite graft materials in a spinal fusion model. *Clin. Orthop.* 328:250-60.

104. Bell R, Beirne OR (1988) Effect of HA, tricalcium phosphate, and collagen on the healing of defects in the rat mandible. *J. Oral. Maxillofac. Surg.* 46:589-94.

105. Takaoka T, Okumura M, Ohgushi H, Inoue K, Takakura Y, Tamai S (1996) Histological and biochemical evaluation of osteogenic response in porous hydroyapatite coated alumina ceramics. *Biomaterials.* 17:1499-505.

106. Yoshikawa T, Ohgushi H, Tamai S (1996) Immediate bone forming capability of prefabricated osteogenic hydroxyapatite. *J. Biomed. Mater. Res.* 32:481-92.

107. Frame JW (1987) Hydroxyapatite as a biomaterial for alveolar ridge augmentation. *Int. J. Oral. Maxillofac. Surg.* 16:642-55.

108. Munting E (1996) The contributions and limitations of hydroxyapatite coatings to implant fixation: A histomorphometric study of load bearing implants in dogs. *Int. Orthop.* 20:1-6.

109. Levine JP, Bradley J, Turk AE, Ricci JL, Benedict JJ, Steiner G, Longaker MT, McCarthy JG (1997) Bone morphogenetic protein promotes vascularization and osteoinduction in preformed hydroxyapatite in the rabbit. *Ann. Plast. Surg.* 39(2):158-68.

110. Reddie AH (2001) Bone morphogenetic proteins: from basic science to clinical applications. *J. Bone Joint Surg.* 83A(Suppl 1, Part 1):S1-S6.

111. Wozney JM, Rosen V, Celeste AJ, Mitsock LM, Whitters MJ, Kriz RW, Hewick RM, Wang EA (1988) Novel regulators of bone formation: molecular clones and activities. *Science.* 242:1528-34.

112. Koempel JA, Patt BS, O'Grady K, Wozney J, Toriumi DM (1998) The effect of recombinant human bone morphogenetic protein-2 on the integration of porous hydroxyapatite implants with bone. *J. Biomed. Mater. Res.* 5:359-63.

113. Noshi T, Yoshikawa T, Dohi Y, Ikeuchi M, Horiuchi K, Ichijima K, Sugimura M, Yonemasu K (2001) Recombinant human bone mophogenetic protein-2 potentiates the in vivo osteogenic ability of marrow/hydroxyapatite composites. *Artif Organs.* 25:201-8.

114. Noshi T, Yoshikawa T, Ikeuchi M, Dohi Y, Ohgushi H, Horiuchi K, Sugimura M, Ichijima K, Yonemasu K (2000) Enhancement of the in vivo osteogenic potential of marrow/hydroxyapatite composites by bovine bone morphogenetic protein. *J. Biomed. Mater. Res.* 52:621-30.

115. Ripamonti U, Ramoshebi LN, Matsaba T, Tasker J, Crooks J, Teare J (2001) Bone induction by BMPs/OPs and related family members in primates. *J. Bone Joint. Surg.* 83-A(Suppl 1):S116-27.

116. Lind M, Overgaard S, Jensen TB, Song Y, Goodman SB, Bunger C, Soballe K (2001) Effect of osteogenic protein 1/collagen composite combined with impacted allograft around hydroxyapatite-coated titanium alloy implants is moderate. *J. Biomed. Mater. Res.* 55:89-95.

117. Oda S, Kinoshita A, Higuchi T, Shizuya T, Ishikawa I (1997) Ectopic bone formation by biphasic calcium phosphate (BCP) combined with recombinant human bone morphogenetic protein-2 (rhBMP-2). *J. Med. Dent. Sci.* 44:53-62.

118. Cranin AN, Satler NM (1984) Human mandibular alveolar ridge augmentation with HA: final report of a five year investigation. 10th Annual Meeting of the Society for Biomaterials. p. 324, Washington, DC.

119. Holmes RE, Wardrop RW, Wolford LM (1988) HA as a bone graft substitute in orthognathic surgery: histologic and histometeric findings. *J. Oral. Maxillofac. Surg.* 46:661-71.

120. Kent JN, Quinn JH, Zide MF, Finger IM, Jarcho M, Rothstein SS (1982) Correction of alveolar ridge deficiencies with nonresorbable HA. *J. Am. Dent. Assoc.* 105:993-1001.

121. Rothstein SS, Paris D, Sage B (1984) Use of durapatite for the rehabilitation of resorbed alveolar ridges. *J. Am. Dent. Assoc.* 109:571-74.

122. Meadows G (2002) Adjunctive use of ultraporous beta-tricalcium phosphate bone void filler in spinal arthrodesis. *Orthopedics.* 25(5 Suppl):S579-84.

123. Szabo G, Suba Z, Hrabak K, Barabas J, Nemeth Z (2001) Autogenous bone versus beta-tricalcium phosphate graft alone for bilateral sinus elevations (2- and 3-dimensional computed tomographic, histologic, and histomorphometric evaluations): preliminary results. *Int. J. Oral. Maxillofac. Implants.* 16:681-92.

124. Muschik M, Ludwig R, Halhubner S, Brursche K, Stoll T (2001) Beta-tricalcium phosphate as a bone substitute for dorsal spinal fusion in adolescent idiopathic scoliosis: preliminary results of a prospective clinical study. *Eur. Spine J.* 10(Suppl 2):S178-184.

125. Russotti GM, Okada Y, Fitzgerald RH, Chao EYS, Gorski JP (1987) Efficacy of using a bone graft substitute to enhance biological fixation of a porous metal femoral component, In: The Hip: proceedings of the 15th open scientific meeting of the Hip Society. p. 120-54.

126. Vedantam R, Ruddlesdin C (1996) The fully hydroxy-apatite-coated total hip implant. *J. Arthroplasty.* 11:534-42.

127. D'Antonio JA, Capello WN, Manley M (1996) Remodeling of bone around hydroxyapatite-coated femoral stems. *J. Bone Joint Surg. Am.* 78:1226-34.

128. D'Antonio JA, Capello WN, Jaffe WL (1992) HA-coated implants: multi-center three-year clinical and radiographic results. *Clin. Orthop.* 285:102-15.

129. D'Antonio JA, Capello WN, Manley MT, Geesink RGT (2001) Hydroxylapatite femoral stems for total hip arthroplasty: 10-13 year follow-up. *Clin. Orthop.* 393:101-11.

130. Hardy DCR, Frayssinet P, Guilhem A, LaFontaine MA, DeLince PE (1991) Bonding of hydroxyapatite-coated prostheses. Histopathology of specimens from four cases. *J. Bone Joint Surg. Br.* 73:732-40.

131. Bloebaum RD, Merrell M, Gustke K, Simmons M (1991) Retrieval analysis of a hydroxyapatite-coated hip prosthesis. *Clin Orthop.* 267:97-102.

132. Bauer TW (1993) The histology of HA-coated implants, In: HA Coatings in Orthopaedic Surgery, Geesink, R. and Manley, M., Editors. Raven Press: New York. p. 305-18.

133. Tonino AJ, Therin M, Doyle C (1999) HA-coated femoral stems. Histology and histomorphometry around five components retrieved at post mortem. *J. Bone Joint Surg. Br.* 81:148-54.

134. Thanner J, Karrholm J, Herberts P, Malchau H (1999) Porous cups with and without hydroxylapatite-trical-cium phosphate coating: 23 matched pairs evaluated with radiostereometry. *J. Arthroplasty.* 14:266-71.

135. Epinette JA, Manley MT, D'Antonio JA, Edidin AA, Capello WN (2003) A 10-Year Minimum Follow-Up of Hydroxyapatite-Coated Threaded Cups: Clinical radiographic and survivorship analyses with comparison to the literature. *J. Arthroplasty.* 18(2): 140-8.

BASIC SCIENCE:
HISTOLOGY
AND EXPERIMENTAL WORKS

1 Hydroxyapatite: from Plasma Spray to Electrochemical Deposition

Paul Serekian, MS

INTRODUCTION

The success of hydroxyapatite (HA) coated implant devices is now well documented, with numerous published studies (1, 2, 3, 4) demonstrating excellent long-term clinical results. Clearly, many of the HA coatings used in earlier clinical studies involving plasma-sprayed HA-coated product were not as consistent in chemistry and mechanical properties as those now found on contemporary prostheses. The overall consistency and quality of HA plasma-sprayed coating on implant surfaces improved soon after their introduction, as early concerns arose regarding adequate bonding properties to the substrate, the sequela of HA debris, and possible osteolysis. Typically, as with the introduction of most new technologies to the orthopedic community, use of HA-coated implants did not increase dramatically until 5 years after regulatory acceptance was granted in the US (1991), and excellent clinical results were reported from a number of studies. Currently in the US, 30% of all cementless hip implants are HA-coated.

The vast majority of HA-coated orthopedic implants introduced in the early 1990's were coated using a plasma spray technique. Yankee (5) *et al.* concluded that plasma spraying HA was the preferred method of coating, as it represented an established baseline of technology, was cost efficient, and reproducible. The particulars of the technique are well documented in the literature (5). Despite the early concerns relating to HA coating delamination, the majority of HA-coated implants with coatings in the thickness range of 40-100 um performed well and proved to be an excellent cementless fixation option. At present, the favorable clinical history with HA-coated hip implants exceeds 12 years, and the majority of the experience is associated with plasma-sprayed HA on non-porous surfaces.

ALTERNATE PROCESSING ADVANCEMENTS

The early experience with HA-coated, non-porous implants proved very successful. However, with the advent of three-dimensional interstitial porous and textured surfaces, a considerable level of interest and focus was directed toward exploring non-line-of-site coating techniques. Attempts to coat beaded porous structures were encumbered by the masking of the outermost layer of beads and restricting the pore size opening for bony ingrowth. Advancements in the area of solution-deposited, electophoretic, ion-beam-assisted deposition (IBAD) provide the capability of uniformly coating three-dimensional porous structures without the restrictions associated with plasma spraying.

All the alternate HA application techniques to be discussed result in coatings that are thinner (ranging 2 μm – 20 μm) than the typical 50 μm thick plasma-sprayed coating. Although in a number of cases the coatings exhibit enhanced mechno-morphological merit, there is little clinical experience with these coatings. A further advantage of the alternative coating techniques is that they require a low temperature environment only. Low temperature processing enables a more predictable and controlled environment for depositing the coating, and eliminates the creation of other calcium phosphates and changes in coating crystallinity.

HYDROXYAPATITE SOLUTION DEPOSITION

There are distinct advantages for near room temperature deposition of apatite coatings that relate to a more chemically integrated and crystallographic consistent coating when compared to plasma spraying. A distinct advantage is the ability to uniformly coat three- dimensional structures, thereby providing a larger surface area for osteoconduction and avoiding coating only substrate surfaces in the direct line of HA particles (as from the plasma gun). Figure 1 depicts the HA coating distribution of solution-deposited versus plasma-sprayed coating on a beaded, two layer porous coating.

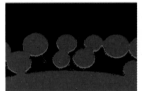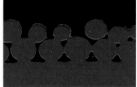

Figure 1 – Solution-deposited vs plasma-sprayed HA on a two layer porous surface.

Although the concept of depositing calcium phosphate coating from an aqueous solution onto a substrate was explored by a number of investigators, the researchers at Norian were the first to successfully demonstrate proof of concept in their laboratory. The coating technique was subsequently licensed by Howmedica and scaled up to production levels. This Howmedica "Peri-Apatite" coating represented the earliest introduction of a commercially proven method for depositing highly crystalline, non-line-of-sight HA on implant surfaces. In this patented process first described by Constantz *et al.* (6, 7), calcium and phosphate ions nucleate and grow into hydroxyapatite crystals on the surface of an implant submerged in supersaturated calcium phosphate solution. The crystals form a near stoichometric HA coating with a typical overall thickness of 20 um. Solution kinetics are controlled by pH, temperature, and ionic concentration of the calcium/phosphate bath. The solution-deposited HA results in an acicular, 100% crystalline structure with a large surface area.

The coating of production quantities of Peri-Apatite HA as described by Zitelli *et al.* (8) takes

place in an automated machine as depicted in Figure 2. The coating tank contains a high calcium phosphate ionic concentration in an aqueous solution in which the implants are submerged and masked in positioned metal fixtures. The precipitation reaction releases acid which is neutralized by the addition of ammonium hydroxide for solution control. The pH of the reaction controls the Ca to P ratio of the HA crystal. The surface area of Peri-Apatite is approximately 1000 times that of HA plasma-sprayed coatings. The significant increase in the surface area is projected to be responsible for the near equivalent resorption rate of the coating to plasma-sprayed coatings, despite the 35% difference in crystallinity. The effects of high temperature (up to 20,000 C) associated with the plasma spray technique result in decreased levels of crystallinity and a chemical transformation of the starting feedstock. HA crystallinity post plasma can be reduced by up to 40%, and the transformation of feedstock typically results in the formation of an amorphous calcium phosphate components, such as brushite, tricalcium phosphate (TCP), and tetra tricalcium phosphate (TTCP). A decrease in crystallinity and the presence of other calcium phosphates associated with more rapid resorption affect the resorption profile of the coating.

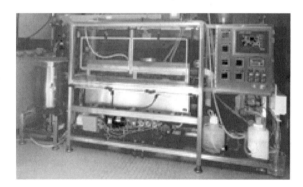

Figure 2 – Peri-Apatite HA coating machine.

There are a number of pre-clinical studies (11-16) that have been published on the Peri-Apatite HA coating. The overall outcomes of the studies demonstrate biocompatibility, efficacy in early time frames in improving fixation of implants to bone, and the absence of adverse tissue reactions. There is also clinical experience with Peri-Apatite beginning in Europe in 1996, Australia in 1997, and the US in 1998 (hip stems).

ELECTROPHORETIC TECHNIQUE

The electrophoretic process fundamentally relies on deposition of electically charged HA particles through a liquid or gel. Recent refinements in the process enable the deposition of sophisticated coating profiles as reflected in size, crystallinity, composition, and morphology. In general, although the electrophoretic process provides the option of depositing non-line-of-sight, thin calcium phosphate coatings, the coatings tend to be irregular and have a relatively weak adherence to the substrate. A more recent technique described by Nie *et al.* (9) uses a electrolytic plasma to augment the electrophoretic process, thereby producing a more predictable, high bond strength coating than that produced by the electrophoretic process alone.

The substrate surfaces to be processed with the plasma assist technique are pretreated for 10 minutes with and oxidation plasma electrolysis technique in order to form a titanium oxide (TiO_2) layer. A transverse section of such a coating consists of a top layer of HA, a middle layer of HA/Ti O_2, and a base layer of TiO_2, with the outermost layer exhibiting equiaxial grains 1/5 the size of typically deposited semi-acicular platelets representative of straight electrophoretic coatings.

Although the plasma assisted HA deposition technique enables the fabrication of denser and higher bond strength coatings compared to electrophoretic coatings, there are no long term data to confirm enhanced tissue response.

ELECTROPHORETIC NANOTECHNOLOGY

The process of depositing nanostructured apatite coatings on implant surfaces by electrophoretic deposit is a relatively new development (17), and provides a number of advantages over plasma spray. "Nano", for the purpose of reference, shall mean a dominant scale length of < 100nm as relates to particle size, grain size, and/or phase. The advantage of working with nano-sized particles/grains of HA as a coating is the extraordinary surface to mass ratio obtained (~ 300m^2/g) compared to the surface-to-mass ratios associated with plasma-sprayed coatings. Thus, whereas the

abstract resorption rate of earlier formulations of calcium phosphates was primarily controlled by crystallinity and chemistry, the advent of nano apatites allows total resorption rates to be achieved in a matter of days.

In general, nanostructured HA provides:
– controlled molecular assembly;
– an enhanced ability to be processed;
– superior material properties.
Typical cluster size is depicted in Figure 3.

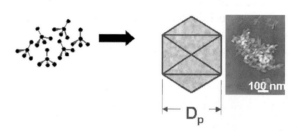

Figure 3

A comparison of the nano HA to conventional HA and periapatite is depicted in Figure 4.

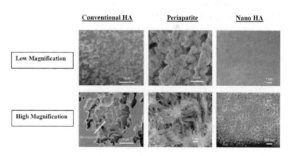

Figure 4

Nano *vs* Conventional Microstructure

Theoretically, nanostructure apatites provide for a level of manipulation and control not possible given the processing restrictions of plasma spraying. The prospect of manipulating the substitution-tolerant crystallographic structure of nanoapatites allows the synthesis of coatings with precise chemistry, ultrafine microstructure, and material properties tailored to applications.

	Bending Strength (Mpa)	Compressive Strength (Mpa)	Fracture Toughness (Mpa•m1/2)
Compact Bone	160	170-193	2-12
Conventional HAP	38-113	120-800	1.0
Nano HA	183	879	> 1

Table 1 – Mechanical properties of nano HA.

The clinical performance of nanostructure apatites on plain and ingrowth surfaces is yet to be demonstrated. It is limited not only by the ability to engineer the chemistry, crystallinity, and assembly to provide a technical platform, but also by the ability to couple growth factors not attainable by plasma spraying techniques. Controlled molecular assembly results in a lower concentration of flaws and flaw size. The overall effect is improved mechanical properties, as shown in Table 1.

ION BEAM ASSISTED DEPOSITED COATINGS (IBAD)

The deposition process is composed of an electron beam bombarding and vaporizing a high purity hydroxyapatite bulk target. At the same time, an argon ion beam is focused on the metal substrate to assist in the deposition of HA. The IBAD deposition of HA on a titanium substrate has been shown by Lin *et al.* (10) to generate tensile bond strengths of 70 MPa. This compares to the tensile bond strength of 51 MPa typically associated with the plasma spray deposition process. The higher bond strengths associated with the IBAD prepared films are seen as a consequence of an atomic intermixing interfacial layer formed by ion dynamic intermixing (10). The interfacial layer is 25 um thick and consists of a transitional structure that includes amorphous HA, amorphous calcium phosphates, amorphous titanium phosphate compounds, and a two-stage gradient of interrupted titanium. It is suggested that a chemical bond forms at the HA/titanium interface as a consequence of the energetic ion bombardment process. The coating thickness associated with the IBAD process is typically in the 2-4 μm range and can be made thicker with extended exposure times (hours). Although IBAD represents a viable methodology with excellent bonding prop-

erties to the substrate, there is no known long term clinical experience with this type of coating.

CONCLUSION

The majority of the clinical experience with HA-coated implants has been with plasma-sprayed coatings and overall, HA-coated hip implants have proven to be a highly effective option for cement-less fixation.

More recently, there has been an emerging level of interest in alternative HA deposition techniques that enable coating of three-dimensional porous structures without the exposure to high temperature processing and its influential effects on spin-off calcium phosphate chemistry and charges in crystallinity effects. Although electrophoretic and IBAD processing techniques offer theoretical and process advantages over plasma spray methods, the clinical experience with the newer deposition methodologies require clinical follow-up for demonstrating equivalence and superiority to plasma-spray applied HA coating.

Reference List

1. Capello WM, D'Antonio JA, Manley MT, Feinberg JR (1998) Hydroxyapatite In Total Hip Arthroplasty, Clinical Results and Critical Issues, *Clin. Orthop.* (355):200-11.

2. Capello WN, D'Antonio JA, Feinberg JR, Manley MT (1997) Hydroxyapatite-Coated Total Hip Femoral Components In Patients Less Than Forty Years Old. Clinical and Radiographic Results after Five to Eight Years of Follow-Up, *J. Bone Joint Surg. Arm.* 79 (7): 1023-9.

3. Geesink RG, Hoefnagels NH (1995) Six Year Results of Hydroxyapatite-Coated Tota Hip Replacement, *J. Bone Joint Surg. Br.* 77:534-47.

4. Garcia Araujo C, Fernandez Gonzalez J, Tonino A, (1998) Rheumatoid Arthritis And Hydroxyapatite-

coated Hip Prostheses: five-year results. J Arthroplasty 13(6): 660-7.

5. Yankee SJ, Pletka BJ, Luckey HA, Johnson WA (1990) Process for Fabricating HA Coatings for Biomedical Applications, Thermal Spray Research and Applications, Proceedings of the T National Thermal Spray Conference, May 20-25, Long Beach, California: 433-8.

6. Constantz BR, Osaka GC (1992) US Patent No. 5164187.

7. Constantz BR (1993) US Patent No. 5188670.

8. Zitelli JP, Higham P (2000), A Novel Method for Solution Deposition of Hydroxyapatite on to Tree Dimensional Porous Metallic Surfaces: Peri-Apatite HA, Mat *Res. Soc. Proc.*, Vol. 599, Materials Research Society.

9. Liu JQ, Luo ZS, Liu FZ, Duuan XF, Peng LM, High Resolution Transmission Electron Microscopy Investigations of a Highly Adhesive Hydroxyapatite Coating/Titanium Interface Fabricated by Ion-Beam-Assisted Deposition, *J. Biomed. Mater. Res.* 52:115-8.

10. Nie X, Leyland A, Matthews A, Juang JC, Melitis EI (2001), Effects of Solution PH and Electical Parameters on Hydroxyapatite Coatings Deposited by a Plasma-Assisted Electropharesis Technique, *J. Biomed. Mater. Res.* 51:612-8.

11. Aberman HM, Tores LC, Baines DP, Villanuerva AR, Constantz R, Hungerford DS, Dumbleton JH (1993) Gap Healing in a Non-Weight Bearing Dog Model: Effectiveness of A Solution Precipitated Apatite Coating, 39th Annual Meeting, Orthopaedic Research Society, p 466.

12. Fagan M, Aberman HM, De Young DJ (1994) Effect Of Precipitated Calcium Phosphate Coating on Bone Fixation of a PCA Canine Hip Stem at Early Time Periods, ASME Advances in Bioengineering, BED-Vol.28, pp. 439-40.

13. Aberman HM, Jones LC, Fagan M, Hungerford DS, Dumbleton JH (1996), The Effectivenss of Peri-Apatite Coatings In Bridging Implant Gaps, 42nd Annual Meeting, Orthopaedic Research Society, p. 526.

14. Aberman HM, Goodman SB, Lalor PA, Fagan M, Dumbleton JH (1996), *In vivo* Biostability of a Solution Precipitated Apatite Coating, 5th World Biomaterials Congress, May 29-June, p. 662.

15. Anderson DE, St. Jean G, Richardson DC, Debowes RM, Roush JK, Lowry SR, Toll DW, Aberman HA, Van Sickle DC, Hoskinson JJ (1997), Improved Osseointeraction of Calcium Phosphate-Coated External Fixation Pins, *Acta Orthop. Scand.* 68, (6) 571-6.

16. Turner AS, Eckhoff DG, Dewell RD, Villanueva AR, Aberman HM (1996), Peri-Apatite-Coated Implants Improve Fixation In Osteopenic Bone, 40th Annual Meeting, Orthopaedic Research Society, New Orleans, p. 41.

17. Private communication with Edward Ahn, PhD.

2   Calcium Phosphate Coatings for Implant Fixation

Ole Rahbek, MD, PhD, Søren Overgaard, MD, PhD and Kjeld Søballe, MD, PhD

INTRODUCTION

It has been predicted that the number of revisions due to mechanical loosening after total hip replacement will increase steadily from year to year due to the increasing number of joint replacements. Unfortunately, results after revision arthroplasty are clearly inferior to those of primary arthroplasty (1). Especially in younger active patients, the conventional prostheses do not live up to expectations and there is widespread concern about the significant risk of failure for these patients (2). These facts have led to increased interest in cementless implant fixation, primarily by means of biological fixation provided by press fit insertion followed by bone ingrowth into a porous surface texture. Clinical retrieval studies of non-cemented metal porous coated hip and knee prostheses have revealed that many of the components were fixed to the skeleton by fibrous tissue ingrowth instead of bony ingrowth (3, 4). For these reasons great efforts have been concentrated on enhancement of bony ingrowth into the non-cemented prosthetic surface. Special interest has focused on hydroxyapatite which has been demonstrated to be successfully coated onto a metal surface using plasma spray technique (5-12).

In 1977, sintered hydroxyapatite (HA) was proved to bond strong with bone (13-15). However, due to the mechanical properties of bulk materials with low resistance to fatigue failure the material was unsuitable for load-bearing application. In 1987, de Groot *et al.* and others published results of plasma sprayed HA-coated bone implants (6, 16-18). It was demonstrated that HA had osteoconductive properties and that mechanical fixation of HA-coated implants were better than uncoated implants during optimal surgical conditions (press fit).

Clinical experience with HA coating is increasing but long-term follow-up remains to be evaluated. However, numerous short-term studies have shown promising results (19-32). Thus studies using roentgen stereophotogrammetric analysis have demonstrated that HA coating is capable of reducing the early migration of both femoral hip and tibial knee components (20, 25, 29-32). In addition, human retrievals have documented good bone apposition suggesting stability between implant and bone (33-37).

Despite the general belief that resorption is necessary for bone bonding to occur, it has been proposed that resorption reduces the bonding strength between implant and substrate and disintegrates the coating. This could lead to delamination and failure of implant fixation and to acceleration of the third body wear process (38-46). Another issue of debate is ; which coating quality is optimum ? Should it stay on the implant surface or should its function only be temporary. In regard to long-term or temporary performance of Ca-P coatings two research direction have been directed. One toward creating more stable coatings to enhance bonding strength between coating and implant and one toward creating more resorbable coatings to increase coating bioactivity (47-57). In addition, currently, HA coatings are available on prostheses with either a grit-blasted and rough or porous substrate surface.

An interesting feature of hydroxyapatite is the possible sealing effect against migration of wear debris in the bone implant interface. The coating of implant surfaces influences the accumulation of wear particles in the bone-implant interface. In cemented arthroplasty migration of wear debris occurs in the implant-cement and bone-cement interface and in fatigue cracks in the cemented mantle leading to localized bone lesions (58, 59). Furthermore, particulate cement originating from the cement mantle is believed to contribute to peri-implant osteolysis (60). In non-cemented arthroplasty is has been hypothesised, that a biological seal is created by the use HA-coated implants. A biological seal has been defined as a seal consisting of host tissue or other bio-active material, which has the potential of healing if defects occur due to mechanical stress (61). In this way a more durable seal as compared to the cemented can be created.

This chapter describes a series of experimental and human studies performed in order to systematically evaluate potential improvements of bone implant fixation using hydroxyapatite (HA) and fluorapatite (FA) coating when subjected to pathological and mechanical conditions mimicking the clinical situation (7-10, 20, 62-65). We also studied factors influencing resorption of the coatings *in vivo*. Furthermore, the effect hydroxyapatite on the periimplant migration of wear debris is reported.

MATERIALS AND METHODS

Models for Implantation

We chose the distal femoral epiphysis in the dog as the implantation site because it contains cancellous bone in order to mimic the clinical practice including presence of a cancellous bone bed and also is affected by arthritic joint changes (66).

The micromotion device consisted of an implantable dynamic device manufactured in titanium alloy (fig. 1a and b), which was inserted into the weight-bearing part of the femoral condyle. When the knee was loaded during gait, load transfer from the tibial part of the knee displaced the implant in the axial direction and tightened the spring. When the leg was unloaded the tightened spring moved the implant back to the initial position. Thus, a controlled movement occurred during each gait cycle. The system was adjusted preoperatively to a stiffness of approximately 14 N/mm with a preload of 0.5 N, the total displacement force being 10 N. The maximal movements in axial direction could be predetermined and limited to the desired amount due to the design of the device.

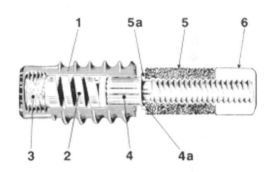

Figure 1a – The unstable device consists of seven components all manufactured from titanium alloy (Ti-6Al-4V) as the porous coated Ti implant. A hollow titanium cylinder (1) with self tapping threads to ensure firm fixation in the bone. A spring (2) is placed inside the cylinder and held in place by a screw (3) at one end. In the other end a titanium piston (4) can move freely in the axial direction. When mounted, the platform (4a) on the piston projects exactly 500 microns over the end of the titanium cylinder. When the implant (5) is screwed onto the threads of the piston and axial load applied on the polyethylene plug (6), the implant will move until it is stopped by reaching the titanium cylinder and the movement is limited to 500 microns. In order to prevent rotation of the piston, one end of the spring is fixed to the piston (4) and the other to the screw (3) which is locked into the titanium cylinder by a small polyethylene plug inserted into the threads of the screw. (From ref (65)).

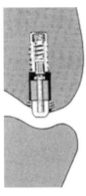

Figure 1b – The dynamic system is inserted into the weight-bearing part of the medial femoral condyle. The polyethylene plug projects above the femoral articular cartilage. When the knee is loaded during gait, load transfer from the tibial part of the knee will displace the polyethylene and the implant in axial direction and tighten the spring. When the leg later is unloaded the tightened spring will move the implant back to the initial position. Thus, a controlled movement will occur during each gait cycle.

Movements of 500 μm and 150 μm were used. Also immobilized implants devices were used without any micromovements.

In study XI and XII a stable implant device was inserted into each femoral distale condyle with a 0.75 mm periimplant gap. The diameter of the PE-plug was reduced in order to allow the access of joint fluid to the periimplant gap. Polyethylene particles were repeatedly injected into the knee joint.

In study VII, the implants coated with HA and FA were inserted in the iliac crest in patients suffering from an acute spinal fracture at the thoracolumbar region. The implants were inserted into trabecular bone in a unloaded 1 mm gap model. A similar implant model was used in study X. The implants were inserted in the medial aspect of the proximal tibia of the dog surrounded by 2 mm gap. The gap was filled with hyaloronic acid mixed with particulate material.

Implants and Coatings

The cylindrical titanium (Ti) plugs were 6.0 mm in diameter with an overall length of 10 mm, consisting of a solid Ti-6Al-4V alloy core with a plasma-sprayed coating of Ti-6Al-4V with a mean pore size of 300 microns. In study IV, V, VII, XI, and XII implants with a grit-blasted surface were also included.

The HA and FA coated implants consisted of analogous titanium porous coated implants on which a layer of spray dried synthetic hydroxyapatite was deposited by plasma spraying technique.

RESULTS AND DISCUSSION

Effects of Hydroxyapatite Coating on Mechanical Fixation and Bone Ingrowth

Obtaining rigid initial stability seems to be one of the major problems in non-cemented endoprosthetic surgery and depends initially on the strength of mechanical interlock between implant and bone achieved during implantation. Several studies have been performed to investigate the stability of hip and knee prostheses immediately after implantation and there is agreement that relative movements between implant and bone occurs in the range of 100-600 µm (67-69). Even when using rigid fixation with screws and pegs, differences in elasticity between bone and the metallic porous material have been shown to result in tangential displacement of 150 µm at the periphery of tibial trays (70).

Moreover, macroscopic motion has been demonstrated at tibial interfaces. In contrast, cemented prostheses have been shown to be more stable (71).

Since the degree of micromotion and its effect on bone tissue is difficult to assess in clinical practice, we found it important to create a dynamic system to study the significance of controlled micromovements between bone and implant.

In the first study I (65), movements of 500 µm were studied and in the next study II (63) 150 µm movements were investigated. Mechanically stable implants functioned as controls and the observation period was 4 weeks.

In both studies, micromovements resulted in a fibrous membrane (fig. 2), whereas variable amounts of bone ingrowth were obtained in mechanically stable implants (fig. 3). Both studies also demon-

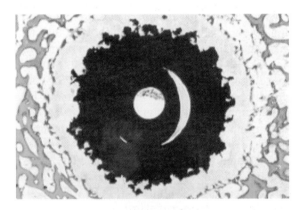

Figure 2 – Photomicrograph from an implant subjected to micromovements showing fibrous tissue around HA coated implant. (Light green, Basic Fuchsin, grounded section, original magnification x6). (From ref. (63)).

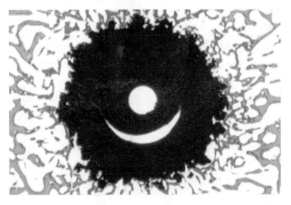

Figure 3 – Photomicrograph from a stable HA coated implant showing bone ingrowth across the initial gap and bone apposition on the implant. (Light green, Basic Fuchsin, grounded section, original magnification × 6) (From ref. (63)).

strated development of islands of fibrocartilage around unstable HA coated implants whereas the membrane predominantly consisted of connective tissue around unstable Ti implants. Results from histomorphometric analysis of the presence of fibrocartilage in the membrane is shown in Table 1.

Fibrocartilage	500 µm movement (I(65))	150 µm movement (VII(63))
Titanium implants	2 (0-9) %	5 (0-20) %
Hydroxyapatite implants	32 (0-100) %	53 (31-88) %

Table 1 – Results from quantitative analysis of presence of fibrocartilage in membranes around Ti and HA coated implants.

Study I (65). *500 µm movements.* Seven mature dogs were used. Push-out test showed that the shear strength of unstable Ti and HA implants was significantly reduced as compared to the corresponding mechanically stable implants (P < 0.01). However, shear strength values of unstable HA coated implants were significantly greater than those of unstable Ti implants (P < 0.01) and comparable to those of stable Ti implants. The greatest shear strength was obtained with stable HA coated implants, which was three-fold increased as compared to the stable Ti implants (P < 0.001) (fig. 4).

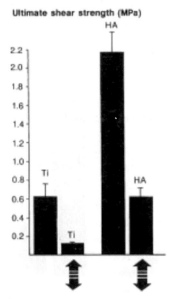

Figure 4 – Results from mechanical test from the 500 µm study. The arrows indicate unstable implants, the two other bars represent stable implants. HA = hydroxyapatite, Ti = titanium. (From ref. (65)).

Quantitative determination of bony ingrowth confirmed the mechanical test except for the stronger anchorage of unstable HA implants as compared to unstable Ti implants, where no difference in bony ingrowth was found. Collagen concentration was significantly higher in membranes around HA coated implants as compared with membranes around Ti implants.

Study II (63). *150 µm movements.* This study comprised 14 mature dogs. Results from the 500 µm study were reproduced regarding presence of fibrocartilage around unstable HA coated implants (Table 2), whereas fibrous connective tissue characterized the membrane around unstable

Obs. Time	4 weeks (65)	4 weeks (63)	16 weeks (64)
Range of motion	500 µm	150 µm	150 µm
Titanium	0.12 (0.01)	0.26 (0.07)	1.8 (0.8)
Hydroxy-apatite	0.63 (0.1)	1.85 (0.4)	4.6 (1.0)

Table 2 – Ultimate shear strength (MPa) of unstable Ti and HA coated implants with different observation time and range of motion. Mean (SEM).

Ti implants. In addition this study revealed a thinner membrane around unstable HA implants compared to unstable Ti implants. A radial orientation of collagen fibers was found in the membrane around unstable HA coated implants whereas a more random orientation was found in most membranes around Ti implants. Shear strength of unstable HA coated implants was significantly greater than that of unstable Ti implants (p < 0.001) but also than that of stable Ti implants (P < 0.05). The greatest shear strength, obtained by stable HA coated implants, was ten-fold higher than that of stable Ti implants (p < 1 × 10⁻⁸) (fig. 5). No significant difference was demonstrated between the amounts of bone apposition on unstable HA and stable Ti implants. The gap-healing capacity around stable HA coated implants increased toward the HA surface and was significantly greater than that of Ti implants.

In conclusion, initial stability of the implant was shown to be a requirement for achieving bone ingrowth (63-65) which is supported by other studies (72-76). However, HA coating seemed to be capable of modifying the fibrous membrane resulting in a stronger fibrous anchorage when subjected to relative motion between bone and implant.

Ultimate shear strength (MPa)

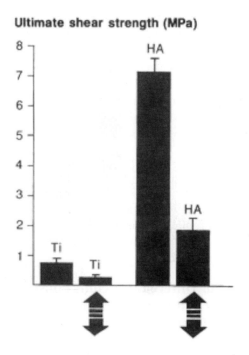

Figure 5 – Results from mechanical test from the 150 μm study. The arrows indicate unstable implants, the two other bars represent stable implants. HA = hydroxyapatite, Ti = titanium. (From ref. (63)).

Magnitude of Motion

The threshold of motion allowing bone ingrowth still is unknown. A dog study showed bone ingrowth and remodeling into non cemented femoral components in THA despite the initial implant motion was as high as 56 μm (77). Burke *et al.* (78) supported our results using another model with controlled movements of 150 μm for 8 hours a day which prevented bone ingrowth and resulted in a dense fibrous tissue layer surrounding the implants. Similar implants with 20 μm movements achieved bone ingrowth indicating that the threshold for bone ingrowth is between 20 and 150 μm movement. These findings seems to be in agreement with Sumner *et al.* (70) showing that bone ingrowth occurs close to the fixation pegs in Ti fiber metal coated tibial components, whereas minor amounts of bone ingrowth was obtained at more peripheral sites of the prosthesis probably due to tangential displacement in the range of 150 μm at the periphery of the tibial tray (79).

Thus, there seems to be a relationship between the magnitude of bone-implant motion and type of interfacial tissue developed. It is therefore inter-

esting to look at the effect of different amounts of movements on implant fixation in our studies (Table 2). An increased fixation strength was obtained with decreased range of motion (500 μm to 150 μm) by both HA and Ti implants and a further increase in fixation when the observation time was extended from 4 weeks to 16 weeks (63-65). Comparing the fixation strength of continuous loaded Ti implants with 16 weeks observation time (1.8 MPa) with those from the 4 weeks study with HA coating (1.85 MPa) equal values were obtained which indicate that fixation of fibrous anchored HA implants is obtained in 1/4 of the time required for the equal fixation of implants without HA coating.

Fibrous Anchorage

It has been suggested that ingrowth of fibrous tissue could be beneficial for energy absorption by providing better distribution of stresses. Longo *et al.* (80) have demonstrated a stable fibrous tissue interface around press fit carbon composite femoral stems in dogs, which obtained clinical results comparable with HA coated stems which were anchored by bone apposition after one year observation period. They concluded that bone bonding of the implant is not essential for implant success. These suggestions are supported by clinical experience where fibrous tissue anchorage is often present in clinical satisfactory prostheses (4). The observation by Ryd (71) who showed significant displacement of clinically stable tibia plateaus in total knee replacements confirm these *in vivo* observations in dogs. According to our results after 4 weeks implantation (63,65) the fibrous membrane around titanium coated implants had almost no capacity of fixation. However, the fibrocartilaginous membrane around unstable HA coated implants was found to be significantly stronger and might be sufficient to dissipate stresses in total joint arthroplasties.

Study III (64). In the two previous studies, (63, 65) a fibrocartilaginous membrane was demonstrated around HA coated implants subjected to micromovements for 4 weeks, whereas fibrous connective tissue predominated around Ti implants. In the present study 14 dogs were used and the long term course of continuous load on fibrous anchored Ti and HA coated implants was studied.

All implants were subjected to 150 μm movements and allowed continuous load for 16 weeks. Histological analysis of implants with continuous load for 16 weeks showed a fibrous membrane around Ti implants, whereas the membrane around HA coated implants was replaced by bone. Push-out test showed inferior fixation of Ti implants compared to HA coated implants (p < 0.001). Bone ingrowth was seven-fold increased in continuously loaded HA implants compared with continuously loaded Ti implants ($P < 1 \times 10^{-2}$).

Reasons for conversion of fibrous membrane to bone around HA coated implants (64) are multifactorial. Theoretically it may be explained by the presence of fibrocartilaginous tissue around HA coated implants as found at 4 weeks which may prepare the gap around the implant mechanically and biologically for later bony anchorage of the implant by endochondral ossification. This explanation seems to be in agreement with the interfragmentary strain theory, (81) stating that the initial presence of fibrous tissue in fracture healing may reduce the strain between the fracture fragments to a level where cartilage can be formed. Presence of fibrocartilage may further reduce the strain to a level where bone can be formed.

Similar presence of bone ingrowth around HA coated implants and fibrous tissue around Ti implants (64) after a longer observation period has been demonstrated in other studies. In a loaded model Manley *et al.* (82) demonstrated that HA coated intramedullary implants were anchored in bone and Ti alloy implants were surrounded by fibrous tissue after 10 weeks. Another weight-bearing model with femoral hemiarthroplasty in dogs (83) showed bone apposition on HA coated grooved macrotextured prostheses, whereas fibrous connective tissue surrounded uncoated control implants after 10 weeks. Geesink *et al.* (6) reported on total hip replacements with HA coating in dogs and found similar differences after observation periods as long as 12 months. Thus, HA coating seems to be efficacious also in a more clinically relevant situation when the implant is subjected to loaded conditions during the entire observation period.

The further course of a persistent fibrous membrane could later lead to loosening of the prosthesis due to bone resorption caused by the presence of macrophages in the membrane. According to Goldring (84) the membrane might be transformed to a "macrophage" membrane initiated by

continuous movement between implant and bone. Such "macrophage" membranes have been described around cemented prostheses (84) to content PGE_2 and collagenase. Presence of these substances may explain the progressive lysis of bone found around both cemented and non-cemented prostheses. In the present studies (63-65) macrophages were present especially around Ti implants which might suggest that these membranes would be able to produce PGE_2 and collagenase. These substances were, however, not quantified because of lack of sufficient membrane material.

Effects of Different Calcium Phosphate Coatings and the Underlying Implant Surface Texture on Mechanical Fixation

Study IV (85) and V (86). The effects of porous-coated versus grit-blasted surface texture of HA-coated implants on mechanical fixation and bone ingrowth and coating delamination were evaluated after 25 weeks and 16 weeks during non weight-bearing and weight-bearing conditions with controlled micromotion of 500 μm, respectively (85, 86). Mechanical testing showed that energy absorption for porous-coated implants was increased 2-3 fold compared with grit-blasted implants, whereas shear stiffness was lower for porous-coated implants (fig. 6). By contrast, ultimate shear strength was at the same level for both implant types. Mechanical fixation was higher for implants inserted into the distal femur compared with the proximal humerus although the observation period was shorter. This might be explained by higher bone density in the distal femur, and moreover, weight-loading might have contributed to enhance fixation.

Macroscopic evaluation of the implant surface after push-out testing revealed that grit-blasted implants had pronounced delamination of the HA coating in contrast to porous-coated implants indicating that the bonding strength of HA on porous-coated implants was greater (fig. 7). Grit-blasted implants had greater bone ingrowth compared with porous-coated implants indicating different surface activities on the implants (Table 3).

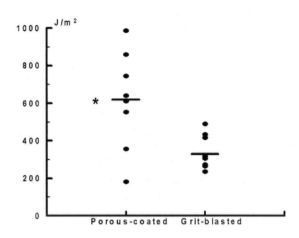
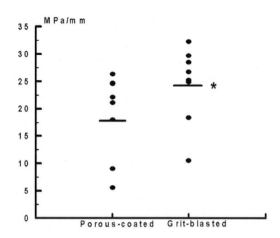

Figure 6 – Push-out test of porous-coated versus grit-blasted hydroxyapatite-coated implants inserted for 25 weeks in a non weight-bearing model. Energy absorption (A) was greater and shear stiffness (B) was lower for porous-coated compared with grit-blasted implants. Solid lines represent mean values, *p < 0.05.

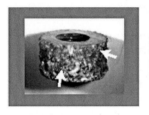
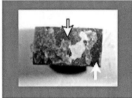

Figure 7 – Macroscopic evaluation after push-out test of porous-coated and grit-blasted implants inserted for 25 weeks A) Porous-coated implants predominantly failed at the hydroxyapatite (HA)-tissue interface. Delamination of the HA coating might have occurred on top of the titanium porous coating (arrows). In contrast Grit-blasted implants B) had pronounced delamination of the HA coating (arrows).

| | Hydroxyapatite-coated implant | |
	Porous-coated	Grit-blasted
Study (89) (n = 8)	48.8 ± 9.1	66.2 ± 11.3 (p < 0.01)
Study (86) (n = 5)	30.1 ± 13.5	44.5 ± 40.4 (NS)

Table 3 – Bone ingrowth/ongrowth to porous-coated and grit-blasted implants in percentage of the total implant surface. Mean ± SD.

The Effect of Underlying Surface Texture

We showed that HA-coated grit-blasted implants had higher bone in/ongrowth than porous-coated implants, but without better mechanical fixation (86, 89). In contrast, energy absorption was higher and shear stiffness was lower for porous-coated suggesting that mechanical fixation of porous-coated implants was stronger than grit-blasted implants. Increased energy absorption was not explained by greater bone ingrowth for porous-coated implants, neither in percentage nor in absolute values. However, it might be explained by the interdigitated bone-implant interface, resulting in a variety of compression, tensile, and shear stresses at the porous surface during push-out testing (90, 91). By contrast, shear stresses overshadow other stresses at the grit-blasted surface. This might also explain why grit-blasted implants had pronounced delamination of the HA coating during push-out testing in contrast to porous-coated implants (fig. 8).

Study VI (87) and VII (88). The effects of HA- versus FA-coated implants on mechanical fixation and bone ingrowth on remodeling were evaluated in a stable weight-bearing model during 25 weeks (87), and the effects on bone ongrowth were evaluated in humans in a non weight-bearing gap model in trabecular bone during 1 year (88). During stable weight-bearing conditions no difference between HA- and FA-coated implants in mechanical fixation and bone ingrowth were demonstrated (87). In humans, however, HA-coated implants had 30% more bone ongrowth than FA-coated implants (79% ± 11.1 *versus* 61% ± 9.8) (p < 0.05) (88).

The effects of HA coating crystallinity on mechanical fixation and bone ingrowth were evaluated in a weight-bearing model with con-

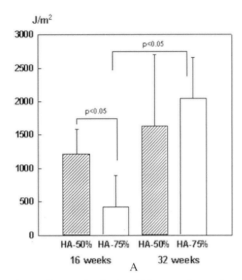
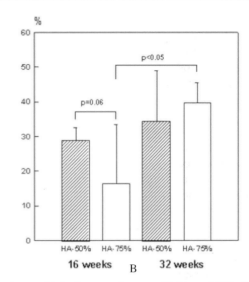

Figure 8 – Mechanical and histomorphometric results of implants with hydroxyapatite crystallinities of 50% (HA-50%) and 75% (HA-75%). Mean, error bar=SD.

A) Energy absorption (J/m²). Energy absorption for HA-50% was increased 3 fold as compared with HA-75% after 16 weeks. After 32 weeks, no difference between HA-50% and HA-75% was shown. HA-75% gained stronger anchorage from 16 to 32 weeks, whereas HA-50% showed no difference from 16 to 32 weeks.

B) Bone ingrowth (%). Bone ingrowth to HA-50% implants was increased 2 fold as compared with HA-75% after 16 weeks. Bone ingrowth to HA-75% implants increased from 16 to 32 weeks while no difference for HA-50% was shown.

trolled micromotion of 250 µm during 16 and 32 weeks (55).

After 16 weeks during controlled micromotion of 250 µm push-out testing showed that ultimate shear strength and apparent shear stiffness were increased 2 fold for HA-50% whereas energy absorption was increased 3 fold compared with HA-75% (fig. 8A). After 32 weeks no difference in mechanical fixation was found. Histology revealed that all HA-50% implants and only four HA-75% implants had bony anchorage after 16 weeks whereas after 32 weeks all implants had bone ingrowth. Bone ingrowth to HA-50% implants was increased 2 fold as compared with HA-75% after 16 weeks whereas no difference was shown after 32 weeks (fig. 8B). Thus, early bone ingrowth seems to be accelerated by low HA crystallinity.

Hydroxyapatite Coating Stability

Generally, for clinical use, none or slow resorption resorbable coatings with high crystallinity have been recommended in order to retain the bonding strength of the coating-implant interface (92). However, this contradicts the statement that the ideal interface between the implant material and surrounding tissue should match the tissue being

replaced. Moreover, HA coating crystallinity has been stated to be one of the most important factors for bioactivity of the HA coating (93). From this point of view the coating should be of low crystallinity with content of carbonate. However, this might weaken the bonding strength between coating and substrate *in vivo*. Since one of the first steps in bonding to the coating involves dissolution of the coating surface, it might be suggested that less crystalline or more resorbable coatings would be more beneficial for early bone ingrowth than high crystalline coatings (51, 56).

We showed that implants coated with low crystalline HA yielded better anchorage after 16 weeks than implants with high crystalline HA coating. This was in accordance with Maxian *et al.* who reported greater strength of grit-blasted implants coated with low crystalline HA after 4 weeks in a non weight-bearing transcortical model (51, 54). The effect diminished after 12 weeks. No effect was shown on implants with a rough surface. These observations might indicate that the effect of crystallinity in the early postoperative period, an observation which also was evident in our study. Low crystalline HA coating did not achieve better anchorage from 16 to 32 weeks whereas the high crystalline coating was stronger fixed after

32 weeks than after 16 weeks. Our results confirmed the hypothesis by de Bruijn *et al.* that rapidly resorbable coatings might be more bioactive than slowly resorbable HA coatings (56). Higher bioactivity of the low crystalline coating might be explained by the physico-chemical nature of the coating in the local micro-environment. A low crystalline coating releases more calcium and phosphate ions than the high crystalline coating due to dissolution and cell mediated resorption enhancing bone formation and bonding (52, 93-95).

Whether or not mechanical fixation of implants with low crystalline coatings will diminish in the long run can be questioned; at present, no data supports this hypothesis for plasma-sprayed HA coatings. On the other hand, reports on TCP coatings *in vivo* have shown inferior fixation strength as compared with HA, most likely due to rapid coating resorption (96, 97). It can be speculated that the bioactivity of an HA coating will reach a maximal level at a certain crystallinity and that there is a balance between bioactivity and interface strength.

Resorption of Hydroxyaoatite and Flourapatite Coatings *in vivo*

Loss of FA and HA coating is most likely caused by to three different mechanisms.

1) *A dissolution* may occur when low pH appears as suggested from *in vitro* studies. (52, 98, 99).

2) *Cell-mediated* resorption has been proved. *in vitro* studies have shown that the osteoclast can create resorption lacunae probably due to low pH at the ruffle border (100-102). In addition, *in vivo* studies have demonstrated that osteoclast-like cells, monocytes, and fibroblasts, and osteocytes might phagocytose ceramics. (100, 103-108).

3) *Mechanical removal and wear* due to micromovemennts might also occur *in vivo* (42, 109).

We have in a series of studies investigated several factors which might affect coating loss *in vivo*.

Coating Related Factors

Study VI (87), VII (88) and VIII (55). Both in dogs and humans, significant loss of HA and FA coatings was found (87, 88). In dogs, a tendency towards greater loss of the HA coating was shown but not significantly (87). In humans no difference in overall coating loss between HA and FA was shown, however, the HA coating was significantly thinner than FA when bone marrow was present

(Table 4) (fig. 9) (88). Interestingly, the HA coating was significantly thicker than FA when bone was present on the coating surface. This suggests that resorption of Ca-P coatings is governed by multiple factors in the local microenvironment.

During controlled micromovements of 250 μm both low (HA-50%) and high (HA-75%) crystalline coatings were significantly reduced compared with non-inserted control implants (55). HA coverage and thickness were significantly more reduced on HA-50% implants than on HA-75% implants after both 16 and 32 weeks demonstrating increased resorption of the low crystalline coating. Interestingly, no further coating loss was shown from 16 to 32 weeks indicating two phases of resorption (see discussion).

| | Coating type | | |
	Hydroxyapatite	Fluorapatite	
Control implants	69.1 ± 2.1	68.4 ± 2.2	p = 0.59
Test implants			
Overall	56.6 ± 5.1	57.0 ± 1.9	p = 0.75
Bone	62.3 ± 2.2*#	59.0 ± 2.1*#	p < 0.01
Bone marrow	39.3 ± 9.9	53.9 ± 2.4	p < 0.001
Fibrous tissue	43.6 ± 13.9	55.9 ± 1.6	p = 0.13

All parameters on test implants were significantly reduced compared with control implants.

* Significant difference in coating thickness between bone and bone marrow for HA and FA coatings.

\# Significant difference in coating thickness between bone and fibrous tissue for HA and FA coatings. No difference in coating thickness between bone marrow and fibrous tissue.

Table 4 – Mean (±SD) thickness (μm) of hydroxyapatite (HA) and fluorapatite (FA) coatings on non-implanted controls and on test implants inserted for 13 ±0.6 months in humans. Coating thickness is presented as an overall value for the total implant and is separated into different tissue types covering the ceramic coating.

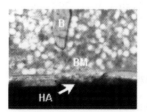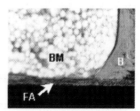

Figure 9 – Histological sections from A) hydroxyapatite- (HA) and B) fluorapatite- (FA) coated implants. The HA coating is thinner than FA in the presence of bone marrow (BM) on the coating surface (arrows) indicating that FA is more stable than HA. B=Bone. Light microscopy, sections stained with light green and basic fuchsin. Original magnification × 100.

Mechanical Factors

Clinically, the mechanical factor might play an important role in loss of ceramic coatings especially during the early postoperative period when micromotion is suspected to occur.

Study IV (85) and IX (108). The effects of micromotion and immobilization of the implants on coating loss was investigated after 16 weeks of implantation (85). HA coverage, absolute surface area and volume were significantly reduced on immobilized implants and further reduced on continuously loaded implants as compared with control implants (fig. 10A and 10B). Continuously loaded implants had 3-fold reduction in coating surface area and volume as compared with immobilized implants. Thus, micromotion seems to accelerate resorption of HA coatings. Completely resorbed coating was partly replaced by bone in direct contact with the implant surface varying from 12 to 36 % (108).

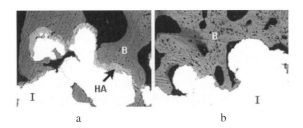

a   b

Figure 10 – Backscattered scanning electron images from a) an immobilized implant (I) and from b) a continuously loaded implant (I)
The hydroxyapatite (HA) coating (arrow) is reduced significantly on the continuously loaded implant as compared with the immobilized implant. Resorbed HA coating on top of the porous coating on the continuously loaded implant is partly replaced by bone (B) in direct contact with the titanium implant surface. Most of the HA coating on the immobilized implant is covered with bone. Note: no signs of delamination of HA coating on the immobilized implant.

Hydroxyapatite Coating Loss

As previously mentioned, three mechanisms may play a role in loss of HA coating *in vivo*, however, solid documentation at the *in vivo* level does not exist in the literature (40, 44, 85, 109, 110). Several factors might affect loss of Ca-P coatings *in vivo*. They can be categorized as coating related, mechanical, biological, and as implant related factors (110). In addition, two phases of coating loss is suggested to occur. *Phase I* with rapid coating loss, and *phase II* with slow loss. During *phase I* the implant is subjected to micromotion and a fibrous tissue membrane with high metabolic activities is developed (111). The fibrous tissue membrane is dominated by fibroblasts and macrophages able to phagocytose HA (65, 103, 107, 108, 112). Because of unstable conditions, low pH is maintained due to inhibited angiogenesis. In addition, fluid flow is increased along the interface leading to accelerated dissolution due to changes in calcium and phosphate concentrations (113, 114). During *phase I,* the low crystalline coating parts will be resorbed leaving the more crystalline coating on the implant surface. In addition, coating crystallinity might eventually increase with time thus possibly contributing to low coating loss in *phase II* (115). *Phase II,* begins by stabilization of the implant when the initially formed fibrous tissue membrane is transformed to bone through endochondral ossification If the implant is not stabilized, phase *I* will continue and complete coating loss might occur.

Significance of Hydroxyapatite Coating Loss

Is it preferable that the HA coating retains on the substrate surface or should the HA coating be resorbed in the long-term run? Ducheyne pointed out that it cannot be reasonably expected that the mechanical function of the HA coating can last for the patient's lifetime and suggested that a coating must necessarily be resorbed (43). Coating loss *in vivo* might be critical first of all for bone ingrowth and secondly for implant fixation. How rapid the HA coating can be resorbed without disturbing bone ingrowth to the implant surface is a balance between release of calcium and phosphate ions and bone formation. The rate of resorption is most likely important for implant fixation, since implants coated with rapidly resorbed coatings like TCP have been found to be inferiorly anchored compared to a slowly resorbed HA coating when applied to a grit-blasted surface (97, 116). This addresses the importance of underlying surface texture. If the coating is completely resorbed, implant fixation is solely provided solely by the metal surface. In that case, a rough or porous-coated surface will probably provide stronger implant fixation than a grit-blasted surface.

Whether HA coating loss can reduce implant fixation when bony anchorage has occurred is doubtful. In the present studies, coating loss did not seem to interfere with bone ingrowth and resorbed coating was partly replaced by bone which suggests firm implant fixation. Coating loss due to extensive delamination might be a severe problem of coating quality and might result in implant loosening. This was, however, not shown in our studies.

The Effect of Hydroxyapatite Particles in the Bone-Implant Interface on the Fixation of the Implant

Study X (117) Unloaded HA implants surrounded by a 2 mm gap were inserted in the proximal part of tibia. The purpose was to investigate the effect of hydroxyapatite and polyethylene (PE) particles around a newly implanted HA-coated implant. One could imagine that HA particles are produced by delamination during the insertion of a HA implant in press fit. Results from the mechanical testing after one month did not show impaired fixation of the implants due to HA particles. Histology showed that particles were incorporated into the bone matrix (fig. 11).

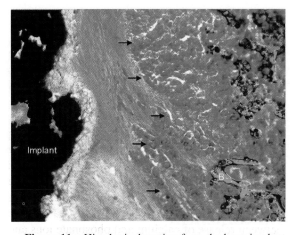

Figure 11 – Histological section from the bone implant interface around a HA implant. HA particles (seen as brown dots) are distributed in a large area (see arrows) in the interface and also incorporated into bone matrix. B = bone. Light microscopy, sections stained with light green and basic fuschin.

The Effect Particulate Hydroxyapatite Particles on Mechanical Fixation

The influence of wear debris on bone healing around orthopaedic implants is debated. Polyethylene (PE) particles have been shown to have a negative effect on osteoblasts (118) as well as net bone formation (119). HA particles have also been shown to have inhibitory effect on osteoblast cultures *in vitro* (120). This study demonstrated that fagocytosable HA particles can be incorporated into bone. Based on mechanical testing no significant effect of HA or PE particles could be found. It can be speculated that the strong osteoconductive effect of the HA coating as seen in previous studies overrides the negative effects of the particulate material on bone formation.

Effects of Hydroxyapatite on the Migration of Wear Debris in the Bone-Implant Interface

It is generally accepted that aseptic loosening of primarily stable implants is caused by wear debris. Wear debris originating mainly from the articulating surfaces migrates to the bone-implant interface and initiates osteolysis. The particulate debris is phagocytosed by macrophages. Hereby the cells are stressed to the secretion of cytokines (interleukin 1β, interleukin 6), prostaglandin E_2 and monocyte activating and chemotatic factor (84, 121-125).

In non-cemented arthroplasty is has been hypothesised, that a biological seal is created by the use HA-coated implants. By preventing the access of wear debris to the bone-implant interface the mechanisms behind aseptic loosening might be inhibited. This hypothesis is supported by several clinical rapports. Distal osteolysis around circumferential HA coated stems is a rare and almost a non-existing finding (126, 127), not even after 12 years follow-up (128). This could indicate that the accumulation of wear debris in the bone implant interface is inhibited.

We have in a series of studies investigated the effect of hydroxyapatite on periimplant migration of polyethylene particles.

Study XI (129) and XII (61). A loaded HA coated implant and a non-coated gritblasted Ti implant was implanted in each distal femoral condyle. The test implant was surrounded by a gap, which was communicating with the joint space, allowing access of joint fluid to the bone-implant interface. PE particles were injected into the joint space repeatedly. This way the continuous release of wear debris into joint fluid was mimicked. After eight weeks only few particles were found around HA coated implants. In contrast periimplant tissue around Ti implants contained large amounts of particles (fig. 12). HA-coated implants had approximately 35% bone ingrowth, whereas Ti implants had virtually no bone ingrowth and were surrounded by a fibrous membrane.

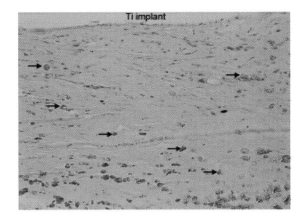

Figure 12 – Histological section showing scattered PE particles (see arrows) in the membrane surrounding a Ti implant. The text: "Ti implant" illustrates the site of the implant before removal. (Oil red O stain).

After 52 weeks huge amounts of PE particles were found around Ti-implants. Mainly in the bone-implant interface. Infiltration of mononuclear inflammatory cells was present around 3 out of 7 Ti implants in relation to PE particles. HA implants had approximately 70 percent bone ongrowth. In contrast, no bone ongrowth was seen on any Ti implants, all being surrounded by a fibrous membrane. The number of PE particles was evaluated semi-quantitatively. We found significantly more PE particles around Ti implants as compared with HA implants ($p < 0.002$). Furthermore the pattern of distribution of particles was completely different for HA coated implants (fig. 13).

The Sealing Effect of HA

Both short and long-term studies show that HA coating of implants is able to inhibit periimplant PE particle migration, by creating a seal of tightly bonded bone to the implant surface. After 52 weeks chronic inflammation was present around Ti implants, but not seen around HA implants. This indicates that HA coating can inhibit or delay the adverse effects of wear debris in the bone implant interface. In contrast, the thin fibrous membrane surrounding the Ti implants contained a huge number

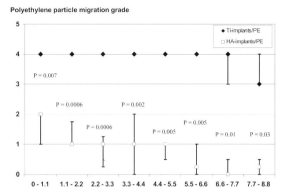

Figure 13 – Median values (n = 7) for PE particles in the interface according to the grading system (61). Error bars = interquartile range. Data grouped in areas (1.1 × 0.75mm) from the juxtaarticular tip of the implant. Presence of PE particles was significantly reduced in all areas around HA coated implants. P-values shown for each area. From reference (61).

of polyethylene particles. Our findings supports the findings by Kraemer who found similar effect of HA in a hemi-arthroplasty model in dogs (130).

The effect of bony anchorage on PE particle migration can be explained by two mechanisms. It acts as a mechanical barrier and it increases implant stability. The transport of wear particles by the pumping of fluid in the unstable interface can therefore be avoided. Our results after 52 weeks indicates that the sealing effect is durable and may be superior to that of a cementmantle, since cracks in the cement is bound to occur with time due to mechanical stress. Bone ingrowth to the HA implants was doubled from 35 to 70 percent in the period between 8 and 52 weeks creating an even stronger seal.

CONCLUSION

HA has in our studies proven to positively modify tissue ingrowth onto a porous surface during stable and unstable mechanical conditions. Micromotion between bone and implant prevented bony ingrowth and resulted in development of a fibrous membrane. HA coating, however, induced a membrane with presence of fibrocartilage, higher collagen concentration, radiating orientation of collagen fibers, and a thinner membrane as compared to Ti implants. After 16 weeks, the membrane around HA coated implants was demonstrated to be replaced by bone even when subjected to continuous load, whereas the membrane around Ti implants persisted.

HA coated grit-blasted implants had higher bone in/ongrowth than porous-coated implants, but without better mechanical fixation. This can be explained by the interdigitated bone-implant interface of the porous coated implants. Shear stresses overshadow other stresses at the grit-blasted surface. Furthermore pronounced delamination of the HA coating during push-out testing was found on grit-blasted implants in contrast to porous-coated implants. Low crystalinity (HA-50%) coating had better anchorage after 16 weeks than implants with high crystalline (HA-75%) coating. The effect on fixation disappeared after 32 weeks. These observations indicate a positive effect of low crystallinity in the early postoperative period.

Both HA and FA coatings are resorbed *in vivo*. Both low crystallinity and micromotion accelerates the loss of HA coating. Whether HA coating loss can reduce implant fixation when bony anchorage has occurred is doubtful. Coating loss did not seem to interfere with bone ingrowth and resorbed coating was partly replaced by bone, which suggests firm implant fixation. However, coating loss addresses the importance of underlying surface texture. A rough or porous-coated surface will probably provide stronger implant fixation than a grit-blasted surface, since implant fixation is solely provided by the metal surface if HA is resorbed completely. Delamination of HA coating may produce HA particles in fagocytozable sizes. Such particles did not impair the fixation of HA coated implants after 4 weeks.

HA coated implants did inhibit the migration of PE particles in the bone-implant interface after 8 and 52 weeks. This effect was due to the bony ingrowth to the HA implants. After 52 weeks 70% of the HA implants were covered by bone. In contrast, a fibrous membrane surrounded the Ti-implants containing huge amounts of PE particles. Some of the membranes had infiltration of chronic inflammatory cells, which may be the beginning of the process of aseptic loosening.

Our experimental work indicates that a circumferential HA coating with low crystallinity on a porous surface may improve the longevity of noncemented implants. HA improves the early fixation of the implant both in stable and unstable situations and has the ability to bridge gaps between implant and bone bed with newly formed bone. The porous surface texture maintains the bony fixation obtained by

the HA even after the HA is resorbed and may protect the HA coating against delamination. The HA coating must be circumferential to seal off the bone implant interface from wear debris dispersed in the joint fluid; thus reducing the effective joint space.

Reference List

1. Overgaard S, Knudsen HM, Hansen LN, Mossing N (1992) Hip arthroplasty in Jutland, Denmark. Age and sex-specific incidences of primary operations. *Acta Orthop. Scand.* 63:536-8.

2. Malchau H, Herberts P (1996) Prognosis of total hip replacement. Scientific Exhibition, AAOS, Atlanta, 22-6.

3. Collier JP, Bauer TW, Bloebaum RD, Bobyn JD, Cook SD, Galante JO, Harris WH, Head WC, Jasty MJ, Mayor MB (1992) Results of implant retrieval from postmortem specimens in patients with well-functioning, long-term total hip replacement. *Clin. Orthop.* 97-112.

4. Cook SD, Thomas KA, Haddad RJ, Jr (1988) Histologic analysis of retrieved human porous-coated total joint components. *Clin. Orthop.* 90-101.

5. de Groot K, Geesink R, Klein CP, Serekian P (1987) Plasma sprayed coatings of hydroxylapatite. *J. Biomed. Mater. Res.* 21:1375-81.

6. Geesink RG, de Groot K, Klein CP (1987) Chemical implant fixation using hydroxyl-apatite coatings. The development of a human total hip prosthesis for chemical fixation to bone using hydroxyl-apatite coatings on titanium substrates. *Clin. Orthop.* 147-70.

7. Søballe K, Hansen ES, Brockstedt Rasmussen H, Hjortdal VE, Juhl GI, Pedersen CM, Hvid I, Bünger C (1991) Fixation of titanium and hydroxyapatite-coated implants in arthritic osteopenic bone. *J. Arthroplasty* 6:307-16.

8. Søballe K, Hansen ES, Brockstedt Rasmussen H, Pedersen CM, Bünger C (1990) Hydroxyapatite coating enhances fixation of porous coated implants. A comparison in dogs between press fit and noninterference fit. *Acta Orthop. Scand.* 61:299-306.

9. Søballe K, Hansen ES, Brockstedt-Rasmussen H, Pedersen CM, Bünger C (1992) Bone graft incorporation around titanium-alloy and hydroxyapatite-coated implants in dogs. *Clin. Orthop.* 282-93.

10. Søballe K, Pedersen CM, Odgaard A, Juhl GI, Hansen ES, Rasmussen HB, Hvid I, Bünger C (1991) Physical bone changes in carragheenin-induced arthritis evaluated by quantitative computed tomography. *Skeletal. Radiol.* 20:345-52.

11. Thomas KA, Kay JF, Cook SD, Jarcho M (1987) The effect of surface macrotexture and hydroxylapatite coating on the mechanical strengths and histologic profiles of titanium implant materials. *J. Biomed. Mater. Res.* 21:1395-414.

12. van B CA, Koerten HK, Hesseling SC, Terpstra RA, de Groot K, Grote JJ (1990) Calcium phosphates

during inflammation. In: *Bioceramics, volume 2* Ed by G Heimke.

13. Jarcho M (1981) Calcium phosphate ceramics as hard tissue prosthetics. *Clin. Orthop.* 259-78.

14. Jarcho M, Kay JF, Gumaer KI, Doremus RH, Drobeck HP (1977) Tissue, cellular and subcellular events at a bone-ceramic hydroxylapatite interface. *J. Bioeng.* 1:79-92.

15. Sun JS, Lin FH, Hung TY, Tsuang YH, Chang WH, Liu HC (1999) The influence of hydroxyapatite particles on osteoclast cell activities. *J. Biomed. Mater. Res.* 45:311-21.

16. Cook SD, Thomas KA, Kay JF, Jarcho M (1988) Hydroxyapatite-coated porous titanium for use as an orthopedic biologic attachment system. *Clin. Orthop.* 303-12.

17. de Groot K, Geesink R, Klein CP, Serekian P (1987) Plasma sprayed coatings of hydroxylapatite. *J. Biomed. Mater. Res.* 21:1375-81.

18. Kay JF, Golec TS, Riley RL (1987) Hydroxyapatite-coated subperiosteal dental implants: design rationale and clinical experience. *J. Prosthet. Dent.* 58:339-43.

19. Geesink RG (1990) Hydroxyapatite-coated total hip prostheses. Two-year clinical and roentgenographic results of 100 cases. *Clin. Orthop.* 39-58.

20. Søballe K, Toksvig Larsen S, Gelineck J, Fruensgaard S, Hansen ES, Ryd L, Lucht U, Bünger C (1993) Migration of hydroxyapatite coated femoral prostheses. A Roentgen Stereophotogrammetric study. *J. Bone Joint Surg. Br.* 75:681-7.

21. Kroon PO, Freeman MA (1992) Hydroxyapatite coating of hip prostheses. Effect on migration into the femur. *J. Bone Joint Surg. Br.* 74:518-22.

22. Furlong RJ, Osborn JF (1991) Fixation of hip prostheses by hydroxyapatite ceramic coatings. *J. Bone Joint Surg. Br.* 73:741-5.

23. Freeman MA, Plante-Bordeneuve P (1994) Early migration and late aseptic failure of proximal femoral prostheses. *J. Bone Joint Surg. Br.* 76:432-8.

24. Capello WN (1994) Hydroxyapatite in total hip arthroplasty: five-year clinical experience. *Orthopedics* 17:781, 792.

25. Karrholm J, Malchau H, Snorrason F, Herberts P, Rorabeck CH, Bourne RB, Laupacis A, Feeny D, Wong C, Tugwell P, Leslie K, Bullas R (1994) Micromotion of femoral stems in total hip arthroplasty. *J. Bone Joint Surg. Am.* 76:156-64.

26. Tonino AJ, Romanini L, Rossi P, Borroni M, Greco F, Garcia-Araujo C, Garcia-Dihinx L, Murcia-Mazon A, Hein W, Anderson J (1995) Hydroxyapatite-coated hip prostheses. Early results from an international study. *Clin. Orthop.* 211-5.

27. Geesink RG, Hoefnagels NH (1995) Six-year results of hydroxyapatite-coated total hip replacement. *J. Bone Joint Surg. Br.* 77:534-47.

28. Rossi P, Sibelli P, Fumero S, Crua E (1995) Short-term results of hydroxyapatite-coated primary total hip arthroplasty. *Clin. Orthop.* 98-102.

29. Onsten I, Carlsson AS, Sanzen L, Besjakov J (1996) Migration and wear of a hydroxyapatite-coated hip prosthesis. A controlled roentgen stereophotogrammetric study. *J. Bone Joint Surg. Br.* 78:85-91.

30. Kienapfel H, Nilsson K, Karrholm J (1995) Analysis of micromotion of porous-coated tibial total knee arthroplasty components. The effect of additional hydroxyapatite coating – a randomized RSA study. Transaction EORS 5, 54.

31. Nelissen RG, Valstar ER, Rozing PM (1998) The effect of hydroxyapatite on the micromotion of total knee prostheses. A prospective, randomized, double-blind study. *J. Bone Joint Surg. Am.* 80:1665-72.

32. Onsten I, Nordqvist A, Carlsson AS, Besjakov J, Shott S (1998) Hydroxyapatite augmentation of the porous coating improves fixation of tibial components. A randomised RSA study in 116 patients. *J. Bone Joint Surg. Br.* 80:417-25.

33. Collier JP, Bauer TW, Bloebaum RD, Bobyn JD, Cook SD, Galante JO, Harris WH, Head WC, Jasty MJ, Mayor MB (1992) Results of implant retrieval from postmortem specimens in patients with well-functioning, long-term total hip replacement. *Clin. Orthop.* 97-112.

34. Søballe K, Gotfredsen K, Brockstedt Rasmussen H, Nielsen PT, Rechnagel K (1991) Histologic analysis of a retrieved hydroxyapatite-coated femoral prosthesis. *Clin. Orthop.* 255-8.

35. Bauer TW, Stulberg BN, Ming J, Geesink RG (1993) Uncemented acetabular components. Histologic analysis of retrieved hydroxyapatite-coated and porous implants. *J. Arthroplasty* 8:167-77.

36. Bauer TW, Geesink RC, Zimmerman R, McMahon JT (1991) Hydroxyapatite-coated femoral stems. Histological analysis of components retrieved at autopsy. *J. Bone Joint Surg. Am.* 73:1439-52.

37. Tonino AJ, Therin M, Doyle C (1999) Hydroxyapatite-coated femoral stems. Histology and histomorphometry around five components retrieved at post mortem. *J. Bone Joint Surg. Br.* 81:148-54.

38. Jarcho M (1992) Retrospective analysis of hydroxyapatite development for oral implant applications. *Dent. Clin. North. Am.* 36:19-26.

39. Maxian SH, Zawadsky JP, Dunn MG (1993) Mechanical and histological evaluation of amorphous calcium phosphate and poorly crystallized hydroxyapatite coatings on titanium implants. *J. Biomed. Mater. Res.* 27:717-28.

40. Jarcho M (1992) Retrospective analysis of hydroxyapatite development for oral implant applications. *Dent. Clin. North. Am.* 36:19-26.

41. Bloebaum RD, Beeks D, Dorr LD, Savory CG, DuPont JA, Hofmann AA (1994) Complications with hydroxyapatite particulate separation in total hip arthroplasty. *Clin. Orthop.* 298:19-26.

42. Campbell P, McKellop H, Park SH, Malcolm AJ (1993) Evidence of abrasive wear particles from hydroxyapatite coated hip prosthesis. Transaction ORS 18, 224.

43. Ducheyne P (1994) Bioactive ceramics. *J. Bone Joint Surg. Br.* 76:861-2.

44. Bauer TW (1995) Hydroxyapatite: coating controversies. *Orthopedics* 18:885-8.

45. Søballe K, Overgaard S (1996) The current status of hydroxyapatite coating of prostheses [editorial]. *J. Bone Joint Surg. Br.* 78:689-91.

46. Frayssinet P, Hardy D, Cartillier JC, Vidalain JP (1996) Calcium phosphate particles are found at the surface of polyethylene inserts implanted in humans. Transaction EORS 6, 39.

47. Dhert WJ, Klein CP, Jansen JA, van der Velde EA, Vriesde RC, Rozing PM, de Groot K (1993) A histological and histomorphometrical investigation of fluorapatite, magnesiumwhitlockite, and hydroxylapatite plasma-sprayed coatings in goats. *J. Biomed. Mater. Res.* 27:127-38.

48. Klein CP, Wolke JG, Blieck-Hogervorst JM, De Groot K (1994) Features of calcium phosphate plasma-sprayed coatings: an *in vitro* study. *J. Biomed. Mater. Res.* 28:961-7.

49. Klein CP, Wolke JG, Blieck-Hogervorst JM, de Groot K (1994) Calcium phosphate plasma-sprayed coatings and their stability: an *in vivo* study. *J. Biomed. Mater. Res.* 28:909-17.

50. Lugschneider E, Weber T, Knepper M (1988) Production of biocompatible coatings of hydroxyapatite and flourapatite. National Thermal Spray Conference, Cincinatti, OH, 332-43.

51. Maxian SH, Zawadsky JP, Dunn MG (1993) Mechanical and histological evaluation of amorphous calcium phosphate and poorly crystallized hydroxyapatite coatings on titanium implants. *J. Biomed. Mater. Res.* 27:717-28.

52. Maxian SH, Zawadsky JP, Dunn MG (1993) *In vitro* evaluation of amorphous calcium phosphate and poorly crystallized hydroxyapatite coatings on titanium implants. *J. Biomed. Mater. Res.* 27:111-7.

53. Dalton JE, Cook SD (1995) *in vivo* mechanical and histological characteristics of HA-coated implants vary with coating vendor. *J. Biomed. Mater. Res.* 29:239-45.

54. Maxian SH, Zawadsky JP, Dunn MG (1994) Effect of Ca/P coating resorption and surgical fit on the bone/implant interface. *J. Biomed. Mater. Res.* 28:1311-19.

55. Overgaard S, Bromose U, Lind M, Bünger C, Søballe K (1999) The influence of crystallinity of the hydroxyapatite coating on the fixation of implants. Mechanical and histomorphometric results. *J. Bone Joint Surg. Br.* 81:725-31.

56. de Bruijn JD, Bovell YP, van Blitterswijk CA (1994) Structural arrangements at the interface between plasma sprayed calcium phosphates and bone. *Biomaterials* 15:543-50.

57. Chou L, Marek B, Wagner WR (1999) Effects of hydroxylapatite coating crystallinity on biosolubility, cell attachment efficiency and proliferation *in vitro*. *Biomaterials* 20:977-85.

58. Crawford RW, Evans E, Ling RS, Murray DW (1999) Fluid flow around model femoral components of differing surface finishes. *Acta Orthop. Scand.* 70[6], 589-95.

59. Anthony PP, Gie GA, Howie CR, Ling RS (1990) Localised endosteal bone lysis in relation to the femoral components of cemented total hip arthroplasties. *J. Bone Joint Surg. Br.* 72:971-9.

60. Horowitz SM, Gonzales JB (1996) Inflammatory response to implant particulates in a macrophage/osteoblast coculture model. *Calcif Tissue Int.* 59:392-6.

61. Rahbek O, Overgaard S, Jensen TB, Bendix K, Søballe K (2000) Sealing effect of hydroxyapatite coating: a 12-month study in canines. *Acta Orthop. Scand.* 71:563-73.

62. Søballe K (1993) Hydroxyapatite ceramic coating for bone implant fixation. Mechanical and histological studies in dogs. *Acta Orthop. Scand. Suppl* 255:1-58.

63. Søballe K (1992) Brockstedt Rasmussen H, Hansen ES, Bünger C: Hydroxyapatite coating modifies implant membrane formation. Controlled micromotion studied in dogs. *Acta Orthop. Scand.* 63:128-40.

64. Søballe K, Hansen ES, Brockstedt Rasmussen H, Bünger C (1993) Hydroxyapatite coating converts fibrous tissue to bone around loaded implants. *J. Bone Joint Surg. Br.* 75:270-8.

65. Søballe K, Hansen ES, Rasmussen HB, Jorgensen PH, Bünger C (1992) Tissue ingrowth into titanium and hydroxyapatite-coated implants during stable and unstable mechanical conditions. *J. Orthop. Res.* 10:285-99.

66. Bünger C (1987) Hemodynamics of the juvenile knee. Joint effusion and synovial inflammation studied in dogs. *Acta Orthop. Scand. Suppl.* 222:1-104.

67. Burke DW, O'Connor DO, Zalenski EB, Jasty M, Harris WH (1991) Micromotion of cemented and uncemented femoral components. *J. Bone Joint Surg. Br.* 73:33-7.

68. Vanderby R, Jr., Manley PA, Kohles SS, McBeath AA (1992) Fixation stability of femoral components in a canine hip replacement model. *J. Orthop. Res.* 10:300-9.

69. Volz RG, Nisbet JK, Lee RW, McMurtry MG (1988) The mechanical stability of various noncemented tibial components. *Clin. Orthop.* 38-42.

70. Sumner DR, Jacobs JJ, Turner TM, Urban RM, Galante JO (1989) The amount and distribution of bone ingrowth in tibial components retrieved from human patients. *Transaction ORS* 14, 375.

71. Ryd L (1986) Micromotion in knee arthroplasty. A roentgen stereophotogrammetric analysis of tibial component fixation. *Acta Orthop. Scand.* Suppl 220:1-80.

72. Aspenberg P, Goodman S, Toksvig Larsen S, Ryd L, Albrektsson T (1992) Intermittent micromotion inhibits bone ingrowth. Titanium implants in rabbits. *Acta Orthop. Scand.* 63:141-5.

73. Cameron HU, Pilliar RM, MacNab I (1973) The effect of movement on the bonding of porous metal to bone. *J. Biomed. Mater. Res.* 7:301-11.

74. Ducheyne P, De Meester P, Aernoudt E (1977) Influence of a functional dynamic loading on bone ingrowth into surface pores of orthopedic implants. *J. Biomed. Mater. Res.* 11:811-38.

75. Pilliar RM, Cameron HU, Welsh RP, Binnington AG (1981) Radiographic and morphologic studies of load-bearing porous- surfaced structured implants. *Clin. Orthop.* 249-57.

76. Pilliar RM, Lee JM, Maniatopoulos C (1986) Observations on the effect of movement on bone ingrowth into porous-surfaced implants. *Clin. Orthop.* 108-13.

77. Zalenski EB, Jasty M, O'Connor DO, Page A, Krushell R, Bragdon C, Russotti GM, Harris WH (1990) Micromotion of porous-surfaced, cementless prostheses followed for 6 months of *in vivo* bone ingrowth in a canine model. Transaction ORS 14, 377.

78. Burke DW, Bragdon CR, O'Connor D, Jasty M, Haire T, Harris WH (1991) Dynamic measurement of interface mechanics *in vivo* and the effects of micromotion on bone ingrowth into a porous surface device under controlled loads *in vivo*. Transaction ORS 16, 103.

79. Yang A, Sumner DR, Choi S, Natarajan R, Andriacchi TP (1990) Direct measurement of micromotion at bone-implant interface: The tibial component in a canine model. *Transaction ORS* 15[233].

80. Longo JA, Magee FP, Mather SE, Yapp RA, Koeneman JB, Weinstein AM (1989) Comparison af HA and non-HA coated carbon composite femoral stems. *Transaction ORS* 14, 384.

81. Perren SM (1979) Physical and biological aspects of fracture healing with special reference to internal fixation. *Clin. Orthop.* 175-196, 9

82. Cook SD, Thomas KA, Kay JF, Jarcho M (1988) Hydroxyapatite-coated titanium for orthopedic implant applications. *Clin. Orthop.* 225-43.

83. Thomas KA, Cook SD, Haddad RJ, Jr., Kay JF, Jarcho M (1989) Biologic response to hydroxylapatite-coated titanium hips. A preliminary study in dogs. *J. Arthroplasty* 4:43-53.

84. Goldring SR, Schiller AL, Roelke M, Rourke CM, O'Neil DA, Harris WH (1983) The synovial-like membrane at the bone-cement interface in loose total hip replacements and its proposed role in bone lysis. *J. Bone Joint Surg. Am.* 65:575-84.

85. Overgaard S, Søballe K, Josephsen K, Hansen ES, Bünger C (1996) Role of different loading conditions on resorption of hydroxyapatite coating evaluated by histomorphometric and stereological methods. *J. Orthop. Res.* 14:888-94.

86. Overgaard S, Lind M, Glerup H, Bünger C, Søballe K (1998) Porous-coated versus grit-blasted surface texture of hydroxyapatite-coated implants during controlled micromotion: mechanical and histomorphometric results. *J. Arthroplasty* 13:449-58.

87. Overgaard S, Lind M, Glerup H, Grundvig S, Bünger C, Søballe K (1997) Hydroxyapatite and fluorapatite coatings for fixation of weight loaded implants. *Clin. Orthop.* 286-96.

88. Overgaard S, Søballe K, Lind M, Bünger C (1997) Resorption of hydroxyapatite and fluorapatite coatings in man. An experimental study in trabecular bone. *J. Bone Joint Surg. Br.* 79:654-9.

89. Overgaard S, Lind M, Rahbek O, Bünger C, Søballe K (1997) Improved fixation of porous-coated versus grit-blasted surface texture of hydroxyapatite-coated implants in dogs. *Acta Orthop. Scand.* 68:337-43.

90. Hong L, Xu HC, de Groot K (1992) Tensile strength of the interface between hydroxyapatite and bone. *J. Biomed. Mater. Res.* 26:7-18.

91. Fujiu T, Ogino M (1984) Difference of bond bonding behavior among surface active glasses and sintered apatite. *J. Biomed. Mater. Res.* 18:845-59.

92. Tofe AJ, Brewster.G.A (1992) Bowerman MA, Muers RNHSM. Hydroxylapatite powders for implant coatings. Characterization and performance of calcium phosphate coatings for implants, 9-15.

93. de Bruijn JD, Flach JS, de Groot K, van Blitterswijk CA, Davies JE (1993) Analysis of the bony interface with various types of hydroxyapatite *in vitro*. *Cells and Materials* 3:115-27.

94. LeGeros P, Orly I, Gregoire M, Daculsi G (1991) Substrate surface dissolution and interfacial biological mineralization. In: *The bone-biomaterial interface* pp 76-88. Ed by JE Davies. Toronto, University of Toronto Press.

95. Gross KA, Berndt CC, Goldschlag DD, Iacono VJ (1997) *In vitro* changes of hydroxyapatite coatings. *Int. J. Oral. Maxillofac. Implants* 12:589-97.

96. Klein CP, Patka P, van der Lubbe HB, Wolke JG, de Groot K (1991) Plasma-sprayed coatings of tetracalciumphosphate, hydroxyl-apatite, and alpha-TCP on titanium alloy: an interface study. *J. Biomed. Mater. Res.* 25:53-65.

97. Lind M, Overgaard S, Bünger C, Søballe K (1999) Improved bone anchorage of hydroxypatite coated implants compared with tricalcium-phosphate coated implants in trabecular bone in dogs. *Biomaterials* 20:803-8.

98. Daculsi G, LeGeros P, Mitre D (1989) Crystal dissolution of biological and ceramic apatites. *Calcif Tissue Int* 45:95-103.

99. Klein CP, Blieck-Hogervorst JM, Wolke JG, de Groot K (1990) Studies of the solubility of different calcium phosphate ceramic particles *in vitro*. *Biomaterials* 11:509-12.

100. De Bruijn JD (1993) Calcium Phosphate Biomaterials: Bone-bonding and Biodegradation properties (Thesis). 1-172. Den Haag, Cip-Data Koninklijke Bibliotheek.

101. Fallon U (1984) Alterations in the pH of osteoclast resorbing fluid reflects changes in bone degradative activity. *Calcif. Tissue Int.* 36:458.

102. Vaes G (1988) Cellular biology and biochemical mechanism of bone resorption. A review of recent developments on the formation, activation, and mode of action of osteoclasts. *Clin. Orthop.* 239-71.

103. Gomi K, Lowenberg B, Shapiro G, Davies JE (1993) Resorption of sintered synthetic hydroxyapatite by osteoclasts *in vitro*. *Biomaterials* 14:91-6.

104. Gregoire M, Orly I, Kerebel LM, Kerebel B (1987) *In vitro* effects of calcium phosphate biomaterials on fibroblastic cell behavior. *Biol. Cell* 59:255-60.

105. Muller-Mai CM, Voigt C, Gross U (1990) Incorporation and degradation of hydroxyapatite implants of different surface roughness and surface structure in bone. *Scanning Microsc.* 4:613-22.

106. Ogura M, Davies JE (2001) Resorption of calcium hydroxyapatite substrata by osteoclast-like cells *in vitro*. In: *Bioceramics* pp 121-126. Ed by W Bonfield, GW Hastings, and KE Tanner. London, Butterworth-Heinemann Ltd.

107. Orly I, Gregoire M, Menanteau J, Heughebaert M, Kerebel B (1989) Chemical changes in hydroxyapatite biomaterial under *in vivo* and *in vitro* biological conditions. *Calcif Tissue Int.* 45:20-6.

108. Overgaard S, Lind M, Josephsen K, Maunsbach A, Bünger C, Søballe K (1998) Resorption of hydroxyapatite and flourapatite ceramic coatings on weight-bearing implants: A quantitative and morphological study in dogs. *J. Biomed. Mater. Res.* 39:141-52.

109. Bauer TW (1993) The histology of HA-coated implants. In: *Hydroxylapatite coatings in orthopaedic surgery* pp 305-318. Ed by R Geesink and MT Manley. New York, Raven Press.

110. Overgaard S (2000) Calcium phosphate coatings for fixation of implants. *Acta Orthop. Scand.* Suppl 279 71:1-74.

111. Buckwalter JA, Glimcher MJ, Cooper RR, Recker R (1996) Bone biology. I: Structure, blood supply, cells, matrix, and mineralization. *Instr. Course Lect.* 45:371-86.

112. van der MJ, Koerten HK (1994) Inflammatory response and degradation of three types of calcium phosphate ceramic in a non-osseous environment. *J. Biomed. Mater. Res.* 28:1455-63.

113. Page M, Hogg J, Ashhurst DE (1986) The effects of mechanical stability on the macromolecules of the connective tissue matrices produced during fracture healing. I. The collagens. *Histochem. J.* 18:251-65.

114. Prendergast PJ, Huiskes R, Søballe K (1997) ESB Research Award 1996. Biophysical stimuli on cells during tissue differentiation at implant interfaces. *J. Biomech.* 30:539-48.

115. Gross KA, Berndt CC (1994) *In vitro* testing of plasmasprayed hydroxyapatite coatings. *J. Mater. Science* 5:219-24.

116. Klein CP, Patka P, Wolke JG, Blieck-Hogervorst JM, de Groot K (1994) Long-term *in vivo* study of plasma-sprayed coatings on titanium alloys of tetracalcium phosphate, hydroxyapatite and alpha-tricalcium phosphate. *Biomaterials* 15:146-50.

117. Rahbek O, Overgaard S, Kold S, Søballe K (2001)The Effect of Particulate Hydroxyapatite and Polyethylene on Mechanical Fixation of Hydroxyapatite Coated Implants. *EORS* June 1-3, :40, 1 A.D.

118. Haynes DR, Hay SJ, Rogers SD, Ohta S, Howie DW, Graves SE (1997) Regulation of bone cells by particle-activated mononuclear phagocytes. *J. Bone Joint Surg. Br.* 79:988-94.

119. Goodman S, Aspenberg P, Song Y, Regula D, Lidgren L (1996) Polyethylene and titanium alloy particles reduce bone formation. Dose-dependence in bone harvest chamber experiments in rabbits. *Acta Orthop. Scand.* 67:599-605.

120. Sun JS, Liu HC, Chang WH, Li J, Lin FH, Tai HC (1998) Influence of hydroxyapatite particle size on bone cell activities: an *in vitro* study. *J. Biomed. Mater. Res.* 39:390-7.

121. Chiba J, Rubash HE, Kim KJ, Iwaki Y (1994) The characterization of cytokines in the interface tissue obtained from failed cementless total hip arthroplasty with and without femoral osteolysis. *Clin. Orthop.* 304-12.

122. Kim KJ, Chiba J, Rubash HE (1994) *in vivo* and *in vitro* analysis of membranes from hip prostheses inserted without cement. *J. Bone Joint Surg. Am.* 76:172-80.

123. Al Saffar N, Revell PA (1994) Interleukin-1 production by activated macrophages surrounding loosened orthopaedic implants: a potential role in osteolysis. *Br. J. Rheumatol.* 33:309-16.

124. Murray DW, Rushton N (1990) Macrophages stimulate bone resorption when they phagocytose particles. *J. Bone Joint Surg. Br.* 72:988-92.

125. Frøkjær J, Deleuran B, Lind M, Overgaard S, Søballe K, Bünger C (1995) Polyethylene particles stimulate monocyte chemotactic and activating factor production in synovial mononuclear cells *in vivo*. An immunohistochemical study in rabbits. *Acta Orthop. Scand.* 66:303-7.

126. Geesink R, Hoefnagels N (1997) Eight years results of HA-coated primary total hip replacement. *Acta Orthop. Belg.* 63 Suppl 1:72-5:72-5.

127. Rokkum M, Brandt M, Bye K, Hetland KR, Waage S, Reigstad A (1999) Polyethylene wear, osteolysis and acetabular loosening with an HA-coated hip prosthesis. A follow-up of 94 consecutive arthroplasties [see comments]. *J. Bone Joint Surg. Br.* 81:582-9.

128. McNally SA, Shepperd JA, Mann CV, Walczak JP (2000) The results at nine to twelve years of the use of a hydroxyapatite-coated femoral stem. *J. Bone Joint Surg. Br.* 82:378-82.

129. Rahbek O, Overgaard S, Lind M, Bendix K, Bünger C, Søballe K (2001) Sealing effect of hydroxyapatite coating on peri-implant migration of particles. An experimental study in dogs. *J. Bone Joint Surg. Br.* 83:441-7.

130. Kraemer WJ, Maistrelli GL, Fornasier V, Binnington A, Zhao JF (1995) Migration of polyethylene wear debris in hip arthroplasties: a canine model. *J. Appl. Biomater.* 6:225-30.

3 Biological Activities of Biomimetic Calcium Phosphate Coatings

Florence Barrere, PhD, Pamela Habibovic, BEng, Klaas DeGroot, PhD

INTRODUCTION

Calcium Phosphate (Ca-P) coated metallic prostheses have been highly successful in orthopedic surgery due to their osteoconductive properties. The osseointegration of orthopedic implants is related to both their surface morphology and the nature of Ca-P coating. On one hand, porous surfaced-implants can enhance bone ingrowth as compared to dense implants *in vivo* (1-3). On the other hand, Ca-P coated implants stimulate the early bone formation onto the implants, as compared to non-coated implants *in vivo* (4-6), and Ca-P coated porous implants enhance bone ingrowth as compared to porous implants (7-9). This bone stimulation is due to the dissolution of the Ca-P coating in the surrounding body fluids and the release of free $Ca2^+$ (10, 11). The osteogenic potential of Ca-P coating is still active in gaps up to 2mm created between the host bone and the Ca-P coated implant (12-14). Ca-P ceramics have also shown osteoinductive properties. For example, some specific Ca-P porous materials induced bone growth in nonosseous environments (15-19). Although the reasons behind osteoinduction by Ca-P remain unclear, osteoinduction strongly depends on the geometry of the material (20), the nature of the implanted Ca-P ceramics (21), and on the microporosity of the implant (22). Such osteoinductive Ca-P biomaterials could be attractive for bone repair in clinics because they may facilitate bone formation by osteogenic cells, especially in revision of hip arthroplasty where press-fit of the implant cannot be always achieved.

So far, the deposition of Ca-P coatings on and in porous material has been incomplete because of the line-of-sight application of the current plasma-spraying coating technique. However, it is nowadays possible to evenly coat porous implants with Ca-P by using the biomimetic route. This biomimetic route is based on the nucleation and growth of Ca-P from supersaturated calcifying solutions called Simulated Body Fluids (SBF) (23). Since the process occurs in aqueous media, it is now possible to coat complex shaped materials. Resulting from the physiological conditions of this technique, diverse Ca-P phases such as Octacalcium Phosphate (OCP) or bone mineral-like carbonated apatite (BCA) that are solely stable at low temperature, can be deposited (24-26). The aim of this paper was to study the biological activity of these novel biomimetic coatings: the *in vitro* and *in vivo* degradation, the osteogenecity in osseous sites and the osteoinductivity. In addition, the benefit of covering uniformly porous implants was evaluated.

PROCESSING BIOMIMETIC CALCIUM PHOSPHATE COATINGS ON IMPLANTS

The formation of Ca-P coatings *via* the biomimetic way is based on the nucleation/crystal growth mechanism occurring in bone mineralization. By tuning the composition of the solution in which the implants are immersed, different Ca-P phases can be deposited as coatings. The composition of all the solutions used in the present study is summarized Table 1.

The presented biomimetic coatings were produced by a two-step procedure. First, the samples were pre-treated by soaking at $37 \pm 1°C$ for 24 h in a Simulated Body Fluid solution concentrated by a factor five (SBF-A, Table 1). The solubility of SBF-A was controlled by supplying carbon dioxide

	Na$^+$	Mg^{2+}	Ca^{2+}	Cl$^-$	HPO$_4^{2-}$	HCO$_3^-$
HBP	142.0	1.5	2.5	103.0	1.0	27.0
SBF	142.0	1.5	2.5	147.8	1.0	4.2
SBF-A	733.0	7.5	12.5	720.0	5.0	21.0
SBF-B	140.4	0.5	2.5	142.9	1.0	2.0
SBF-C	140.4	–	3.1	142.9	1.86	–

Table 1 – Composition in mM of Human Blood Plasma (HBP), regular SBF solution
and the various soaking solutions (SBF-A, SBF-B and SBF-C).

gas at 0.2 bars prior to immersion of the plates (27, 28). Second, the pre-coated samples were divided into two groups. Each group was soaked in a second calcifying supersaturated solution in order to grow a Ca-P coating. One group was soaked in the metastable solution SBF-B for 24 h at 50ºC, (see chapter by Habibovic et al.) in order to grow a coating 65% crystalline, with a carbonate apatite structure close to bone mineral structure (26)

(fig. 1a, 1b). This coating was therefore named bone-like carbonated apatite (BCA) coating. The other group was soaked in the supersaturated solution SBF-C for 48 h at 37ºC in order to grow an 100% crystalline octacalcium phosphate coating (OCP, Ca$_8$(HPO$_4$)$_2$(PO$_4$)$_6$.5H$_2$O) (24) (fig. 1c, 1d). The coating thickness was approximately of 20-30 μm, for both the OCP and BCA coatings.

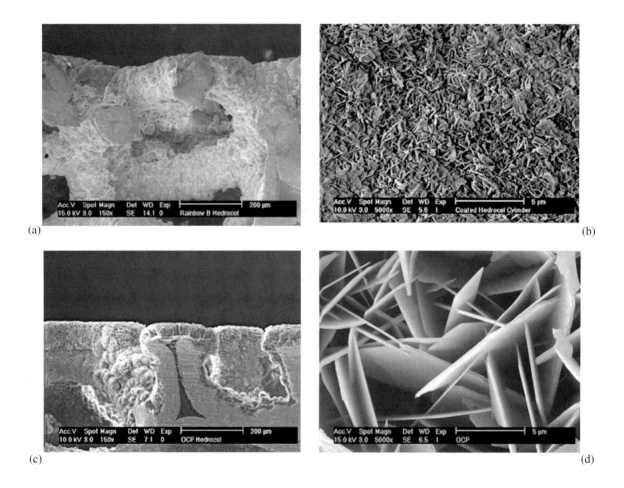

(a)

(b)

(c)

(d)

Figure 1 – ESEM photos of Ta implant coated with BCA at (a) magnification x150,
(b) at magnification x 5000), and with OCP (c) at magnification x 150, (d) at magnification x 5000.

DEGRADATION OF THE BIOMIMETIC CALCIUM PHOSPHATE COATINGS *IN VITRO* AND *IN VIVO*

In order to evaluate the physico-chemical and biological events occurring when the OCP and BCA coated implants, a degradation study was performed *in vitro* and *in vivo*. *In vitro,* coated and non-coated samples were soaked in a physiological medium (α-MEM) buffered at pH = 7.3 and incubated at 37°C. *In vivo,* subcutaneous implantation in male Wistar rats was performed. For both *in vitro* and *in vivo* the investigation time was 1, 2 and 4 weeks.

In vitro degradation of OCP and BCA coatings

Bare, OCP coated and BCA coated Ti6Al4V plates ($10 \times 10 \times 1mm^3$) were immersed into α-MEM. The bare Ti6Al4V plates did not show any surface modification after any immersion time in α-MEM. After 2 weeks of immersion in α-MEM, the biomimetic OCP coating was covered by a dense thin layer (fig. 2b). After 4 weeks, the OCP coating appeared denser due to a thickening of each initial crystal that suggests a horizontal binding between the OCP crystals through the whole thickness of the coating (fig. 2c). Additionally, the OCP coating became thinner when immersion time was longer. The infrared spectra (IR) of the OCP coating versus immersion in α-MEM time showed changes in the coating structure (fig. 3).

After 2 weeks of immersion in α-MEM, the phosphate vibration bands located at of the initial OCP coating became less sharp and less numerous as shown in figure 3, indicating a decrease in crystallinity. In addition, carbonate bands appeared indicating the formation of a carbonated apatitic phase among the OCP phase. The position of CO_3^{2-} bands indicated that CO_3^{2-} groups replaced PO_4^{3-} and OH^- groups, suggesting an AB-carbonated apatitic phase. After 4 weeks of immersion in the medium, only two large phosphate bands

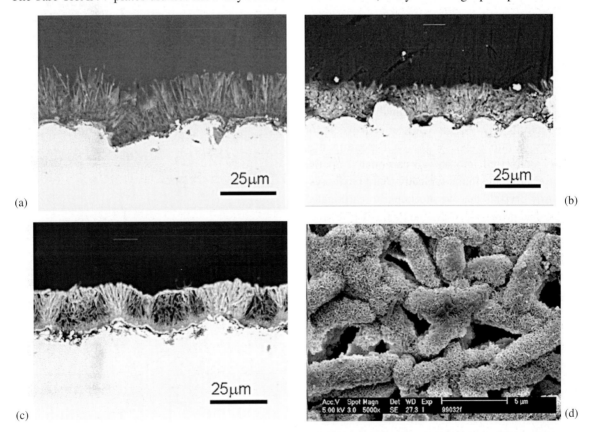

(a)   (b)   (c)   (d)

Figure 2 – OCP coating: (a) BSEM photo of the initial OCP coating, (b) BSEM photo after 2 weeks of immersion in α-MEM, (c) BSEM photo after 4 weeks of immersion in α-MEM, (d) ESEM photo after 4 weeks of immersion α-MEM. ESEM photos magnification x 5000.

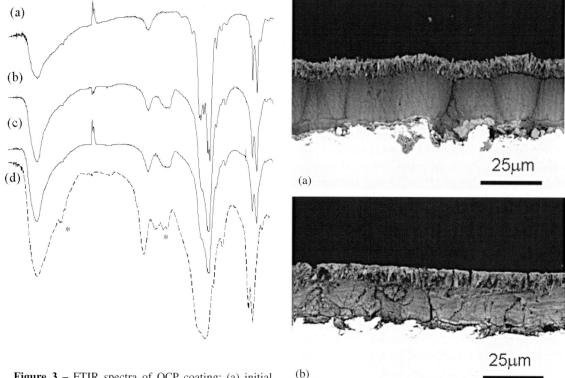

Figure 3 – FTIR spectra of OCP coating: (a) initial coating, (b) *in vitro* after 2 weeks of immersion, (c) *in vitro* after 4 weeks of immersion, and (d) *in vivo* after 4 weeks of implantation. (*) Bands attributed to organic compounds.

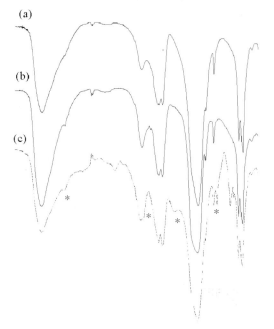

Figure 4 – BSEM photos of BCA coating: (a) initial coating, (b) after 4 weeks of immersion.

remained, and CO_3^{2-} bands remained similar to the IR spectrum at 2 weeks. Thus, after 4 weeks of immersion into α-MEM, the OCP coating was totally converted into an AB-carbonated apatite coating. From the initial typically sharp OCP crystals, tiny crystals that we attributed to carbonated apatite had grown sideward and on the detriment to OCP phase (fig. 2).

With regard to BCA coating, after 4 weeks of immersion in α-MEM, the dense layer exhibited cracks that might be due to a long hydration time followed by drying. On the top of this dense layer the crystals appeared slightly denser than the initial top crystal layer (fig. 4b). In addition, the coating became thinner overtime. The IR spectrum recorded after 4 weeks into α-MEM was accurately similar to the initial BCA coating (fig. 5a, 5b). Therefore, the soaking of BCA coated Ti6Al4V plates into α-MEM affected the coating morphology but not its structure, which remained composed of carbonated apatitic crystals.

Figure 5 – FTIR spectra of BCA coating: (a) initial coating, (b) *in vitro* after 4 week of immersion, and (c) *in vivo* after 4 weeks of implantation. (*) Bands attributed to organic compounds.

In vivo degradation of OCP and BCA coating

In order to assess the biological degradation of OCP and BCA coatings, coated Ti6Al4V plates were subcutaneously implanted in 12 male Wistar rats, for 1, 2 and 4 weeks of survival period. As negative control, bare Ti6Al4V plates were implanted. After retrieving and embedding in poly-methylmethacrylate blocks, sectioning, and staining with 1% methylene blue and 0.3% fuchsin, the histological slides of the implants did not reveal any systemic toxic effects or inflammatory reaction could be observed. No significant foreign body giant cell reaction was noted in any of the evaluated sections. Light microscopy showed no signs of particulate debris or coating delamination. In addition, the coating did not disappear *in vivo*. The entire titanium alloy surface was still covered with a uniform coating after 1, 2 and 4 weeks implantation under the skin.

The IR spectra of the OCP coating after 4 weeks of implantation time exhibit changes in structure (fig. 3d). Similarly to the *in vitro* study, OCP evolved into carbonated apatite. Additionally, three other bands appeared corresponding to aliphatic C-H and amine N-H vibrations, that suggests the incorporation of proteins or amino-acids while the initial OCP coating was converted into a carbonated apatitic coating.

On the other hand, the carbonate apatitic structure of BCA coating remained apparently unchanged (fig. 5c). However, like previously observed for OCP coating, after 4 weeks of implantation, the aliphatic C-H vibration bands were observed, in addition to three other bands, which were not detected in the implanted OCP coatings. Since these bands do not correspond to any phosphate or hydrogenophosphate bands or amines, they should be assigned to any other unidentified organic compounds. For both coatings, organic compounds from the surrounding body fluids were incorporated into the coating during the subcutaneous implantation.

Comparison between the degradation *in vitro* and *in vivo*

After embedding in a polymethylmethacrylate block, the implants were cross-sectioned in their middle. A cross section picture of the Ca-P coating on Ti6Al4V plate, obtained by backscattering electronic microscopy (BSEM) (fig. 2 and 4), was used to determine the Ca-P coating two-dimensional (2-D)-surface area with an image analysis software (VIDAS).

Week	OCP Coating area (μm^2)	BCA coating area (μm^2)
Week 0	884 ± 54	501 ± 28
Week 1	773 ± 43	545 ± 51
Week 2	777 ± 317	579 ± 36
Week 4	776 ± 42	602 ± 235

Table 2 – Coating surface area in μm^2 before (week 0) and after one, two and four weeks of subcutaneous implantation. The measurements have been performed on BSEM pictures (magnification x 40) of cross-sections. The given values are absolute.

Table 2 represents the evolution of the measured surface area of both coating versus implantation time. The measurement of the cross-sectioned surface area of the coating indicated a decrease of 100 μm^2 after 1 week of subcutaneous implantation. Thereafter, for 2 and 4 weeks, the 2D-surface area did not evolve, remaining at approximately 775 μm^2. On the other hand, the morphology of OCP coating did not evolve after 1, 2 and 4 weeks of implantation. In contrast to the *in vitro* study, the coating kept its sharp crystals *in vivo*. In the case of BCA coating, the morphology of the cross-sectioned samples after 1, 2 and 4 weeks did not change overtime. However, the 2D-surface area of the coating slightly increased with time. This suggested a calcification of the coating by mineral ions contained in the surrounding body fluids.

GAP HEALING MODEL APPLIED ON BIOMIMETIC CALCIUM PHOSPHATE COATED POROUS IMPLANTS

The biomimetic route allows the covering of complex shaped materials, such as porous implants. The advantage of uniformly applying either OCP or BCA coating was evaluated in a gap-healing model. In a defect of 7mm in diameter created in the lateral and medial condyle of both femurs (left and right) of Dutch milk goats, two bare and four coated (two OCP and two BCA) porous tantalum (Ta) implants were inserted for each implantation time (12 and 24 weeks). The cylinders (5mm in diameter, 10mm in length) were held centered by placing o-ring Teflon spacers of 1mm in thickness on each end of the plug.

	Gap healed	Direct bone contact	Bone in the center
Bare Ta	0/2	0/2	0/2
OCP Ta	0/2	2/2	2/2
BCA Ta	0/2	2/2	0/2

Table 3 – Bone incidence in the porous implants in the gap (1mm) created in the femoral condyle of goats.

The Teflon washers created a 1mm gap surrounding the implant. For each goat, four implantation sites were used in total. The porous Ta is a porous material fabricated by chemical vapor infiltration of pure tantalum onto a highly porous vitreous carbon skeleton. The porous structure possessed 70 to 75% porosity and a regular array of interconnecting pores averaging 400 to 500 µm. Table 3 summarizes the bone incidence of the gap-healing implantation in the femoral condyle.

Bare Tantalum (Ta) Cylinders

After 12 weeks of implantation, the original margins of the drill hole were still visible. At the drill margins of the trabeculae, newly formed bone could be seen. Bare Ta implants showed columns of bone growth towards the implant, but bone was confined along the Teflon spacers and the outer perimeter of the implant. A fibrous tissue was observed between the newly formed bone and the Teflon spacer, as well as between the newly formed bone and the walls of the pores. The rest of the implant was mainly filled by fat cells and by fibrous tissues (fig. 6a).

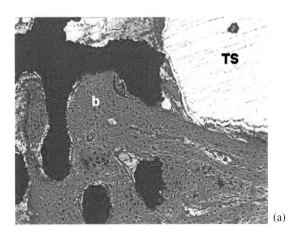

(a)

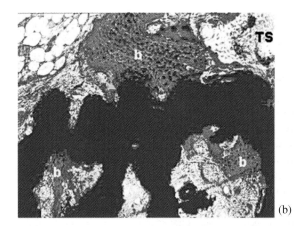

(b)

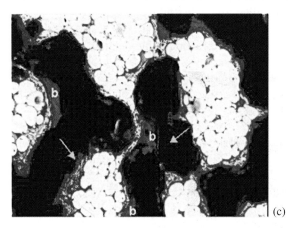

(c)

Figure 6 – Porous Ta cylinders after 12 weeks of implantation in femoral condyle (gap-healing model). Magnification × 100. Arrows indicate the remaining coating. (a) Bare Ta: de novo bone (b) was only observed at the vicinity of the Teflon spacer (TS); (b) BCA coated Ta; (c) OCP coated Ta.

BCA-coated Tantalum (Ta) Cylinders

After 12 weeks of implantation, light microscopy of the two BCA coated implants showed similar features compared to bare Ta cylinders: new bone formed in the gap between the cortical bone and the implants, and bone reached the implants only along the Teflon spacers (Figure 6b). Additionally, BCA coating had almost completely disappeared. The coating could be rarely detected in the pores of the implant, and in some parts, it was integrated with *de novo* bone. Bone was in direct contact with Ta cylinders. No evidence of bone in the center of the implant could be detected. The rest of the implant was filled mainly by fat cells and fibrous tissue.

OCP coated Ta cylinders

After 12 weeks of implantation, light microscopy of the 2 OCP coated implants showed bone growth along the Teflon spacers towards the implant. The original margins of the drill hole were still visible. In contrast with BCA coating, OCP coating could still be detected after 12 weeks of implantation, and newly formed bone was also present in the center of the Ta implants (fig. 6c). BSEM revealed that OCP coating was integrated in the newly formed bone (fig. 7a, 7b). In fig. 7b, OCP crystals were visible and they were completely interlocked in *de novo* bone. The rest of the porous implant was filled mainly with fat cells and fibrous tissues.

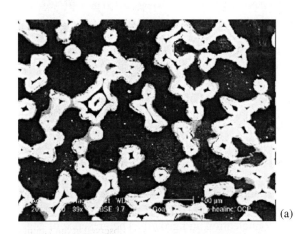

(a)

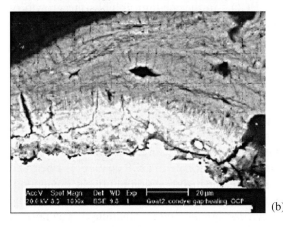

(b)

Figure 7 – BSEM photo of bone in the center of OCP coated Ta implanted in the femoral condyle (gap-healing model). (a) at magnification × 40, (b) at magnification × 1000: note the bonding between OCP and bone, the OCP crystals are interlocked with ectopic bone. White areas correspond to the tantalum pore walls (Ta), The dark grayish areas correspond to ectopic bone (b), and the light gray layer represents OCP coating (black arrow).

OSTEOINDUCTION OF OCP COATED POROUS IMPLANTS

With regard to the intramuscular study, 8 porous Ta and 8 dense Ti6Al4V cylinders (5mm in diameter and 10mm in length) were implanted in for a survival period of 12 and 24 weeks. Both lateral back muscles (left and right) of each Dutch milk goat were used. In each side, two bare and two coated metal implants (OCP or BCA) were inserted according to a defined implantation scheme. Table 4 summarizes the bone incidence of the intramuscular implantations.

	12 weeks	24 weeks
Bare Ti6Al4V	0/4	0/4
OCP Ti6Al4V	1/4*	1/4*
Bare Ta	0/4	0/4
OCP Ta	3/4	0/4

Table 4 – Bone incidence after intramuscular implantation in goats. (*) bone was detected in the cavity of the Ti6Al4V cylinder, and not on the outer surface.

OCP coated and bare Ti6Al4V cylinders

After 12 and 24 weeks, OCP coating dissolved extensively, and remained in few random areas after 12 weeks of implantation. Fibrous tissue covered the Ti6Al4V implants. In two cases, one at 12 weeks and on at 24 weeks, histology showed ectopic bone formed in the inner cavity of the Ti6Al4V cylinders (fig. 8).

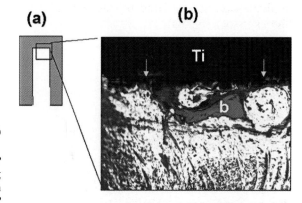

Figure 8 – (a) Design of the Ti6Al4V cylinder implants. (b) ectopic bone (b) formed in the cavity of the Ti6Al4V cylinder, as shown by light microscopy (× 200). The yellow arrows point out the remaining OCP coating.

OCP coated and bare Ta cylinders

After 12 and 24 weeks of implantation, the OCP coating had completely disappeared. Three out of four OCP-coated Ta implants exhibited bone in the pores after 12 weeks implantation (fig. 9). BSEM

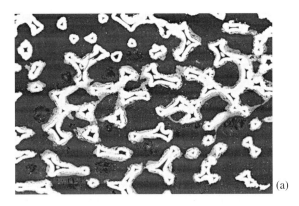

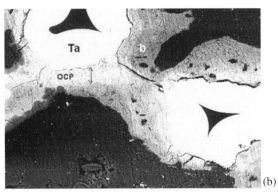

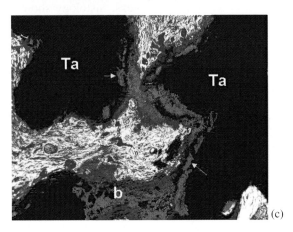

Figure 9 – OCP coated Ta explanted after 12 weeks from muscle of goats: a) BSEM (x25), b) BSEM (x250). White areas: tantalum pore walls (Ta), the dark grayish areas: ectopic bone (b), and the light gray layer: OCP coating (black arrow), c) light microscopy (x100). The arrows indicate the remaining OCP coating.

images indicated that bone was in direct contact with Ta substrate without the intervention of fibrous tissue. However, in some places the OCP coating could be visible as an integrated layer in de novo bone. Bone was formed in the interior of the implants, and in several parts of the porous implants. After 24 weeks of implantation, two coated Ta implants exhibited a random purple filling in the pores similar to bone stained in similar conditions. However, no bone cells-like could be detected, suggesting the presence of a calcified matrix.

DISCUSSION

In vitro and *in vivo* degradation of OCP coating

It is clear that the OCP coating transforms overtime into a carbonate apatitic structure *in vitro* and *in vivo*. This evolution can be attributed to the effect of the salts contained in α-MEM such as Mg^{2+}, Ca^{2+}, HPO_4^{2-} and HCO_3^- ions. *In vitro* OCP-to-carbonate apatite transformation must result from an interfacial dissolution-reprecipitation mechanism. Once immersed into α-MEM, Ca^{2+} and HPO_4^{2-} ions must be liberated from the surface to the medium. At the vicinity of the OCP coating, supersaturation in α-MEM is reached, resulting to Ca-P nucleation and growth. The presence of Mg^{2+} and HCO_3^- in the medium inhibits the growth of the OCP phase and favors the formation of poorly crystallized carbonate apatite (25).

Irrespective to the continuous dissolution *in vitro*, OCP coating partially dissolved after 1 week of implantation, and thereafter remained stable for 2 and 4 weeks of implantation while being converted into carbonate apatite from the first week on. This initial dissolution of OCP can result from a thermodynamic instability in body fluids due to an initial lack of carbonate in OCP coating. Further, in a later stage, the incorporation of organic compounds could reduce the dissolution rate, as it has been shown for bovine serum albumin co-precipitated into a similar biomimetic OCP coating (29).

In vitro and in vivo *degradation of BCA coating*

With regard to BCA coating our analysis indicated that the mineral structure did not change. However, we hypothesize that a dissolution-precipitation mechanism could have taken place as crystal morphology has changed with immersion time in α-MEM. After implantation, BCA coating contained organic compounds, which were either incorporated or adsorbed. *In vivo*, the BCA coating grew continuously over implantation period. Since histology did not reveal any bone formation, this growth can be interpreted as a surface calcification of the BCA coating from the body fluids. Our *in vivo* data are in accordance with Heughebaert *et al.* who quantified a similar calcification with sintered HA ceramics (30), whereas a weight loss occurred for sintered carbonate apatite (31). This suggests that the processing of the material, and therefore the microstructure and composition have a great influence on its stability *in vivo*.

Similarities and differences between OCP and BCA degradation

The biomimetic OCP and BCA coatings have a relatively comparable behavior both *in vitro* and *in vivo*. Initially, a partial dissolution takes place followed by the reprecipitation of a carbonated apatitic layer. In our study, this layer is detected in bone cell-free environment, and its formation results from a purely physicochemical process. However, *in vivo*, OCP partially dissolves, whereas BCA calcifies. Three parameters can explain this *in vivo* dissimilarity.

Influence of proteins

IR spectra of both coating displayed the presence of organic compounds. These compounds were incorporated or adsorbed in both implanted coatings. Even if we could not identify namely the interacting organic compounds, it is clear that they were not identical for the two coatings. IR spectra of implanted OCP exhibited an amino group band that can be reasonably attributed to proteins, whereas IR spectra of implanted BCA did not exhibit this band, suggesting that BCA did not incorporate proteins. This observation is in accordance with Johnsson *et al.* (32) who have shown that OCP and BCA have specific and distinct affinities for other compounds present in body fluids. These various compounds might promote or prevent dissolution. Besides direct interactions (adsorption or incorporation) between organic compounds and Ca-P, the sole presence of organics

in the medium can influence the Ca-P stability. For example, serum albumin present in the medium interacts with free Ca^{2+}, enhancing HA dissolution (33, 34). Thus, the cocktail of numerous organic and inorganic compounds present in the body fluids and their specific interactions with BCA or OCP can drastically influence the dissolution behavior of the implanted Ca-P phase.

Influence of microstructure

It is microscopically clear that OCP and BCA coating have different microstructures. The OCP coating is composed of large vertical crystals exhibiting a great open structure to the surrounding body fluids, whereas the BCA exhibits smaller and denser crystals. Since a greater surface is exposed to the body fluid, one might expect a higher reactivity between OCP coating and its environment, than for BCA coating. Specific surface area measurements were not performed in this study because such analysis requires the scrapping off the coating, and thereby the exposed surface morphology would have been markedly modified, misleading the interpretation of the data. On the other hand, BCA crystallinity is significantly lower than OCP, due to the distortions and deficiencies created by the incorporation of carbonate in the apatitic lattice (35). This lower crystallinity would suggest a faster dissolution of BCA compared to OCP.

Physicochemical aspect

In addition to the comparison of crystallinity, we have to compare two different crystal lattices. Under physiological conditions apatite is thermodynamically more stable than OCP, suggesting in theory a higher dissolution rate for OCP than for apatite. In summary, this dissolution study has shown a competition between two different Ca-P phases OCP and BCA, exhibiting a great *versus* small microstructure, a crystalline *versus* less-crystalline structure, and a more thermodynamically stable *versus* less thermodynamically stable structure. All of these features markedly influence the dissolution behavior, as already mentioned previously for dissolution rate determination in saline solutions (36). Although α-MEM and body fluids are more complex than saline solution in term of composition, microstructure, crystallinity and thermodynamics, the dissolution behavior of OCP and BCA coatings seems to be also the result of a combination of those parameters.

Similarities and differences between OCP and BCA osteogenicity

When OCP-coated, BCA-coated, and bare Ta were implanted in a gap of 1mm in the condyle, marked distinctions could be noted between the three sorts of implant. First, contact could be established between newly formed bone and Ta along the Teflon spacer. Direct bone contact could be noted for BCA and OCP coated Ta, whereas a fibrous tissue layer was often detected between the bare implant and the newly formed bone. Therefore, Ca-P coating allowed a direct bonding between the implant and the hosting bone. In all the cases OCP-coated, BCA-coated and bare Ta, the gap of 1mm was not healed, whereas bone was detected in the center of the OCP coated porous implant. Due to the high interconnectivity of Ta, one cannot confirm that bone present in the center of the implant does not have a direct contact with host bone.

Further, OCP coated Ta could induce bone in nonosseous sites, as reported in the present results and discussed below. Therefore, one can think that bone formed in the center of the implant is not necessarily connected with the host bone. Nevertheless, this observation suggests that OCP coating has a markedly higher osteogenic potential than BCA coating. In relation to this osteogenecity difference, one could note that BCA coating had completely disappeared, whereas OCP coating remained partially after 12 weeks of implantation in trabeculae. The faster degradation observed for BCA coating is contradictory with the results of the subcutaneous implantation in rats described above, although the environmental conditions a significantly different between the two studies.

When Ta implants are inserted in femoral condyles, one must consider the strong influence of bone marrow cells. In a bony environment, the resorption of the coating depends strongly on the osteoclastic activity, ruled by the physicochemistry of the Ca-P coating (37, 38, 39). The more soluble Ca-P is, the less osteoclastic activity is (38, 39). In the case of OCP and BCA coatings, Leeuwenburgh *et al.* have shown that resorption pits had extended more on BCA coating *in vitro* (37). Therefore, osteoclastic activity may be higher *in vivo* in the case of BCA than for OCP coating. A too fast osteoclastic resorption of BCA could therefore affect bone formation onto BCA coated Ta.

On the other hand, the initial microstructure of the two coatings is markedly different, as mentioned previously. The relatively rough microstructure of OCP coating might influence positively bone formation, whereas the relatively smooth BCA might influence negatively bone formation, as already reported by Yuan *et al.* (22). Independently of the material, cell adhesion, morphology and orientation are strongly affected by the implant roughness and surface physics and chemistry (40-48). Redey et al. have shown that a difference in surface energy between a HA substrate and a type A carbonated apatite could influence significantly the early osteoblastic adhesion *in vitro*, while surface roughness of both material was similar (41). Although the two substrates evolved into a type AB carbonated apatite in the culture medium with time, and despite a similar final cell growth on the two materials, the authors observed differences in the kinetics of cell attachment. The relatively high-energy HA substrate accelerated cell attachment and spreading as compared to the low-energy type A carbonated apatite.

In addition, for a similar surface chemistry and roughness, the bigger the HA crystallite were, the higher the response of the osteoblasts was (46). These two aforementioned studies could explain our experimental observations: the large OCP crystals may favor osteoblastic activity, and the presence of carbonate in BCA may decrease its surface energy, inhibiting the early osteoblasts response towards BCA. Besides surface energy considerations, Knabe et al related a relative inhibition of osteoblasts growth *in vitro* with a relatively high phosphate-ion release (47, 48). This observation is quite in accordance with the present study: OCP has an atomic calcium to phosphorus ratio (Ca/P) of 1.33, whereas BCA has a Ca/P = 1.60 (36). In addition BCA dissolves faster than OCP in the condyle, therefore a higher phosphate-ion release with BCA coating than with OCP coating.

Osteoinductivity of OCP coating

With regard to the intramuscular implantation in goats, it appears that OCP coating can induce bone formation in a nonosseous site. First, bare materials - Ti6Al4V and Ta cylinders – did not lead to ectopic bone formation. Second, OCP coated porous structure induced bone formation, either in the Ta pores, or in the inner cavity of the Ti6Al4V cylinder, but not on flat substrates such as Ti6Al4V cylinders.

From these observations, two conditions seem to be required to induce ectopic bone formation: 1) the presence of a Ca-P coating, and 2) the architecture of the implant. These two conditions are simultaneously mandatory. Within porous implants, the sole surface composition of the pore walls rule the formation or not of bone. Vice versa, dense flat OCP coated implants did not lead to any bone formation, whereas in the cavity of the Ti6Al4V cylinder, bone could be found apparently formed following the intramembranous ossification route (49). According to the BSEM imaging, OCP alone was not detected on the surface of the pores, indicating that the coating dissolves in contact with body fluids. On the other hand, OCP was fully integrated in the newly formed bone, without intervention of fibrous tissues. In other areas where bone is present, no OCP coating could be detected, suggesting that OCP coating was completely resorbed. Bone was in direct contact with Ta material.

Osteoinduction by porous Ca-P ceramics can be attributed to 1) the incorporation and concentration of Bone Morphogenetic Proteins (BMPs) by Ca-P crystals (49-51), 2) a low oxygen tension in the central region of the implant triggering the pericytes of microvessels to differentiate into osteoblasts, 3) a rough surface produced by the 3D microstructure causing the asymmetrical division of mesenchymal cells that would produce osteoblasts, 4) the surface charge of the substrate triggering cell differentiation, 5) the bone-like apatite layer formed in vivo that recognize mesenchymal cells, or 6) the local high level of free Ca^{2+} provided by the Ca-P material that triggers cell differentiation and bone formation (49).

In our experiments, as the presence of Ca-P and of a porous structure are two simultaneously required conditions for bone induction, the proposals 3), 4) and 5) concerning the rough 3D-microstructure, the surface charge and the bone-like apatite recognition cannot be the sole parameters. Otherwise, bone could have been induced on the OCP coated dense Ti6Al4V cylinders, and not only in the cavity of the Ti6Al4V implants. Incorporation of BMPs (proposal 1), and the presence of Ca^{2+} (proposal 6) are also expected from a flat and smooth substrate such as OCP coated Ti6Al4V, as observed under the skin of rats for OCP coated Ti6Al4V plates.

We hypothesize that OCP reacts also dynamically towards the surrounding body fluids: exchanging Ca^{2+} and HPO_4^{2-} and interacting with organic compounds in the muscle of goats. Bone Morphogenetic Proteins (BMPs) for example, could possibly interact with the OCP coated porous Ta cylinders. Since porous Ta cylinders have a much greater specific surface area than dense Ti6Al4V cylinder, the quantity of free Ca^{2+} is much higher for a porous substrate than for a dense one. In relation to the specific surface area of the implant, the possible interaction sites with BMPs must exist to a greater extent in the case of a porous cylinder than in the case of a dense one. The level of BMPs and free Ca^{2+} are highly critical in the osteoinduction phenomenon.

On the other hand, bone also formed in the cavity of the Ti6Al4V cylinder, which suggests that the confinement is also a critical factor. In a confined site, the amount free Ca^{2+} released from OCP coating may remain quite stable, and may be high enough to trigger cell differentiation and bone formation (proposal 6). Therefore, it appears in the present study that the primary condition for inducing ectopic bone could be a quite stable critical level of free Ca^{2+}, which can be achieved in the pores of Ta.

Bone formation is, however, limited in time. After 24 weeks of implantation, no bone was observed in the four explanted Ta. Ectopic bone could be detected solely in the cavity of one Ti6Al4V cylinder. However, in two out of four cases, a calcified matrix was detected in the pores. It is clear that bone does not continuously grow as function of time. As no more bone is detected on the 24-weeks implants, we can suggest that bone induced by OCP coating degraded with time. This resorption could be related to an interruption of Ca^{2+} supply from OCP coating because of its complete dissolution. The implant being in a nonosseous site cannot benefit of a continuous differentiation into bone cell to pursue bone formation. On the other hand, the encapsulation of the implant by fibrous tissue could limit the flow of surrounding body fluids into the porous implant. This could lead to the degradation of the newly formed bone, which could be attributed to the calcified matrix observed in two porous implants after 24 weeks.

CONCLUSION

The biomimetic OCP and BCA coatings show similarities in their *in vitro* and *in vivo* behavior. Whatever their environment, simulated physiological fluids or natural body fluids, the surfaces of these materials interact dynamically. A carbonated apatite formed on the coated plates *in vivo* and *in vitro*. However, subcutaneously, OCP and BCA coatings incorporate distinct organic compounds, and OCP dissolved partially at the first week of implantation, whereas BCA calcified. In the femoral condyle, bone was detected in the center of OCP coated porous implants, whereas bone formed solely at the vicinity of the BCA coated porous implants. In the muscle, the presence of OCP coating in a macroporous structure induced ectopic bone formation. The nature of the Ca-P coating influenced markedly the biological activity of Ca-P coated implants via the microstructure, the dissolution rate, the chemistry, and the physics of their surface. As a consequence of these specific factors, the osteogenecity of OCP and BCA coating was markedly influenced.

Reference List

1. Overgaard S, Lind M, Glerup H, Bünger C, Søballe K (1998) Porous-coated versus grit-blasted surface texture of hydroxyapatite-coated implants during controlled micromotion: mechanical and histomorphometric results. *J. Arthroplasty* 13:449-58.

2. Simmons CA, Valiquette N, Pilliar RM (1999) Osseointegration of sintered porous-surfaced and plasma spray-coated implants: An animal model study of early postimplantation healing response and mechanical stability. *J. Biomed. Mater Res.* 47:127-38

3. Deporter DA, Watson PA, Pilliar RM, Chipman ML (1990), Valiquette N. A histological comparison in the dog of porous-coated vs. threaded dental implants. *J. Dent. Res.* 69:1138-45.

4. Jansen JA, van der Waerden JPCM, Wolke JGC, de Groot K (1991) Histologic evaluation of the osseous adaptation to titanium and hydroxyapatite-coated titanium implants. *J. Biomed. Mat. Res.* 25:973-89.

5. Dhert WJA, Klein CPAT, Jansen JA, van der Velde EA, Vriesde RC, Rozing PM, de Groot K (1993) A histological and histomorphometrical investigation of fluoroapatite, magnesiumwhitlockite, and Hydroxylapatite plasma-sprayed coatings in goats. *J. Biomed. Mat. Res.* 27:127-38.

6. Klein CPAT, Wolke JGC, de Blieck-Hogervorts JMA, de Groot K (1994) Calcium Phosphate plasma-sprayed coatings and their stability: an in vivo study. *J. Biomed. Mat. Res.* 28:909-17.

7. Cook SD, Thomas KA, Dalton JE, Kay JF (1991). Enhanced bone ingrowth and fixation strength with hydroxyapatite-coated porous implants. *Semin. Arthroplasty* 2:268-79.

8. Pilliar RM, Deporter DA, Watson PA, Pharoah M, Chipman M, Valiquette N, Carter S, De Groot K (1991) The effect of partial coating with hydroxyapatite on bone remodeling in relation to porous-coated titanium-alloy dental implants in the dog. *J. Dent. Res.* 70:1338-45.

9. Cook SD, Enis J, Armstrong D, Lisecki E (1992) Early clinical results with the hydroxyapatite-coated porous LSF Total Hip System. *Dent. Clin. North Am.* 36:247-55.

10. Geesink RG, de Groot K, Klein CP (1988) Bonding of bone to apatite-coated implants. *J. Bone Joint Surg. Br.* 70B: 17-22.

11. Hanawa T, Kamira Y, Yamamoto S, Kohgo T, Amemyia A, Ukai H, Murakami K, Asaoka K (1997) Early bone formation around calcium-ion-implanted titanium inserted into rat tibia. *J. Biomed. Mater Res.* 36:131-36.

12. Sakkers RJB, Dalmeijer RAJ, Brand R, Rozing PM, van Blitterswijk CA (1997) Assessment of bioactivity for orthopedic coatings in a gap healing model. *J. Biomed. Mat. Res.* 36:265-73.

13. Søballe K, Hansen ES, Brockstedt-Rasmussen, Bunger C (1991) Gap healing enhanced by hydroxyapatite coatings in dog. *Clin. Orthop.* 272:300-307.

14. Clemens JAM, Klein CPAT, Vriesde RC, Rozing PM, de Groot K (1998) Healing of large (2mm) gaps around calcium phosphate-coated bone implant: a study in goats with a follow up of 6 months. *J. Biomed. Mat. Res.* 40:341-49.

15. Yamasaki H (1990) Ectopic bone formation around porous hydroxyapatite ceramics in the subcutis of dogs. *Japan J. Oral Biol.* 32:190-92.

16. Yuan H, de Bruijn JD, Yang Z, de Groot K, Zhang X (1998) Osteoinduction by calcium phosphates. *J. Mater Sci. Mater Med.* 9:717-21.

17. Vargervik K (1992) Critical sites for new bone formation. Bone grafts & bone substitute :112-20.

18. Ripamonti U (1991) The morphogenesis of bone in replicas of porous hydroxyapatite obtained from conversion of calcium carbonate exoskeletons of coral. *J. Bone & Joint Surg.* 73A:692-703.

19. Zhang X (1991) A study of porous blocks HA ceramics and its osteogenesis. Bioceramics and the Human Body:408-15.

20. Magan A, Ripamonti U (1996) Geometry of porous hydroxyapatite implants influences osteogenesis in baboons (Papio ursinus). *J. Craniofac. Surg.* 7:71-8.

21. Yuan H, de Bruijn JD, Li Y, Feng Z, Yang K, de Groot K, Zhang X (2001) Bone formation induced by Calcium phosphate ceramics in soft tissue of dogs: a comparative study between a-TCP and b-TCP. *J. Mater Sci. Mater Med.* 12:7-13.

22. Yuan H, Kurashina K, de Bruijn JD, Li Y, de Groot K, Zhang X (2000) A preliminary study on osteoinduction of two kind of calcium phosphate ceramics. Biomaterials 20:1283-90.

23. Kokubo T, Kushitani H, Sakka S, Kitsugi T, Yamamuro T (1990) Solutions able to reproduce *in vivo* surface-

structure changes in bioactive glass-ceramics A-W3. *J. Biomed. Mat. Res.* 24:721-34.

24. Barrère F, Layrolle P, van Blitterswijk CA, de Groot K (2001) Biomimetic Calcium Phosphate coatings on Ti6Al4V: Growth study of OCP. *J. Mater. Sci. Mater. Med.* 12:529-34.

25. Barrère F, Layrolle P, van Blitterswijk CA, de Groot K (1998) Biomimetic Calcium-Phosphate Coatings on Ti6Al4V: a Crystal Growth Study of Octacalcium Phosphate and Inhibition by Mg^{2+} and HCO_3^-. *Bone* 25:107S-11S.

26. Habibovic P, Barrère F, van Blitterswijk CA, de Groot K and Layrolle P (2002) Biomimetic Hydroxyapatite coating on metal implants. *J. Am. Ceram. Soc.* 85:517-22.

27. Barrère F, van Blitterswijk CA, de Groot K, Layrolle P (2002) Influence of ionic strength and carbonate on the Ca-P coating formation from SBFx5 solution. *Biomaterials* 23:1921-30.

28. Barrère F, van Blitterswijk CA, de Groot K, Layrolle P (2002) Nucleation mechanism of Ca-P coating formed from SBFx5 solution: influence of magnesium. *Biomaterials* 23:2211-20.

29. Liu Y, Layrolle P, van Blitterswijk CA, de Groot K (2000) Incorporation of proteins into biomimetic hydroxyapatite coatings. *Bioceramics* 13:71-4.

30. Heughebaert M, LeGeros RZ, Gineste M, Guihlem A, Bonel G. (1988) Physicochemical characterization of deposits associated with HA ceramics implanted in nonosseous sites. *J. Biomed. Mater. Res. Appl. Biomat.* A3:257-68.

31. Barralet J, Akao M, Aoki H, Aoki H (2000) Dissolution of dense carbonate apatite subcutaneously implanted in Wistar rats. *J. Biomed. Mater. Res.* 49:176-82.

32. Johnsson MSA, Paschalis E, Nancollas GH (1991) Kinetics of mineralization, demineralization, transformation of calcium phosphates at mineral and protein surface. In: Davies JE, editor. The Bone-Biomaterial interface. Toronto, Canada: University of Toronto Press, p. 68-75.

33. Radin S, Ducheyne P, Bethold P, Decker S (1998) Effect of serum proteins and osteoblasts on the surface transformation of a calcium phosphate coating: a physicochemical and ultrastructural study. *J. Biomed. Mater. Res.* 39:234-43.

34. Bender SA, Bumgardner JD, Roach MD, Bessho K, Ong JL (2000) Effect of protein on the dissolution of HA coatings. *Biomaterials* 21:299-305.

35. Rey C, Collins B, Goehl T, Dickson IR, Glimcher MJ (1989) "The carbonate environement in bone mineral: a resolution-enhanced fourier transform infrared spectroscopy study". *Calcif. Tissue Int.* 45:157-64.

36. Barrere F, Stigter M, Layrolle P, van BlitterswijkCA, de Groot K (2000) *In vitro* dissolution of various Calcium-Phosphate coatings on Ti6Al4V. *Bioceramics* 13: 67-70.

37. Leeuwenburgh S, Layrolle P, Barrère F, de Bruijn J, Schoonman J, van Blitterswijk CA, de Groot K (2001) Osteoclastic resorption of biomimetic calcium phosphate coatings *in vitro*. *J. Biomed. Mat. Res.* 56:208-15.

38. Doi Y, Iwanaga H, Shibutani T, Moriwaki Y, Iwayama Y (1999) Osteocalstic responses to various calcium phosphates in cell cultures. *J. Biomed. Mater. Res.* 47: 424-33.

39. Yamada S, Heymann D, Bouler JM, Daculsi G (1997) Osteoclastic resorption of calcium phosphate ceramics with different hydroxyapatite/b-tricalcium phosphate ratios. *Biomaterials* 18:1037-41.

40. Boyan BD, Hummert TW, Dean DD, Schwartz Z (1996) Role of material surfaces in regulating bone and cartilage cell response. *Biomaterials* 17:137-46.

41. Redey SA, Nardin M, Bernache-Assolant D, Rey C, Delannoy P, Sedel L, Marie PJ (2000) Behavior of human osteoblastic cells on stoechiometric hydroxyapatite and type A carbonate apatite: role of surface energy. *J. Biomed. Mat. Res.* 50: 353-64.

42. Chou L, Firth JD, Uitto VJ, Brunette DM (1998) Effects of titanium substratum and grooved surface topography on metalloproteinase-2 expression in human fibroblasts. *J. Biomed. Mat. Res.* 39:437-45.

43. Lampin M, Warocquier-Clerout, Legris C, Degrange M, Sigot-Luizart MF (1997) Correlation between substratum roughness and wettability, cell adhesion and cell migration. *J. Biomed. Mat. Res.* 36:99-108.

44. Anselme K (2000) Osteoblast adhesion on biomaterials. *Biomaterials* 21: 667-81.

45. Eisenbarth E, Meyle J, Nachtigall W, Breme J (1996) Influence of the surface structure of titanium materials on the adhesion of fibroblasts. *Biomaterials* 17: 1399-403.

46. Ong JL, Hoppe CA, Cardenas HL, Cavin R, Carnes DL, Sogal A, Raikar GN (1998). Osteoblast precursor cell activity on HA surfaces of different treatments. *J Biomed Mat Res* 39: 176-83.

45. Knabe C, Gildenhaar R, Berger G, Ostapowicz W, Fitzner R, Radlanski RJ, Gross U (1887). Morphological evaluation of osteoblasts cultured on different calcium phosphate ceramics. *Biomaterials* 18: 1339-47.

48. Knabe C, Driessens FCM, Planell JA, Gildenhaar R, Berger G, Reif D, Fritzner R, Radlanski RJ, Gross U (2000) Evaluation of calcium phosphates and experimental calcium phosphate bone cements using osteogenic cultures. *J. Biomed. Mat. Res.* 52: 498-508.

49. Yuan H (2001) Osteoinduction by Calcium Phosphates, PhD thesis, Leiden University,The Netherlands.

50. Ripamonti U (1996) Osteoinduction in porous hydroxyapatite implanted in ectopic sites of different animal models *Biomaterials* 17:31-5.

51. Yuan H, Zou P, Yang Z, Zhang X, de Bruijn JD, de Groot K (1998) Bone morphogenetic protein and ceramic-induced osteogenesis. *J. Mat. Sci. Mat. Med.* 9: 717-21.

4   Histology and Fate of Bioactive Coatings

Thomas W. Bauer, MD, PhD and Satoshi Takikawa, MD, PhD

INTRODUCTION

Many previous studies have demonstrated the osteo-conductive, biocompatible nature of hydroxyapatite coatings (1-16), numerous clinical reports have demonstrated safety and efficacy of bioactive coatings on joint implants components from different manufacturers (17-28), and several recent studies have illustrated the histology of HA-coated implants obtained at revision arthroplasty or autopsy (29-33), but questions persist concerning the long term consequences of HA-coatings, the most appropriate texture beneath the coating, and the influence of drugs that alter bone remodeling on coating efficacy and durability. The basic science behind hydroxyapatite coatings, technical aspects concerning its composition and application, and clinical results with the use of HA-coated total joint implants are included elsewhere in this volume. The purpose of this chapter is to describe the basic histology of the interface between HA-coated devices and bone, as well as the fate of coatings and the potential consequences of coating loss.

Mechanisms of Osteoconduction

Many animal studies have demonstrated bone apposition to hydroxyapatite *in vivo* (1, 7-13, 15, 16) (fig. 1 and 2). Bone apposition appears to occur as early as three weeks (34, 35), and at least one study showed greater than 90% bone apposition at 96 weeks (35). There appear to be at least two fundamental mechanisms responsible for these bioactive properties. First, calcium ions are thought to dissolve from the amorphous component of the coating, and then precipitate on the surface, probably as a carbonated apatite of low crystalline order (3, 36-40). This crystallization process is thought to

serve as a nidus for subsequent crystal growth. Second, hydroxyapatite has been used for decades in column chromatography because it avidly binds pro-

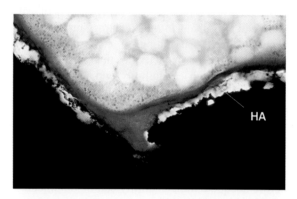

Figure 1 – HA-coated, textured titanium alloy femoral implant from a canine study at 26 weeks. There is extensive bone apposition without intervening fibrous membrane and the adjacent bone marrow is histologically normal.

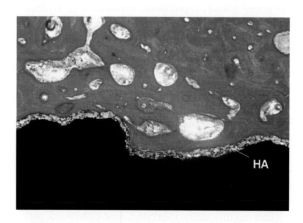

Figure 2 – HA-coated femoral implant from a canine total hip study at 1 year. There appears to be no degradation of this highly crystalline hydroxyapatite coating at one year, but in this optical field there is essentially 100% bone apposition. Coatings of lower crystallinity are rarely intact after 1 year *in vivo*.

teins (41-45). It seems likely that endogenous growth factors and cytokines are bound to the hydroxyapatite shortly after the implant is inserted *in vivo*. These proteins are probably gradually released, much as they are released from normal bone mineral during the course of bone remodeling. Although not yet experimentally tested, it is likely that the microporosity of the coating may influence the diffusion and binding of these proteins, and hence the biology of subsequent coating resorption and remodeling.

Coating durability and bioactivity can be influenced by several different factors, including the purity, crystallinity, calcium/phosphate ratio, density, bond strength, and thickness of the coating as well as the presence of substitutions in the apatite structure (14, 15, 46-53). Because initial crystal growth is thought to involve precipitation of calcium and phosphate onto the coating surface, it has been speculated that coatings of increased solubility might show greater bioactivities than sintered coatings of very high crystallinity and relatively low solubility. While this remains a topic of study, the excellent clinical results reported for femoral implants with highly crystalline HA coatings suggest that increasing coating solubility is unlikely to offer clinically significant advantages, and may pose some disadvantages if the coating dissolves before adequate initial stability can be obtained.

Influence of Alendronate on Early Fixation

As noted above, rapid bone apposition to hydroxyapatite coatings contributes to early implant fixation, but long term implant stability is influenced by bone remodeling around implants. Alendronate (4-amino-1hydroxybutylidene-1,1-bisphosphonate sodium) is an inhibitor of bone resorption that is being used to treat many patients with osteoporosis and other skeletal disorders. Because bone remodeling is thought to be initiated by osteoclastic bone resorption, it is appropriate to consider the potential consequences of alendronate on early fixation of HA-coated implants. However, a recent canine total hip arthroplasty study showed that alendronate neither significantly inhibited, nor enhanced early bone apposition to HA-coated devices (54) (fig. 3).

As discussed above and elsewhere in this volume, the biocompatibility and osteoconductive properties of calcium phosphate coatings have been well established. Controversial aspects now concern: 1) the

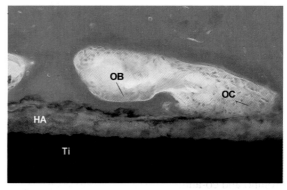

Figure 3 – HA-coated femoral implant from a canine study at 12 weeks. There is extensive bone apposition to the HA-coating, but the space indicates an area of active bone remodeling. Osteoblasts, as well as a single probable osteoclast are evident.

mechanisms of coating loss, 2) optimum physiochemical properties of the coating, 3) long term consequences of coating loss, and 4) optimum substrate texture beneath the coating.

Mechanisms of Coating Loss

We have hypothesized four mechanisms whereby HA can be lost from the surface of implants: 1) osteoclastic resorption of the coating as part of normal bone remodeling, 2) delamination, 3) dissolution at neutral pH, and 4) abrasion (46).

Resorption by Osteoclasts

We have previously described cells with morphologic features consistent with osteoclasts adjacent to HA-coatings (29) (fig. 4). Other authors have

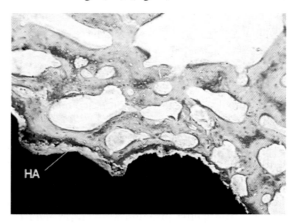

Figure 4 – Photograph of an HA-coated femoral stem at 4 weeks in a canine treated with alendronate. Alendronate inhibits osteoclast activity, but was no difference in bone apposition was evident when compared to animals not receiving alendronate.

also described osteoclasts adjacent to HA-coated implants (32, 55). In addition, recent laboratory studies have shown that osteoclasts in cell culture are capable of resorbing synthetic HA materials (56, 57). The presence of new bone immediately adjacent to the metal substrate in the absence of HA coatings in areas of anticipated load transfer also suggest that the process of bone and HA resorption probably occurs, at least in part, based on Wolff's law, but the ways in which load influence remodeling is controversial. For example, Tonino and co-authors reported the histological and histomorphometric results of clinically successful hydroxyapatite-coated cementless acetabular components that were retrieved at autopsy (32). All of the cups showed bone ongrowth, with a mean bone-implant contact of 36.5 ± 13.5%. Degradation of the hydroxyapatite coating by osteoclasts was observed. They concluded that cell-mediated hydroxyapatite resorption is the most likely mechanism for loss of the hydroxyapatite coating, and that the extent of bone ongrowth was independent of the amount of residual hydroxyapatite.

Based in part on additional studies of HA-coated femoral components retrieved at autopsy (33), Tonino and co-workers further suggested that areas of increased mechanical load were likely to show greater hydroxyapatite resorption due to a higher rate of bone remodeling at that site when compared with areas of the implant that transmit a lower mechanical load. On the other hand, our observations of clinically satisfactory hydroxyapatite-coated femoral and acetabular implants retrieved at autopsy reveal hypertrophy of bone and preservation of the hydroxyapatite in areas of expected load transfer, with preferential resorption of bone and hydroxyapatite in areas of the implant not active in load transmission (29, 30, 58). For example, our study of hydroxyapatite-coated threaded acetabular cups showed relative bone hypertrophy and preservation of the hydroxyapatite over the peaks of some of the threads, a site expected to transmit mechanical load, with absent bone apposition and absent hydroxyapatite in the valleys between threads, an area not expected according to the hypothesis of Tonino *et al.* (32).

We speculate that the extent of bone apposition and hydroxyapatite preservation is highest where the implant transmits load to the cortex. We tend to see bone hypertrophy and hydroxyapatite preservation along the medial and anterior aspects of hydroxyapatite-coated femoral stems where the implant is relatively close to the cortex, while the posterior and lateral stem surfaces show less hydroxyapatite preservation and less bone apposition.

Dissolution of hydroxyapatite coatings in the acid environment created by osteoclasts represents one mechanism of coating loss, but some retrieved implants seem to demonstrate more hydroxyapatite loss than would be expected if osteoclast resorption were the only mechanism of coating degradation. Additional possible mechanisms of coating loss include dissolution at neutral pH, delamination, and abrasion.

Delamination

Bonding of the plasma-sprayed coating to the substrate is important, and is influenced by many factors, including the texture of the substrate as well as the processing conditions and composition of the coating. Using high-resolution electron spectroscopic imaging, Filliaggi, Coombs and Pilliar 59 suggested significant phosphate diffusion into the metal to a depth of 25nm, possibly along grain boundaries. While the binding of HA to the substrate is primarily mechanical, these observations suggest that a chemical interaction may also play a role in the bonding of HA coatings to titanium substrates.

Although certainly representing a significant theoretical problem, we have identified coating delamination only rarely, primarily in animal specimens. When present, the delaminated coating is usually surrounded by bone, and is not associated with a foreign body giant cell reaction, histiocytic proliferation, fibrosis or osteolysis. For example, we have identified delamination of the hydroxyapatite in a canine total hip prosthesis that was retrieved by Dr. RGT Geesink at post mortem, ten years after total hip arthroplasty. In this clinically satisfactory specimen, the delaminated hydroxyapatite became surrounded by bone, resembling a bone-graft substitute material rather than an abrasive particle (fig. 5). Delamination of an implant coating is theoretically undesirable, but in this canine hip, delamination did not lead to implant loosening or to accelerated polyethylene wear (46).

It should be noted that some published photographs said to represent delamination in fact are almost certainly due to artificial cracking occurring during histologic processing. Acting more like a bone graft substitute, we do not believe that delaminated fragments of HA are a significant cause of

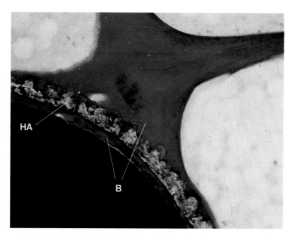

Figure 5 – Delaminated HA-coating from a canine femoral stem, 10 years after total hip arthroplasty. This highly crystalline coating showed good durability and maintained osteoconductivity even after 10 years *in vivo*. After delaminating from the substrate, the HA attained the attributes of a bone graft substitute. (Canine experimental model performed by Dr. RGT Geesink).

bone resorption or implant abrasion. If extensive delamination occurred in the immediate post-operative period, then mechanical loosening could result, but we have no evidence that this is a significant clinical problem at this time.

Dissolution at neutral pH

We expect synthetic HA coatings to dissolve at the very acid pH created by osteoclasts, but some coatings also appear to dissolve at neutral pH. It is difficult to consistently manufacture perfect coatings of high HA content and high crystallinity. Our previous experimental studies suggest that coatings with increasing proportions of non-HA calcium phosphates or lower crystalline moieties will show increased solubility at neutral pH, and it is possible that some of the implants clinically retrieved that show focal HA loss after only a few weeks or months *in vivo* may have had somewhat more soluble coatings. One of the consequences of increased coating solubility appears to be the release of smaller granules containing HA crystals of higher density into the adjacent tissue. The presence of granules of HA within macrophages adjacent to femoral stems in animals treated with alendronate (54) provides additional evidence of mechanisms of coating dissolution that are independent of osteoclasts. Interestingly, some manufacturers have suggested that increased coating solubility is desirable. While this occurs to some extent with all coatings, granules are increased

with coatings of increased solubility. Nevertheless, these granules do not appear to be associated with osteolysis and are almost certainly dissolved within the phagolysosomes of marrow macrophages.

Abrasion

If an implant does not achieve initial fixation, then the coating may become damaged by simple abrasion. We have received several implants in which adjacent pieces of bone graft caused abrasion of the coating. This emphasizes the importance of good clinical judgment and technique in implant insertion. HA coatings will not in themselves assure fixation of a device that is inappropriately designed or inserted.

Long Term Consequences of Coating Loss

Potential loss of calcium phosphate coatings may have implications concerning both implant fixation and debris formation.

Implant Fixation: It is reasonable to suspect that if gross delamination were to occur before adequate bone remodeling had developed around an implanted stem, then mechanical stability might be compromised. The excellent clinical results thus far reported for HA-coated femoral components suggests that this is not a significant problem at this time. As long as the HA loss is associated with normal bone remodeling, then fixation will be largely dependent upon the specific properties of the implant itself, *e.g.,* it's shape and stiffness. Implants which by their design poorly transmit load to the femoral cortex are less likely to maintain fixed after HA resorption than implants of superior design.

Consequences of Particulate Hydroxyapatite: As noted above, particles of HA are commonly identified within histiocytes adjacent to implants. Nevertheless, these cells do not appear to proliferate into the large sheets of histiocytes commonly associated with polyethylene-induced osteolysis and osteolysis has not been a significant problem in the available clinical series of HA-coated femoral component. Because lysosomal pH within macrophages is close to 4.8 (60-63), phagocytosed HA particles are likely to be dissolved within the cytoplasm of macrophages without inducing a clinically important inflammatory reaction.

Could particulate HA accelerate polyethylene wear by acting as third body debris? Many different types of particles migrate into the joint space and may increase polyethylene wear, including particles of bone cement or barium sulfate, fragments of bone, and loose metal beads and wires. It is appropriate to be concerned about three body wear induced by HA particles, but evidence to date suggests that this is not a significant clinical problem. To assess this question more directly, we previously used laser profilometry to compare the extent of surface abrasion on modular heads obtained from implants coated with HA with those from cemented and uncemented implants without HA (64). The results showed surface roughness greater than manufacturer specifications in all groups of modular heads, but the cobalt-chrome alloy heads from the HA-coated group showed significantly less surface roughness and less deep scratches than the heads from either the porous or uncemented group. While three body wear appears to be a significant problem in total hip arthroplasty, it appears to be no more of a problem with HA-coated devices than with porous or cemented implants (64).

Optimum Substrate Texture

A wide variety of implant surfaces are utilized for bone ingrowth fixation of prosthetic devices (fig. 6). In spite of several decades of research, the optimum surface texture for total joint replacement is unclear. We recently used a canine model to test the *in vivo* response to three different surface modifications: Arc-deposited CP titanium, Arc-

deposited CP titanium post-treated with an apatitic blast, and Arc-deposited CP-titanium with a 50 µm thick plasma sprayed coating of highly crystalline hydroxyapatite (65). The Arc-deposited CP-titanium with hydroxyapatite group resulted in significantly more bone apposition at both 12 weeks (41.5%) and 24 weeks (65.5%) when compared to Arc-deposited CP titanium group (15.5%) and Arc-deposited CP titanium post-treated with an apatitic blast group (31.5%). The Arc-deposited implants in this study yielded adequate unsatisfactory mechanical stability and relatively prominent fibrous membranes. We speculate that small metal asperities on the un-blasted Arc-deposited surface interfered with bone apposition resulting in implants nearly surrounded by fibrous tissue. Bone apposition was improved by removing the asperities using an apatitic blasting step, producing a surface texture that was macroscopically rough, but microscopically relatively smooth. The efficacy of HA was further demonstrated by even greater bone apposition to the apatitic blasted ARC-deposited titanium surface coated with hydroxyapatite (65).

Many surgeons are attracted to the concept of HA coatings applied to porous surfaces, but there have been technical problems with applying hydroxyapatite to porous coatings using plasma spraying. Nevertheless, some experimental studies have shown good bone ingrowth into beads or fiber metal surfaces coated with various calcium phosphate preparations (15, 66, 67), and recent electrochemical deposition methods have allowed hydroxyapatite coatings to be precipitated onto surfaces with three-dimensional porosity (48). From a practical standpoint, it will be difficult for any new implant design to improve upon the clinical results currently available for HA coatings applied to carefully designed grit-blasted titanium femoral components, but hydroxyapatite coated, three-dimensionally porous surfaces might be desirable for implants subjected to tensile loads, such as portions of the acetabulum.

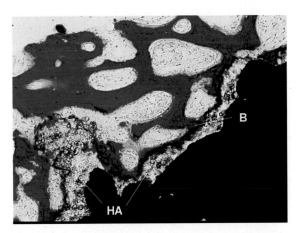

Figure 6 – Bone apposition to an HA-Coated SecurFit® acetabular component removed for dislocations 4 weeks after insertion. After only 4 weeks there is extensive bone apposition to this HA-coated, textured metal surface.

Reference List

1. Al Hertani W, Waddell JP, Anderson GI (2000) The effect of partial *versus* full hydroxyapatite coating on periprosthetic bone quality around the canine madreporic femoral stem. *J. Biomed. Mater. Res.* 53: 518-24.

2. Cook SD, Thomas KA, Kay JF, Jarcho M (1988) Hydroxyapatite-coated titanium for orthopedic implant applications. *Clin. Orthop.* 232: 225-43.

3. Daculsi G, LeGeros RZ, Nery E, Lynch K, Kerebel B (1989) Transformation of biphasic calcium phosphate ceramics *in vivo*: ultrastructural and physicochemical characterization. *J. Biomed. Mater. Res.* 23:883-94.

4. Ducheyne P, Hench LL, Kagan A, 2nd, Martens M, Bursens A, Mulier JC (1980) Effect of hydroxyapatite impregnation on skeletal bonding of porous coated implants. *J. Biomed. Mater. Res.* 14:225-37.

5. Geesink RG, de Groot K, Klein CP (1987) Chemical implant fixation using hydroxyl-apatite coatings. The development of a human total hip prosthesis for chemical fixation to bone using hydroxyl-apatite coatings on titanium substrates. *Clin. Orthop.* 225:147-70.

6. Geesink RG, de Groot K, Klein CP (1988) Bonding of bone to apatite-coated implants. *J. Bone Joint Surg. Br.* 70:17-22.

7. Karabatsos B, Myerthall SL, Fornasier VL, Binnington A, Maistrelli GL (2001) Osseointegration of hydroxyapatite porous-coated femoral implants in a canine model. *Clin. Orthop.* 392:442-9.

8. Moroni A, Caja VL, Egger EL, Trinchese L, Chao EY (1994) Histomorphometry of hydroxyapatite coated and uncoated porous titanium bone implants. *Biomaterials* 15:926-30.

9. Overgaard S, Bromose U, Lind M, Bunger C, Soballe K (1999) The influence of crystallinity of the hydroxyapatite coating on the fixation of implants. Mechanical and histomorphometric results. *J. Bone Joint Surg. Br.* 81:725-31.

10. Overgaard S, Lind M, Glerup H, Grundvig S, Bunger C, Soballe K (1997) Hydroxyapatite and fluorapatite coatings for fixation of weight loaded implants. *Clin. Orthop.* 336:286-96.

11. Overgaard S, Soballe K, Josephsen K, Hansen ES, Bunger C (1996) Role of different loading conditions on resorption of hydroxyapatite coating evaluated by histomorphometric and stereological methods. *J. Orthop. Res.* 14:888-94.

12. Rahbek O, Overgaard S, Lind M, Bendix K, Bunger C, Soballe K (2001) Sealing effect of hydroxyapatite coating on peri-implant migration of particles. An experimental study in dogs. *J. Bone Joint Surg. Br.* 83:441-7.

13. Schreurs BW, Huiskes R, Buma P, Slooff TJ (1996) Biomechanical and histological evaluation of a hydroxyapatite-coated titanium femoral stem fixed with an intramedullary morsellized bone grafting technique: an animal experiment on goats. *Biomaterials* 17:1177-86.

14. Soballe K (1993) Hydroxyapatite ceramic coating for bone implant fixation. Mechanical and histological studies in dogs. *Acta Orthop. Scand.* Suppl 255:1-58.

15. Tisdel CL, Goldberg VM, Parr JA, Bensusan JS, Staikoff LS, Stevenson S (1994) The influence of a hydroxyapatite and tricalcium-phosphate coating on bone growth into titanium fiber-metal implants. *J. Bone Joint Surg. Am.* 76:159-71.

16. Walenciak MT, Zimmerman MC, Harten RD, Ricci JL, Stamer DT (1996) Biomechanical and histological analysis of an HA coated, arc deposited CPTi canine hip prosthesis. *J. Biomed. Mater. Res.* 31:465-74.

17. Capello WN (1994) Hydroxyapatite in total hip arthroplasty: five-year clinical experience. *Orthopedics* 17:781-92.

18. D'Lima DD, Walker RH, Colwell CW, Jr (1999) Omnifit-HA stem in total hip arthroplasty. A 2- to 5-year followup. *Clin. Orthop.* 363:163-9.

19. Donnelly WJ, Kobayashi A, Freeman MA, Chin TW, Yeo H, West M, Scott G (1997) Radiological and survival comparison of four methods of fixation of a proximal femoral stem. *J. Bone Joint Surg. Br.* 79:351-60.

20. Epinette J-A, Edidin AA (1997) Hydroxyapatite-coated unicompartmetal knee replacement. A report of five to six years' follow-up of the HA unix tibial component. In: Cartier P, Epinette J-A, Deschamps G, Hernigou P, eds. Unicompartmental Knee Arthroplasty. Paris, France: Expansion Sientifique Francaise 243-59.

21. Geesink RG, Hoefnagels NH (1995) Six-year results of hydroxyapatite-coated total hip replacement. *J. Bone Joint Surg. Br.* 77:534-47.

22. Geesink RGT (2002) Osteoconductive coatings for total joint arthroplasty. *Clin. Orthop.* 395:53-65.

23. Karrholm J, Malchau H, Snorrason F, Herberts P (1994) Micromotion of femoral stems in total hip arthroplasty. A randomized study of cemented, hydroxyapatite-coated, and porous-coated stems with roentgen stereophotogrammetric analysis. *J Bone Joint Surg Am* 76:1692-705.

24. Kay RM, Kabo JM, Seeger LL, Eckardt JJ (1994) Hydroxyapatite-coated distal femoral replacements. Preliminary results. *Clin. Orthop.* 302:92-100.

25. McPherson EJ, Dorr LD, Gruen TA, Saberi MT (1995) Hydroxyapatite-coated proximal ingrowth femoral stems. A matched pair control study. *Clin. Orthop.* 315:223-30.

26. Rokkum M, Reigstad A (1999) Total hip replacement with an entirely hydroxyapatite-coated prosthesis: 5 years' follow-up of 94 consecutive hips. *J. Arthroplasty* 14:689-700.

27. Rothman RH, Hozack WJ, Ranawat A, Moriarty L (1996) Hydroxyapatite-coated femoral stems. A matched-pair analysis of coated and uncoated implants. *J. Bone Joint Surg. Am.* 78:319-24.

28. Tanzer M, Kantor S, Rosenthall L, Bobyn JD (2001) Femoral remodeling after porous-coated total hip arthroplasty with and without hydroxyapatite-tricalcium phosphate coating: a prospective randomized trial. *J. Arthroplasty* 16:552-8.

29. Bauer TW, Geesink RC, Zimmerman R, McMahon JT (1991) Hydroxyapatite-coated femoral stems. Histological analysis of components retrieved at autopsy. *J. Bone Joint Surg. Am.* 73:1439-52.

30. Bauer TW, Stulberg BN, Ming J, Geesink RG (1993) Uncemented acetabular components. Histologic analysis of retrieved hydroxyapatite-coated and porous implants. *J. Arthroplasty* 8:167-77.

31. Hardy DC, Frayssinet P, Bonel G, Authom T, Le Naelou SA, Delince PE (1994) Two-year outcome of hydroxyapatite-coated prostheses. Two femoral prostheses retrieved at autopsy. *Acta Orthop. Scand.* 65:253-57.

32. Tonino A, Oosterbos C, Rahmy A, Therin M, Doyle C (2001) Hydroxyapatite-coated acetabular components. Histological and histomorphometric analysis of six cups retrieved at autopsy between three and seven years after successful implantation. *J. Bone Joint Surg. Am.* 83-A:817-25.

33. Tonino AJ, Therin M, Doyle C (1999) Hydroxyapatite-coated femoral stems. Histology and histomorphometry around five components retrieved at post mortem. *J. Bone Joint Surg. Br.* 81:148-54.

34. Bloebaum RD, Merrell M, Gustke K, Simmons M (1991) Retrieval analysis of a hydroxyapatite-coated hip prosthesis. *Clin. Orthop.* 267:97-102.

35. Hayashi K, Uenoyama K, Matsuguchi N, Sugioka Y (1991) Quantitative analysis of *in vivo* tissue responses to titanium-oxide- and hydroxyapatite-coated titanium alloy. *J. Biomed. Mater. Res.* 25:515-23.

36. Cleries L, Fernandez-Pradas JM, Morenza JL (2000) Bone growth on and resorption of calcium phosphate coatings obtained by pulsed laser deposition. *J. Biomed. Mater. Res.* 49:43-52.

37. Cleries L, Fernandez-Pradas JM, Sardin G, Morenza JL (1998) Dissolution behaviour of calcium phosphate coatings obtained by laser ablation. *Biomaterials* 19:1483-7.

38. Hyakuna K, Yamamuro T, Kotoura Y *et al.* (1991) Surface reactions of calcium phosphate ceramics to various solutions. *J. Biomed. Mater. Res.* 25:515.

39. Paschalis EP, Wikiel K, Nancollas GH (1994) Dual constant composition kinetics characterization of apatitic surfaces. *J. Biomed. Mater. Res.* 28:1411-8.

40. Radin SR, Ducheyne P (1993) The effect of calcium phosphate ceramic composition and structure on in vitro behavior. II. Precipitation. *J. Biomed. Mater. Res.* 27:35-45.

41. Gorbunoff MJ, Timasheff SN (1984) The interaction of proteins with hydroxyapatite. III. Mechanism. *Anal. Biochem.* 136:440-5.

42. Kilpadi KL, Chang PL, Bellis SL (2001) Hydroxylapatite binds more serum proteins, purified integrins, and osteoblast precursor cells than titanium or steel. *J. Biomed. Mater. Res.* 57:258-67.

43. Moreno EC, Kresak M, Hay DI (1984) Adsorption of molecules of biological interest onto hydroxyapatite. *Calcif. Tissue Int.* 36:48-59.

44. Moss B, Rosenblum EN (1972) Hydroxylapatite chromatography of protein-sodium dodecyl sulfate complexes. A new method for the separation of polypeptide subunits. *J. Biol. Chem.* 247:5194-8.

45. Ripamonti U, Yeates L, van den Heever B (1993) Initiation of heterotopic osteogenesis in primates after chromatographic adsorption of osteogenin, a bone morphogenetic protein, onto porous hydroxyapatite. *Biochem. Biophys. Res. Commun.* 193:509-17.

46. Bauer TW (1993) The histology of HA-coated implants. In: Geesink RGT, Manley MT, eds. Hydroxyapatite Coatings in Orthopaedic Surgery. NY: Raven Press Ltd., 305.

47. Dhert WJ, Klein CP, Jansen JA, van der Velde EA, Vriesde RC, Rozing PM, de Groot K (1993) A histological and histomorphometrical investigation of fluorapatite, magnesiumwhitlockite, and hydroxylapatite plasma-sprayed coatings in goats. *J. Biomed. Mater. Res.* 27:127-38.

48. Ducheyne P, Radin S, Heughebaert M, Heughebaert JC (1990) Calcium phosphate ceramic coatings on porous titanium: effect of structure and composition on electrophoretic deposition, vacuum sintering and *in vitro* dissolution. *Biomaterials* 11:244-54.

49. Klein CP, Driessen AA, de Groot K, van den Hooff A. (1983) Biodegradation behavior of various calcium phosphate materials in bone tissue. *J. Biomed. Mater. Res.* 17:769-84.

50. Maxian SH, Zawadsky JP, Dunn MG (1993) *In vitro* evaluation of amorphous calcium phosphate and poorly crystallized hydroxyapatite coatings on titanium implants. *J. Biomed. Mater. Res.* 27:111-7.

51. Soballe K, Toksvig-Larsen S, Gelineck J, Fruensgaard S, Hansen ES, Ryd L, Lucht U, Bunger C (1993) Migration of hydroxyapatite coated femoral prostheses. A Roentgen Stereophotogrammetric study. *J. Bone Joint Surg. Br.* 75:681-7.

52. van Blitterswijk CA, Bovell YP, Flach JS *et al.* (1993) Variation in hydroxyapatite crystallinity:Effects on interface reactions. In: Geesink RGT, Manley MT, eds. Hydroxyapatite Coatings in Orhtopaedic Surgery. NY: Raven Press Ltd, 33-47.

53. van Blitterswijk CA, van den Brink J, Bovell YP *et al.* (1994) *In vitro* assessment of bone/HA interactions: Effect of crystallinity. *Proc. Soc. Biomat.* 17:432.

54. Mochida Y, Bauer TW, Akisue T, Brown PR (2002) Alendronate does not inhibit early bone apposition to hydroxyapatite-coated total joint implants. A preliminary study. *J. Bone Joint Surg. Am.* 84:226-35.

55. Overgaard S, Lind M, Josephsen K, Maunsbach AB, Bunger C, Soballe K (1998) Resorption of hydroxyapatite and fluorapatite ceramic coatings on weight-bearing implants: a quantitative and morphological study in dogs. *J. Biomed. Mater. Res.* 39:141-52.

56. Doi Y, Iwanaga H, Shibutani T, Moriwaki Y, Iwayama Y. (1999) Osteoclastic responses to various calcium phosphates in cell cultures. *J. Biomed. Mater. Res.* 47:424-33.

57. Yamada S, Heymann D, Bouler JM, Daculsi G (1997) Osteoclastic resorption of calcium phosphate ceramics with different hydroxyapatite/beta-tricalcium phosphate ratios. *Biomaterials* 18:1037-41.

58. Bauer TW (2001) Commentary and perspective. *J. Bone Joint Surg.* JBJS.ORG; June.

59. Fallon MD (1984) Alterations in the pH of osteoclast resorbing fluid reflects changes in bone degradative activity. *Calcif. Tissue Int.* 36:458.

60. Geisow MJ (1984) Fluorescein conjugates as indicators of subcellular pH. A critical evaluation. *Exp. Cell Res.* 150:29-35.

61. Heilmann P, Beisker W, Miaskowski U, Camner P, Kreyling WG (1992) Intraphagolysosomal pH in canine and rat alveolar macrophages: flow cytometric measurements. *Environ. Health Perspect.* 97:115-20.

62. Nyberg K, Johansson U, Johansson A, Camner P (1991) Phagolysosomal pH and location of particles in alveolar macrophages. *Fundam. Appl. Toxicol.* 16:393-400.

63. Ohkuma S, Poole B (1978) Fluorescence probe measurement of the intralysosomal pH in living cells and the perturbation of pH by various agents. *Proc. Natl. Acad. Sci. USA,* 75:3327-31.

64. Bauer TW, Taylor SK, Jiang M, Medendorp SV (1994) An indirect comparison of third-body wear in retrieved hydroxyapatite-coated, porous, and cemented femoral components. *Clin. Orthop.* 298:11-8.

65. Togawa D, Bauer TW, Mochida Y *et al. (*2001) Bone Apposition to three femoral stem surfaces in canine total hip arthroplasty. *Trans. Soc. Biomat.* 24:251.

66. Burr DB, Mori S, Boyd RD, Sun TC, Blaha JD, Lane L, Parr J (1993) Histomorphometric assessment of the mechanisms for rapid ingrowth of bone to HA/TCP coated implants. *J. Biomed. Mater. Res.* 27:645-53.

67. Cook SD, Thomas KA, Dalton JE, Volkman TK, Whitecloud TS, 3rd, Kay JF (1992) Hydroxylapatite coating of porous implants improves bone ingrowth and interface attachment strength. *J. Biomed. Mater. Res.* 26:989-1001.

5   What is the Function and Fate of the HA Coating in Cementless HA-coated Hip Prostheses?

Histology and histomorphometry around eight hip prostheses retrieved at post mortem between 3 and 9 years after successful implantation

Alfons Tonino, MD, PhD, Kees Oosterbos, MD, Ali Rahmy, MD, M. Thèrin, MD

INTRODUCTION

The effective fixation surface of numerous cementless hip components typically consists of either porous-coating (beads or wires), a titanium plasma-sprayed surface, diverse sintered surface textures, or of bioactive ceramic coatings such as hydroxyapatite (HA) or tricalcium phosphate (TCP). In essence, all effective fixation surfaces, including bone-cement, can be considered to be a rough surface ideally suitable for biological fixation. For cementless components, primary fixation is mechanical and dependent on physical interlock between the components and the pelvic or femoral bone. Secondary fixation is biological and is achieved with osseointegration at the implant-bone interface by way of bone ongrowth or ingrowth to the substrate. When hydroxyapatite is used as an intermediary, bone apposition proceeds without formation of a fibrous interface (1-6). However, for long term stability, it is essential that this direct bond between implant and bone is maintained, even after complete hydroxyapatite resorption.

Experiments in dogs and human autopsy retrievals showed that hydroxyapatite coating resorption is accelerated by loading of the implants (7, 8). However, histomorphometry around hydroxyapatite-coated stems has already shown that the percentage of bone ongrowth to the implant was almost constant, regardless of the amount of hydroxyapatite residue (8). Recent outcomes of clinical series seem to acknowledge this long term stability in hydroxyapatite coated implants (9-14). However, where radiographic and clinical findings are unreliable in predicting exact ingrowth or ongrowth of bone, only histology and histomorphometry in human autopsy retrievals after a long period of successful implantation can give the answers about the relationship between hydroxyapatite resorption and persistence of implant osseointegration, or about the morphology and exact location of polyethylene induced osteolysis.

The purpose of this study of eight clinically succesfull hydroxyapatite-coated hip prostheses, retrieved at post mortem between 3 and 9 years after insertion, was to document the extent and pattern of bone apposition in relation to the hydroxyapatite coating and implantation time. At the same time, the tissue reactions on detected particles (titanium, polyethylene, and hydroxyapatite) were studied. Four hypotheses were tested.

The first hypothesis was that when hydroxyapatite-resorption is determined by the rate of bone remodeling, it must be assumed that hydroxapatite residue is less in the acetabulum than in the femur because of the higher bone turn over in the acetabulum (15). If the HA residue is indeed mainly determined by the rate of bone remodeling, then in older patients it will be resorbed faster because of their higher level of negative bone remodeling.

The second hypothesis was that the percentage of bone-implant contact is independent of the amount of hydroxyapatite residue. This hypothesis is based on the idea that the amount of long term bone apposition or osseointegration is mainly dependent on component characteristics and local bone density rather than on a resorbable coating.

The third hypothesis was that the empty screw holes in the metal cup not only promote ingress of polyethylene particles, but also are a risk factor in the so-called fluid pressure theory (16, 17, 18). The fourth hypothesis was that, as in clinical series (9-14), no linear or distal osteolysis around the stem is noted on the serial radiographs. Therefore, it must be assumed that the proximal femoral canal must be circumferential sealed by bone ongrowth, which inhibits ingress of polyethylene particles into the implant-bone interface.

PATIENTS AND METHODS

Eight primary total hip arthroplasties were performed at the same institution. The femoral stems (ABG; Stryker, Newbury, UK) were made of titanium alloy (Ti6A14V) with the proximal third coated with HA on a macro-relief surface (fig. 1). The metal cup was made of the same alloy and totally coated with HA (fig. 1). The diameter of the cobalt-chrome (CoCr) head was 28mm in all cases. To improve adhesion, the HA coating was applied by a plasma spray torch under a vacuum onto a sublayer of titanium. The coating had a HA content of more than 90% with a porosity of less than 10% and a Ca:P ratio of 10:6. The crystallinity was 100% before coating and more than 75% after. The grain size was 20 to 50mm, and the strength of the tensile bond was 62 to 65 Mpa. The thickness of the hydroxyapatite layer was 60 ± 30mm. The roughness of the cup was RA = 9 ± 2,5mm after sandblasting, RA ± 8,5 ± 2,5mm after titanium spraying, and finally, RA 5 ± 1mm after hydroxyapatite coating. All patients had uneventful THA procedures and died from causes unrelated to hip diseases. Cup sizes ranged from 46 to 58. Two spikes (but no screws) were used for initial rotational stability (fig.1).

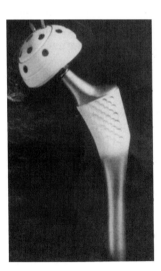

Figure 1 – The hydroxyapatite ABG hip system.

Specimen Preparation

All eight patients had given written consent for prosthetic retrieval at autopsy. The prostheses and surrounding bone were collected at post mortem,

immersed in buffered formalin for seven days, then in 70% ethanol for 24 hours. Photographs and radiographs of the samples were taken. Three gross segments (1.0cm thick), were cut corresponding to DeLee and Charnley (19) zones for the acetabular cup (fig. 2), and three gross sections were cut for the femur corresponding to the Gruen zones, with the proximal Gruen zones 1-7 subdivided into another three sections (fig. 3). Each segment was

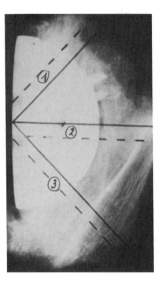

Figure 2 – The retrieved acetabulum and cup of Case 8. Three segments were cut, corresponding to the three zones delineated by DeLee and Charnley. Five sections were cut from each segment for qualitative histological and quantitative histomorphometric analysis.

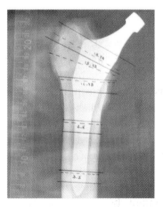

Figure 3 – The retrieved femur and stem of Case 7. Segments were cut, corresponding to the zones delineated by Gruen. The metaphyseal zone 1-7 was subdivided into another three segments. Five sections were cut from each segment for qualitative histological and quantitative histomorphometric analysis.

embedded en bloc in a PMMA resin, and five 20 µm sections were cut from each segment using the technique of Donath and Bienner (20). The sections were stained for qualitative histology (paragon staining, a combination of basic fuschin and toluidine blue) and quantitative histomorphometry. A biopsy of the joint pseudocapsule was taken, embedded in paraffin and prepared for light microscopy using Masson trichrome staining.

Specimen Analysis

We used a Polyvar microscope (Reichert-Jung, Vienna, Austria) for qualitative analysis and an Axioskop microscope (Carl Zeist, Munnich, Germany) equipped with a colour image analysing system (SAMBA ; Technology, Grenoble, France) for quantitative analysis. The quantitative morphometric evaluation of the surrounding bone tissue (bone-implant contact and bone density) was performed on four areas for each cup section (fig. 4)

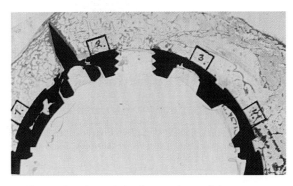

Figure 4 – One of the five sections of the cup, corresponding to zone II of DeLee and Charnley of Case 4. The histomorphometric analysis was performed on four areas for each section. Areas 1 through 4 are shown. The central hole to the right of area 2 is covered by a thin bridge of bone that may have inhibited the ingress of polyethylene particles.

and 7 areas for each metaphyseal femoral section (fig. 5). The surfaces of these areas varied from 10 to 12mm (2). They were scanned, reduced and stored before reconstruction of the image. Sixteen microscopic fields (4x4 fields) were necessary to scan the whole surface of each area. Each pixel of the reduced image represented 61 µm (2) of the section. Implant, bone, and lacunae, including all soft tissues, were successively identified, and their respective surfaces and contacts with the implant were measured. For each of the acetabular and femoral areas the total implant perimeter, the percentage of implant covered by bone, the relative

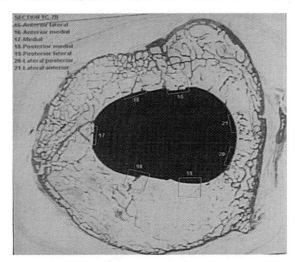

Figure 5 – Qualitative and quantitative evaluation of the surrounding bone tissue was performed on seven areas for each metaphyseal section. This is section 1C-7B of Case 3.

bone density in the vicinity of the implant, the total percentage of residual coating, and the coating thickness were measured. Bone implant contact was defined as direct ongrowth of bone to the hydroxyapatite coating or to the titanium surface without hydroxyapatite and is synonymous with the amount of osseointegration. Bone density was defined as the percentage of the surface of the measured field covered by bone. The means and standard deviations were calculated for each section. We performed statistical analysis using the Spearman test (correlations for rank data) and the Mann-Whitney Rank Sum tests and Paired t-test. P-values less than 0.01 were considered significant. The pathologist (MT) was blinded regarding the clinical results of the investigated components. The histomorphometric parameters for the femoral component of cases 1, 2, 3, 4 and 6 were previously reported (8) as were the histomorphometric parameters for the acetabular component of cases 1, 2, 3, 4, 6, and 7 (21).

RESULTS

The patient details and the results are shown in Table 1. With the exception of Case 5, where the pelvis fractured at retrieval and for which the cup is not included in the study, all cups and stems were stable fixed in the acetabulum and femur at post-mortem and surrounded by a thick white-yellow coloured pseudocapsule.

Table 1 – Details of and Findings in the 8 Cases.

	1	2	3	4	5	6	7	8
Gender	F	M	F	M	M	F	F	F
Age at THA in years	63	65	81	58	72	66	86	73
Diagnosis	OA	OA	OA	OA	OA	OA	OA	RA
Time from implantation (yr)	3.3	5.2	5.4	5.7	6.1	6.2	6.6	8..3
Weight (kg)	85	65	52	50	65	75	65	50
Heigth (m)	1.39	1.69	1.60	1.52	1.66	1.63	1.60	1.55
Merle d'Aubigné score	18	18	18	15	18	18	18	18
Harris score	100	100	97	90	100	100	95	100
Cause of death	Cardiac arrest –	Cerebral haemorrhage	Cardiac arrest –	Cardiac arrest –	Cerebal haemorrhage	Aortic-aneurysm	Pancreatitis	Lung carcinoma
Previous surgery	–	Femoral osteotomy	–	–	Contra lateral THA	–	–	–
Clinical comments	Not active	Active	Active	Not active Down's syndrome	Active	Active	Active	Active
Alignment cup	45°	49°	45°	55°	55°	45°	45°	45°
Alignment stem	Neutral	Neutral	4° valgus	Neutral	4° varus	2° varus	Neutral	Neutral
Distal Femoral fill	Complete	Un complete	Uncomplete	Complete	Uncomplete	Uncomplete	Uncomplete	Complete

Bone-ongrowth (%) and extent of residual HA coating (%) on retrieved cups

DeLee/Charnley zones								
I	47^{28}	36^{19}	9^{3}	60^{12}	–	41^{7}	40^{0}	$38^{1..5}$
II	25^{24}	32^{17}	23^{5}	50^{12}	–	35^{1}	39^{0}	29^{0}
III	59^{26}	38^{24}	27^{3}	38^{14}	–	40^{0}	14^{0}	27^{0}
Mean	44^{26}	35^{20}	21^{4}	49^{13}	–	39^{3}	31^{0}	$31^{0.5}$

Bone-ongrowth (%) and extent of residual HA coating (%) on retrieved stems

Gruen zones								
1A-7A	51^{15}	48^{12}	25	61^{50}	37^{11}	36^{5}	33^{3}	6^{0}
1B-7B	40^{68}	54^{20}	25	45^{68}	35^{18}	52^{7}	12^{2}	40^{10}
1C-7B	39^{83}	67^{31}	42	48^{77}	37^{14}	49^{11}	21^{8}	$36^{5.6}$
Mean	44^{56}	56^{21}	31^{5}	51^{65}	37^{14}	46^{8}	22^{3}	28^{5}

	1	2	3	4	5	6	7	8
Bone femur	44	56	31	51	37	46	22	28
implant acet. contact	44	35	21	49	–	39	31	31
Extent of femur	56	21	5	65	14	8	3	5
residual acet.	26	20	4	13	-	3	0	0,5
				HA coating				

Radiography

All seven cups showed radiographic osseointegration from the beginning. The alignment of the cups was between 45° and 55° without any migration or change of position during follow-up. Radiolucent lines, osteolytic reactions, or other bone reactions were never detected during follow-up. However, the postmortem radiograph of the acetabulum and cup of Case 3 showed some bone osteolysis at the rim of the cup, especially in DeLee and Charnley zone I. This case has already been reported (8). Radiography showed the stem filling the diaphysis completely in cases 1, 4, and 8 where a modest diaphyseal thickening was noted at the two year follow-up, with formation of a reactive line at the tip of the stem. This line vanished between the third and fourth year of follow-up, when the distal part of the stem also became osseointegrated (bonded). When the stem did not fill the medullary canal, as in cases 2, 3, 5, 6 and 7, at six months a reactive line had already developed around the distal part of the stem extending a little upwards into Gruen zones 3 and 5. In these cases endosteal bone apposition was marked at Gruen zone 2 and 6 extending later into Gruen zone 3 and 5 as a sign of distal stem osseointegration. No subsidence or migration of any stem was observed. All patients showed slow but progressive bone resorption in Gruen zones 1 and 7 with rounding of the calcar. In Case 3 a small cyst near the calcar was noted at the 5 year follow-up. All 8 stems showed radiographic stem osseointegration proximally at first, and distally as time progressed.

Histology

The pseudocapsule was mostly composed of a thick and dense fibrous tissue, focally infiltrated by an inflammatory component, and covered by a pluri stratified synovial-like layer. In Case 2, numerous metallic debris could be detected both close to the surface and more deeply within the membrane (8), which showed a white-yellow colour. Polyethylene particles with an obvious inflammatory component were detected in Cases 2 and 7, but in very modest numbers, while in Case 3, an abundant polyethylene particle-induced inflammatory reaction was noted (21). Hydroxyapatite debris was never seen in the pseudocapsule.

In the acetabular sections, all implants were surrounded by numerous bridges of lamellar trabecular bone perpendicular to the implant (fig. 4) rather than thin trabeculae spread on the surface. The hydroxyapatite coating appeared thin, irregular, and almost completely resorbed in areas where bone marrow reached the interface (fig. 6). Even after almost complete hydroxyapatite resorption (Cases 6, 7 and 8), bone tissue could be observed directly on the surface of the metal subtrate along with bone marrow cells without any interposition of connective tissue (fig. 7). The overall osseointegration was highly significant for all cases. The bone implant contact percentages were highest at the rim of the cups and on the top of the spikes.

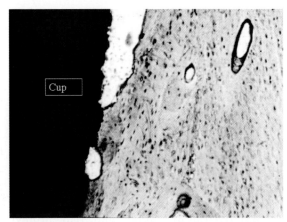

Figure 6 – Case 2. Detail of cup section DeLee-Charnley zone II. The HA coating is thin, irregular and almost completely resorbed in areas where bone marrow reached the interface (8X).

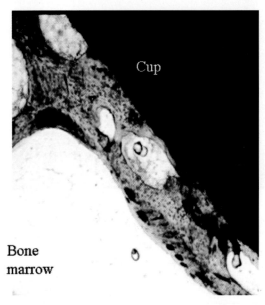

Figure 7 – Case 8. Detail of cup section DeLee-Charnley zone I. Only 1% of the HA coating is left on the surface of the cup, but 38% of the surface is covered by bone ongrowth (8X).

In the femoral sections, the same histological picture was seen. Seven implants showed microscopic evidence of strong metaphyseal osseointegration, i.e., an extensive direct bond between the HA (or the prosthesis) and the bone without any fibrous or inflammatory interface (fig. 8). The surrounding bone tissue at the metaphyseal part of all stems was mature trabecular bone with low remodeling activity. The bone trabeculae were regularly observed spreading directly on the implant surface (fig. 9). The surrounding marrow was histologically normal in all sections (fig. 7, 8, and 9). Only in Case 3 had a progressive histological loosening due to PE particle-related osteolysis begun, starting form the proximal metaphyseal Gruen section 1A-7A down to Gruen zone 1B-7A (8). This debonding process had not yet reached the Gruen zones 1C-7B (fig. 5).

In the upper diaphyseal sections of Gruen zones 2 and 6, the dominant histological appearance in all cases was that of bone apposition, endosteal bone apposition in cases where the stem did not fill the diaphysis, and also modest periosteal bone appositions when there was full diaphyseal fill from the beginning. No intermediate

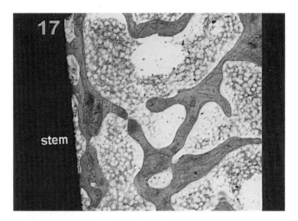

Figure 8 – Case 6. Femoral section 1C-7B. Still 11% of the Ha coating is present and 47% of bone ongrowth. No fibrous interface and normal bone marrow (8X).

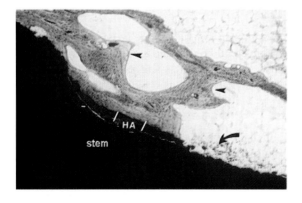

Figure 9 – Case 4. Femoral section 1A-7A. There is nearly complete resorption of the HA coating where it is in contact with the bone marrow (arrow). Also some low remodeling activity is observed (arrowheads). There is no fibrous interface (28X).

fibrous layer formation was noted in any patient. As in the metaphysis, all stems were also bonded in this area.

In the lower diaphyseal sections of Gruen zones 3 and 5, all cases showed signs of recent remodeling and new bone apposition resulting from osseointegration of the distal part of the stem. No PE debris was ever detected in the Gruen zones 3 and 5. Instead, direct bone contact with microscopic osseointegration of the distal part of the stem was observed in all cases.

Particles

Three types of particles were observed: metal, hydroxyapatite, and polyethylene. On the acetabular side, metal particles were rarely seen. This observation contrasted with nearly all metaphyseal sections, where metallic particles were most frequently observed in combination with some HA granules in areas where there was HA coating resorption. However, there was hardly any foreign body reaction or inflammatory response, except for Case 3, at the two upper metaphyseal levels, where metallic particles were also noted at the interface of section level 2-6. Also, in Case 6, some lacunae with conglomerates of metallic particles were noted at Gruen zone 3-5.

Hydroxyapatite granules were sporadically observed in the bone marrow, but only close to the coated surface and without any inflammatory or adverse reaction. Where bone ongrowth onto the coating occurred, no loose hydroxyapatite particles were noted. No signs of hydroxyapatite coating dissolution, abrasion, or delamination could be detected in any section. When HA debris was present, it was seen adjacent to the metaphyseal part of the stem only and was never found distal to the level of the coating. No significant inflammatory response was ever seen near the HA granules, but occasionally osteoclasts or macrophages were seen phagocytosing the HA granules, indicating the excellent biocompatibility of the HA coating. At autopsy in cases 6, 7, and 8, hardly any HA debris could be detected with microscopy in the areas where most of the HA coating was gone. No HA debris was observed on the acetabular side in any case.

Most screw holes exhibited numerous shiny polyethylene particles under polarised light. However, in half of the holes a dense, collagenous membrane or a bony bridge (fig. 4) filled the screw holes and seemed to contain the particles. However, in the other half, the particles were associated with more or less pronounced bone resorption activity and the beginning of debonding around that particular hole; they occasionally appeared to indicate the beginning of cystic osteolysis (21).

In Case 3, polyethylene particles with associated inflammatory tissue reaction were present in profusion, especially in the area of DeLee and Charnley I, where osteolysis with diminished bone implant contact was most prominent. But other other sections of Case 3 also showed some debonding at the rim of the cup or originating at some empty screw-holes (21).

On the stem side, PE particles with an associated inflammatory tissue reaction were only present in Case 3 at the two proximal metaphyseal levels. Further down at Gruen levels 1B-7C, 2-6 and 3-5, no evidence of PE induced osteolysis was observed, but normal percentages (Table 1) of bone ongrowth were prominent. None of the other cases showed PE particles except for Case 6, where a small focus of PE particles was noted at section 1B-7C only, without an inflammatory tissue reaction around it.

Histomorphometry

The average percentage of bone-implant contact for the retrieved cups was 35.9 ± 13.3%. No significant difference was noted between the bone implant contact ratios for the three DeLee and Charnley sections (Table 2). The predominant areas of bone implant contact were near the rim of the acetabular cup and also around the spikes (fig. 4 and 7). With the limited numbers available, the mean bone implant contact percentages of the acetabular bone and metaphyseal bone of the femur in the same patient did not differ significantly, but was always higher for the femur, except for Cases 7 and 8 (Table 1). Nevertheless, in the three oldest patients (Cases 3, 6 and 7) the bone density

was lowest, as was to be expected, and the bone implant contact percentage was lowest.

On the femoral side, evidence of bone contact was seen on almost all sides, but was particularly marked on the anterior side. In the metaphyseal region for each section, direct bone-implant contact correlated highly with the presence of the coating. In this region, the bone density measured in the immediate vicinity of the implant was always larger at the anterior and medial sides compared to the posterior and lateral sides. The overall bone-implant contact in the metaphysis was between 22 to 56% of the total surface. The bone contact and bone density increased along the stem toward the distal region.

Hydroxyapatite Coating

No significant differences were noted between the hydroxyapatite parameters for the three DeLee and Charnley zones (Table 2). The two cups with the longest time of implantation hardly showed any hydroxyapatite residue. With the exception of cases 1 and 4 (not active patients), the percentage of hydroxyapatite residue for the cup and the stem in each patient were of the same order. On the whole, the extent of the hydroxyapatite coating of the cup was always lower than on the metaphyseal part of the femur, indicating a higher rate of bone remodeling on the acetabular side.

The appearance of the coating was non-uniform. In the first four cases, it was thick and regular in areas covered by bone (fig. 6), and thin, irregular, or partly or fully absorbed in those areas, which were covered by bone marrow. However, in the last three patients, such features didn't exist. Additionally, with these cups, in the areas of normal bone-implant contact, virtually no hydroxyapatite residue could be detected (fig. 7). Nevertheless, in these three patients, the percentage of bone ongrowth was between 31% and 39% of the measured surfaces (Table 1).

Table 2 – Means and Standard Deviations of the Measured Bone and Hydroxyapatite Parameters.

	DeLee and Charnley Zones		
	I	II	III
Bone implant contact (%)	38.8 ± 16.8	34.0 ± 9.9	36.0 ± 14.9 ns
Bone area (%) (standard for bone density)	19.8 ± 7.6	14.0 ± 2.5	19.3 ± 7.3 ns
Extent of HA residue (%)	11.5 ± 10.5	9.8 ± 9.5	11.1 ± 11.9 ns
Thickness of HA residue (mm)	22.3 ± 12.6	22.3 ± 13.7	20.6 ± 12.9 ns

Correlations

Because of partial polyethylene-induced debonding of the cup in Case 3, this case was excluded for calculation of correlations. The measured bone and coating parameters were matched according to age at death and length of implantation time. The numbers were too small for valid statistical analysis, but a possible relationship between the bone apposition percentages and bone area according to age was noted. A slow but progressive resorption of the hydroxyapatite coating in relation to time of implantation was obvious.

DISCUSSION

This study is the first to show long term histology and histomorphometry in hydroxyapatite coated acetabular cups and stems in the human, coming from one centre, operated by one surgeon and reviewed by one pathologist.

Role of Osseointegration

Six of these seven clinically successful acetabular autopsy specimens showed complete lack of fibrous membranes, suggesting that each of these implants was mechanically stable. However, in Case 3, where a polyethylene-laden granulomatous tissue reaction had caused partial debonding, the cup was still mechanically stable. Bone ongrowth was consistent in contrast with the results of retrieved porous coated acetabular components, where sometimes there is no bone ingrowth into the porous coating at all (22-25). The mean amount of bone implant contact for the cup was 35.9% ±13.3%, which is somewhat higher than was shown by Pidhorz *et al.* (24) who reported a mean extent of bone of 29.7% at the interface of eleven porous coated acetabular cups retrieved at autopsy after an average of 41 months of implantation. But the extent of bone at the outer layer of a porous coating is not synonymous with ingrowth of bone into the porous coating, which is believed to be mainly responsible for the fixation of the component. Pidhorz *et al.* (24) reports 12.1 ± 8.2% of ingrowth of bone into the porous coating of the retrieved acetabular cups, while Bloebaum *et al.* (26) reports 12 ± 6%.

Even in the three specimens (Cases 6, 7, and 8) where the hydroxyapatite coating had nearly or completely disappeared, the percentage of bone ongrowth to the substrate was still between 31%-39% for the cup. This is in accordance with Overgaard *et al.* (27) who, in a canine cortical bone model using weight loaded hydroxyapatite coated implants, found that completely resorbed hydroxyapatite coating was replaced by 36% ± 6.0% of bone in direct contact with the implant. But in a non weight bearing trabecular bone canine model, Overgaard *et al.* (28) observed that only one fifth of the surface with complete resorption of the hydroxyapatite coating was replaced by newly formed bone. The mean amount of bone ongrowth in the proximal femur of our cases ranged between a somewhat broader scale (22% and 56%), which is in line with 20%-67% of bone ongrowth reported by Carlsson *et al.* (29) for hydroxyapatite coated and grit-blasted titanium implants with an average roughness of Ra = 3.1 μm inserted for three months proximally in human arthritic tibiae. But these authors also reported that smooth titanium implants with an average roughness of Ra = 0.9 μm, inserted at the same spot for the same time, were only fibrous encapsulated. So not only loading, but also the roughness of the hydroxyapatite coating itself and of the substrate texture has a profound impact on amount of bone ongrowth. Further animal experiments showed that also tightness of surgical fit, implantation site, bone type, and time of implantation can play a role in the quality and percentage of bone ongrowth (30, 31). But in our cases, only time of implantation and personel characteristics like age, body weight, level of actvity and amount of bone stock differed. All eight cases showed good medium-term fixation by osseointegration as well as for the stem and the acetabular cup. The almost complete loss of HA, as seen in Cases 6, 7, and 8, did not seem to jeopardize long term fixation or osseointegration. Nevertheless, the amount of bone implant contact of cases 7 and 8 was substantially lower for the cup as well as the stem, but no significant correlation between the amount of osseointegration and the density of the periprosthetic bone could yet be established, as was also seen in the experiments of Eckhoff, Turner and Aberman (32). Their study in sheep showed that generalised age-related involution of bone did not effect the quality or quantity of the osseointegration of the implant of the distal femur. This finding supports our earlier radiological observations in rheumatoid patients (33) that the amount of periprosthetic bone is not a decisive factor in determining the quality of bone-implant osseointegration. Nevertheless, the nearly complete loss of HA in Cases 6, 7, and 8 does point to the importance of the surface texture of the metal, especially in the light of long-term fixation.

It should be noted that, where implant fixation is securely provided by the metal surface when hydroxyapatite coating is completely resorbed, it is clear from our cases that a minimum of 20% of bone implant ongrowth for this cup is still sufficient to maintain reliable implant fixation.

Mechanism of Loss of HA Coating

The analysis of the specimens of the first five cases confirmed our previous findings (8) and those of Overgaard *et al.* (34) that less resorption of the coating was seen when bone was present at the coating surface. In contrast, when bone marrow was present at the interface, nearly all hydroxyapatite was resorbed. However, in the specimens of the last three cases where the implant functioned somewhat longer, no such phenomenon was observed. Also, in areas with full bone-implant contact, the HA coating had vanished. For this phenomenon, two theories are suggested (4, 34); (a) direct disintegration of the hydroxyapatite into the extra cellular fluid (a non cell mediated process), and (b) a cell mediated hydroxyapatite resorption (a process in which hydroxyapatite is disintegrated by osteolastic enzymes into smaller granules, which are then phagocytised and broken down by diverse kinds of cells (27). We think there are more convincing arguments for the theory of cell mediated hydroxyapatite resorption triggered by bone remodelling. First, we know that older patients have augumented negative bone remodelling (bone resorption), and indeed Cases 7 and 8 showed the lowest hydroxyapatite residue. Another argument is the observation that in each patient the hydroxyapatite coating residue was always less at the acetabular side where it is known that bone turnover is higher than in the femur irrespective of loading (15). But the most persuasive argument was the histological observation itself of factual degradation of the hydroxyapatite layer by osteoclasts.

The fate of the hydroxyapatite coating in the medium and long-term, especially in relation to long-term implant fixation, continues to be of great interest for surgeons and manufactures alike. This is the more so since animal studies have always been concerned with short and medium periods of implantation. In a human experimental study in trabecular bone, Overgaard *et al.* (34) estimated the hydroxyapatite resorption rate at approximately 20% of the coating thickness per year. They suggested that, in the clinical situation with weight bearing, micromotion, and eventual access of joint fluid into the extended joint space, the resorption may be accelerated. To the best of our knowledge of literature regarding autopsy retrievals or animal experiments, only one paper by Tonino *et al.* (8), regarding human autopsy femoral retrievals, has noted that the percentage of implant fixation by bone was independent of the amount of hydroxyapatite residue. This observation could be acknowledged again for the seven acetabular retrievals described here. On the one hand it conforms the view of many authors (1-14, 21, 27-29, 31, 33, 34), that a hydroxyapatite coating offers early, reliable and augmented bone ongrowth with improved fixation. On the other hand, it is our opinion that it is the design and the substrate texture that will mainly determine the longevity of the prosthesis in the end, after all hydroxyapatite is resorbed. The design, because it influences mostly the periprostetic bone remodelling pattern and the surface texture, because it influences so greatly the amount of on- or ingrowth of bone.

In contrast to other studies (35, 36, 37), where hydroxyapatite debris had given inflammatory response or loose hydroxyapatite granules had generated third body wear, this study could hardly show any loose hydroxyapatite granules away from the coating. Only once could direct degradation of the hydroxyapatite layer by osteoclasts and subsequent resorption by macrophages be observed. These observations do emphasize that the quality of the hydroxyapatite coating is of paramount importance, as is the process of applying it to the substrate. The specific up to 300mm thick hydroxyapatite coating used by Morscher *et al.* (37) is noted for two negative aspects. First, the method of hot-pressing hydroxyapatite granules with grain sizes of 125 to 250 µm to the subtrate is not a reliable method for coating stability, and second, it is known from experiments that thicker hydroxyapatite coatings have considerably poorer mechanical properties with increased risk of hydroxyapatite abrasion or delamination (38, 39). Up until now, the procedure of applying a thin hydroxyapatite coating (± 60 µm) by plasma sprayed torch under vacuum gives the most reliable adhension to the substrate with the least chance of delamination.

Osteolysis

While it has been shown that short periods of oscillating fluid pressure directed at an osseointegrated titanium-bone interface may lead to osteolysis (16, 17, 18), it is also obvious that the pressure gradient through a large hole is much less than through a small hole. When we look again to Case 3, where debonding osteolysis was mainly seen in DeLee and Charnley zone 1, this fluid pressure theory therefore may give the explanation for the precise location of the observed osteolysis, not only in our Case 3, but even more clearly in the cases shown by Manley *et al.* (40). Their figures also showed high rates of osteolysis (7%-11%) in zone 1 for the cups with the small holes, regardless of hydroxyapatite coating, while the threaded cup with only one large central hole showed osteolysis (2%) in zone 2 only. As in our series in six of the seven observed cups, no polyehylene-laden bone resorbing membrane was observed at the articular margins of the implant. Therefore, it must be assumed that the polyethylene wear particles found around the empty screw holes could not have migrated from the periphery of the cup but must have been generated directly from the back surface of the liner. Also, Bauer *et al.* (41) in a short term histologic analysis of retrieved hydroxyapatite-coated acetabular cups observed that empty screw holes were not completely covered with bone. With the fluid pressure theory, the potential for spreading polyethylene wear debris through the empty screw holes of the cup into the accetabular bone is obvious, and by that it acknowledges the theory of the extended joint space as formulated by Schmalzried *et al.* (42). Both theories are showing the pathways that allow particles from the back surface of the liner to migrate through the screw holes into the open reamed acetabular bone. At the femoral side, polyethylene-induced osteolysis was noted in Case 3 only and in the two most proximal metaphyseal levels only. The morphology of this osteolysis was cystic and not linear.

In conclusion, it has become clear that a plasma-sprayed hydroxyapatite coating with high crystallinity and a thickness of ± 60 µm enhances fast biological fixation of the implant by way of bone ongrowth while allowing only slow resorption depending on the rate of bone remodelling, which is mainly related to patient characteristics such as activity, age, and length of implantation time. Higher bone turnover in the acetabulum than in the proximal femur could be acknowledged, as hydroxyapatite residue was always less in the acetabulum. An important finding was the absence of foreign body reaction, inflammatory response, and delamination of this specific ceramic coating, which was chemically stable with very reliable bonding strength to the substrate. In spite of total hydroxyapatite coating resorption, the percentage of bone-implant contact remained stable within a certain range that seems sufficient for long term stability. The important role of the texture of the substrate in this respect can not be overemphasized. Screw holes are hazardous, not only for ingress of polyethylene wear debris, but also because they may play a major role in osteolysis caused by oscillating joint fluid pressures. As no signs of any linear osteolysis around the stem were found histologically, it has become very obvious that circumferential bone ongrowth around the stem, especially at the most proximal metaphyseal level, is sealing the interface from ingress of polyethylene particles. This observation is sustained by the high amount of bone implant contact at this particular level.

Note: The authors wish to thank the editorial board of the British and the American Journal of Bone and Joint Surgery for granting permission to use some formerly published data. The histlogy and histomorphometry were done at Biomatech SA, ZI de l'Islon Rue Pasteur, 38670 Chasse sur Rhone, France.

Reference List

1. Geesink RGT, Groot de K and Klein CPAT (1988) Bonding of Bone to apatite-coated implants. *J. Bone Joint Surg.* 70-B:17-22.

2. Soballe K, Hansen ES, B-Rasmussen H, Pedersen CM and Bünger C (1990) Hydroxyapatite coating enhances fixation of porous coated implants. A comparison between press fit and non-interference fit. *Acta Orthop. Scand.* 61(4):299.

3. Hardy DCR, Frayssinet P, Guilhem A, Lafontaine MA and Delince PE (1991) Bonding of hydroxyapatite-coated femoral prosthese. Histopathology of specimens from four cases. *J. Bone Joint Surg.* 73-B:732-40.

4. Bauer TW, Geesink RCT, Zimmerman R and McMahon JT (1991) Hydroxyapatite-coated femoral stems. Histological analysis of components retrieved at autopsy. *J. Bone Joint Surg.* 73-A: 1439-52.

5. Maistrelli, GL, Mahomed, N, Garbuz, D, Fornasier, V, Harrington IJ and Binnington A (1992) Hydroxyapatite coating on carbon composite hip implants in dogs. *J. Bone Joint Surg.* 74-B: 452-6.

6. Bloebaum RD, Bachus KN, Rubman MH and Dorr LD (1993) Postmortem comparative analysis of titanium and hydroxyapatite porous-coated femoral implants retrieved from the same patient. A case study. *J. Arthroplasty*, 8:203-11.

7. Overgaard S, Søballe K, Josephsen K, Hansen ES and Bünger C (1996) Role of different loading conditions on resorption of hydroxyapatite coating evaluated by histomorphometric and stereological methods. *J. Orthop. Res.* 14:888-94.

8. Tonino AJ, Thèrin M and Doyle C (1999) Hydroxy-apatite-coated femoral stems. Histology and histomorphometry around five components retrieved at post mortem. *J. Bone Joint Surg.* 81-B:148-54.

9. Geesink RGT and Hoefnagels NHM (1995) Six-year results of hydroxyapatite-coated total hip replacement. *J. Bone Joint Surg.* 77-B:534-47.

10. Capello WN, D'Antonio JA, Manley MT and Feinberg JR (1998) Hydroxyapatite in total hip arthroplasty. Clinical results and critical issues. *Clin. Orthop.* 355: 200-11.

11. Tonino AJ, Rahmy AIA and The International ABG Study Group (2000) The hydroapatite-ABG hip system. 5-7 Years results from an international multicentre study. *J. Arthroplasty*, 15:274-82.

12. Oosterbos C, Rahmy A, Tonino AJ (2001) Hydroxy-apatite-coated hip prostheses followed up for five years. *Int. Orthop.* 25:17-21.

13. McNally SA, Sheppard JAN, Mann CV, Walczak JP (2000) The results at nine to twelve years of the use of a hydroxyapatite coated femoral stem. *J. Bone Joint Surg.* 82-B 378.

14. D'Antonio JA, Capello WN, Manley MT, Geesink R (2001) Hydroxyapatite femoral stems for total hip arthroplasty. *Clin. Orthop.* 393, 101-1.

15. Dempster DW (1995) Bone remodeling. In: Osteoporosis. Edited by B. Lawrence Riggs and C. Joseph Melton III Philadelphia Lippincot-Raven, 67-91.

16. Vis van der HM, Aspenberg P, Kleine de R, Tigchelaar W. and Noorden van CJF (1998) Short periods of oscillating fluid pressure directed at a titanium-bone interface in rabbits lead to bone lysis. *Acta Scand. Orthop.* 69:5-10.

17. Vis van der HM, Aspenberg P, Marti RK, Tighelaar W and Noorden van CJF (1998) Fluid pressure causes bone resorption in a rabbit model of prosthetic loosening. *Clin. Orhop.* 350:201-8.

18. Aspenberg P and Vis van der H (1998) Migration, particles, and fluid pressure. A discussion of causes of prosthetic loosening. *Clin. Orthop.* 352:75-80.

19. DeLee JG and Charnley J (1976) Radiological demacration of cemented sockets in total hip replacement. *Clin. Orthop.* 121:20-32.

20. Donath K and Bienner G (1982) A method for the study of undecalcified bones and teeth with attached soft tissues: the Sage-Schliff (sawing and grinding) technique. *J. Oral. Pathol.* 11:318-26.

21. Tonino AJ, Oosterbos C, Rahmy A, Therin M, Doyle C (2001) Hydroxyapatite coated acetabular components. *J. Bone Joint Surg.* 83-A; 817-b25.

22. Collier DE, Mayor MB, Chae JC, Suprenant VA, Suprenant HP and Dauphinais LA (1988) Macroscopie and microscopic evidence of prosthetic fixation with porous-coated materials. *Clin. Orthop.* 235:173-80.

23. Summer DR, Jasty M, Jacobs JJ, Urban RM, Bragdon CR, Harris WH and Galante JO (1993) Histology of porous-coated acetabular components. *Acta Orthop. Scand.* 64(6): 619-26.

24. Pidhorz LE, Urban RM, Jacobs JJ, Sumner DR. and Galante JO (1993) A quantative study of bone and soft tissues in cementless porous-coated acetabular components retrieved at autopsy. *J. Arthroplasty*, 8:213-25.

25. Cook SD, Thomas KA, Barrack RL and Whitecloud III TS (1992) Tissue growth into porous-coated acetabular components in 42 patients. Effects of adjunct fixation. *Clin. Orthop.* 283:163-70.

26. Bloebaum RD, Mihalopoulus NL, Jensen JW. and Dorr LD (1997) Postmortem analysis of bone growth into porous-coated acetabular components. *J. Bone Joint Surg.* 79A:1013-22.

27. Overgaard S, Lind M, Josephsen K, Maumbach AB, Bünger C and Søballe K (1998) Resorption of hydroxyapatite and fluorapatite ceramic coatings on weight-loaded implants. *J. Biomed. Mater. Res.* 39:141-52.

28. Overgaard S, Lind M, Rahbek O, Bünger C. and Søballe K (1997) Improved fixation of porous-coated versus grit-blasted surface texture of hydroxyapatite-coated implants in dogs. *Acta Orthop. Scand.* 68: 337-43.

29. Carlsson L, Regnér L, Johansson C, Gottlander M. and Herberts P (1994) Bone response to hydroxyapatite-coated and commercially pure titanium implants in the human arthritic knee. *J. Orthop. Res.* 12: 274-85.

30. Cook SD, Thomas KA, Dalton JE, Volkman TK, Whitecloud III TS and Kay JF (1992) Hydroxyapatite coating of porous implants improves bone ingrowth and interface attachment strength. *J. Biomed. Mater. Res.* 26:989-1001.

31. Dhert WJA, Klein CPAT, Jansen JA, Velde van der EA, Vries de RC, Rozing PM and Groot de KA (1993) Histological and histomorphometrical investigation of fluorapatite, magnesiumwhitlocktite, and hydroxylapatite plasma-sprayed coatings in goats. *J. Biomed. Mater. Res.* 27:127-38.

32. Eckhoff DG, Turner AS (1995) Abermann HM Effect of age on bone formation around orthopaedic implants. *Clin. Orthop.* 312:253-60.

33. Garcia Araujo C, Fernandez Gonzalez J, Tonino AJ (1998) Rheumatoid arthritis and hydroxyapatite coated hip prosthesis. *J. Arthroplasty*, 6:666.

34. Overgaard S, Søballe K, Lind M. and Bünger C (1997) Resorption of hydroxyapatite and fluorapatite coatings in man. An experimental study in trabecular bone. *J. Bone Joint Surg.* 79-B:654-9.

35. Bloebaum R and Dupont J (1993) Osteolysis from a press-fit hydroxyapatite-coated implant. A case study. *J. Arthroplasty*, 8:195-202.

36. Bleobaum R, Beeks D, Dorr LD, Savory CG, DuPont JA and Hofmann AA (1994) Complications with hydroxyapatite particulate separation in total hip arthroplasty. *Clin. Orthop.* 298:19-26.

37. Morscher EW, Hefti A and Aebi U (1998) Severe osteolysis after third-body wear due to hydroxyapatite particles from acetabular cup coating. *J. Bone Joint Surg.* 80B: 267-72.

38. Wang BC, Lee TM, Chang E. and Yang CY (1993) The shear strength and the faillure mode of plasma-sprayed hydroxyapatite coating to bone: The effect of coating thickness. *J. Biomed. Mater. Res.* 27:1315-27.

39. Dávid A, Eitenmüller J, Muhr G, Pommer A, Bär HF, Ostermann PAW and Schildhauer TA (1995) Mechanical and histological evaluation of hydroxyapatite-coated, titanium-coated and grit-blasted surfaces under weight-bearing conditions. *Arch. Orthop. Trauma. Surg.* 114: 112-8.

40. Manley MT, Capello WN, D'Antonio JA, Edidin AA and Geesink RGT (1998) Fixation of acetabular cups without cement in total hip arthroplasty. A comparison of three different implant surfaces at a minimum duration of follow-up of five years. *J. Bone Joint Surg.* 80-A:1175-84.

41. Bauer TW, Stulberg BN, Ming J and Geesink RGT (1993) Uncemented acetabular components Histologic analysis of retrieved hydroxyapatite-coated and porous implants. *J. Arthroplasty*, 8:167-77.

42. Schmalzried TP, Jasty M and Harris WH (1992) Periprosthetic bone loss in total hip arthroplasty: polyethylene wear debris and the concept of the effective joint space. *J. Bone Joint Surg.* 74-A:849-63.

6 Biomimetic Hydroxyapatite Coatings

Pamela Habibovic, BEng, Florence Barrère, PhD, Klaas de Groot, PhD

INTRODUCTION

The combination of high mechanical strength of metals with the osteoconductive properties of calcium phosphates results in hydroxyapatite (HA) coatings on titanium implants being widely used in orthopedic surgery. The most popular method to coat titanium implants with an HA coating is plasma-spraying. Earlier investigations have shown that these coatings can successfully enhance clinical success to < 2% failure rate after 10 years (1). Despite excellent clinical performances, the plasma-spray process is limited by intrinsic drawbacks. For instance, this line-of-sight process takes place at high temperatures. The process is, therefore, limited to thermally stable phases like HA; the incorporation of growth factors that stimulate bone healing is impossible. Moreover, this process cannot provide evenly distributed coatings on porous metal surfaces.

Recently, other techniques such as electrophoretic deposition (2), sputter deposition (3), and sol-gel (4) have been studied to improve the quality of coatings. Nevertheless, the deposition of apatite coatings from simulated body fluids (SBFs) offers the most promising alternative to plasma spraying and other coating methods. The biomimetic approach has four main advantages. First, it is a low temperature process applicable to any heat-sensitive substrate including polymers (5). Second, it forms bone-like apatite crystals that have high bioactivity and good resorption characteristics (6). Third, it is evenly deposited on, or even into, porous or complex implant geometries (7). Finally, it can incorporate bone-growth-stimulating factors.

This biomimetic approach consists of soaking metal implants in simulated body fluids at a physiological temperature and pH. Apatite coatings have successfully been formed by the immersion of chemically pretreated substrates such as glasses, metals, and polymers in metastable SBFs (8-10). Although SBF mimics the inorganic composition, pH and temperature of human blood plasma, it is unknown whether these conditions are optimal for a coating process. Indeed, a thin apatite layer has previously been obtained on pretreated substrates by using long immersion time (i.e., 7-14 days) with daily refreshment of SBFs (11-13). The difficulty results from the metastability of SBF. The process requires replenishment and a constant pH to maintain supersaturation for apatite crystal growth. As a result of the low solubility product of HA and the limited concentration range for the metastable phase, this operation is extremely difficult and might lead to local precipitation or uneven coatings. Such an intricate and long process can hardly be applicable in the coating prostheses industry.

This study describes a new biomimetic route for coating titanium alloy and porous tantalum in a few hours with thick, uniform hydroxyapatite layers. Thereby, no chemical pretreatment of the substrate is needed. Our process takes advantage of the higher solubility of calcium phosphate in acidic conditions and its precipitation at a neutral pH. A weak gaseous acid, CO_2, is used to decrease the pH, allowing much higher ionic concentrations for SBFs. While CO_2 gas is naturally released from the solution, the pH and, therewith, saturation, are slowly and uniformly increased. Therefore, carbonate-containing HA crystals precipitate on the implants.

EXPERIMENTAL PROCEDURE

Materials

The biomimetic coatings were applied on two different materials: Ti6Al4V plates (20mm × 20mm

× 1mm) and porous tantalum cylinders (Ø 5mm × 10mm). The adhesion strength of the coating is dependent on the mechanical interlock of the biomimetic HA coating and the implant surface (14-15). For optimal coating, an average surface roughness of 3.5mm is required. This surface roughness on the Ti6Al4V plates was obtained *via* grit blasting, using corundum particles with a particle size of 595-841 micrometers under a pressure of 4 bars.

The porous tantalum implants were manufactured by chemical vapor infiltration of pure tantalum onto a highly porous vitreous carbon skeleton. The porosity of the structure was approximately 75 %, and the average size of the interconnected pores was 450mm.

Before coating, the implants were ultrasonically cleaned for 15 minutes in acetone, ethanol (70 %), and demineralized water.

Coating Solutions

The coating process consisted of two steps. In the first step, the heterogeneous nucleation of a thin and amorphous calcium phosphate layer on the metal surface was obtained. During the second step, the growth of a thick and crystallized apatite coating on the implants was favored because of the lower Mg^{2+} and HCO_3^- contents.

The SBF-A and the SBF-B solutions (Table 1) were prepared according to Kokubo's SBF solution,[16] excluding the TRIS-buffer, K^+ ions, and SO_4^{2-} ions. In the first-step solution, the SBF-A was 5 times more concentrated in NaCl, $MgCl_2.6H_2O$, $CaCl_2.2H_2O$, $Na_2HPO_4.2H_2O$ and $NaHCO_3$ than Kokubo's SBF solution. SBF-B solution had the same composition as the SBF-A solution but, as explained earlier, the contents of inhibitors of crystal growth (*i.e.*, Mg^{2+} and HCO_3^- were lower (Table 1). All salts (reagent grade;

Merck, Darmstadt, Germany) were precisely weighed (± 0.01g) and dissolved in demineralized water under a supply of CO_2 gas at a flow of 650 L/min for 20 minutes and stirred at a speed of 250 rounds per minute (rpm).

The pH evolution was studied as a function of time in the coating solutions SBF-A and SBF-B. As a reference, the pH development in time was studied in a solution containing NaCl at a concentration of 683mM in demineralized water.

Coating Process

All experiments were performed in a 7L bioreactor (Applikon Dependable Instruments, Schiedam, The Netherlands) (fig. 1).

The implants were first soaked in a SBF-A solution for 24 hours to seed the metal surface with calcium phosphate nuclei. During this process, the temperature was kept at 37°C, and the solution was stirred at 250 rpm. To exchange CO_2 gas from the solution with air, a top aeration at a flow of 450 mL/min was performed. Moreover, air was added through the solution (flow 500 mL/min) after the pH had reached a value of 7.1. At the end of the process, the coated samples were cleaned with demineralized water and dried in air overnight. Then, the implants were soaked for another 48 hours in a SBF-B solution under crystal growth conditions. Temperature was maintained at 50°C and the stirring speed at 250 rpm. The same aeration system was used as described above. During this process, two samples were removed from the solution after 1, 2, 3, 4, 5, 6, 7, 8, 24, and 48 hours, respectively. Finally, the coated samples were cleaned with demineralized water and dried in air overnight. At the end of both processes, the solutions were filtered through Whatman filter paper No. 5. The precipitate was collected and dried overnight at 50°C.

	Ion concentration (mM)							
	Na^+	K^+	Ca^{2+}	Mg^{2+}	Cl^-	HPO_4^{2-}	HCO_3^-	SO_4^{2-}
HBP	142.0	5.0	2.5	1.5	103.0	1.0	27.0	0.5
SBF	142.0	5.0	2.5	1.5	148.8	1.0	4.2	0.5
SBF-A	714.8	–	12.5	7.5	723.8	5.0	21.0	–
SBF-B	704.2	–	12.5	1.5	711.8	5.0	10.5	–

Table 1 — Inorganic composition of human blood plasma (HBP), simulated body fluid (SBF) and coating solutions SBF-A and SBF-B.

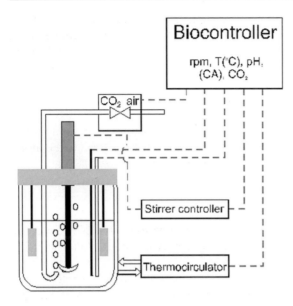

Figure 1 —Bioreactor for biomimetic coating of the metal implants.

Chemical and Structural Characterization of the Coatings

All samples were first investigated macroscopically. After gold-sputtering, the coated samples were observed microscopically using an environmental scanning electronic microscope apparatus equipped with a field emission gun (ESEM-FEG) at an accelerating voltage of 10 keV, coupled with energy-dispersive X-Ray analysis (EDAX) to check for any calcium-phosphate coating. The thickness of the coating was determined using an Eddy-current (electromagnetic) test method (17). Both coating and precipitate were investigated by Fourier transform infrared spectroscopy and X-ray diffraction. X-Rays were produced by a monochromatic source (Cu Kα, $\lambda = 1.54$ Å, 30 kV, 15 mA). All the XRD patterns were recorded at the same conditions (scan range: $2q = 3.00 - 60.00°$; scan speed: $2.00°$/min; scan step: $0.02°$). The crystallinity of the coating (18) and the calcium phosphate ratio (19) were determined. Both coatings and precipitate have similar FTIR spectra and XRD patterns. For convenience, analyses were performed on the precipitate.

RESULTS

pH Study

Comparing the pH-curves *versus* time in the NaCl reference solution and the SBF-A and SBF-B solu-

tions, it was observed that the initial pH of the NaCl reference was significantly lower (3.7) than the initial pH values of SBF-A and SBF-B solutions (5.8 and 5.7, respectively). The end pH of NaCl reference (6.6) after 24 hours was lower as well (pH_{end} SBF-A= 8.3; pH_{end} SBF-B = 7.9). Moreover, the pH of the NaCl reference and SBF-A solution increased progressively from the beginning to the end of the process, while during the process in the SBF-B solution, a drop in the pH was observed.

Coating Process

After 24 hours of soaking in the SBF-A solution, the implants were covered with a calcium phosphate film with a thickness of approximately 3 μm. The ESEM photographs showed that this calcium phosphate layer was uniformly deposited on the Ti6Al4V surface (fig. 2a). The coating was dense and consisted of globules. This thin coating exhibited some cracks, probably formed during the drying process of the coated samples. The EDAX spectrum (not shown) indicated calcium and phosphate peaks, with minute traces of magnesium and sodium. Small peaks of the Ti6Al4V substrate were also detected. The FTIR spectrum of the precipitate and coating (fig. 3a) showed featureless phosphate and carbonate bands. Intense and broad bands assigned to oxygen-hydrogen stretching and bonding were observed at 3,435 and 1,642cm^{-1}, respectively. Moreover, three bands at 868, 1,432 and 1,499cm^{-1} corresponded to the CO_3 groups. Finally, the one-component band at 560 and 1,045cm^{-1} showed the presence of PO_4. This FTIR spectrum is characteristic of carbonated amorphous calcium phosphate. The XRD pattern of the SBF-A precipitate (fig. 4a) corroborates the FTIR results, showing only the halo characteristic of an amorphous phase.

The immersion process in the SBF-B solution was used to develop a second coating layer on the seeded Ti6Al4V surface that resulted from the first coating process. During the immersion process in the SBF-B solution, the pH and coating thickness development were studied (fig. 5). The pH of the solution at the beginning of the process stabilized at 5.7. During the first 4 hours of the process, the pH increased progressively until a value of 6.2. Then, after 4 hours, a drop of 0.4 pH units occurred. After this drop, the pH started increasing again, and reached a value of 8.2 after 24 hours.

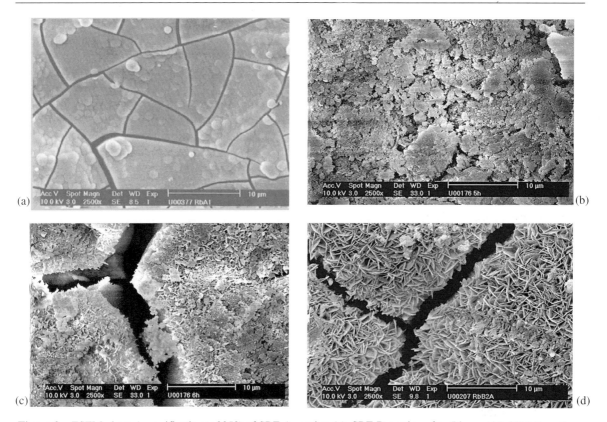

Figure 2. —ESEM photo (magnification × 2250) of SBF-A coating (a), SBF-B coating after 5 hours (b), SBF-B coating after 6 hours (c) and SBF-B coating after 24 hours (d) on Ti-alloy plate.

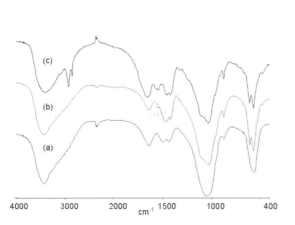

Figure 3. — Infra - red spectra of SBF-A coating (a), SBF-B coating (b) and bone (c).

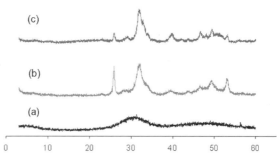

Figure 4 — XRD patterns of SBF-A coating (a), SBF-B coating (b) and bone (c).

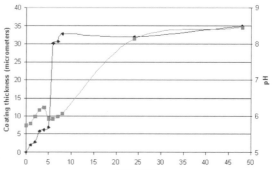

Figure 5 — pH (n) and coating thickness (♦) *versus* immersion time in SBF-B solution.

The pH elaboration of the solution was followed until 48 hours, and the final pH was 8.9.

During the first 4 hours of the process, the solution remained clear, and the thickness of the second coating layer grew very slowly (*i.e.*, ≤ 1.5 µm/h). During the drop in the pH, the precipitation occurred in the solution. After the pH drop, the coating thickness started increasing significantly along with the rise in the pH. After between 5 and 6 hours of the immersion, the coating thickness grew to approximately 30 µm, after which it remained constant after up to 48 hours of soaking.

The ESEM photographs of the titanium implants after 5 and 6 h of immersion (figs 2b and 2c) show many differences. After 5 hours, the metal was covered with loose calcium phosphate particles. The surface looked rough, without any visible crystals, and the thickness of the calcium phosphate layer was locally different. After 6 hours of immersion, the coating thickness was 30 µm. In this case, the whole metal surface was homogeneously covered with a well-formed, bluish coating consisting of globules with some tiny crystals. The coating contained many wide cracks. After 24 hours of soaking, the thickness of the coating did not change significantly in comparison to the coating after 6 hours of soaking. However, the coating looked more homogeneous and denser (fig. 2d), the cracks were much narrower, and the surface consisted of well-formed crystals of 1 to 3 µm in size.

As explained earlier, the EDAX spectrum of the coating from the SBF-A solution showed high calcium and phosphate peaks, and lower magnesium, sodium and titanium peaks. The EDAX spectrum of the coating after 5 hours of soaking in the SBF-B solution showed lower calcium and phosphate peaks and a higher titanium peak, suggesting partial dissolution of the amorphous coating. The magnesium peak was also lower, indicating a difference in the amount of magnesium ions in the coating obtained from the SBF-A and SBF-B solutions. After 6 hours of soaking in the SBF-B solution, an increase in phosphate and calcium peaks and a decreased titanium peak corroborated the growth of the coating. Finally, the EDAX spectrum of the coating after 24 hours of soaking showed very high calcium and phosphate peaks, while the titanium peak was not visible anymore.

The ESEM photograph of the surface of porous tantalum cylinders after 24 hours of immersion in SBF-B solution (fig. 6) indicates that the porous structure was homogeneously covered with a crys-

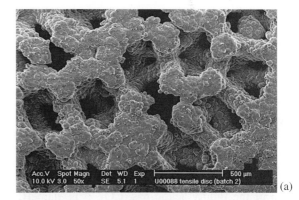

(a)

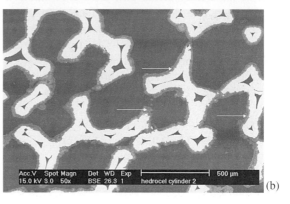

(b)

Figure 6—ESEM photo (magnification × 50) of SBF-B coating on surface (a) and cross-section (b) of porous Ta-cylinders; white arrows indicate coating.

talline calcium phosphate coating. On the cross-sectional surface (fig. 6b), a coating was also visible on the inside of the implant. All pores were well-coated with a thick calcium phosphate layer.

The FTIR spectrum of the precipitate from the SBF-B solution, gathered between 400 and 4,000cm^{-1} (fig. 3b), exhibited the characteristics of a carbonated apatite type A-B. The bands at 3,435 and 1,640cm^{-1} corresponded to oxygen-hydrogen groups. CO_3 group bands were observed at 1,493, 1,417 and 872cm^{-1}, whereas bands at 1,061, 599, and 563cm^{-1} were assigned to PO_4/HPO_4 groups. The XRD pattern exhibited broad diffraction lines (Figure 4B). The position and intensities of these diffraction lines indicated an apatitic structure. The peak at $2\theta = 32.1°$ corresponded to the overlapping of (211), (112), (300), and (202) diffraction peaks. Moreover, the peak at $2\theta = 25.8°$, corresponding to the (002) diffraction plane, indicated that SBF-B precipitate consisted of small apatitic crystals. The crystals had a size of 2-3 µm. The crystallinity of the precipitate was 75% and its calcium phosphate ratio was 1.67.

Previously published results (20) showed that the final apatite coating is well- adhered to the Ti6Al4V substrate, and that no coating delamination or spalls were observed during the scratch test.

DISCUSSION

The results of the experiments show that highly-concentrated solutions can be obtained by the addition of the mildly acidic gas, CO_2. It is, namely, well-known that the solubility of calcium phosphate salts increases with the decrease of pH[21]. Dissolution of CO_2 gas results in a pH decrease caused by the formation of carbonic acid H_2CO_3 (reaction 1), after which the acid immediately dissociates in the HCO_3^- and CO_3^{2-} species (reactions 2 and 3).

$$CO_2 + H_2O \leftrightarrow H_2CO_3 \quad (1)$$
$$H_2CO_3 + H_2O \leftrightarrow HCO_3^- + H_3O^+ \quad (2)$$
$$HCO_3^- + H_2O \leftrightarrow CO_3^{2-} + H_3O^+ \quad (3)$$

When CO_2 gas gradually releases from the solutions, the pH slowly increases again. In the case of the NaCl reference, the pH increases progressively from the start of the process until the finish, slowly approaching the pH of water (6.5). The presence of HCO_3^- and HPO_4^{2-} ions in SBF solutions, together with the CO_2 and HCO_3^- ions that are formed during the dissolution of CO_2 gas (reactions 2 and 3), leads to the formation of a buffered solution. This might explain the fact that the initial pH values of the SBF-A and SBF-B solutions were higher than that of the NaCl reference. During the processes in the SBF-B solution, a drop in the pH was observed simultaneously with the start of precipitation in the solution. This drop of the pH may be explained by the start of the precipitation of crystalline phase according to the reaction (4).

$$10Ca^{2+} + 6PO_4^{3-} + 2OH^- \leftrightarrow Ca_{10}(PO_4)_6(OH)_2 \quad (4)$$

Because of the decreased amount of OH^- ions in the solution, a pH drop was observed. After precipitation, CO_2 gas continued to release from the solution. Therefore, the pH increased progressively until the end of the process.

In the SBF-A solution, more HCO_3^- species were present in comparison with the SBF-B solution (Table 1). Therefore, the buffering capacity of CO_2/HCO_3^- couple was higher. This might explain a slightly higher initial pH and the absence of pH drop during the process in the SBF-A solution, in comparison with the process in the SBF-B solution.

Another factor that may influence the pH evolution during the coating process is the amount of the NaCl species, i.e., the ionic strength of the solution (22). The rate of the CO_2 release from the solution is higher in case of low ionic strength, followed by a higher pH increase. This causes an early and sudden precipitation in the solution. Consequently, the supersaturation of the solution is markedly lowered, and less ionic species are available in the solution for the calcium phosphate nucleation on the substrate. Moreover, there is an inverse relationship between the calcium phosphate concentration and the pH at which precipitation occurs: the lower the concentration, the higher the precipitation-pH (21).

As previously described, a 3 μm thick amorphous layer of carbonated calcium phosphate was obtained on the metal sample by immersion in the SBF-A solution. *In vivo* experiments performed by our group [unpublished results] showed that this amorphous coating was too thin to be able to enhance osteointegration of the implants. Moreover, earlier *in vitro* dissolution experiments[23] showed that, at both an acidic and neutral pH, amorphous carbonated calcium phosphate dissolves markedly faster than other calcium phosphate coatings (i.e., Octacalcium Phosphate (OCP), Carbonated Apatite (CAp) and HA).

Bone formation on biomimetic calcium phosphate coatings results from the dynamic interactions between several physicochemical parameters and the body fluids. The initial structure, the microstructure, the crystallinity, and the surface morphology of calcium phosphate all influence the dissolution rate and the interaction with organic compounds and cells. *Vice versa*, the organic compounds and cells present in the body fluids influence the degradation and dissolution rate, and consequently, the final surface morphology and structure of the calcium phosphates (24). According to the literature and our experience, a coating that successfully enhances osteointegration of metal implants needs to be thick and crystallized enough to accommodate the bone healing process. Preliminary experiments were performed in order to grow a crystalline coating on metal surface without immersion in the SBF-A solution. By immersing cleaned Ti6Al4V directly into the SBF-B solution, a loose and nonuniform layer was obtained, which shows the relevance of amorphous precoating. That is why our biomimetic coating consists of two steps.

Immersion of the implants in a SBF-A solution is necessary for seeding the metal surface with calcium phosphate nuclei. During this nucleation process, calcium phosphate seeds are precipitated in the solution and on the metal surface. Some of these nuclei can dissolve in the solution and some can expand in size. Homogeneous nucleation (precipitation) occurs spontaneously in the solution and can proceed by other seeds that are formed in the meantime. Heterogeneous nucleation, on the other hand, takes place on the metal surface. Both, homogenous and heterogeneous nucleation are in competition during the process in the SBF-B solution. However, nuclei are energetically more stable on the seeded metal surface than in the solution. It is, therefore, essential to provide the metal surface with a thin and uniform primer calcium phosphate layer for subsequent growth of the final coating. The kinetics of the process in SBF-A solution were reported in detail by Barrère *et al.* (25).

After reaching their critical size, seeds can start growing into crystals. The nucleation and growth kinetics of the crystal depend on the temperature, pH, composition, and saturation of the solution. Calcium and phosphate ions are responsible for the formation of the calcium phosphate layer on the metal surface, while magnesium and carbonate ions favor heterogeneous nucleation rather than crystal growth. As presented in Table 1, the SBF-B solution has the same composition as the SBF-A solution, but the contents of Mg^{2+} and HCO_3^- ions are lower. Due to the lower amounts of these so-called crystal growth inhibitors (26-33), a crystalline apatite phase is formed and a drop in the pH is observed at the start of precipitation by immersion in the SBF-B solution. Moreover, a smaller amount of HCO_3^- ions, compared to the SBF-A solution, decreases the buffering capacity of the CO_2/HCO_3^- couple; hence, variations in the pH can be observed. With a lower amount of Mg^{2+} in the SBF-B solution, the calcium phosphate precipitation is accelerated, and the growing coating becomes more crystallized. Earlier research (34-37) proved that crystal growth from a supersaturated solution occurs quickly. This can explain the fact that, within 1 h, the coating thickness grows by 25 μm. Because of precipitation and crystal growth, the amount of calcium and phosphate in the solution decreases. One hour after the start of precipitation, the contents of the calcium and phosphate are too low for further growth. Between the end point of crystal growth and the end of the process, there is equilibrium between the amount of calcium and phosphate in the coating and in the solution. However, the coating might dissolve and reprecipitate onto the surface, resulting in a more homogeneous and denser coating at the end of the process.

As mentioned previously, a dense, adherent film is formed because of the heterogeneous nucleation on the metal surface. However, it is very difficult to prevent loose precipitate in the solution from sticking to the metal surface. This means that both phenomena contribute to film growth, but to a different extent.

There is a difference in the calcium/phosphate ratio between natural calcified tissues (enamel, dentine, and bone) and the biomimetic coatings. The calcium/phosphate ratio of the natural calcified tissues is approximately 1.60, depending on many parameters such as age, sex, bone sites, etc. (38). The biomimetic coating has a calcium/phosphate ratio of 1.67 ± 0.02, as determined after calcination at 1 000°C by XRD and FTIR. In the case of the biomimetic coating, small amounts of magnesium and sodium can substitute for calcium in the HA lattice, lowering the calcium/phosphate ratio. However, carbonate is able to substitute for phosphate, which results in the transformation of HA into CAp and increases the calcium/phosphate ratio. Because the second effect is much stronger, the overall effect is a higher calcium/phosphate ratio compared to bone.

The FTIR spectra (fig. 3) and the XRD patterns (fig. 4) show the similarities in composition and structure between our biomimetic coating and bone. An earlier report of an experiment with osteoclast-enriched mouse bone marrow cell cultures on different coatings (6) showed that numerous resorption lacunae, characteristic of osteoclastic resorption, were found on carbonated apatite after cell culture. In the case of OCP coating, no pits could be found. The results obtained indicated that biomimetic calcium phosphate coatings are easily resorbed by osteoclasts *in vitro*. This phenomenon corresponds to full integration into the human body of biomimetically coated implants. On the contrary, conventional plasma-sprayed coatings may delaminate and release large sintered particles that are not easily degraded by cells (39). The last results might indicate that our biomimetic coatings are markedly more bioactive than plasma-sprayed coatings. However, additional *in vivo* research is necessary to confirm these expectations.

CONCLUSION

The formation of thick and homogeneous calcium phosphate coatings on Ti6Al4V implants and porous tantalum substrates is possible by using a biomimetic method consisting of two steps. By this method, the coating is produced within a few hours and without any chemical pretreatment. The first step of the process results in the formation of a thin, amorphous coating, which ultimately leads to the fast precipitation of 30 ± 10mm thick dense Ca-P coating in the second step of the process. The formation of this coating is strongly related to Mg^{2+} content. The evolution of the pH during the coating process is dependent on the ionic strength of the solution (i.e., the amount of NaCl), and the amount of HCO_3^- ions that, together with the present CO_2, buffer the solution. The final coating closely resembles bone mineral. The biomimetic coating applied on dense and porous orthopedic implants should enhance bone apposition and bone ingrowth, leading to a fast and stable osteointegration of prostheses.

References List

1. Havelin LI, Engesaeter LB, Espehaug B, Furnes O, Lie SA and Vollset SE (2000) The Norwegian Arthroplasty Register, 11 Years and 73,000 Arthroplasties. *Acta Orthop. Scand.* 71(4):337-53.

2. Ducheyne P, van Raemdonck W, Heughebaert JC and Heughebaert M (1986) Structural Analysis of Hydroxyapatite Coatings on Titanium, *Biomaterials* 7(2):97-103.

3. Ong JL, Lucas LC, Lacefield WR and Rigney ED (1992) Structure, Solubility and Bond Strength of Thin Calcium Phosphate Coatings Produced by Beam Sputter Deposition. *Biomaterials* 13(4):249-54.

4. Ben-Nissan B, Chai CS and Gross KA (1997) Effect of Solution Aging on Sol-Gel Hydroxyapatite Coatings. *Bioceramics* 10:175-8.

5. Du C, Klasens P, de Haan RE, Bezemer J, Cui FZ, de Groot K and Layrolle P (2002), Biomimetic Calcium Phosphate Coatings on PolyActive® 1000/70/30: *J. Biomed. Mater. Res.* (United States), 59(3):535-46.

6. Leeuwenburgh S, Layrolle P, Barrère F, Schoonman J, van Blitterswijk CA and de Groot K (2001) Osteoclastic Resorption of Biomimetic Calcium Phosphate Coatings *in vitro. J. Biomed. Mater. Res.* (United States), 56(2):208-215.

7. Layrolle P, van der Valk C, Dalmeijer R, van Blitterswijk CA and de Groot K (2000) Biomimetic Calcium Phosphate Coatings and Their Biological Performances. *Bioceramics* 13: 391-4.

8. Wen HB, Wolke JGC, de Wijn JR, Cui FZ and de Groot K (1997) Fast Precipitation of Calcium Phosphate Layers on Titanium Induced by Simple Chemical Treatment. *Biomaterials* 18:1471-8.

9. Kim HM, Miyaji F, Kokubo T, Nakamura T (1996) Preparation of Bioactive Ti and its Alloys via Simple Chemical Surface Treatment. *J. Biomed. Mater. Res.* 32:409-17.

10. Yamada S, Nakamura T, Kokubo T, Oka M, Yamamura T (1994) Osteoclastic Resorption of Apatite Formed on Apatite- and Wollastonite-Containing Glass-Ceramic by a Simulated Body Fluid. *J. Biomed. Mater. Res.* 28:1357-63.

11. Li P, Kangasniemi I, de Groot K and Kokubo T (1994) Bonelike Hydroxyapatite Induction by a Gel-Derived Titania on a Titanium Substrate. *J. Am. Ceram. Soc.* 77:1307-12.

12. Peltola T, Patsi M, Rahiala H, Kangasniemi I and Yli-Urpo A (1998), Calcium Phosphate Induction by Sol-Gel-Derived Titania Coatings on Titanium Substrates *in vitro. J. Biomed. Mater. Res.* 41:504-10.

13. Li P and Ducheyne P (1998) Quasi-Biological Apatite Film Induced by Titanium in a Simulated Body Fluid. *J. Biomed. Mater. Res.* 41:341-48.

14. Leitao E, Barbosa MA and de Groot K (1987) Influence of Substrate Material and Surface Finishing on the Morphology of the Calcium-Phosphate Coating. *J. Biomed. Mater. Res.* 36:85-90.

15. Thomas KA and Cook SD (1985) An Evaluation of Variables Influencing Implant Fixation by Direct Bone Apposition. *J. Biomed. Mater. Res.* 19:875-901.

16. Kokubo T, Kushitani H, Sakka S, Kitsugi T and Yamamuro T (1990) Solutions Able to Reproduce *in vivo* Surface-Structure Changes in Bioactive Glass-Ceramics A-W3, *J. Biomed. Mater. Res.* 24:721-34.

17. ASTM E 376 (1996) "Standard Practice for Measuring Coating Thickness by Magnetic-Field or EDDY-Current (Electromagnetic) Test Methods".

18. ASTM STP 1196 (1994) "Characterization and Performance of Calcium Phosphate Coatings for Implants".

19. NF S94-066 (French standard 1998) "Determination quantitative du rapport Ca/P de phosphates de calcium"

20. Barrère F, Layrolle P, van Blitterswijk CA and de Groot K (1999) Physical and Chemical Characteristics of Plasma-Sprayed and Biomimetic Apatite Coating. *Bioceramics* 12:125-28.

21. Elliot JC (1994) in Structure and Chemistry of the Apatites and Other Calcium Orthophosphates, edited by Elsevier (Amsterdam The Netherlands).

22. Barrère F, Layrolle P, van Blitterswijk CA and de Groot K (2001), Influence of NaCl and HCO3 on the Biomimetic Ca-P Coating Process from SBFx5 Solution, Submitted to Biomaterials.

23. Barrère F, Stigter M, Layrolle P, van Blitterswijk CA and de Groot K (2000) *in vitro* Dissolution of Various Calcium-Phosphates Coatings on Ti6Al4V. *Bioceramics* 13:67-70.

24. Barrère F (2002) Biomimetic Calcium Phosphate Coatings, Physicochemistry and Biological Activity, PhD Thesis, Enschede, The Netherlands.

25. Barrère F, Layrolle P, van Blitterswijk CA and de Groot K (2000) Fast Formation of Biomimetic Ca-P Coatings on Ti6Al4V. *Mat. Res. Soc. Symp. Proc.* 599:135-40.

26. Newesely H (1961) Changes in Crystal Types of Low Solubility Calcium Phosphates in Presence of Accompanying Ions, *Arch. Oral Biol.*, Special Supplement 6, 174-80.

27. Tomazic B, Tomson M and Nancollas GH (1975) Growth of Calcium Phosphates on Hydroxyapatite Crystals: The Effect of Magnesium. *Arch. Oral Biol.* 20:803-08.

28. Salimi MH, Heughbaert JC and Nancollas GH (1985) Crystal Growth of Calcium Phosphates in the Presence of Magnesium Ions. *Langmuir* 1:119-22.

29. Eanes ED and Rattner SL (1980) The effect of Magnesium on Apatite Formation in Seeded Supersaturated Solutions at pH=7.4. *J. Dent. Res.* 60:1719-23.

30. Boskey AL and Posner AS (1974) Magnesium Stabilization of Amorphous Calcium Phosphate: A Kinetic Study. *Mat. Res. Bull.* 9:907-16.

31. Nancollas GH, Tomazic B and Tomson M (1976) The Precipitation of Calcium Phosphate in the Presence of Magnesium. *Croatia Chemica Acta* 48:431-38.

32. Chikerur NS, Tung MS and Brown WE (1980) A Mechanism for Incorporation of Carbonate into Apatite, Calcif, Tissue. *Int.* 32:55-62.

33. Bachara BN and Fisher HRA (1969) The Effect of Some Inhibitors on the Nucleation and Crystal Growth of Apatite, Calcif. *Tissue Res.* 3:348-57.

34. Füredi-Milhofer H, Brecevic LJ and Purgaric B (1976) Crystal Growth and Phase Transformation in the Precipitation of Calcium Phosphates. *Faraday Discuss. Chem. Soc.* 61:184-90.

35. Koutsoukos P, Amjad Z, Tomson MB and Nancollas GH (1980), Crystallization of Calcium Phosphates: A Constant Composition Study. *J. Am. Chem. Soc.* 102:1553-7.

36. van Kemenade M and de Bruyn PL (1987) A Kinetic Study of Precipitation from Supersaturated Calcium Phosphate Solutions. *J. Colloid and Interface Sci.* 118:564-85.

37. Kohman GT (1963) Precipitation of Crystals from Solution, in: The Art and Science of Growing Crystals, edited by Gilman, John Wiley and sons, London, p.152-62.

38. LeGeros R (1991) In: Calcium Phosphates in Oral Biology and Medicine, Karger, Basel, Switserland, 109-27.

39. de Bruijn JD, Flach JS, Leenders H, van den Brink J and van Blitterswijk CA (1992) Degradation and Interface Characteristics of Plasma-Sprayed Coatings with Different Crystallinities. *Bioceramics* 5:291-98.

7 Combination of HA and Bisphosphonate Coating to Control the Bone Remodeling Around the Orthopedic Implant

Dominique P. Pioletti, PhD, Bastian Peter, BSc, Lalao R. Rakotomanana, PhD, Pascal Rubin, PhD and Pierre-François Leyvraz, MD

INTRODUCTION

The peri-implant osteolysis following a total joint arthroplasty (TJA) is responsible for the majority of orthopedic implant loosening (1). Failure rates of hip arthroplasty can exceed 30% after 15 years for patients younger than 50 years old (2). A revision surgery where the old implant is replaced by a new one is then performed. Joint disorders treated with TJA can reasonably be expected to give satisfactory results for 20 to 30 years with an initial and revision surgery. No subsequent procedure can be performed in a routine manner. The actual trend is to propose TJA to younger patients with the caveat that a second surgery is likely to be required.

The peri-implant bone resorption is caused either by stress shielding (3) or by inflammatory reaction induced by wear particles (4). Besides the improvement of the material and wear properties of the implant, a new therapy using a systemic treatment with drugs targeting osteolysis, e.g., bisphosphonates (5), has been recently considered. However, the systemic use of drugs presents drawbacks such as important side effects (e.g., throat or stomach ulcers for bisphosphonates (6)) or difficulties in determining the appropriate dosage. These problems could limit the use of the pharmacological therapy in controlling the peri-implant bone remodeling.

In order to solve those problems, we suggest a new view of the use of implants. The implants would not only be a structural support but also a local drug delivery system. To realize this innovative concept, the stem of a cementless implant could be coated with a carrier e.g., hydroxyapatite combined with a drug e.g., bisphosphonate (7), which would enable local control of bone remodeling.

In the present study, we numerically investigate the concept of an implant used as a drug delivery system. We modified an existing model developed by our group for calculation of bone density around an implant during remodeling (8, 9). The effects of drugs were accounted for by locally modifying bone remodeling parameters. We also evaluated the advantage of a partial in comparison to a full stem-biocoating. This last point is motivated by the fact that the peri- implant bone density is uneven. The optimal control of bone remodeling in the implant surrounding could be best achieved by a partial biocoating.

MATERIALS AND METHODS

Biomechanical Bone Remodeling Model

To relate the bone adaptation to the mechanical stress environment, it has been proposed e.g. (9-13) to link the relative density evolution $d\phi/dt$ to the mechanical stimulus ψ applied to the bone by a piecewise linear evolution relation. In this kind of description, an equilibrium zone, where bone neither resorbs nor densifies is delimited by two threshold stimuli ψ_r and ψ_d while v_r and v_d are respectively the slopes of the resorption and densification rates *versus* ψ. The equation describing the bone adaptation behavior can be generally expressed by e.g. (9):

$$\frac{d\phi}{dt} = \begin{cases} v_r(\psi - \psi_r) & \psi < \psi_r \\ 0 & \psi_r \leq \psi \leq \psi_d \\ v_d(\psi - \psi_d) & \psi > \psi_d \end{cases} \quad \text{(Eq. 1)}$$

Model of Bisphosphonate Effect on Bone Remodeling

Bisphosphonates such as aledronate received daily have been shown to continuously increase patients bone mineral density (BMD) (14). This increase in BMD was due at least in part to an increase of the degree of mineralization of bone structural unit (BSU) induced by the marked slowing of bone turnover (15). Indeed, this kind of treatment did not impair bone mineralization and did preserve the biomechanical properties of the bone (16). Bisphosphonate has been shown to inactivate osteoclasts, which then undergo apoptosis, resulting in reduced bone resorption, lower bone turnover, and a positive bone balance (17,18). It was then hypothesized that a reduced turnover increases the life span of BSU and leads to a more mature bone in which most units approach at least a normal level in their degree of mineralization (15). The lower bone turnover allows the secondary mineralization to be achieved and maintained resulting in an increase bone mineral density (19). Bisphosphonate such aledronate seems then to reduce bone resorption and bone turnover. Based on these considerations, the effects of bisphosphonate could be taken into account by affecting the values of the resorption parameters such as v_r or ψ_r, but not the formation parameters such as v_d and ψ_d, in the model described previously. More specifically, we propose to model the effect of bisphosphonate in the biomechanical description proposed by stating that the reduction of bone resorption can be accounted for by decreasing the value of v_r, while the reduction of bone turnover can be accounted for by decreasing the value of ψ_r. We assume that there is no effect of bisphosphonate on the bone formation parameters. This point has been confirmed recently (16).

The effect of bisphosphonate on bone resorption parameters v_r and ψ_r, was modeled by transforming the two resorption parameters in functions depending on the drug effect.

$$v_r(\kappa) = v_r \cdot \kappa$$
$$\psi_r(\kappa) = \psi_r \cdot \kappa$$

(Eq. 2)

The factor κ is a value between 0 and 1 which is defined for each location in the bone and can be dependent upon the drug concentration or other biological properties. The implementation of the drug altered relative density evolution $d\phi/dt$ has been achieved by using a set of parameters and calculated with (Eq. 1). The dependencies of the parameters and upon κ will have to be experimentally determined. For the present study, this dependency has been arbitrarily set to a linear relation (Eq. 2).

Application to Hip Arthroplasty

Geometry and FEM

The three-dimensional geometry of a proximal femur was reconstructed from CT slices. The initial bone density distribution corresponds to the density distribution as it has been measured just after implantation of a THR implant. Then, a finite element model of the bone-implant system was obtained with a 3D mesh generator (20). The FE mesh was based on 8-node isoparametric elements. The evolution equation was iteratively solved by custom- made software REM (9) driving ABAQUS (Hibbitt, Karlsson, & Sorensen Inc., Newpark, USA) analysis program. The forces used to simulate muscle action on the head of the implant have been experimentally determined (21-23).

Global Drug Application

In order to validate the concept of biocoating, three different sets of simulation were used. The parameters were set so as to decrease bone resorption. The first case called Fullcoat 1 was a simulation run with

$$\psi_r(\kappa = 0.5) = \frac{\psi_r}{2}$$

(Eq. 3)

The second one called Fullcoat 2 was a simulation run with

$$v_r(\kappa = 0.5) = \frac{v_r}{2}$$

(Eq. 4)

The third one called Fullcoat 3 was a simulation run with

$$\psi_r(\kappa = 0.5) = \frac{\psi_r}{2}$$
$$v_r(\kappa = 0.5) = \frac{v_r}{2}$$

(Eq. 5)

In all three cases, any other parameter was left at the standard values of v_r, ψ_r, v_d, and ψ_d.

Local Drug Application

For the study of local drug effect, $v_r(\kappa)$ and $\psi_r(\kappa)$ were varied at the same time in certain regions of the femur, as shown in Figure 1 and (Eq. 5).

The parts of the femur that are not designated by the arrows use the standard values of v_r, ψ_r, v_d and ψ_d.

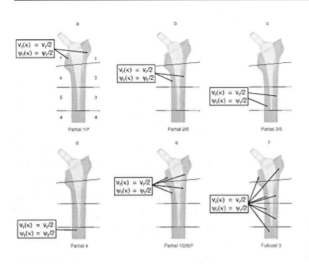

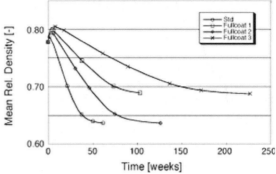

Figure 2 – Evolution of the relative density in time for four cases being Standard (Std), 50% decreased (Fullcoat 1), 50% decreased (Fullcoat 2), 50% decreased and (Fullcoat 3).

Figure 1 – Description of the different modeled coatings in reference to the 7 Gruen zones (detailed in a) taken as pairs (1/7, 2/6, 3/5 and 4).

Remodeling Parameter Values

The numerical values used in this study have been experimentally determined (9, 24, 25)

$$v_r = 2.800 \ week^{-1} \quad \psi_r = 7.5 \cdot 10^{-3}$$
$$v_d = 0.805 \ week^{-1} \quad \psi_d = 3.0 \cdot 10^{-2} \quad \text{(Eq. 6)}$$

A simulation of the bone remodeling using these values was performed for reference and was defined as standard (Std).

RESULTS

Global Drug Application

The three coated implants showed a higher density than the standard implant (fig. 2). The Fullcoat 1 and Fullcoat 3 ended up with higher densities than the standard implant, whereas Fullcoat 2 reaches equilibrium with the same density than the standard case. All three full coatings needed longer times to reach equilibrium than the standard case corresponding then to a decreased rate of bone turnover. Decreasing ψ_r was more effective to slow down bone resorption than decreasing v_r.

For all Gruen zones and at any time, the density was higher in the Fullcoat 3 case compared to the standard (Figure 3). The most marked differences were located in zones 1 and 7 with a density 1.5 time higher than in Std after 50 weeks. The resorption rate $d\phi/dt$ was 2.2 times higher in the standard case than in the Fullcoat 3 case. When locally observing the density evolution (fig. 2), it was

noted that the biggest difference between the standard case and Fullcoat 3 was found in the Gruen zones 1, 2, 6 and 7. The density of the zones 3, 4 and 5 was slightly higher in the Fullcoat 3 case than in the standard case.

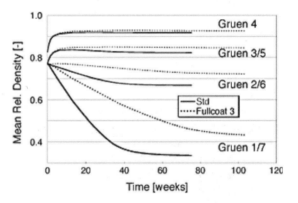

Figure 3 – Comparison of the mean density temporal evolution between the Std coating and Fullcoat 3.

Local Drug Application

In order to demonstrate the advantage of a partial biocoating concept, one global coating (Fullcoat 3) was compared with three partially coated implants (Partial 1/7, Partial 2/6 and Partial 1/2/6/7).

The cases Partial 1/7, Partial 2/6 and Partial 1/2/6/7 resulted in a lower mean density than Fullcoat 3 (fig. 4). Results have shown that the cases Partial 3/5 and Partial 4 reach almost the same equilibrium density as the standard while the other three keep a higher density than the standard case.

A comparison of bone density between Fullcoat 3 or Partial 1/7 with the standard case was performed by calculating the bone density difference

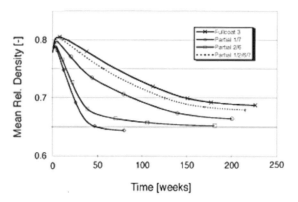

Figure 4 – Comparison of the relative density evolution between local and global drug use.

for each node (fig. 5). In both coating cases, most nodes have a higher density than in the standard case. The Partial 1/7 case reached a higher density in Gruen zones 1 and 7 compared to the Fullcoat 3 case. The fully coated implant case induced a bone slightly denser in the medial proximal bone next to the implant and in the lateral proximal outer region of the bone. The main difference resided in the zones 2 and 6, in particular in the lateral region next to the implant, where the bone around the full coating is 10% denser as in Partial 1/7. In the regions 3/5 and 4, the fully coated implant resulted also in a denser bone as compared to a partial coating. In all cases, the denser bone was mainly located in lateral part and the higher increases were next to the implant.

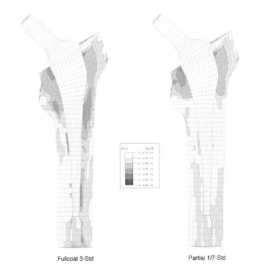

Figure 5 – Spatial density variation of Full coating and partial coating compared to Std. Dark zone represents the highest difference in bone density while clear zone represents slight difference.

DISCUSSION

There is a need to increase the life span of hip implants especially for younger patients. To this end, Shanbhag (5) studied the inhibition of wear debris mediated osteolysis in a canine total hip arthroplasty model by oral use of a bisphosphonate (alendronate sodium). Despite promising results, the systemic use of bisphosphonates bears some dangers like throat damage or ulcer (6). Therefore we propose to coat the implant with a combination of hydroxyapatite and a drug as bisphosphonate to create a local delivery system. This allows to control the bone remodeling around the implant. The basic underlying assumption is that decreasing the bone resorption in the early stage following a TJA could considerably increase the stability of the implant resulting in a longer implant service life. In the present study, we tested this hypothesis by extending a bone remodeling model for analyzing the effect of a drug coated on the implant surface.

The decrease of the two resorption parameters of the model ψ_r and v_r were effective in increasing the mean bone density around the implant. However only the variation of ψ_r enables maintenance of higher mean density up to the equilibrium state. The influence of decreased v_r lies mainly in delaying bone resorption. For example, in order to reach a density $\phi = 0.65$, it took 40 weeks with a standard implant, 75 weeks with a decreased v_r (Fullcoat 2) while for the two cases Fullcoat 1 (ψ_r decreased) and Fullcoat 3 (ψ_r and v_r decreased) the density stayed always above 0.65 (fig. 2).

By comparing the evolution of the mean density (fig. 2), for the couples Std-Fullcoat 2 and Fullcoat 1-Fullcoat 3, the observed effect of a decreased v_r is to increase the time to reach the equilibrium density. The consequence of this is that at the same moment in the remodeling process (for example week 50), the coating inducing a decreased v_r generated a bone of higher density around the implant. This leads to the conclusion that the ideal drug would be one that decreases ψ_r in order to reach a higher equilibrium density and decreases v_r in order to reach the equilibrium by keeping the highest possible density during the remodeling process.

The distal part of the implanted femur tends to increase its mean density with time (fig. 3) which has been associated to the stress-shielding problem (26). In the Fullcoat as in the Partial cases, the model indicated that the distal parts of the implanted bone (zones 3, 4 and 5) were denser than in the initial case whereas the proximal part of the bone (zone 1, 2, 6 and 7) resorbed. This leads to a situation which is biomechanically unfavorable to the stability of the bone-implant system (27). Those observations lead to the concept of partial biocoating.

Since the densification of the distal zones (3, 4 and 5) is not desirable, partial coatings were applied to the zones (1, 7) and (2, 6) and (1, 2, 6 and 7). Interestingly, in all three partial coatings, the density in the modified zone was higher than in the same zone for the full biocoating. This result favoured the use of a local coating compared to a full coating for the two reasons that first a higher bone density is obtained in the needed regions and second no decrease of bone resorption is induced in the distal part of the implant where an over densification already took place.

Two clinical studies related the use of partially coated implants. McAuley (28) showed that in the case of an anatomical medullary locking hip implant, the full coating results in less bone loss in the proximal femur but a density increase in the distal part of the femur. But the authors admit themselves that those results are probably particular to the design of this implant. Rosenthall (29) compared the density evolution in all Gruen regions around Multilock implants where, some were proximally coated with hydroxyapatite while the others were not coated. They could show that in any Gruen zone and at almost any moment, the density was higher in the proximally coated implant. These two studies illustrate the conflicting results that can be obtained *in vivo*. This fact highlights the usefulness of a numerical model to estimate the influence of different implants on the peri-implant bone remodeling.

The model used constant values to simulate the effect of the drug. The decrease of drug activity over time or the diffusion of drug in the bone were not accounted for. These effects could modify the calculated bone density. The diffusion of the drug in the bone will be measured in an experimental study and incorporated in the developed model. Regarding the decrease of drug activity, this effect is less important for bisphosphonate as it has been shown that this drug is not degraded during its stay in the body (7).

Acknowledgements

This work was supported by Leenaards Foundation Grant #309.

Reference List

1. Clarke IC, Campbell P, Kossovsky N (1992) Debris-mediated osteolysis-A cascade phenomenon involving motion, wear, particulates, macrophage induction, and bone lysis. In: St. John KR (ed.) Particulate debris from medical implants: mechanisms of formation and biological consequences, ASTM STP 1144. American Society for testing and materials, Philadelphia, pp. 7-26.

2. Amstutz H, Dorey FJ, Finerman GAM (1998) The cemented T-28/TR-28 prosthesis. In: Finerman GAM, Dorey FJ, Grigoris P, McKellop HA (eds.) Total hip arthroplasty outcomes. Churchill Livingston, New York, pp. 55-63.

3. Huiskes R (1987) Finite element analysis of acetabular reconstruction. Noncemented threaded cups. *Acta Orthop. Scand.* 58:620-5.

4. Friedman RJ, Black J, Galante JO, Jacobs JJ, Skinner HB (1993) Current concepts in orthopaedics biomaterials and implant fixation. *J. Bone Joint Surg.* 75-A(7):1086-109.

5. Shanbhag AS, Hasselman CT, Rubash HE (1997) The John Charnley Award. Inhibition of wear debris mediated osteolysis in a canine total hip arthroplasty model. *Clin. Orthop.* (344):33-43.

6. Elliott SN, McKnight W, Davies NM, MacNaughton WK, Wallace JL (1998) Alendronate induces gastric injury and delays ulcer healing in rodents. *Life Sci.* 62:77-91.

7. Fleisch H (1995) Bisphosphonates in bone disease, from the laboratory to the patient, 1 ed., vol. 1. The Parthenon Publisching Group, pp. 176.

8. Terrier A, Rakotomanana RL, Ramaniraka AN, Leyvraz PF (1997) Adaptation Models of Anisotropic Bone. *Comput. Methods Biomech. Biomed. Engin* 1:47-59.

9. Terrier A (1999) Adaptation of bone to mechanical stress: theoretical model, experimental identification and orthopaedic applications Physics. EPFL, Lausanne, pp. 175.

10. Beaupre GS, Orr TE, Carter DR (1990) An approach for time-dependent bone modeling and remodeling-application: a preliminary remodeling simulation. *J. Orthop. Res.* 8:662-70.

11. Carter DR (1984) Mechanical loading histories and cortical bone remodeling. *Calcif. Tissue Int.* 36(Suppl 1):S19-24.

12. Cowin SC, Sadegh AM, Luo GM (1992) An evolutionary Wolff's law for trabecular architecture. *J. Biomech. Eng.* 114(1):129-36.

13. Huiskes R, Weinans H, Grootenboer HJ, Dalstra M, Fudala B, Slooff TJ (1987) Adaptive bone-remodeling theory applied to prosthetic-design analysis. *J. Biomech.* 20(11-12):1135-50.

14. Liberman UA, Weiss SR, Broll J, Minne HW, Quan H, Bell NH, Rodriguez-Portales J, Downs RW, Jr., Dequeker J, Favus M (1995) Effect of oral alendronate on bone mineral density and the incidence of fractures in postmenopausal osteoporosis. The Alendronate Phase III Osteoporosis Treatment Study Group. *N. Engl. J. Med.* 333(22):1437-43.

15. Meunier PJ, Boivin G (1997) Bone mineral density reflects bone mass but also the degree of mineralization of bone: therapeutic implications. *Bone* 21(5):373-7.

16. Chavassieux PM, Arlot ME, Reda C, Wei L, Yates AJ, Meunier PJ (1997) Histomorphometric assessment of the long-term effects of alendronate on bone quality and remodeling in patients with osteoporosis. *J. Clin. Invest.* 100(6):1475-80.

17. Fleisch H (1996) The bisphosphonate ibandronate, given daily as well as discontinuously, decreases bone resorption and increases calcium retention as assessed by 45Ca kinetics in the intact rat. *Osteoporos Int.* 6(2):166-70.

18. Odan GA, Martin TJ (2000) Therapeutic approaches to bone diseases. *Science* 289(5484):1508-14.

19. Boivin G, Meunier PJ (1999) How do bone resorption inhibitors increase bone mineral density? *Rev. Rhum. Engl. Ed.* 66(11):534-7.

20. Rubin PJ, Leyvraz PF, Aubaniac JM, Argenson JN, Esteve P, de Roguin B (1992) The morphology of the proximal femur. A three-dimensional radiographic analysis. *J. Bone Joint Surg. Br.* 74(1):28-32.

21. Crowninshield RD, Brand RA (1981) A physiologically based criterion of muscle force prediction in locomotion. *J. Biomech.* 14(11):793-801.

22. Davy DT, Kotzar GM, Brown RH, Heiple KG, Goldberg VM, Heiple KG, Jr., Berilla J, Burstein AH (1988) Telemetric force measurements across the hip after total arthroplasty. *J. Bone Joint Surg. Am.* 70(1):45-50.

23. Goldberg VM, Davy DT, Lotzar GL, Heiple KG, Brown RH, Berilla J, Burstein AH (1988) *In vivo* hip forces. Non-cemented total hip arthroplasty. In: Fitzgerald R (ed.) *In vivo* hip forces. Non-cemented total hip arthroplasty. Raven Press, New York, pp. 251-6.

24. Nauenberg T, Bouxsein ML, Mikic B, Carter DR (1993) Using clinical data to improve computational bone remodleing theory. 39th Meeting Orthopaedic esearch Society, San-Fransisco.

25. Rubin CT, Lanyon LE (1985) Regulation of bone mass by mechanical strain magnitude. *Calcif. Tissue Int.* 37(4):411-7.

26. Van Rietbergen B, Huiskes R, Weinans H, Sumner DR, Turner TM, Galante JO (1993) ESB Research Award 1992. The mechanism of bone remodeling and resorption around press-fitted THA stems. *J. Biomech.* 26(4-5):369-82.

27. Weinans H, Huiskes R, Grootenboer HJ (1994) Effects of fit and bonding characteristics of femoral stems on adaptive bone remodeling. *J. Biomech. Eng.* 116(4):393-400.

28. McAuley JP, Sychterz CJ, Engh CA, Sr. (2000) Influence of porous coating level on proximal femoral remodeling. A postmortem analysis. *Clin. Orthop.* (371):146-53.

29. Rosenthall L, Bobyn JD, Tanzer M (1999) Bone densitometry: influence of prosthetic design and hydroxyapatite coating on regional adaptive bone remodelling. *Int. Orthop.* 23(6):325-9.

8 Coating of Titanium with Hydroxyapatite by Laser Surface Powder Cladding: Exploratory Results

Pascal Deprez, PhD, Philippe Hivart, PhD

INTRODUCTION

Numerous procedures for the coating of metallic implants with hydroxyapatite (HA) exist (1). Indeed, HA close to bone tissue is often used as implant material but is seldom employed alone because having poor mechanical properties. Among these methods, high temperature processes are widespread. HA powder is heated to high temperatures and deposited on the metallic substrate. At present, the most current industrial application is plasma spraying. Laser surface treatments are an attractive alternative to that technology (2). On the face of it, the principle is similar: a powder heated by the laser beam forms on a substrate a mechanically bonded layer when cooling. The porosity of the HA layer can be also optimised as regards its easiness of substitution by bone tissue when implanted in a body. Indeed, it is a function of the power density, the pulse duration, the pulse energy, the coverage coefficient and the nature of the ambient gas of the laser. However, the advantages over plasma spraying are important, from a basic technical point of view as much as for its possibilities.

The first great basic advantage is that the laser technology does not need any surface preparation such sandblasting or undercoating before coating, so it does not lead to pollution problems. Moreover, the small diameter of the laser beam allows a homogeneous treatment of complex surfaces; it does not lead to localised overthickness. It does not need masking, and it allows the coating of only the necessary surface. During coating, the heat affected zone of the substrate remains thin without cooling the piece. Due to the implementation, the coated part is never completely heated at the same time. At present, the precision and the reproducibility of the laser treatment are also significant advantages.

The ability of substituting laser technology for plasma spraying technology for a similar coating treatment is known, but the possibilities of laser for the production of new materials with specific properties are more widespread. Three main points may be here considered: modification of the characteristic of the surface of the substrate, modification of the layer, and creation of intermediate layer. The surface of the substrate can be modified. It is enough to notice the classical wave effect, or the possibility of changing the roughness, and the porosity layer using laser parameters previously detailed. Others modifications (structure, composition) can be also realised.

For instance, a previously created HA layer can be treated in order to modify porosity, surface roughness, structure, or even composition (3).

Finally, the melting of the surface of the substrate when depositing the heated HA leads to its insertion and to the formation of an intermediate layer. This latter is therefore a compound of HA in a titanium matrix, and it could be comparable to a composite ceramic-metal. That technology is called laser powder cladding, which is discussed in this chapter.

A laser powder cladding method has been developed for the deposition of hydroxyapatite onto titanium alloy, Ti6Al4V. In a high temperature coating process, the misfit of the thermal expansion coefficients of Ti6Al4V and HA (about 60%) leads to residual tensile stresses in HA during cooling. It usually produces cracks in the ceramic that weaken the layer and decrease its bonding to the substrate (4). The main goal is avoid cracks in the ceramic. The process is studied and implemented. Examinations are made in order to identify possible cracks and to study the interface. The heat affected zone is determined. Having shown the feasibility, complementary studies are planned and expected results are discussed.

EXPERIMENTAL PROCEDURE

The chosen metallic substrate to be coated is titanium alloy that contains 6% aluminium and 4% vanadium in weight (Ti6Al4V). The coated samples are plates, whose length, width and thickness are 50, 20, and 1mm, respectively. Pure commercial hydroxyapatite $Ca_{10}(PO_4)_6(OH)_2$ is used in powder form.

In the chosen process, cladding materials are delivered by either preplacing a powder bed (HA) on the substrate, or blowing the powder into the molten pool. In the latter, a laser beam is directly irradiated on the titanium alloy substrate. In this case, it is difficult to obtain a molten pool because of the high reflectivity of titanium to laser. One of the ways to reduce reflectivity is to put the HA powder on the titanium alloy, because it has a much lower reflectivity. Accordingly, the preplaced powder method was employed in the present exploratory work.

A pulsed Nd :YAG laser (wavelength λ = 1.06μm) is used (commercial reference : Laser Application LAP4000). Its mean power is 400W. The laser beam pulse has a multi mode power repartition. The waist of the laser beam is about 420μm at the surface of the substrate. The treatment velocity is about 120μm/min^{-1}. Different irradiation conditions are studied by changing the laser parameters in the following domains: pulse energy, 1.5 – 3J ; pulse frequency, 10-20Hz, and pulse duration,1.6 – 3ms. Nitrogen is used as a shielding gas at low pressure under a constant flow rate of 5 l.min^{-1}.

The deposited HA powder on the plate is covered by a piece of glass to avoid projections that prevent a homogeneous treatment and disturb the control of the layer thickness. The transparent glass has no other influence on the result. Figure 1 shows the process principle. The surface is then swept by the laser beam and irradiated by laser spot delivered at the chosen frequency. The lap of two successive passes is about 50%. Optical and SEM examinations of surface and of the laser treated specimens are conducted.

RESULTS

Numerous experimental series allow an approach of the optimum setting of the laser processing parameters. They are selected to ensure a uniform induced structure and to minimise the heat affected zone and the cracks in the HA layer. The cohesion at the interface is visually appreciated and so it only concerns detachment problems. According to the above criteria the optimum laser processing conditions used in this study are: pulse energy, 2.5J ; pulse frequency, 10Hz ; pulse duration, 1.6ms, and waist / powder surface distance : 2mm.

The cross-sections in Figures 1 and 3 show the laser effect on the substrate. The melted zone is about 300μm. The heat affected zone is about 10μm on average. The lower and upper limits of these zones show a wave effect. Localised insertions of HA are clearly visible in the melted zone till its bottom (fig. 3). They are more or less regularly spaced in the titanium.

A HA layer is formed on the titanium (fig. 1). Its average thickness is about 450μm. Figure 3 shows that there is a continuity with the insert. Micrographically, the whole does not present any cracks or problem of cohesion. Tilted SEM micrographies (figs 4 and 5) allow the examination of both surface and section of the HA layer. No characteristic major cracks may be seen while the porosity is clearly shown. The average diameter of porosity is about 0.1mm. The HA layer is very homogeneous.

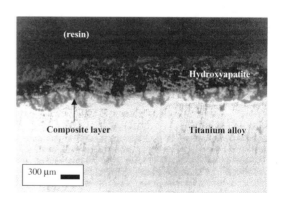

Figure 2 – Optical micrography of coating of (hydroxyapatite) on titanium alloy by laser powder cladding (cross-section).

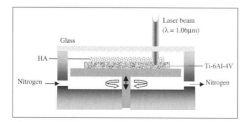

Figure 1 – Experimental apparatus.

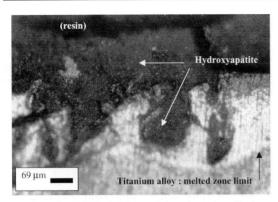

Figure 3 – Optical micrography of coating (hydroxyapatite) on titanium alloy by laser powder cladding (cross-section, detail).

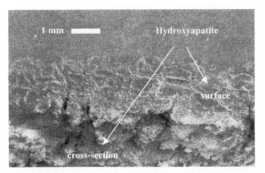

Figure 4 – SEM micrography of coating (hydroxyapatite) on titanium alloy by laser powder cladding (tilted cross-section, detail).

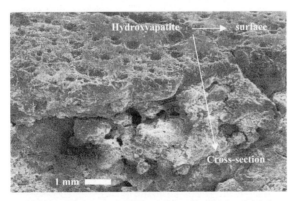

Figure 5 – SEM micrography of coating (hydroxyapatite) on titanium alloy by laser powder cladding (tilted cross-section, detail).

DISCUSSION

The heterogeneity in substrate topography results from the non-uniform laser beam energy spatial distribution. Therefore, the higher energy concentration at the center of the laser spot leads to steeper thermal gradients and higher cooling and solidification rates. The rapidly-solidified central zone is much more refined and smooth compared to the boundary zone. But the cracking tendency in this zone due to the high residual tensile-stress fields induced by laser treatment (thermal and solidification stresses) does not appear on the micrographies. The laser works on pulse mode; added to the non-uniformity, it leads to the wave effect. Moreover, during laser-substrate interaction, a part of the molten material is ejected, forming "lips" surrounding the central melt-zone after subsequent solidification.

The quick cooling is driven by mechanisms of conduction (heat transfer to the substrate) and convection (heat transfer occurs with relative mass transfer into the molten pool). It leads to the insertion of HA in the melted zone. It generates a composite layer made of ceramic HA in titanium matrix. Its thickness is comparable with the HA layer thickness. This new intermediate layer could be responsible of the minimization of the cracks. Indeed, its thermal expansion coefficient is probably between those of Ti6Al4V and HA. It would allow an accommodation that would avoid the formation of cracks by allowing residual tensile stresses to relax during cooling.

The intermediate layer probably plays a major part in the bonding of HA layer on the titanium substrate. Indeed, the continuity between the inserted HA and the superficial HA layer makes each laser pulse during coating correspond to a cramping point. The bonding should be more important than only the mechanical bonding to the roughness. Moreover, it was shown (5) that the laser treatment creates a porous surface that apparently allows the HA to key-in to the metallic substrate. Of course, it is also expected that the bonding of bone tissue after HA resorption would be greater. The good porosity of the created HA layer, opening to the outside interface, will facilitate the colonization by the bone tissue till the metallic surface.

It must be noticed that the composite intermediate layer is not created from a third material. Possible pollution such as with alumina use (6) is then avoided. Moreover, the adaptation of the thermal expansion coefficient of titanium to HA for instance by alloying (7) is not necessary.

When the HA powder pre-deposited on the titanium is irradiated by the laser beam, only the part located near the focal point of the beam is treated.

This point is close enough to the substrate to melt it. Therefore, the upper part is not affected and remains in powder form, being removed after the treatment. The coating thickness does not simply depend on the initial HA powder deposited on the surface. Different thickness of HA layer can be created by successive laser passes until the powder is exhausted, or until the desired thickness is reached. The obtained results show that the final HA layer is homogeneous and it can not be dissociated.

CONCLUSION

Micrographically studied results of the application of laser powder cladding to the coating of titanium by hydroxyapatite show that this process is an interesting alternative to existing techniques for making HA coatings, like plasma spraying. The cross-sections show that a 300μm thick composite layer formed by HA inserted into Ti6Al4V is created during the laser treatment. Its thermal characteristics are probably intermediate between those of HA and titanium; it could explain that no major cracks were noted. It would play as a thermomechanical accommodation layer.

Moreover, there is continuity between the inserted HA and the superficial HA layer that would contribute to cramp this coating to the metallic substrate.

The HA layer is quite homogeneous and 450μm thick. The porosity is 0.1mm diameter but it can be modified by changing laser parameters to allow a better colonisation by bone tissue. This latter will be cramped into the titanium substrate after having replaced the inserted HA.

This exploratory work is based on micrographic study. A complete study is beginning at present. The mechanical part of this study aims mainly to characterise the bonding of the HA layer onto the titanium substrate when the chemical one is to determine the created compounds. Particularly possible modifications of HA (new phases, Ca/P ratio, etc.) or the emergence of new compounds must be brought to the forefront, completed by an accurate determination of the heat affected zone. The quantification of the physical characteristics of the compounds is also essential. Density, hardness and thermal characteristics are principle concerns, but a particular interest is taken in the study of the porosity. Indeed, the confirmation of interconnections between the pores is fundamental for the planned biomedical application. Other important data are expected from a microstructural study. More generally stresses, microcracking, and interfaces must be highlighted. The whole will be completed by an in-vitro biological study.

This pre-study shows that laser processes are worth being studied in detail and developed. The observed advantages lead to think that the laser powder cladding should be an interesting improvement in the field of biomaterials.

Acknowledgement

The authors thank Dr A. Deffontaines, head of Centre d'Application des Lasers Flandres Artois (CALFA, University of Artois, France) for his support and Pr. J. Crampon of the Laboratoire du Solide et des Propriétés de l'État Solide (LSPES, ESA CNRS 8008, University of Lille, France) for his assistance.

Reference List

1 Brès E and Hardouin P (1998) Calcium phosphate materials fundamentals. Sauramps Medical Ed., Montpellier-France.

2 Garcia-Sanz FJ, Mayor MB, Arias JL, Pou J and Leon B (1997) Hydroxyapatite coatings: a comparative study between plasma-spray and pulsed laser deposition techniques. Journal of materials science. *Materials in Medicine*, Vol. 8, No. 12, pp. 861-5.

3 Cheang P, Khor KA, Teoh LL and Tam SC (1996) Pulsed laser treatment of plasma-sprayed hydroxyapatite coatings. *Biomaterials,* Vol. 17, pp. 1901-4.

4 Huaxia J and Marquis PM (1993) Effect of heat treatment on the microstructure of plasma sprayed hydroxyapatite coating. *Biomaterials*, Vol. 14, pp. 64-8.

5 Sampathkumaran U, De Guire M and Wang R (2001) Hydroxyapatite coatings on titanium. *Advanced Engineering Materials*, Vol. 3, No. 6, pp. 401-5.

6 Bonel G (1998) Hydroxyapatite biomaterials: industrial and clinical aspects; evolution of the conceptions. in *Calcium phosphate materials fundamentals*. Sauramps Medical Ed., Montpellier-France, pp. 9-24.

7 Breme J, Zhou Y and Groh L (1995) Development of a titanium alloy suitable for an optimized coating with hydroxyapatite. *Biomaterials*, Vol. 16, pp. 239-44.

9 Finite Element Analysis in Bioactive-coated Tibial Components

Nobuyuki Yoshino, MD, PhD, Shinro Takai, MD, PhD, Sadami Tsutsumi, PhD

INTRODUCTION

The stability of the components is vital for successful, long-term results of total knee arthroplasty (TKA). The loosening of the tibial component is more common than that of the femoral component. Therefore, methods to improve the fixation of the tibial component have been continually developing. Roentgenstereometric analysis (RSA) has shown that early migration can predict loosening of tibial component (1, 2). In cemented TKA, initial postoperative migration occurs as a result of the operative trauma, such as thermal bone necrosis from cementing or sawing. In cementless TKA, initial instability may be due not only to operative trauma from sawing, but also to irregularities of the cut surface. To fill the gap between component and cut surface, bioactive coating or clay, such as hydroxyapatite (HA) or tri-calcium phosphate (TCP), was developed. Some animal studies have shown that hydroxyapatite coating (3) or clay (4) enhances the fixation of unstable cementless implants. In clinical studies, some authors showed successful use of bioactive coated implants (5, 6). However, some authors reported early failure due to separation of the coating (7).

The objective of the present study is to assess the effectiveness of bioactive coating with tibial components. For this objective, finite element method (FEM) was employed for four different modalities of fixation with the same stem-type design, 1) rigid interface, 2) rigid interface only at tibial tray, 3) early stage of bioactive coating, and 4) fibrous fixation.

MATERIALS & METHODS

The two-dimensional FEM was performed to study the stress distribution in the proximal tibia under loaded conditions. Figure 1 shows FEM models. Figure 1a is assumed to be the condition with rigid osseous ingrowth or good cement-bone integration between the tibial component and cancellous bone (rigid fixation model). Figure 1b is assumed to be the condition with rigid osseous ingrowth or good cement-bone integration between the tibial tray and cancellous bone, with fibrous fixation between the tibial stem and cancellous bone (partial rigid fixation model). Figure 1c is assumed to be the condition of early stage of a bioactive-coated tibial component (bioactive coating model). Figure 1d is assumed to be the condition with fibrous fixation between the tibial component and cancellous bone (fibrous fixation model). In the models 1b, 1c, and 1d, gap elements were used to represent early bone ingrowth or fibrous fixation. The difference between early bone ingrowth and fibrous fixation was the material property of the gap elements. The material properties of cancellous bone, cortical bone, UHMWPE, metal (Co-Cr-Mo) and gap elements are shown in Figure 2. Figure 3 shows the material properties of cancellous bone, which were derived from previously reported numerical

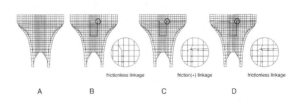

Figure 1 – Finite element mesh.
a) Rigid fixation model with complete interface bonding along the implamt.
b) Partial rigid fixation model with complete interface bonding along the tibial tray, and with fibrous fixation between tibial stem and cancellous bone.
c) Bioactive coated model.
d) Fibrous fixation model.

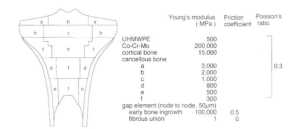

Figure 2 – Material properties.

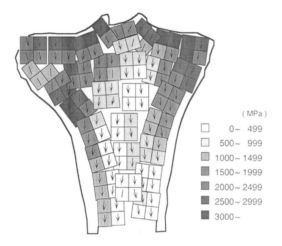

Figure 3 – Distribution of the Young's modulus and mean trabecular orientation of the cancellous bone.

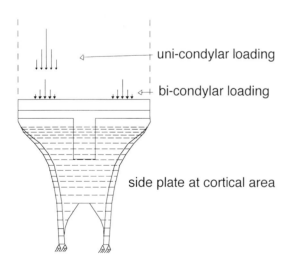

Figure 4 – Loading and boundary conditions.
a) Bi-condylar loading.
b) Uni-condylar loading.

analysis of a soft X-ray photo of the sliced proximal tibia (8). Figure 4 shows the loading and boundary conditions.

There are two loading conditions, one is bi-condylar (neutral) loading, and the other is uni-condylar (varus or valgus) loading. Totally 600N was applied in 10 steps in each condition. In all models, the distal ends of model were constrained in X-Y direction. To consider hoop stress and to make a two-dimensional model quasi three-dimensional model, side plates (spanning elements) were applied at the cortical bone area (9). On the models with gap elements, two truss elements for stability of models (Young's modulus is 10^{-6}MPa) were applied on medial and lateral upper end of tibia to avoid dispersion of analysis.

RESULTS

Figure 5 shows von Mises' equivalent stress distribution with a 20X magnified deformity under bi-

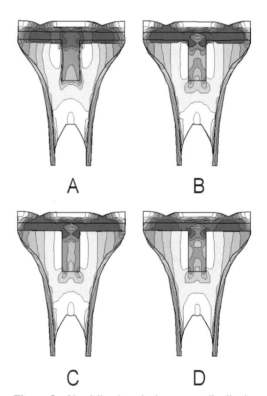

Figure 5 – Von Mises' equivalent stress distribution under bi-condylar loading.
a) Rigid fixation model.
b) Partial rigid fixation model.
c) Bioactive coated model.
d) Fibrous fixation model.

condylar loading. The stress distribution pattern is similar among the four models. The stress around the tip of the stem in a bioactive coating model and fibrous fixation model is slightly larger then that of a rigid fixation model. The von Mises' equivalent stress of the elements beneath the tibial component were also similar among the four models.

Figure 6 shows von Mises' equivalent stress distribution with a 20X magnified deformity under uni-condylar loading. Stress sharing of the unloaded side in a partial rigid fixation model and bioactive coating model was larger than that in rigid fixation model. In the fibrous fixation model, stress sharing of the unloaded side was not seen and lift-off of the component, which leads to the teeter-totter phenomenon, was noted.

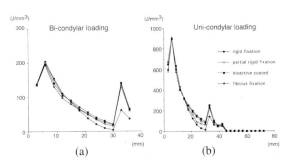

Figure 7 – Strain energy density
of the elements beneath the implants.
a) Bi-condylar loading.
b) Uni-condylar loading.

rule of remodeling in FEM analysis (10, 11). SED of the bioactive coated model and that of the fibrous fixation model are almost same. SED of the elements beneath the stem in these two models were higher than those in rigid fixation and partial rigid fixation models. SED of the elements beneath the tibial tray of unloaded area in rigid fixation model was lower than that of other three models.

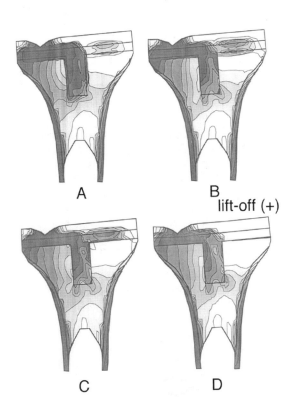

Figure 6 – Von Mises' equivalent stress distribution
under uni-condylar loading.
a) Rigid fixation model.
b) Partial rigid fixation model.
c) Bioactive coated model.
d) Fibrous fixation model.

Figure 7 shows strain energy density (SED) of the elements beneath the tibial components. SED is thought to be one of the parameters to decide the

DISCUSSION

The tibial components fixed without cement have shown larger migration than the corresponding cemented components when analyzed with RSA (12, 13). To augment the fixation of uncemented components, bioactive coating has been developed. However, the evaluation of bioactive coating is still under debate. Some RSA studies showed that micromotion of hydroxyapatite-coated tibial components fixed without cement was similar to that of cemented components (14, 15). Contrary to these reports, other authors reported that the hydroxyapatite coating might offer an advantage over a simple porous costing for tibial component fixation, but is no better than cemented fixation (12). Thus, the advantage of hydroxyapatite coating over the cementless fixation without coating has been established, but the advantage over the cement fixation is still unclear. Hydroxyapatite coating may differ with respect to composition, crystallinity, porosity, thickness, and to what substrate it is applied. Standardization of these factors should be approached by both medical and engineering fields.

FEM is frequently used for analyses of load transfer and stress patterns in bone/implant structures to assess the adequacy of the prosthetic design and position. The commonly applied FEM models assume complete interface bonding and are descriptive of idealized configurations. These linear analyses were substantially equivalent to the clinical results, such as the superiority of metal-backed implants (16, 17), wide contact area (18), and so forth. To our knowledge, in 1977, Svensson et al. firstly studied the cement/bone interface loosening (19), and in 1984, Brown *et al.* first reported the use of non-linear contact element in the analysis of natural adult hip (20). Since then, many FEM studies used the contact element ("gap element") for analyzing not only the problems between the faced bone in the joints, but also the problem between the bone/implant interface. In these studies, the contact elements between the faced articular cartilage in the joints were established on the basis of the results from experimental studies of articular cartilage. However, the a decision on the interface condition between bone and implants has not been achieved so far, because the precise material property of the interface substance can not be obtained experimentally.

The results of von Mises equivalent stress distribution in the present study showed that there was little difference among the four different modalities of fixation methods. The results of SED in the present study also showed that there was little difference among the four different modalities of fixation methods, even the difference between the rigid fixation model (identical model) and fibrous fixation model (initial loosening model). The factors influencing the results in FEM analysis include geometry, division of elements, loading condition, boundary condition, interface condition, etc. We used the practicably optimum condition, for example the division of elements after convergency test, usage of side plate, detailed material properties of cancellous bone, etc. (21). Therefore, we thought that the little differences in our results occurred because of the difficulty of the reproduction in interface areas. It would be impossible to compose the cut tibial surface precisely. Furthermore, in the non-linear numerical analysis, making the decision about the interface condition is one of the most difficult problems, because the precise material property of the interface substance can not be obtained experimentally, as mentioned above. Other FEM studies of femoral prosthesis, which dealt with the remodeling process, also

could not show the advantage of the hydroxyapatite coating (22). Therefore, the advantage of the bioactive coating should be evaluated by long-term clinical results, because it could not be reasonably assessed by numerical analysis.

Reference List

1. Ryd L, Albrektsson BEJ, Carlsson L, Dangsgård F, Herberts P, Lindstrand A, Regnér L, Toksvig-Larsen S (1995) Roentgen stereophotogrammeric analysis as a predictor of mechanical loosening of knee prosthesis. *J. Bone Joint Surg.* 77B:377-83.

2. Grewal R, Rimmer MG, Freeman MAR (1992) Early migration of prostheses related to long-term survivorship. Comparison of tibial components in knee replacement. *J. Bone Joint Surg.* 74B:239-42.

3. Søballe K, Hansen ES, Brocksted-Rasmussen H, Bünger C (1991) Gap healing enhanced by hydroxyapatite coating in dogs. *Clin. Orthop.* 272:300-7.

4. Maruyama M (1995) Hydroxyapatite clay used to fill the gap between implant and bone. *J. Bone Joint Surg.* 77B:213-8.

5. Regnér L, Carlsson L, Kärrholm J, Herbert P (1998) Ceramic coating improves tibial component fixation in total knee arthroplasty. *J. Arthroplasty* 13:882-9.

6. Toksvig-Larsen S, Jorn LP, Ryd L (2000) Lindstrand A: Hydroxyapatite-enhanced tibial prosthetic fixation. *Clin. Orthop.* 370:192-200.

7. NilssonKG, Cajander S, Kärrhorm J (1994) Early failure of hydroxyapatite-coating in total knee arthroplasty. A case report. *Acta Orthop. Scand.* 65:212-4.

8. Yoshino N, Inoue N, Watanabe Y, Yamashita F, Hirasawa Y, Hirai T, Katayama T (1992) Stress Analysis of the Proximal Tibia after Total Knee Arthroplasty with a Finite Element Method. In: Niwa S, Perren SM, Hattori T (eds) Biomechanics in Orthopedics. Springer-Verlag Tokyo,Tokyo, pp. 253-62.

9. Hampton SJ, Andriacchi TP, Galante JO, Belytscheko TB (1976) Analytical approach to the study of stresses in the femoral stem of total hip prostheses. Proceedings 29th ACEMB, Boston, 32:1.

10. Carter DR (1987) Mechanical loading history and skeletal biology. *J. Biomech.* 20:1095-109.

11. Huiskes R, Weinans H, Grootenboer HJ, Dalstra M, Fudala B, Slooff TJ (1987) Adaptive bone-remodeling theory to prosthetic-design analysis. *J Biomech.* 20:1135-50.

12. Önsten I, Nordqvist A, Carlsson ÅS, Besjakov J, Shott S (1998)Hydroxyapatite augmentation of the porous coating improves fixation of tibial components. A randomized RSA study in 116 patients. *J. Bone Joint Surg.* 80B: 417-25.

13. Nilsson KG, Kärrhorm J (1993) Increased varus-valgus tilting of screw-fixed knee prostheses: stereoradiographic study of uncemented versus cemented tibial components. *J. Arthroplasty* 8: 529-40.

14. Nelissen RGHH, Valstar ER, Rozing PM (1998) The effect of hydroxyapatite on the micromotion of total knee arthroplasty. *J. Bone Joint Surg.* 80-A. 1665-72.

15. Nilsson KG, Kärrhorm J, Carlsson L, Dalén T (1999) Hydroxyapatite coating versus cemented fixation of the tibial component in total knee arthroplasty. Prospective randomized comparison of hydroxyapatite-coated and cemented components with 5-year follow-up using radiostereometry. *J. Arthroplasty* 14:9-20.

16. Lewis JL, Askew MJ, Jaycox DP (1982) A comparative evaluation of tibial component designs of total knee prostheses. *J. Bone Joint Surg.* 64A:129-35.

17. Murase K, Crownishield RD, Pedersen DR, Chang T-S (1982) An analysis of tibial component design in total knee arthroplasty. *J. Biomech.* 16:13-22.

18. Garg A, Walker PS (1986) The effect of the interface on the bone stresses beneath tibial components. *J. Biomech.* 19:957-67.

19. Svensson NL, Valliappan S, Wood RD (1977) Stress analysis of human femur with implanted Charnley prosthesis. *J. Biomech.* 10:581-88.

20. Brown TD, DiGiola AM (1984) A contact-coupled finite element analysis of the natural adult hip. *J. Biomech.* 17:437-48.

21. Yoshino N, Takai S, Hirasawa Y, Tsustsumi S, Murase K (1996) Establishment of conditions in finite element analysis of the tibia replaced by prosthesis. *J. Jpn Soc. Clin. Biomech.* 17:23-27 (in Japanese).

22. Huiskes R. Weinans H (1994) Biomechanical aspects of hydroxyapatite coatings on femoral hip prostheses. In: Epinett JA, Geesink RGT (eds) Hydroxyapatite coated hip and knee arthroplasty. Expansion scientifique francaise, Paris, pp. 41-50.

BIOACTIVE COATINGS:
CLINICAL WORKS

1   Current Status of Bioactive Coatings in Japan

Shunsuke Fujibayashi, MD, PhD, Takashi Nakamura, MD, PhD

INTRODUCTION

Bone defects often appear in the orthopedic clinical arena after tumor resections, infectious osteolysis, trauma, and at donor sites after bone harvest or revision surgery in procedures such as arthroplasty. The repair of large bone defects is a challenging problem for orthopedic surgery. For the stabilization of unstable segments, including the pseudoarthrosis of long bone or spinal disorders, autograft or allograft bone or ceramics are usually used for augmentation between the unstable segments.

Most artificial materials implanted into bone defects are encapsulated by a fibrous tissue that isolates them from the surrounding bone. However, ceramics (1), such as glasses in the Na_2O-CaO-SiO_2-P_2O_5 system (Bioglass®), sintered hydroxyapatite ($Ca_{10}(PO_4)_6(OH)_2$), and glass ceramics containing apatite and wollastonite ($CaO \cdot SiO_2$), bond to living bone. These ceramics are widely used clinically, but cannot be used at sites experiencing high load, such as femoral and tibial bones, because their fracture toughness is not as high as that of human cortical bone. Metallic materials, such as titanium and its alloys, can be used under high load conditions because of their biocompatibility and high fracture toughness, but are bioinert and do not bond to living bone (2, 3).

The main methods used to anchor these implants to recipient bone include cement fixation with polymethylmethacrylate (PMMA) glue, or mechanical interlocking through a microporous layer. Unfortunately, through these methods, the clinical lifetime of the implants may be less than a decade, owing to their poor bone-bonding strength.

A total hip prosthesis with a porous surface is thought to bear the body weight primarily *via* the porous layer. A ceramic coating is a recommended means of enhancing bone tissue formation around, and into, the prosthetic surface, thereby helping to establish a mechanical anchor. Recently, several investigators have reported that a hydroxyapatite (HA) coating promotes direct bonding (4-7). Although many good clinical results with plasma-sprayed HA coatings have been reported, there have been several problems with its porosity, low fatigue strength, degradation, and delamination during long-term implantation, and with its weak adherence to the metallic substrate during implantation. Furthermore, when hydroxyapatite is plasma-sprayed onto the porous layer of the prosthesis, the possibility exists that occlusion of the surface pores and a change in the surface pore size, porosity, and thickness may occur.

AW glass ceramic is one of the bioactive ceramics developed at Kyoto University in 1982 (8, 9). Approximately 60,000 AW glass ceramic implants, including an iliac spacer, a vertebral prosthesis, an intervertebral spacer, an interlaminae spacer and a bone defect filler (fig. 1) (Cerabone® AW, Nippon Electric Glass Co., Otsu, Japan), have been used for the treatment of approximately 45,000 patients during the past decade in Japan, with satisfactory results. Cerabone® AW is able to directly bond to bone tissue within a shorter implantation time than synthetic HA, and its mechanical strength is greater than that of synthetic HA and human cortical bone.

We attempted to combine AW glass ceramic with titanium alloy implants to further accelerate the bone-bonding process of the implants, and to improve the bone-bonding strength. In cases where AW glass-ceramic was coated only into the deeper part of the pores, alterations in the surface pore size, porosity, and thickness did not occur.

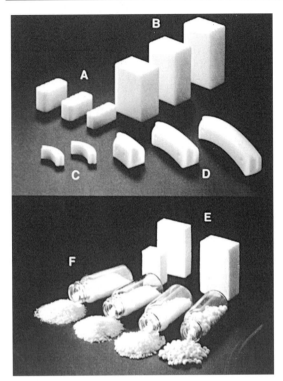

Figure 1 – Cerabone AW: intervertebral spacer (A), artificial vertebrae (B), interlaminae spacer (OLE3) (C), iliac spacer (D), porous block (E), and bone filler (F).

Recently, another approach has been developed to improve bone–titanium bonding. Kokubo *et al.* showed that, after a combination of an alkali and a heat treatment, bone-like apatite forms on the surface of the titanium in simulated body fluid (SBF) (10). In studies of the bone-bonding mechanism of bioactive ceramics, it was shown that the essential requirement for artificial materials to bond to living bone is the formation of bone-like apatite (11). All the bioactive ceramics form an apatite layer on their surfaces in the living body. As the composition and structure of this apatite layer are very similar to those of bone mineral, the cells do not recognize it as a foreign material, and hence bone-producing cells (osteoblasts) preferentially proliferate and differentiate, rather than the fibrous tissue-producing cells (fibroblasts), on the bone-like apatite layer. As a result, the surrounding bone can come into direct contact with the bone-like apatite layer without forming fibrous tissue. When this occurs, a tight chemical bond forms between the bone mineral and the surface apatite to reduce the interface energy between them. The NaOH and heat treatments produce a uniform amorphous sodium titanate layer on the surface of titanium.

The sodium titanate induces formation of bone-like apatite in the SBF very soon after immersion.

Other research on the surface modification of titanium metal has been reported. Hanawa *et al.* reported on Ca^{2+}-implanted titanium (12, 13). The calcium ions were implanted into titanium with an energy of 18 keV. In *in vivo* experiments, more new bone was formed on the Ca^{2+}-treated side than on the untreated side. In addition, the bone made partial contact with the Ca^{2+}-treated surface. Ohtsuki *et al.* demonstrated that titanium becomes bioactive after a surface chemical treatment using an $H_2O_2/TaCl_5$ solution (14, 15). Commercially-available pure metallic titanium was chemically treated at 60°C for 24 h with H_2O_2 solutions containing various metals. Apatite deposited on the specimens treated with $H_2O_2/TaCl_5$ and $H_2O_2/SnCl_2$ solutions. Basic Ti-OH groups in titania hydrogel layers located on their surfaces were responsible for the apatite nucleation and growth. In addition, anatase titania gel layers were found to be bioactive, as they formed deposits of apatite incorporating carbonate ions in SBF.

In this review, we have focused on both bioactive glass coating and bioactive titanium. The results of research and clinical applications are reviewed and discussed.

BIOACTIVE GLASS COATING

Preparation of Bioactive Glass Coatings

We attempted to combine AW glass ceramic with titanium alloy implants to further accelerate the bone-bonding process of the implants and to improve the bone-bonding strength. As it appeared difficult to bind them chemically, the AW glass ceramic was mechanically coated over the surface of the titanium alloy implants in a very thin layer, using the dipping method in two ways: full coating and bottom coating. The full coating method did not improve the interfacial shear strength, but the bottom coating method significantly improved the shear strength compared with titanium plasma spray-coated titanium alloy implants. This difference is probably be due to the fact that the AW glass ceramic full-coated layer achieves direct bonding to bone, even though the mechanical strength of the porous titanium surface filled with bone tissue is stronger than that of AW glass ceramic.

With the bottom coated implants (fig. 2), the AW glass ceramic enhances bone ingrowth, and rapidly achieves direct mechanical anchoring with the pores at the implant surface, and bonds directly with the AW glass ceramic layers at the bottom of the pores.

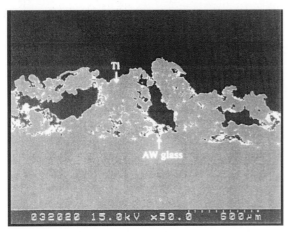

Figure 2 – Scanning electron microscope photograph of the cross-section of a porous layer with an AW bottom coating. The bright areas indicate the AW coating layer.

Animal Experiments Under Load-Bearing Conditions (Simulating Knee Arthroplasty) (16)

Three kinds of implants were prepared. 1) *Uncoated alumina ceramic implant*: a trapezoid alumina ceramic implant ($7 \times 10 \times 5$mm) with smooth surfaces. Each test piece had a small hole near the articular surface to provide an anchor to the jig used in the pull-out test. 2) *Titanium plasma spray-coated titanium alloy implant:* a titanium alloy implant of the same shape and size as above was prepared, and its side recess was plasma spray-coated with pure titanium. The recess was first plasma spray-coated with pure titanium, and then diffusion bonding and heat treatment at 1050°C were performed to bond the pure titanium firmly to the titanium alloy implant. The pore size of the coated layer was, on average, 380µm, and the porosity was 56 – 60% with an average of 58%. 3) *Titanium plasma spray-coated and AW glass ceramic-coated titanium alloy implant:* the titanium plasma spray-coated titanium alloy implant described above, was further coated on its side recess with AW glass ceramic using the dipping method with subsequent removal of the superficial AW glass ceramic (bottom coating). The AW glass

ceramic coating was so thin that the pore size of the coated surface remained almost unchanged.

The three types of implant described above were implanted in both the femoral condyles of adult mongrel dogs using the press-fit method. The animals were sacrificed 4, 8, or 24 weeks after surgery. Pull-out mechanical tests (fig. 3) and histological examinations were performed at each time for each group.

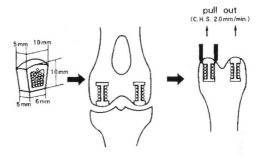

Figure 3 – Schematic drawings of the implant, implantation, and pull-out tests.

The results of the pull-out tests revealed that the AW glass ceramic bottom coating had the highest shear strength at all times, and that these values were statistically significant (fig. 4). Histological observations revealed that bone had gradually grown into the pores and, especially with the AW glass ceramic-coated implants, the maturation of trabecular bone and its direct contact were significantly advanced. These results indicated that when the AW glass ceramic was coated only in the bottom of pores of the titanium plasma spray-coated implants, then the bone-bonding process was accelerated and the bone-bonding strength was markedly improved.

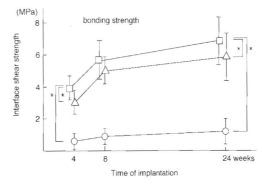

Figure 4 – Results of the pull-out tests for uncoated alumina ceramic implants (O), titanium plasma spray-coated titanium alloy implants (Δ), and titanium plasma spray-coated and AW glass ceramic-coated titanium alloy implants (□).(*): $p < 0.05$

Animal Experiments Under Load-Bearing Conditions (Simulating Hip Arthroplasty) (17)

Two types of cementless total hip prosthesis were studied in canine models. The femoral head was made of zirconia ceramic, 12 mm in diameter. The straight-stemmed, collared femoral component, was made of Ti-6Al-2Nb-1Ta, and had porous surfaces on the anterior and posterior proximal parts. The hemispherical acetabular component measured 20 mm in outer diameter, with four fixative screws. A 2-mm thick polyethylene liner provided the articulation with the femoral head. Both femoral and acetabular components were coated with plasma-sprayed titanium. In both components, the pores in the deep layer of one group were further coated with AW-glass ceramic using the dipping method, with subsequent removal of the superficial AW glass-ceramic to open the pores in the porous surface. The control group had the same components without any AW coating. The average pore size was 350μm, the porosity 60%, and the thickness of the porous layer of 700μm was identical in both groups.

Fifty dogs underwent unilateral total hip replacements, and were sacrificed 1, 3, or 6 months after surgery. The femoral and the acetabular components were evaluated mechanically and histologically.

After one month, the detaching load and bone ingrowth of the AW glass-ceramic coated femoral and acetabular components were higher than those of the control implants (Tables 1 and 2). However, there was no difference between the two groups at

Table 1 – The detaching load (N) of the femoral component. Mean ± SD

	1 month	3 months	6 months
AW Group	1 041 ± 206a	1514 ± 325	1815 ± 287a
Control group	671 ± 153b	1410 ± 259b	1691 ± 300b

a, b $p < 0.05$

Table 2 – The detaching load (N) of the acetabular component. Mean ± SD

	1 month	3 months	6 months
AW Group	299 ± 62a	583 ± 107a, c	720 ± 89a
Control group	197 ± 75b	274 ± 116b	617 ± 72b, c

a, b, c $p < 0.05$

3 and 6 months (fig. 5). Thus, the AW glass-ceramic enhanced the early phase in the cementless implant fixation process.

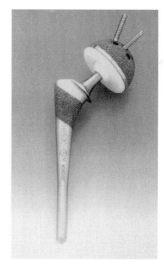

Figure 5 – A new cementless artificial hip joint system made of titanium alloy. The acetabular cup and proximal portion of the femoral component were porous coated using the plasma-spray method combined with AW bottom coating.

In this experiment, bone growth into the deepest part of the porous layer had already occurred at one month, even though the AW glass-ceramic was no longer present. Thus, the AW glass-ceramic enhanced bone ingrowth, and implant fixation by mechanical anchoring was achieved without any degradation of the ceramic. An AW glass-ceramic coating on the deeper part of the porous layer can lead to earlier implant fixation time, and thereby shorten the period of load-protection.

Clinical Application

A new type of cementless hip prosthesis was developed, and has been used clinically with success (fig. 5) (K-MAX ABC HIP® System, Kobe Steel Ltd., Kobe, Japan). As described above, the plasma-sprayed porous coated portions were treated with an additional AW glass ceramic bottom coating to enhance bone ingrowth. About 1 500 prostheses have been implanted for the treatment of hip disorders in Japan during the period 1996 to 2000.

Overall, according to our initial clinical trial data, the results were excellent. Radiographically, no femoral component was either definitely or probably loose. No side effect relating to the prosthesis was observed. These results indicate that the new cementless hip prosthesis is safe and reliable for the reconstruction of the hip joint.

Figure 6 shows a retrieved implant because of a femoral shaft fracture from the result of a postoperative accidental fall at seven months. Massive ingrown bone had bonded to the AW coated porous surface of the implant.

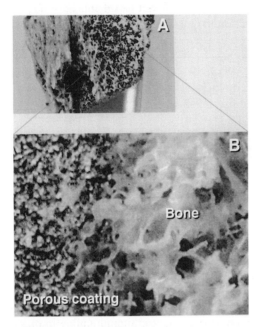

Figure 6 – The coated portion of a retrieved implant at seven months postoperative (A). Massive bone bonding has occurred at the porous surface (B).

BIOACTIVE TITANIUM

Formation of Functional Groups on Titanium Metal (18)

Chemical treatment of the surface of titanium metal is an established procedure to change a bioinert surface into a bioactive one. Titanium metal is simply immersed in aqueous NaOH solution, and subsequently heat treated to form sodium titanate on its surface. This sodium titanate overlayer is integrated onto the titanium surface through functionally graded properties, which are gradually altered without causing any phase discontinuity. The formation of Ti-OH surface functional groups via ion exchange of the Na^+ ion in the sodium titanate with the H_3O^+ ion in the fluid and the induction of apatite nucleation by the Ti-OH, causes the spontaneous growth of the apatite nuclei, consuming the calcium and phosphate ions

in the fluid, as shown in Figure 7. Figure 8 shows the bone-like apatite formations induced on a titania gel in an SBF.

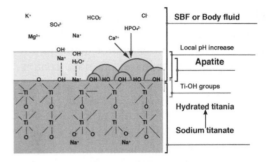

Figure 7 – A schematic representation of apatite formation on titanium metal subjected to the NaOH and heat treatments in a simulated body fluid or body environment.

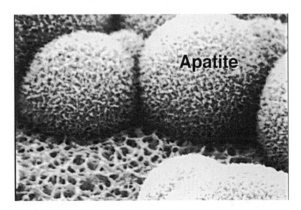

Figure 8 – Scanning electron microscope photograph (5000 ×) of the surface of titanium metal soaked in a simulated body fluid for three days after the treatment with 5.0 M NaOH at 60°C for 24 h, and heat treated at 600°C for 1 h.

For example, when commercially-pure titanium metal is exposed to 5 M NaOH at 60°C for 24 hours, a thin porous surface layer is formed, as shown in Figure 9. The sodium titanate hydrogel has a graded structure with a 1μm thickness. This gel layer is, however, so soft that it can be scratched with a dia-

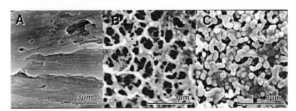

Figure 9 – Scanning electron microscope photographs (7000 ×) of the surfaces of titanium substrates: (A) before treatment, (B) after treatment with 5.0 M NaOH at 60°C for 24 h, (C) the same NaOH treatment and subsequent heat treatment at 600°C for 1 h.

mond needle under a load as small as 5 grf. The gel layer is stabilized as a fairly dense layer by heat treatment at 600°C for 1 h, as shown in Figure 9-C. This amorphous layer is so hard that it is not scratched even under a load as high as 20 grf.

These results mean that the bioactive surface layer is graded as a function of the depth toward the substrate and, therefore, it is not a coating.

Application for Titanium Alloys (19, 20)

As described, titanium metal can be made bioactive by surface chemical and thermal treatments. In the clinical arena, some titanium alloys, which possess superior mechanical properties, are often used for implants. Using the same scheme of NaOH and heat treatments, titanium alloys such as Ti-6Al-4V, Ti-6Al-2Nb-Ta and Ti-15Mo-5Zr-3Al have been shown to form functionally-graded bioactive sodium titanate on their surface, and these treated substrates form a dense and uniform bone-like apatite layer on their surface in a SBF. The present chemical and thermal surface treatment can be applied not only pure titanium metal, but also to some titanium alloys. This treatment can be applied to all existing titanium and titanium alloy implants.

Surface Stability of Bioactive Titanium *in vitro* (21)

The *in vitro* bonding strength of the apatite layer formed on titanium metals to substrates in the SBF were examined under tensile stress, and compared with those of apatite layers formed on Bioglass 45S5-type glass, dense sintered hydroxyapatite, and glass-ceramic AW, which are already used clinically. The NaOH-treated titanium metals showed a higher bonding strength of the apatite layer to the substrates than all the examined bioactive ceramics; this was maximized by heat treatments at 500 and 600°C. The adhesive strength of the apatite layer to the titanium substrate exceeded 30MPa, and it was also shown to have a graded interface on the metal substrate. The bioactive metals thus obtained are believed to be useful as bone substitutes, even under load-bearing conditions.

Mechanical Properties of Bioactive Titanium Metal (22)

The mechanical properties of bioactive titanium metal prepared from NaOH and heat treatments

were evaluated by tensile strength and fatigue tests, and compared with those of untreated titanium metal. The bioactive titanium metal showed tensile and yield strengths, reduction area and elongation, and fatigue behavior almost equal to those of the untreated metal (fig. 10). These results show that the surface NaOH and heat treatments have no adverse effect on the mechanical properties of the metal.

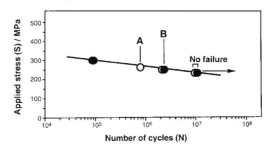

Figure 10 – S–N curves of the untreated (A), and the NaOH- and heat-treated (B) titanium metals.

Application for Microporous Structure (23)

A microporous titanium surface layer is often formed on titanium and titanium alloy implants for the fixation of the implants to bone *via* bony ingrowth into the porous structure. The NaOH and heat treatments produce a uniform amorphous sodium titanate layer on the surface of the porous titanium (figs. 11-A and 11-B). The sodium titanate induces a bone-like apatite formation in an SBF early on in the soaking period, whereby the apatite layer grows uniformly along the surface and cross-sectional microtextures of the porous titanium (fig. 11-C). Such a bioactive microporous layer on an implant is expected not only to enhance bony ingrowth into the porous structure, but also to provide a chemical integration with bone *via* apatite formation on its surface in the body.

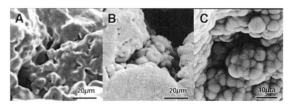

Figure 11 – Scanning electron microscope photographs of the surfaces of the porous titanium layer: (A) before treatment, (B) after treatment with 5.0M NaOH at 60°C for 24 h and heat treatment at 600°C for 1 h, and (C) (OLE4)after soaking in a simulated body fluid for seven days.

Bonding of Titanium Metal and Its Alloys to Living Bone (An *in vivo* Study)

The chemically surface-treated titanium metal was investigated in a number of animal models, revealing promising results toward clinical applications.

Evaluation in Rabbit Tibia (Non-Load-Bearing Condition) (24, 25)

Detaching test (26)

A rectangular-shaped titanium plate (15 × 10 × 2mm) was implanted into the metaphyses of the tibiae of rabbits. The titanium plates were implanted in a frontal direction, perforating the tibia, and protruding from the medial to lateral cortex. Following euthanasia of the rabbits, the segments of the proximal tibial metaphyses containing the implanted plates were harvested and prepared for the detaching test (fig. 12). Traction was applied vertically to the implant surface at a crosshead speed of 35mm/min using an Instron-type autograph through specially-designed hooks holding the bone–plate–bone construct. The detaching failure load was measured when the plate was detached from the bone. If the plate was detached before the test, the failure load was defined as "0 kgf". When a tensile stress was applied to their interfaces, the treated metals required a much higher load than the untreated metals to produce a fracture at the interface, and the difference between them increased with increasing time after the implantation (fig. 13).

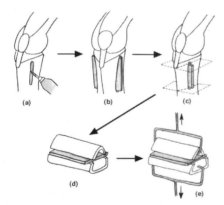

Figure 12 – Schematic drawings of the preparation of a rabbit tibial bone for the detaching test. (a) Making a bony hole at the medial cortex of the tibial metaphyses. (b) Insertion of the titanium plate into the tibia. (c) Cutting the tibia at the proximal and distal ends of the plate. (d) The bone-plate-bone construct. (e) Applying tensile load by holding the anterior and posterior cortices until detachment.

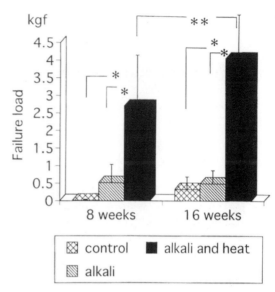

Figure 13 – Results of the detaching test. Failure loads (mean ± standard deviation). (*): $p < 0.001$. (**): $p < 0.05$.

Histological Examination at the Bone-Implant Interface

The bone to implant interface of undecalcified specimens was examined after the detaching test using scanning electron microscopy and surface stained microscopy. On being implanted into tibia of rabbit, the rectangular specimen of the chemically – and thermally – treated titanium metal and alloys (Ti-6Al-4V, Ti-6Al-2Nb-1Ta, and Ti-15Mo-5Zr-3Al) bonded directly to the bone (fig. 14-A). Meanwhile, the untreated implants had an intervening layer of fibrous tissue between the bone and the plate (fig. 14-B). Surface analysis of the titanium plate after the detaching test demonstrated that mature bone was well integrated with the porous structure of the treated surface (fig. 15).

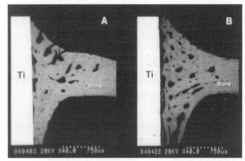

Figure 14 – Backscattered scanning electron microscope photographs of a bone–implant interface at eight weeks after implantation. A) NaOH- and heat-treated group, and (B) the non-treated group.

These findings indicate that the avulsion occurred not at the interface between the bone and implant, but in the bone.

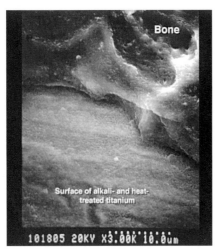

Figure 15 – Scanning electron microscope photograph of the surface of an NaOH⁻ and heat-treated titanium plate after the detaching test at 24 weeks after surgery. Mature bone is directly bonded, and well-integrated into the treated titanium.

Evaluation in the Femoral Canal (Simulating Hip Arthroplasty) (27)

On being implanted into the medullary canal of a femur, a cylindrical rod, 5mm in diameter and 25mm long, of alkali- and heat-treated titanium metal was completely covered with surrounding bone within 12 weeks. This is in contrast to the untreated metal. The treated metal required a much higher load for it to be pulled out from the medullary canal. At 12 weeks, fracture occurred not at the interface between the metal and the bone, but in the bone. Analysis, from confocal scanning laser micrographs, of the cross-sections showed that calcein-labeled areas were recognized at the surface of the titanium metal rod in the treated group. This finding indicates that apatite or new bone had formed on the surface of the treated titanium.

Bone Ingrowth into the Microporous Structure (Dog Femora) (28)

Porous titanium implants were prepared. A pure titanium rod, 4.6mm in diameter and 13mm long, was coated with pure titanium particles to a thickness of 0.7mm using the plasma-spraying technique. Three types of implants were manufactured from this porous implant. The control implant was

a porous titanium rod, and the other two implants were one with an additional AW-bottom coating and one subjected to the alkali and heat treatments. The implants were inserted hemi-transcortical fashion into the bilateral femora of dogs. At four and 12 weeks, the bone-bonding strengths were examined using the push-out test, and bone growth into the pores was evaluated histologically. At four weeks, the alkali- and heat-treated porous titanium showed higher shear strengths than the other two groups. At 12 weeks, there was no significant deference between the bonding strengths of the three groups, presumably because the strength of the mechanical interlocking was superior to that of chemical bonding by this time. Histologically, the direct bone contact with the implant surface was significantly higher in the alkali- and heat-treated group than in the other two groups (fig. 16).

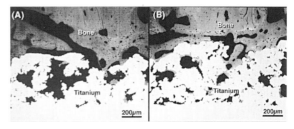

Figure 16 – Backscattered scanning electron microscope photographs of the cross-sections of (A) untreated, and (B) NaOH- and heat-treated porous titanium metals implanted in a canine femur for eight weeks.

When the titanium metal has a porous surface structure, the newly grown bone can penetrate into the pores uniformly. This occurs in the case of the alkali- and heat- treated samples; that is, the alkali and heat treatments can provide porous titanium implants with faster stable fixation. This alkali- and heat-treated porous titanium may be useful in clinical situations, for example, with cementless hip or knee arthroplasty.

Enhancement of Bioactive Ability

We have seen that titanium metal and alloys have bioactive surfaces after chemical and heat treatments. However, the bioactive ability of such treated titanium is inferior to those of AW glass ceramics and other bioactive ceramics. For clinical applications, it is necessary to enhance the bioactive ability to the level of those of other bioactive ceramics. Recently, it was revealed that a sodium removal stage introduced between the alkali and heat treatment processes accelerates the bioactive ability of alkali- and heat-treated titanium (29). In an *in vitro* study, titania gels with different concentrations of Na_2O or CaO were prepared using the sol-gel method, and heat-treated at different temperatures. Their apatite-forming abilities were examined in an SBF, and discussed in terms of their composition and structure. A titania gel formed the apatite on its surface in an SBF, where it assumed an anatase-like structure, irrespective of the composition. This indicates that a specific anatase structure of the titania gel is effective for apatite formation on its surface in a body environment.

In an *in vivo* study (30), sodium removal enhanced the bone-bonding strength of bioactive titanium at four and eight weeks after surgery. However, its bone-bonding strength was inferior to that of conventional alkali- and heat-treated titanium at 16 and 24 weeks. Histological examinations carried out after the detaching test revealed breakage of the treated layer in the sodium-free alkali- and heat-treated titanium group (fig. 17). These phenomena can be explained by sodium removal accelerating the *in vitro* and *in vivo* bioactivity of the bioactive titanium, and achieving faster bone-bonding because of its anatase surface structure. However, this means the loss of the surface's graded structure, as the complete removal of sodium decreases the adhesive strength of the treated layer to the titanium substrate. That is, a surface-graded structure is an essential condition to stabilize the porous structure of bioactive titanium and to achieve tight bonding.

Clinical Applications of Bioactive Titanium Metal and Its Alloys

As described above, there is some room for improvement in the bioactivity and surface stability of bioactive titanium. Bioactive metals have a high fracture toughness, as well as a high bone-bonding ability. Therefore, they are expected to be useful as bone substitutes, even under load-bearing conditions such as in hip and knee joints, the spine, and tooth roots. The advantages of bioactive titanium are its simple manufacturing process and cost benefits compared with HA plasma spray coating and other methods. Another advantage of this titanium surface treatment is its thin, strong bioactive layer. The treated layer is approximately 1μm thick, which is much thinner than commercially-available HA coatings. As this thin bioactive layer does not change the surface morphology of the implants, including screws and porous structures, this coating technique can be applied to all existing implants with precise surface structures.

Clinical trials of bioactive titanium alloys for application in hip joints have already begun. It is expected that a hip joint made of bioactive metal will be securely fixed to the surrounding bone for a long period.

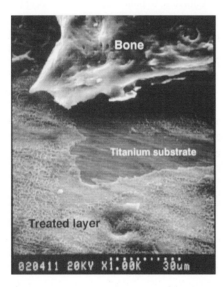

Figure 17 – Scanning electron microscope photograph of the surface of a sodium-free alkali- and heat-treated titanium plate after the detaching test at eight weeks after surgery. Breakage of the porous structure of the treated layer is evident.

Reference List

1. Ducheyne P, Qiu Q (1999) Bioactive ceramics: the effect of surface reactivity on bone formation and bone cell function. *Biomaterials* 20(23-24), 2287-303.

2. Head WC, Bauk DJ, Emerson RH Jr (1995) Titanium as the material of choice for cementless femoral components in total hip arthroplasty. *Clin. Orthop.* 311, 85-90.

3. Lester DK (1997) Microscopic studies of human press fit titanium hip prostheses. *Clin. Orthop.* 341, 143-50.

4. Yee AJ, Kreder HK, Bookman I, Davey JR (1999) A randomized trial of hydroxyapatite coated prostheses in total hip arthroplasty. *Clin. Orthop.* 366, 120-32.

5. McNally SA, Shepperd JA, Mann CV, Walczak JP (2000) The results at nine to twelve years of the use of a hydroxyapatite-coated femoral stem. *J. Bone Joint Surg. Br.* 82(3), 378-82.

6. Geesink RG, Hoefnagels NH (1995) Six-year results of hydroxyapatite-coated total hip replacement. *J. Bone Joint Surg. Br.* 77(4), 534-47.

7. Moroni A, Toksvig-Larsen S, Maltarello MC, Orienti L, Stea S, Giannini S (1998) A comparison of hydroxyapatite-coated, titanium-coated, and uncoated tapered external-fixation pins. An *in vivo* study in sheep. *J. Bone Joint Surg. Am.* 80(4), 547-54.

8. Kokubo T (1993) A/W glass-ceramic: Processing and properties. An introduction to Bioceramics, ed. By LL Hench and J Wilson, *World Sci.*, Singapore, p. 75-88.

9. Yamamuro T (1993) A/W glass-ceramic: Clinical application An introduction to Bioceramics, ed. By LL Hench and J Wilson, World Sci., Singapore, p. 89-103.

10. Kokubo T (1996) Spontaneous formation of bonelike apatite layer on chemically treated titanium metals *J. Am. Ceram. Soc.* 79(4), 1127-9.

11. Kokubo T, Kushitani H, Sakka S (1990) Solutions able to reproduce *in vivo* surface-structure changes in bioactive glass-ceramic A-W. *J. Biomed. Mater. Res.* 24, 721-34.

12. Hanawa T, Kamiura Y, Yamamoto S, Kohgo T, Amemiya A, Ukai H, Murakami K, Asaoka K (1997) Early bone formation around calcium-ion-implanted titanium inserted into rat tibia. *J. Biomed. Mater. Res.* 36(1), 131-6.

13. Hanawa T, Kon M, Ukai H, Murakami K, Miyamoto Y, Asaoka K (1997) Surface modifications of titanium in calcium-ion-containing solutions. *J. Biomed. Mater. Res.* 34(3), 273-8.

14. Ohtsuki C, Iida H, Hayakawa S, Osaka A (1997) Bioactivity of titanium treated with hydrogen peroxide solutions containing metal chlorides. *J. Biomed. Mater. Res.* 35(1), 39-47.

15. Wang XX, Hayakawa S, Tsuru K, Osaka A (2000) Improvement of bioactivity of H(2)O(2)/TaCl(5)-treated titanium after subsequent heat treatments. *J. Biomed. Mater. Res.* 52(1), 171-6.

16. Yamamuro T, Takagi H (1991) Bone bonding behavior of biomaterials with different surface characteristics under load-bearing condition. Bone Biomaterials Interface (Ed. Davis JE) Toronto Univ, Toronto 406-14.

17. Ido K, Matsuda Y, Yamamuro T, Okumura H, Oka M, Takagi H (1993) Cementless total hip replacement Bioactive glass ceramic coating studied in dogs. *Acta Orthop. Scand.* 64(6), 607-12.

18. Kim HM, Miyaji F, Kokubo T, Nishiguchi S, Nakamura T (1999) Graded surface structure of bioactive titanium prepared by chemical treatment. *J. Biomed. Mater. Res.* 45(2), 100-7.

19. Kim HM, Miyaji F, Kokubo T, Nakamura T (1996) Preparation of bioactive Ti and its alloys via simple chemical surface treatment. *J. Biomed. Mater. Res.* 32(3), 409-17.

20. Kim HM, Takadama H, Kokubo T, Nishiguchi S, Nakamura T (2000) Formation of a bioactive graded surface structure on Ti-15Mo-5Zr-3Al alloy by chemical treatment. *Biomaterials* 21(4), 353-8.

21. Kim HM, Miyaji F, Kokubo T, Nakamura T (1997) Bonding strength of bonelike apatite layer to Ti metal substrate. *J. Biomed. Mater. Res.* 38(2), 121-7.

22. Kim HM, Sasaki Y, Suzuki J, Fujibayashi S, Kokubo T, Matsushita T, Nakamura T (2000) Mechanical properties of bioactive titanium metal prepared by chemical treatment Bioceramics Vol.13 Trans Tech Pub, Switzerland p. 227-30.

23. Kim HM, Kokubo T, Fujibayashi S, Nishiguchi S, Nakamura T (2000) Bioactive macroporous titanium surface layer on titanium substrate *J. Biomed. Mater. Res.* 52, 553-7.

24. Nishiguchi S, Nakamura T, Kobayashi M, Kim HM, Miyaji F, Kokubo T (1999) The effect of heat treatment on bone-bonding ability of alkali-treated titanium. *Biomaterials* 20(5), 491-500.

25. Nishiguchi S, Kato H, Fujita H, Kim HM, Miyaji F, Kokubo T, Nakamura T (1999) Enhancement of bone-bonding strengths of titanium alloy implants by alkali and heat treatments. *J. Biomed. Mater. Res.* 48(5), 689-96.

26. Nakamura T, Yamamuro T, Higashi S, Kokubo T, Ito S (1985) A new glass-ceramic for bone replacement: evaluation of its bonding ability to bone tissue *J. Biomed. Mater. Res.* 19, 631-48.

27. Nishiguchi S, Kato H, Fujita H, Oka M, Kim HM, Kokubo T, Nakamura T (2001) Titanium metals form direct bonding to bone after alkali and heat treatments. *Biomaterials* 22(18), 2525-533.

28. Nishiguchi S, Kato H, Neo M, Oka M, Kim HM, Kokubo T, Nakamura T (2001) Alkali- and heat-treated porous titanium for orthopedic implants. *J. Biomed. Mater. Res.* 54(2), 198-208.

29. Uchida M, Kim HM, Kokubo T, Fujibayashi S, Nakamura T (2002) Effect of water treatment on the apatite-forming ability of NaOH-treated titanium metal. *J. Biomed. Mater. Res.* 63(5), 522-30.

30. Fujibayashi S, Nakamura T, Nishiguchi S, Tamura J, Uchida M, Kim HM, Kokubo T (2001) Bioactive titanium: effect of sodium removal on the bone-bonding ability of bioactive titanium prepared by alkali and heat treatment. *J. Biomed. Mater. Res.* 56(4), 562-70.

2   Radiological Assessment and Predictive Meaning of Bone Remodeling in Cementless Implants

Philippe Massin, MD and Jean-Alain Epinette, MD

INTRODUCTION

This chapter deals with several kinds of radiographic changes that are currently observed following insertion of a cementless femoral component in total hip arthroplasty. This includes bone modeling and particle-induced osteolysis.

Bone modeling we define as the reaction of the host bone to the mechanical stress provoked by the implantation of a metallic implant. In fact, insertion of a stiff stem into the intramedullary canal of the femur greatly alters the stress patterns of the bone. In the intact loaded femur, the level of stresses supported by the cortical bone decreases from the proximal part down to the mid shaft. Conversely, this gradient is reversed in the implanted femur (26, 27). Bone modeling is more apparent around cementless stems. Its formal description dates back to the 1990s, with the publication of a radiographic score by CA Engh and Ph Massin (14). Later on, JA Epinette and RGT Geesink (15), based on their observations of long-term results obtained with hydroxyapatite (HA)-coated implants, felt it necessary to adapt this score, because bone modeling was found to be milder around this new generation of stems. This is why they proposed the ARA score.

Bone modeling develops secondarily to the fixation of living structures to an inert material. It appears during the first two years following the operation, and generally settles down thereafter (14). It is dependant on the quality of the bone fixation, which may be more or less successful. The success of this so-called "biologic" or "secondary" fixation is highly related to the stability of the initial or "primary" fixation achieved at surgery.

Radiographic changes that are currently observed around cementless implants include also another kind of bone resorption called osteolysis, which can extensively destroy bone. Such a phenomena is explained by a biological process induced by a cellular reaction to wear debris that comes from either a joint space where it has accumulated (bearing surfaces, *etc.*), or from some other aspect of the metallic implant (e.g., local fretting mechanism). Unlike bone modeling, which suggests bone growth in the medullary canal toward the implant surface, osteolysis always results in bone destruction (8,30).

The purpose of the current chapter is to assess the predictive value of these radiographic changes on implant fixation. A failure of fixation can proceed from 2 mechanisms, either a failure of the biologic fixation, leading to implant instability, or from the destruction of a previously stable fixation by an extensive osteolysis (22).

In surgical practice, the decision process at revision surgery may be greatly improved by a better understanding of the bone resorption mechanism. If the radiographic appearance of bone modeling is optimal, the development of severe osteolytic lesions should lead to revision of only the damaged bearings and replacement of them by new ones without removing the implants that are still solidly fixed to their bony support. Eventually, zones of bone lysis can be grafted. Conversely, if the radiographic appearance of bone modeling suggests the failure of implant osteointegration, the entire prosthesis must be revised.

In the following article, the term "porous-coated" refers to porous metallic surfaces that are not covered with HA, while the term HA-coated refers to any porous surfaces covered with HA. The term "macroporous" applies to any coating featuring macrostructures (beads, mesh, *etc.*), while "microporous" applies to grit-blasted surfaces. By extension, the term "coating" generally refers to any surfaces that eventually become ingrown by bone, whereas "smooth" surfaces can only reach a state of bone contact or bone apposition, with no microinterlocking between the bone and the metal.

Bone Modeling: How it Works

The radiographic appearance of bone modeling depends on the prosthetic design, the surface finish of the stem, the difference between the stiffness of the implant and of its bone support, and finally, on the stability of the bone-implant interface.

The Prosthetic Design

An adequate prosthetic design is mandatory if a successful primary mechanical fixation is to be achieved. A stable initial fixation requires an adaptation of the geometry of the implant to the shape of the medullary canal. It can be obtained by filling the metaphysis, thus achieving a proximal bone contact with a variable amount of press-fit. This kind of fixation can be improved by the use of a collar, or by retention of the neck according to M. Freeman (16). In contrast, a distal fixation requires a diaphyseal press-fit.

A proximal fixation is expected to respect the physiologic gradient of the bone stresses, thus reducing the bone modeling. Due to the conical shape of the metaphysis, and consequently of the proximal aspect of a well-designed stem, the primary fixation is optimized by the load. The self-impaction mechanism of a so-called "taper slide" stem helps decrease the shear stresses at the bone-metal interface, while increasing the compression stresses. According to the Wolff's laws, compressive stresses preserve or increase the bone density.

Conversely, a diaphyseal press fit is expected to deeply alter the gradient of bone stresses, by "shielding" the metaphysis, thus inducing an over-stated bone modeling of the surrounding bone. Using cylindrical implants to match the femoral isthmus increases the shear and the tensile stresses at the bone-metal interface, and is likely to provoke disuse osteoporosis of the adjacent bone.

Stem Surface Finish

The type of surface finish interferes with the bone modeling process because it alters the stresses at the bone-metal interface. Two types of surface finish currently used are the rough surface-finish

corresponding to "macrostructured" surface, and the smooth surface finish corresponding to a "microstructured" surface.

Macrostructures are of different types, such as madrepore, porous-coating with 250 to 400 micrometers diameter pores, or fibermesh (fig. 1). There are several different methods for fixing the beads or the mesh to the implant, such as high-temperature sintering, diffusion bonding, or plasma-spray. With this type of surface finish, biologic fixation is achieved by "bone ingrowth" or "fibrous ingrowth" into the pores of an irregular surface. This results in an intimate bond between the metal and the bone called microinterlocking. If this type of interconnection between the inert material and the bone happens to develop, the stiffer material (i.e., the metallic stem) supports the majority of the load. Thus, the less stiff material (i.e., the surrounding bone), is "stress and strain protected" or stress-shielded (12). Such a firm bond between two materials of different stiffness results in shear and tensile stresses at the bone-metal interface. The bone reaction involves a more or less important loss of bone density and a higher level of porosity (sponginess-like phenomenon), at least in the portion of the bony structure adjacent to the osseointegrated macrostructured surface (12, 19).

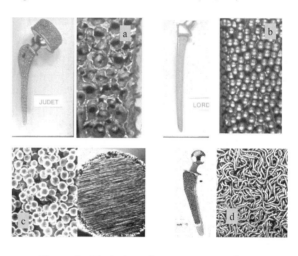

Figure 1 – Evolution of macroporous surfaces:
a) The Judet madreporic prosthesis
b) The minimadreporic Lord prosthesis
c) The sintered porous coated implants (AML prosthesis)
d) The Titanium fiber mesh (Harris Galante prosthesis)

In contrast, a smooth or microstructured surface allows some micromotion at the bone-metal interface, which will not jeopardize bone growth at the metal surface if the micromovements do not exceed one hundred microns (32). Should an optimal bone contact be achieved, the transmission of the load from the metal to the bone is less dependent on the difference in stiffness between the bone and the metal. Rather, it is related to the design of the prosthesis (18). The level of the compressive stresses tends to increase, while the level of the shear stresses (tangential to the interface) and of the tensile stresses (perpendicular to the interface) tends to decrease. Bone modeling is less pronounced.

Gradient of Stiffness Between Bone and Metallic Implant

The higher is the difference in stiffness between the bone and the implant, the more severe the bone modeling. This situation of stress shielding leads to a long-lasting decrease in bone density.

The implant stiffness depends primarily on the modulus of elasticity of its constituting alloy. Thus, titanium (Ti) has a lower modulus of elasticity than cobalt chromium (CoCr). Because the modulus of elasticity of titanium is closer to that of cortical bone, it is more suitable for cementless fixation (26). In addition, the stiffness of the implant increases with the cube of its caliber (12).

The bone stiffness also varies with its modulus of elasticity. The cortical bone has a higher modulus of elasticity than the cancellous bone. Like the stem, the stiffness of the femur is related to the caliber of its diaphysis and also to the thickness of its cortices. Thus two extreme situations can be described (12). On one hand, a large stem may be required if one has to implant the osteoporotic femur of an elderly female patient who has a wide medullary canal and thin cortices. In such a case, bone modeling is expected to be severe. On the other hand, a small implant should fit in a strong femur of a young patient with a narrow canal and thick cortices. Because the gradient in stiffness between the bone and the implant is lower, bone modeling is likely to be mild (19).

In fact, all kinds of in-between situations may be encountered. Precise information regarding specifications of both the alloy and the type of the metallic substrate is critical for assessing the features of bone modeling.

Type of Biological Anchorage

In the great majority of hip replacements performed with the currently available devices, biologic fixation results in a firm bond between the bone and the metal, with an intimate contact between the two structures. However, secondary stabilization of the stem by the biologic fixation can be incomplete, or may eventually fail. In these latter cases, intervening fibrous tissue grows between the bone and the metal. It may even encompass the entire implant with a fibrous encapsulation. Sufficient stability of the implant can eventually be obtained, but clinical failures are more likely to occur with this type of fixation.

When the bone has grown toward the metallic surface, a stable fixation is achieved, and bone modeling generally develops in the first postoperative year. It can be severe if a large, porous-coated, press-fitted stem is implanted in osteoporotic bone. In contrast, it is mild or barely noticeable on standard films if a less rigid grit-blasted stem of small caliber (titanium alloy, small size) is implanted with a metaphyseal press-fit in a highly dense bone with thick cortices.

In the case of a fibrous encapsulation, the stability of the implant depends on the thickness and of the density of the fibrous layer. Its most characteristic radiographic feature takes place at the bone-metal interface: it is the radiolucent space, whose width correspond to the thickness of the fibrous layer. Usually, bone modeling is very different, because there is no firm bond between the metal and the bone. In these cases, bone modeling depends on both the design of the implant and of its stability.

In the case of a loose fibrous encapsulation, the stem tends to subside and to rotate. The upper part of the femur withstands stresses that are similar or even higher than those supported by an intact femur. Subsidence of collared implants produces high compression stresses at the calcar, which can far exceed the bone strength and eventually lead to bone necrosis and bone resorption (10, 13). Thus, in contrast to the bony fixation, fibrous encapsulation results in calcar densification.

Description of The Radiographic Patterns of Bone Remodeling

Lucent Lines and Reactive Lines

The description of the so-called "radiolucencies" is often confusing, because it is used for the description of various radiographic patterns of bone modeling such as "the radiolucent space", or "radiopaque lines". Actually, both aspects are usually combined, and the radiopaque line delimits the radiolucent space, allowing it to be visible.

Moreover, the term "radiolucencies" is frequently used for characterizing different patterns, involving opposed histologic phenomena. In the English semantics, the term "radiolucency" is used according to its descriptive meaning, i.e., lower bone density as compared to the adjacent bone. This refers to a visual impression of contrast, and one must be very cautious in trying to interpret it. Sometimes it results from a cortical cancellization, which tends to develop in elderly female osteoporotic patients at the metal-bone interface (21, 24). The term "neo-canal" was even used to explain this kind of bone modeling around cemented stems (9).

Radiolucencies are also observed in the cases of a more or less stable implant surrounded by fibrous tissue. It generally takes the radiographic appearance of a thin, regular space of constant width, delimited by a thin dense line, surrounding the prosthetic stem or the cement mantle. When the radiolucent space remains stable and parallel to the implant surface, secondary fibrous stabilization is likely to have occurred (fig. 2). If the width of the

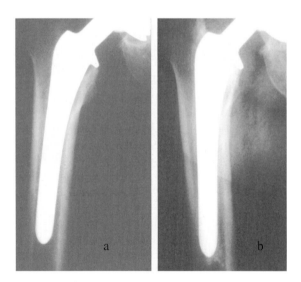

Figure 2 – Example of a stable fibrous encapsulation of a smooth Titanium cementless stem at 2 years (AP view). Note the condensation of the calcar, the radiolucency at the shoulder of the prosthesis, the pedestal below the tip of the stem.

space happens to exceed 2 or 3 mm, the secondary stabilization of the implant becomes questionable. Should the radiolucent space appear divergent to the metallic surface, the implant is likely to migrate, and should be considered unstable (fig. 3).

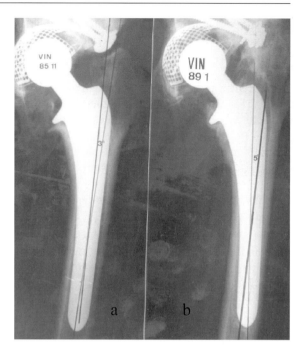

Figure 3 – In this case, the fibrous encapsulation has failed to stabilize the implant. The implant has migrated continuously from the postoperative status (3a) over the 2 first postoperative year (3b) with a varus tilt of the stem. Supero- lateral and infero-medial radiolucencies have developed and look divergent. The collar is embedded by dense bone. This is a definite failure of the biologic fixation.

Histologic analysis reveals a more or less well-organized layer of fibrous tissue in relation to the degree of instability. In the most favorable cases, the layer of fibrous tissue is dense and formed with concentric layers of fibroblasts (25). The fibrous layer is delineated by a line of edging bone formation corresponding to the radiopaque line (fig. 4). This pattern should be associated with a negative score in regard to implant stability, because it is significantly correlated with the occurrence of implant migration. In particular, it has a poor prognosis if located in regard to a coated surface, or if it encompasses the all implant.

"Reactive lines" have a different meaning. However, at first glance, they are difficult to differentiate from lucent lines. They consist of a thin, dense line approximately 1 mm away from the implant surface, parallel to it, with regular and identical bone density on either side of the line. Hence, they look similar to the lucent lines ; however, their evolution is different. Over the years, these reactive lines may thicken progressively and reach the metal. Such reactive lines are currently observed at the distal smooth portion of proximally coated stems (fig. 5).

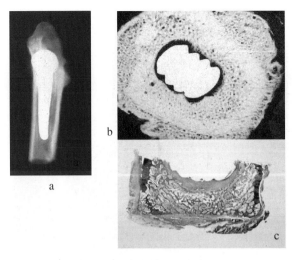

Figure 4 – From a canine study (Massin *et al.*, Int Orthop, 1991): Histology of the radiolucent line around a smooth cementless femoral.

a) Radiographic aspect of the radiolucent space

b) Microradiography showing the bone ingrowth into the medullary canal

c) Histologic aspect of the radiolucent space corresponding to a layer of fibrous tissue delimited by a front of active ossification

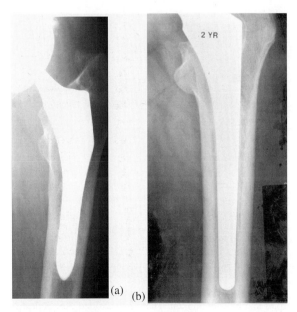

Figure 5 – Radiographs showing the aspect of the bone modeling around two HA-coated implants, i.e., ABG stem (5a) and HA Omnifit stem (5b) having with respectively 8 and 2 years of follow-up. The clinical result is excellent. Bone trabeculae are visible between the femoral cortex and the metal, with a ascendant direction. On the lefthand side, bone trabeculae are visible at the tip of the stem, suggesting complete implant osteointegration. Calcar modeling is mild. On the right handside, a reactive line surrounds the distal smooth part of the stem. There is no pedestal.

Histologically, the dense line corresponds to an active ossification front with thick osseous and dense trabecular bays, scattered with numerous osteoblasts. The space between this dense line and the implant is filled in by bone of lesser density, so that the radiopaque line appears like a neocortex within the medullary canal (9). This scenario supposes that the stem has been initially stabilized by the growth of the bone. Actually, they correspond to a late densification of the cancellous bone, which has enveloped the distal extremity of the stem.

One way to explain these lines consists of assimilating them to a line of microfractures, resulting from the persistence of important strains in the bony structure in contact with the smooth portion of a fully osteointegrated stem (15).

Remodeling of the Calcar at the Medial Metaphyseal Cortex

Although remodeling can be more or less pronounced, it is almost a constant phenomenon around intramedullary femoral implants, whatever the type of their fixation (cementless or cemented). Calcar modeling corresponds to 2 different radiographic patterns, calcar atrophy, and the calcar loss of density or calcar cancellization. It can be difficult to distinguish from the calcar resorption due to osteolysis.

Atrophy corresponds to either a loss of thickness of the medial metaphyseal cortex or to a loss of height of the calcar. Sometimes it is mild and takes the aspect of a simple "round-off" of the medial cortex. Its meaning is different, whether it is combined with a loss of bone density or with bone condensation.

Cancellization of the calcar corresponds to a loss of bone density at the medial metaphyseal cortex (fig. 6). It generally arises when facing an adjacent porous-coated area of the implant surface. If the bone has grown into the porosity of that surface, the calcar area becomes stress and strain protected, because the majority of the load is supported by the implant. The extent of this bone loss is directly related to the extent of the coated area. This loss of bone density becomes apparent on standard radiographs if it exceeds 40% of the bone mass. This "stress-shielding" aspect is typically predominant in the proximal areas of the femur, because the difference of stiffness between the implant and the femur is the greatest at that level.

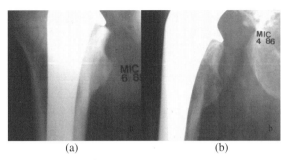

(a)   (b)

Figure 6 – Radiographs showing a mild calcar modeling below the collar of a smooth Titanium implant (6a: postop; 6b: 4 years postoperatively). There is no radiolucency at other portion of the bone implant interface. The implant has remained stable and the clinical result is optimal.

Implant stiffness is high because it generally concerns the part of the stem with the largest caliber, the stiffness of the femur is low because the thickness of the cortical bone is thinner proximally than distally. Conversely, the gradient in stiffness between the implant and the bone decreases progressively from the metaphysis to the diaphysis, while the caliber of the stem decreases and the thickness of the cortices increases.

Engh and Massin (14) have considered the cancellization of the calcar as a sign highly predictive of bony ingrowth. They found it to have a high level of specificity for bone fixation. However, it is also true that an absence of calcar cancellization does not necessarily mean the absence of bone ingrowth. In fact, it is milder with grit-blasted implants, particularly if they are manufactured from a alloy with a low modulus of elasticity.

Condensation of the calcar has a different meaning, and suggests increased compressive stresses (fig. 7). It is sometimes related to an instability of the stem, which tends to subside. If the stem is supplied with a collar, compressive stresses are amplified below the collar. These stresses can exceed the bone strength and provoke bone necrosis. In extreme cases in which the stem is grossly unstable, a paradoxical aspect of calcar hypertrophy can even be observed. In theses cases, which correspond to impending failures of implant fixation, the collar appears embedded in ectopic ossifications (figs 3 and 8). It is not uncommon to note a lucent line in zone 6 of Gruen, just below the calcar. Hence, condensation of the calcar can be considered highly predictive of fibrous fixation, whether stable or unstable (10, 14).

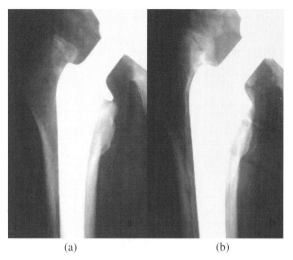

(a)   (b)

Figure 7 – Radiographs showing the calcar condensation below the collar of a smooth Titanium implant, which displayed an early migration, before being stabilized (7a: postop film; 7b: 5 years postoperatively). Note the radiolucency at the shoulder of type implant. This bone modeling suggests a secondary fibrous stabilization of the implant.

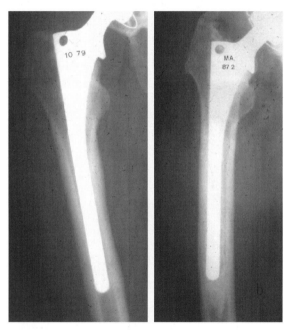

Figure 8 – Example of a pedestal developed below the tip of an unstable implant. The stem subsided. The pedestal is connected with an infero-medial radiolucency suggesting a varus tilt of the implant.

Endosteal Ossification

Endosteal ossifications or "spot welds" consist of areas of dense bone growing within the medullary canal, bridging the gap left between the cortical bone and the implant surface. Therefore, they are particularly visible at these spots where the implant does not contact the femoral cortex. There are currently observed at the level of the implant surface where the porous coating stops. Spot welds also delimit the upper portion of the femoral cortex, which has been stress shielded from the distal portion, which has conserved its original density (fig. 9).

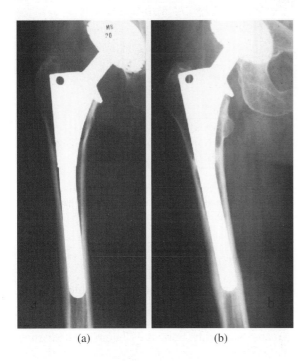

(a)   (b)

Figure 9 – Radiographs showing spot-welds at the junction between the porous coated area and the smooth distal portion of a cementless AML stem. Note the density and the hypertrophy of the cortices around the smooth portion of the stem, attesting of a complete bone osteointegration (9a: postop film ; 9b: 6 years postoperatively).

This pattern of bone modeling typically results from the change of regimen in bone stresses. Above the spot welds, i.e., adjacent to the porous surface, compressive stresses are shielded from the bone, whereas shear stresses predominate. Below the spot welds, compressive stresses are transmitted from the implant to the bone, whereas shear stresses tend to vanish. With grit-blasted stems, bone modeling is less apparent and spot-welds can be absent.

Histologically, these endosteal ossifications correspond to bays of dense bone tissue. Engh and Massin (14) considered endosteal ossifications as a

sign highly predictive of bone ingrowth. However, the absence of spot welds does not necessarily the absence of bone ingrowth.

Bone Remodeling at the Tip of the Stem

The pedestal is an endosteal bone formation that grows below the tip of the stem. It can be compared to a plug, which obstructs, more or less completely, the medullary canal. If it is complete, it takes a symmetrical aspect. If not, it is asymmetric. Its superior limit looks like the bottom of an egg, and is well delineated from the rest of the canal.

We interpret the pedestal as a local reaction to overall instability of the stem. In some cases, the pedestal is connected to radiolucencies encompassing the distal portion of the stem. In these cases, the pedestal should be considered as an attempt of the host to limit the subsidence of an otherwise unstable implant. So, it has a poor predictive value in regard to bone fixation. Generally, the stem is definitively unstable (fig. 9). Rarely, the pedestal may eventually disappear, should a proximal fixation of the stem by bone become secondarily successful (mainly seen with HA-coated implants) (fig. 10).

In other cases, the pedestal comes in contact with the tip of the stem with no intervening radiolucency. In these cases, one may consider that a distal bone fixation of the stem has occurred, whereas fixation of the proximal portion by bone has failed. Eventually, proximal radiolucencies may be present, in contrast with the density and the thickening of the distal cortex (fig. 11). We call this kind of pedestal a "stable pedestal", in contrast to the former aspect, which is called an "unstable pedestal".

Finally, the pedestal must be distinguished from a distal spot weld in these extensively coated implants with no smooth distal portion. Like spot welds, it delimits the shielded portion of the femur, which is solidly connected to the porous coating, from the lower femur below the tip of the stem, which sustains physiologic stresses and strains.

Thus, interpreting the pedestal in terms of stem stability can raise some difficulties. With partially coated implants, the absence or the resorption of a pre-existing pedestal is highly suggestive of successful bone growth at the coated portion of the stem. With extensively coated implants, a pedestal combined with distal radiolucencies, suggest definite failure of the biologic fixation. It must be distinguished from a spot-weld embedding the tip of

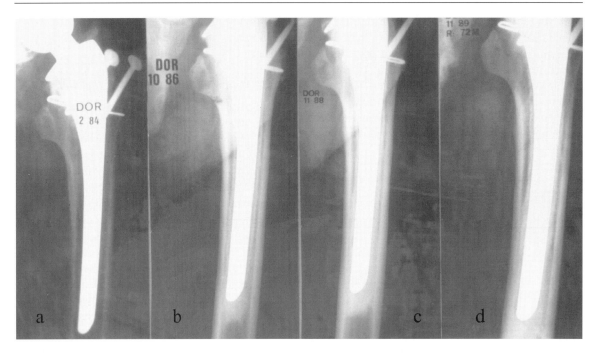

Figure 10 – Radiographs showing a secondary late stabilization of a smooth cementless Titanium implant by bone over years from 10a to 10d. Note that the implant has subsided. The calcar is dense and has embedded the collar. The radiolucencies have finally disappeared, leaving place to a bone osseointegration of the whole implant.

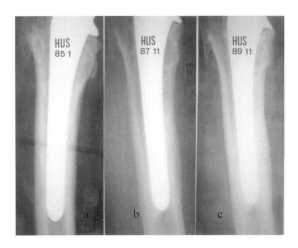

Figure 11 – Example of a radiolucency surrounding a smooth Titanium cementless femoral prosthesis. However, the lucencies do not reach the pedestal and stop at some distance form the tip of the stem. Distal cortices have thickened and a pedestal has grown below the tip of the stem, attesting to the successful host response to stabilize the implant. Calcar modeling is absent. The implant is stable and fixed mainly at a distal level. The pedestal belongs to the category "stable" (11a: postop film; 11b: 2 years postop; 11c: 4 years postoperatively).

the stem that, on the contrary, suggests complete implant osteointegration.

Cortical Hypertrophy

Cortical hypertrophy is an external thickening of the cortex, symmetrical or not, without any periostitis or reaction of the adjacent soft tissues. It produces a smoothly bordered "bump" that disrupts the contour of the femur. We distinguish two aspects of different significance in terms of implant stability. In the first aspect, the cortical hypertrophy is isolated, asymmetric, and involves the distal lateral Gruen zone 3. Generally, this pattern is combined with divergent lucent lines onto the medial distal and lateral proximal zones of the bone implant interface. They indicate a varus tilt of the stem. In such a case, the lateral cortical hypertrophy provides evidence of abnormal compressive stresses at the lateral and distal aspects of the stem. Typically, it is associated with a condensation of the calcar. It is related to some degree of implant instability.

The second aspect consists of a symmetric cortical hypertrophy around the distal portion of the stem. Sometimes it is asymmetric, but it involves the distal and medial aspect of the metal bone interface (zone 5 of Gruen), corresponding to the portion of the femoral cortex which is submitted to compression under physiological load. We believe that it is explained by an optimal bone fixation of the distal portion of the stem. It is a response of the bone to the transmission of the load from the implant to the femoral cortex. It can be associated with a "stable" pedestal, if the proximal coated portion has not been ingrown by bone (fig. 11). There is no pedestal when the stem has been completely osteointegrated.

In conclusion, the aspect of the bone modeling depends on the type of the biologic fixation around the implant (fibrous or bony), and is consequently correlated to the stability of the stem (34). Should bone fixation occur, the intensity of the bone modeling is related to the specifications of the implant (stiffness, constituting alloy), and to the quality of the bone support (degree of osteoporosis). If present, these patterns can be combined so as to form two opposite characteristic aspects. If the bone has grown in a macroporous surface, a proximal loss of bone density is associated with endosteal ossifications and, eventually, with a distal cortical hypertrophy. However, there is no pedestal below the tip of the stem, and no lucent line at the bone metal interface (fig. 12). Conversely, if the implant has been encapsulated by fibrous tissue, an increase in the calcar density is often associated with extensive lucent lines along the coated areas of the stem surface, and with a pedestal below the tip of the stem. Moreover, a certain amount of implant migration can be observed (fig. 8).

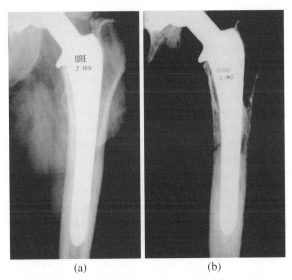

(a)   (b)

Figure 12 – Typical aspect of stress-shielding at 5 years around a smooth cementless implant. The diaphyseal cortices are dense and thick, whereas the proximal portion of the bone has almost vanished. There is no radiolucency. Complete bone osteointegration is very likely (12a: postop; 12b: at 5 years).

Biological Response to Wear Debris

The particle-induced bone resorption is sometimes difficult to recognize from the loss of bone density due to bone modeling, particularly in its subliminal aspect. In fact, it can take the form of an insidious radiolucent space that widens progressively. On the contrary, it is easy to identify when it takes the form of an extensive pseudo-tumoral bone cyst completely empty of any bony substance, with smooth and rounded limits.

Their location is not related to changes in bone stresses, but rather to the dissemination of wear debris (23). This migration is induced by mechanical phenomena. The contraction of the muscles about the hip increases the intra-articular pressure, which in turn propels the intra-articular fluid toward the bone metal interface, should this interface be permeable for some reason. Moreover, opposite stresses are successively supported by the stem during the gait (compressive and tensile stresses), which may result in a pumping mechanism at the bone metal interface (31).

Osteolysis can develop at the proximal aspect of the femur, close to the joint space, in which wear debris logically accumulate. Due to the migration of the particles, osteolysis can also take place at remote portions of the bone metal interface.

Proximal osteolysis was described for more than 20 years with cemented stems by Blaker and Charnley (4). These authors called it "cavitation" of the calcar. It is also currently observed into the cancellous bone of the greater trochanter (fig. 13). While calcar osteolysis progresses slowly, the progression of trochanteric osteolysis is rather rapid and extensive. Proximal osteolysis tends to grow toward the more distal portion of the femur (35), and may affect the entire bone metal interface. Usually, this type of bone resorption looks like a radiolucent space. However, while the radiolucency in relation to a fibrous interposition is well delineated from the adjacent bone, the radiolucency in relation to osteolysis has an irregular contour, realizing a characteristic aspect called "scalloping".

Distal osteolysis can be either isolated or associated with proximal osteolysis. It is explained by the migration of wear debris at some aspects of the implant surface that have remained free from bone growth. Logically, distal osteolysis is rarely observed with proximally coated implants ingrown by bone on the entirety of their circumference (11,

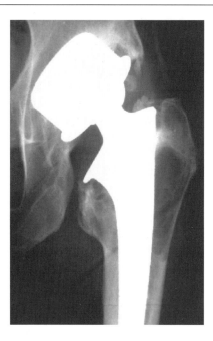

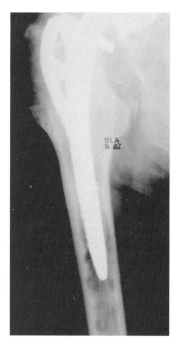

Figure 13 – Example of an extensive osteolysis in the greater trochanter. Note the wear of the polyethylene measured by the upper displacement of the center of the head in the metallic shell.

Figure 14 – Radiographic appearance of a Judet madreporic prosthesis at 11 years of follow-up. Example of an osteolysis developing at the tip of the stem, whereas the rest of the bone implant interface remains intact. The implant is stable with more than 10 years of follow-up. Note the aspect of "scalloping" surrounding the tip of the stem.

29). However, distal osteolysis can be associated with positive signs of bone modeling for bone fixation (20), because these signs appear as soon as some bone has grown into the pores of the macrostructure at some place on the implant surface, even if the rest of it remains uninvolved in the process (fig. 14).

Histologically, osteolytic cysts are filled with a lumpy, whitish tissue that is sometimes combined with fibrous tissue. Bony areas surrounding the cavity demonstrate an inflammatory reaction, with accumulation of numerous macrophagic cells, histiocytes, or giant multinuclear cells. If polyethylene debris are present, microscopic examination in polarized light can show birefringent particles located into the macrophagic cells, corresponding to polyethylene debris. Centrifugation of membranes obtained at revision surgery or from specimens retrieved at autopsy revealed that most of these debris had a submicron size (23). Optical microscopy allows visualization of particles of larger size, extra cellular, migrating between the trabecular bays into the medullary spaces of the cancellous bone. Metallic debris can also be present and are sometimes predominant (1). The question of hydroxyapatite debris leading to early wear of polyethylene (5) remains controversial. In fact,

the presence of hydroxyapatite debris detached from the coating of the prosthesis itself has not been confirmed. Moreover, the long term observation of HA-coated implants has not revealed unusual wear (2, 28).

Osteolytic lesions progress as long as the bearings remain in place. Exchange of the bearings stops the osteolytic process. The cysts formed prior to revision do not heal spontaneously, so grafting at the time of revision is suitable to reconstruct the defects (3). Usually, osteolysis is a delayed process, which rarely appears before the seventh postoperative year. To our knowledge, no precise data support the hypothesis that osteolysis would be more frequent in case of fibrous fixation compared to the bony fixation (11). However, the faster progression of polyethylene particulates along smooth surfaces compared to the coated ones has been shown experimentally (7). Thus, it is logical to observe a lower rate of distal osteolysis with circumferentially coated implants.

Osteolysis is a destructive process that theoretically jeopardizes fixation of the implant in the long run, should it extend to all the ingrown areas at the implant surface. This is why revision of the implant should be considered in the early steps of the process, whether symptomatic or not. Some aspects of this phenomenon are particularly worrying. Distal osteolysis is rapidly destructive, because it weakens the femoral cortices. Proximal osteolysis in the greater trochanter extends rapidly and jeopardizes the healing of an eventual trochanterotomy required to facilitate the revision procedure.

Calcar osteolysis is slower and can be observed for many years with no need for revision. The decision for revision is not urgent and is based upon the extent of the osteolysis along the coated areas. However, it must be emphasized that standard films tend to underestimate the gravity of the bone destruction. Actually, they are not sufficient to assess precisely the volume of the osteolysis. At the very least specific, oblique views are required. Scanograms are of great help for assessing the circumferential extent of the osteolytic process.

Assessment of the Implant Stability

Implant stability is related to the quality of the implant fixation by the biologic process. Implant migration in the early postoperative period, if it occurs, is probably the most important sign to predict the long term durability of implant fixation (17).

The stability of the implant depends first on the type of the biologic fixation, second on the design of the implant, and third on the presence of osteolytic lesions that might jeopardize the biologic fixation.

Gross measurements of the vertical migration of femoral implants on standard comparable films allows to describe three scenarios (13). In the first case, there is no measurable migration. The primary implant fixation is optimal, and was relayed by secondary bone fixation. This fixation is very likely to be a long lasting one. In fact, when positive signs of bone ingrowth have appeared on the one-year postoperative film, no cases of late migration have been to date reported.

In the second case, an early but moderate migration occurs, but it is rapidly followed of a delayed but durable stabilization. This late stabilization is generally due to a late but tight fibrous encapsulation (6). More rarely, but possible, with HA-coated stems, a delayed stabilization by bone ingrowth can occur (33).

In the third scenario, the implant subsides continuously over the first 2 postoperative years with no delayed stabilization. The bone response of the host, which is more or less intense, has failed to stop the implant subsidence. A pedestal is frequently developed, connected with circumferential and eventually divergent radiolucencies. These cases must be considered as definitive failures of the biologic fixation.

A fourth scenario must be evoked, although it remains to date rather theoretical: the late destruction of the bone ingrowth by an extensive osteolytic process. Usually, osteolysis starts around the proximal part of the implant and grows distally. To date, stem breakage precedes complete loosening. It takes place at the junction between the loosened proximal portion and the still solidly fixed distal portion of the stem. Revision procedures are usually complicated, because the distal portion of the stem is difficult to remove from the diaphysis (22).

CONCLUSION

Radiographic changes observed around cementless implants involve different processes. The appropriate assessment of these radiologic changes allows better understanding of their causes and eventually provides ways to treat them adequately. Due to the improvements afforded by the widespread use of hydroxyapatite in cementless arthroplasty, the incidence of fibrous encapsulation or of unstable fixations has decreased; presently, a stable bony fixation can be routinely obtained.

The proximal bone loss in relation to the bone modeling process can be minimized using implants with a lower modulus of elasticity and with microporous surfaces. Thus, intense bone modeling has become unusual, and bone destruction should be mainly attributed to an osteolytic reaction. In fact, a higher frequency of particle-induced osteolysis must be expected, and it is important to assess precisely this phenomenon, because it can lead to possible revision of an otherwise asymptomatic patient.

When it is possible, the confrontation between histologic data obtained from specimens retrieved at autopsy and the clinical and radiographic pre-mortem data of the same patient is probably the best way to improve our knowledge and understanding of the biologic phenomena around cementless implants.

Reference List

1. Meunier A, Christel P, Sedel L, Witwoet J, Blanquaert D (1990) Influence du module d'élasticité des tiges fémorales de prothèses totales de hanche et de la collerette sur la répartition des déformations du fémur. *Int. Orthop.* 14:67-73.

2. Oh I, Harris WH (1978) Proximal strain distribution in the loaded femur. An *in vitro* comparison of the distributions in the intact femur and after insertion of different hip-replacement femoral components. *J. Bone Joint Surg.* 60-A:75-85.

3. Engh CA, Massin P, Suthers KE (1990) Radiologic assessment of the biologic fixation of porous surfaced femoral components. *Clin. Orthop.* 257:107-28.

4. Epinette JA (1995) Hydoxyapatite-Coated Omnifit Stems in Primary Hip Replacement Surgery: Seven Years Experience in Cahiers d'Enseignement de la Sofcot, n° 51 (English Volume), "Hydroxyapatite Coated Hip and Knee Arthroplasty", pp. 215-26. Paris, Expansion Scientifique Française.

5. Carlsson AS, Gentz C, Linder L (1983) Localised bone resorption in the femur in mechanical failure of cemented total hip arthroplasties. *Acta Orthop. Scand.* 54:396-402.

6. Santavirta S, Hoikka V, Eskola A, Konttinen YT, Paavilainen T, Tallroth K (1990) Agressive granulomatous lesions in cementless total hip arthroplasties. *J. Bone Joint Surg.* 72-B: 980-4.

7. Letournel E (1987) Failures of biologically fixed devices: causes and treatment. In Capello W (Ed.): The Hip. Proceedings of the Fifteenth Open Scientific Meeting of the Hip society. St. Louis, C.V. Mosby, 318-50.

8. Freeman MAR (1986) Why resect the neck? *J. Bone Joint Surg.* 68-B:346-49.

9. Engh CA, Bobyn JD (1988) The influence of stem size and extent of porous coating on femoral bone resorption after primary cementless arthroplasty. *Clin. Orthop.* 231:7-28.

10. Huiskes R, Weinans H, Van Rietbergen B (1992) The relationship between stress shielding and bone resorption around total hip stems and the effects of flexible materials. *Clin. Orthop.* 274:124-34.

11. Soballe K, Hansen ES, Rasmussen HB, Jorgensen P, Bünger C (1992) Tissue ingrowth into titanium and HA-coated implants during stable and unstable mechanical conditions. *J. Orthop. Res.* 10:2285-99.

12. Huiskes R (1990) The various stress patterns of press-fit, ingrown, and cemented femoral stems. *Clin. Orthop.* 261:28-38.

13. Duparc J, Massin P (1992) 2-6 year results of cementless total hip replacement using smooth cementless femoral components 203 consecutive cases. *J. Bone Joint Surg.* 74-B, 251-56.

14. Engh CA, Massin P (1989) Cementless total hip replacement using the AML stem. Results using a survivorship analysis. *Clin. Orthop.*, 249: 141-58.

15. Kwong LM, Jasty M, Mulroy RD, Maloney WJ, Bragdon C, Harris WH (1992) The Histology of the radiolucent line *J. Bone Joint Surg.* 74-B:67-73.

16. Maloney WJ, Jasty M, Burke WD, O'Connor DO, Zalenski EB, Bragdon C, Harris WH (1989) Biomechanical and histologic investigation of cemented total hip arthroplasties. A study of autopsy-retrieved femurs after *in vivo* cycling. *Clin. Orthop.* 249:129-40.

17. Collier JP, Bauer TW, Bloebaum RD, Bobyn JD, Cook SD, Galante JO, Harris WH, Head WC, Jasty MJ, Mayor MB, Sumner DR, Whiteside LA (1992) Results of implant retrieval from postmortem specimens in patients with well-functioning long-term total hip replacement. *Clin. Orthop.* 274:97-112.

18. Massin P, Badelon O, Cavagna R, Bocquet L, Duparc J (1991) Radiological and histological observations in smooth cementless femoral implants in canine hip joint arthroplasty. *Intern. Orthop.* 15:299-303.

19. Sumner DR, Galante JO (1992) Determinants of stress shielding: design *versus* materials *versus* interface. *Clin. Orthop.* 274:202-12.

20. Maloney WJ, Smith RL (1995) Periprosthetic osteolysis in total hip arthroplasty: the role of particulate wear debris. *J. Bone Joint Surg.* 77-A:1448-61.

21. Schmalzried TP, Jasty M, Harris WH (1992) Periprosthetic bone loss in total hip arthroplasty. Polyethylene wear debris and the concept of the effective joint space. *J. Bone Joint Surg.* 74-A:849-63.

22. Blacker GJ, Charnley J (1978) Changes in the upper femur after low friction arthroplasty. *Clin. Orthop.* 137:15-23.

23. Tanzer M, Maloney WJ, Jasty M, Harris WH (1992) The progression of femoral cortical osteolysis in association with total hip arthroplasty without cement. *J. Bone Joint Surg.* 74-A:404-10.

24. Emerson RH, sanders SB, Head WC, Higgins L (1999) Effect of circumferential plasmaspray porous coating on the rate of femoral osteolysis after total hip arthroplasty. *J. Bone Joint Surg.* 81-A:1291-8.

25. Rahbek O, Obergaard S, Lind M, Bendix K, Bunger C, Soballe K (2001) Sealing effect of hydroxyapatite coating on peri-implant migration of particles. An experimental study in dogs. *J. Bone Joint Surg.* 83-B:441-7.

26. Jasty MJ, Floyd WE, Schiller AL, Goldring SR and Harris WH (1986) Localized osteolysis in stable non-septic total hip replacement. *J. Bone Joint Surg.* 68-A: 912-9.

27. Agins HJ, Bansal NW, Salvati EA, Wilson PD, Pellici PM, Bullough PG (1988) Metallic Wear in Failed Titanium-Alloy Total Hip Replacements. A histopathological and quantitative analysis. *J. Bone Joint Surg.* 70-A:347-56.

28. Bloebaum RD, Zou L, Bachus KN, Shea KG, Hofman AA, Dunn HK (1997) Analysis of particles in acetabular components from patients with osteolysis. *Clin. Orthop.* 338:109-18.

29. Bauer TW, Taylor SK, Jiang M, Medendorp SV (1994) An indirect comparison of third-body wear in retrieved hydroxyapatite coated porous and cemented femoral components. *Clin. Orthop.* 298:11-18.

30. Önsten I, Carlsson AS, Sanzen L, Besjako J (1996) Migration and wear of a hydroxyapatite coated hip prosthesis. *J. Bone Joint Surg.* 78-B:85-91.

31. Benson ER, Christensen CP, Monesmith EH, Gomes JS, Bierbaum BE (2000) Particulate bone grafting of osteolytic femoral lesions around stable cementless stems. *Clin. Orthop.* 381:58-67.

32. Bobyn JD, Jacobs JJ, Tanzer M, Urban RM, Aribinbi R, Sumner DR, Turner TM, Brooks CE (1995) The susceptibility of smooth implant surfaces to periimplant fibrosis and migration of polyethylene wear debris. *Clin. Orthop.* 311:21-39.

33. Freeman MAR, Plante Bordeneuve P. Early migration and late aseptic failure of proximal femoral prostheses. *J. Bone Joint Surg.* 76-B:432-8.

34. Bobyn JD, Engh CA, Pilliar R (1987) Histological comparison of biological fixation and bone modeling with canine and human porous coated hip prostheses. In: Lemons JE (ed). Quantitative characterization and performance of porous implants for hard tissue applications (Ed ASTM STP 953) American Society for Testing and Materials, Philadelphia, 185-206.

35. Soballe K, Hansen ES, Brockstedt-Rasmussen H, Bunger C (1993) Hydroxyapatite coating converts fibrous tissue to bone around loaded implants. *J. Bone Joint Surg.*, 75-B:270-8.

3 The Extent of Hydroxyapatite Coating: Proximal *versus* Full Coating with Customs Stems Using Compacted Bone Preparation

Jean-Noël A. Argenson, MD, Pierre-Paul Ettore, MD and Jean-Manuel Aubaniac, MD

INTRODUCTION

Numerous experimental and clinical studies have shown the effectiveness of hydroxyapatite coating in providing rigid biological fixation of femoral components (1-3). In comparative studies, Rothman *et al.* (4), found no clinical or radiographic differences between hydroxyapatite and non-hydroxyapatite coated stems after 2.2 years average follow-up. However, McPherson *et al.* (5), in a similar matched pair study reported accelerated bone remodeling characterized by proximal cancellous hypertrophy with hydroxyapatite-coated stems compared with porous-coated stems. Clinically, Ciccotti *et al.* (6) reported less thigh pain with hydroxyapatite augmented stems at 6 month follow-up evaluation. Kärrholm *et al.* (7), recorded less stem subsidence after 2 years with hydroxyapatite-coated stems, similar to the results of Donnelly *et al.* (8), who reported a better survival rate at 5 to 6 years with hydroxyapatite-coated stems compared with the survival rate of press-fit stems. The effect of bone ingrowth and osteolysis of the extent of porous coating on a femoral component of a single design was studied by Engh *et al.* (9-11). However, the clinical and radiographic effects of varying the extent of hydroxyapatite on a femoral component of one design has not been evaluated.

The present study was done to compare the clinical and radiographic findings that result when one cementless femoral stem design is coated with hydroxyapatite in two different ways, fully-coated, and proximally-coated. The primary implant design goals were to achieve proximal fixation by intimate metaphyseal bone contact, to increase primary stability by using a collar, and to avoid thigh pain and stress shielding by incorporating a reduced distal stem diameter. The stem was implanted in two groups of patients who were followed up for a minimum of 2 years. One group received an implant that was proximally-coated with hydroxyapatite. The second group received the identically designed implant fully-coated with hydroxyapatite. It was not a prospective randomized study because the two types of coatings came into use sequentially, but during their respective times, they were implanted on an unselected basis into all patients having cementless total hip arthroplasty.

MATERIALS AND METHODS

Between January 1990 and January 1995, 598 consecutive cementless hip arthroplasties were performed in 558 patients. All patients who received cementless hip arthroplasty during this time were included in the study, whereas patients who received cemented stems, chosen by the two surgeons on the same criteria (bone quality or etiology) were excluded. Five hundred twenty-one patients with 556 hip arthroplasties were available for follow-up, leaving 37 unavailable for follow-up. Thirty-five patients could not be located, and two patients had died.

The first 280 hip arthroplasties were performed using stems proximally-coated with hydroxyapatite. The following 276 hip arthroplasties were performed using stems fully-coated with hydroxyapatite. Average follow-up in the proximal hydroxyapatite group was 52 months (range, 2-6 years) and in the full hydroxyapatite group, 38 months (range, 2-5 years). The demographic data for the two groups are presented in Table 1.

Parameter	Proximal hydroxy-apatite	Full hydroxy-apatite
Age (years)		
Mean	56.5	58.3
Range	17-91	18-81
Standard deviation	13.7	13.2
Gender		
Male	124	138
Female	135	124
Weight (kgs)		
Mean	71.5	69.7
Range	39-123	46-109
Etiology		
Osteoarthritis	108	110
Dysplasia	38	46
Avascular necrosis	34	33
Congenital dislocation of the hip	31	27
Malunion	18	16
Previous osteotomy	14	12
Hip fusion	7	4
Rhumatoid arthritis	7	9
Others	23	19

Table 1 – Proximal hydroxyapatite *versus* full hydroxyapatite control demographics and etiology.

The two groups were similar statistically regarding gender, weight, age, and diagnosis. Sixty-eight patients (26.3%) in the proximal hydroxyapatite group were younger than 50 years of age when the arthroplasty was performed. Sixty-three (24%) patients in the full hydroxyapatite group were younger than 50 years. Osteoarthritis was the primary reason for surgery in 38.6% of patients in the proximally-coated hydroxyapatite group and for 39.9% of patients in the fully hydroxyapatite-coated group. Developmental dysplasia of the hip was the etiology for 11.1% of patients in the proximally hydroxyapatite-coated group and for 9.8% of patients in the fully hydroxyapatite-coated group. Twelve percent of patients in both groups had avascular necrosis.

Cementless custom femoral components (Symbios, Yverdon, Switzerland) designed using computed tomography and made using computer-aided manufacturing techniques were inserted in all the patients. The customization technique reproduced the intramedullary and extramedullary anatomy of the involved femurs. The metaphyseal portion of the stem was designed to achieve intimate proximal fit. The stem was tapered and designed to rest against dense, preserved cancellous bone that was impacted by a smooth, custom broach with identical dimensions to the final implant. The femoral neck was designed to reestablish a normal neck offset and anteversion angle.

The prosthesis was made of titanium (Ti) alloy ($Ti_6 Al_4 V$). For the fully hydroxyapatite-coated version of the stem, the surface consisted of a porous Ti alloy onto which hydroxyapatite was applied. In the proximal hydroxyapatite group, the porous Ti alloy and hydroxyapatite were applied to the proximal 2/3 surface area of the stem which corresponded in length to the proximal half part of the stem, as shown in Figure 1. In the full hydroxyapatite group, the porous Ti alloy covered the proximal 2/3 of the stem and the hydroxyapatite covered the entire stem. The coatings were applied by using atmospheric plasma spray techniques. The porous pure Ti coating had a porosity of 35% and a roughness (peak to peak) between 150 and 325µm. The porous layer thickness was 300µm ± 10µm. The hydroxyapatite coating had a porosity

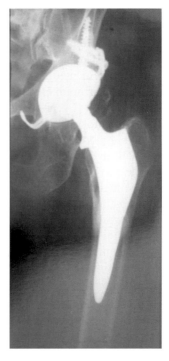

Figure 1 – The characteristic radiographic findings seen at a 5-year follow-up, for proximally hydroxyapatite-coated stems include distal radiolucencies around the distal uncoated part of the stem and both cortical and endosteal hypertrophy at the junction of the coated and uncoated part of the stem.

of 10%, a crystallinity index of 70% ± 10%, a Ca/P rate of 1.667 ± 0.002, and a thickness of 75μm ±25μm. The prosthetic head was a 28mm Zr head available in four lengths (Symbios).

Surgery was performed by the same senior surgeons in both groups. An anterolateral surgical approach (Watson-Jones) was used in all patients except those requiring an osteotomy of the greater trochanter (hip fusion takedowns and severe congenital dislocation of the hip). A hemispheric, hydroxyapatite-coated acetabular metal backed ultra-high molecular weight polyethylene component, fixed distally by a hook in the obturator foramen and proximally by screws (Centroïd, Symbios) was used in all cases. Prophylactic antibiotics were given intravenously at the start of the procedure and continued for 48 hours. Low molecular weight heparin, started on the evening of surgery, and continued for 40 days was used for thromboembolic prophylaxis. All patients began walking the day after surgery. Weight bearing was protected with two crutches for 6 weeks.

Clinical and radiologic follow-up was performed every 3 months for the first year after surgery and annually thereafter. Patients were asked to rank their feelings about the results as : enthusiastic, satisfied, no change, or disappointed. Results were recorded as acceptable (enthusiastic, satisfied) or unacceptable (no change or disappointed). Clinical results were measured using the Harris hip score (12). Any type of thigh pain regardless its type or intensity after 1 year was assessed separately and recorded as present or absent. Length of time in a rehabilitation center and recovery of activity (work of home activity for nonworkers) also were recorded. The clinical and radiological evaluation was performed by a physician independent from the senior operating surgeon.

Radiographic results were determined from anteroposterior (AP) and frog lateral radiographs, obtained at latest follow-up. Correction factors for magnification were calculated for each radiograph on the basis of the ratio of the measured diameter of the prosthetic head to the actual known diameter (13). Preoperatively the anatomy of the proximal femur was studied and the canal flare index was classified as normal, stovepipe, and champagne fluted according to Noble *et al.* (14). The repartition was similar in the two groups with 64% *versus* 62% of normal femurs, 28% of champagne fluted femurs in both groups, and 8% *versus* 10% of stovepipe femurs. Femoral component position was assessed

using a fixed point of reference on the prosthesis (lateral proximal shoulder) and on the femur (tip of the greater trochanter or either lower point of the lesser trochanter in osteotomy cases). Subsidence of 3 mm or more was recorded. The axis of the femur was located between the isthmus and a line tangent to the greater trochanter. The axis of the prosthesis was located between the tip of the prosthesis and a line tangent to the shoulder of the prosthesis. Component orientation was designated as neutral if the centerlines of the component and femur were within 2° of each other. Ectopic bone formation was evaluated according to the classification of Brooker *et al.* (15). The Gruen *et al.* (16), interface analysis was used to measure endosteal new bone, radiolucent lines, calcar modification, cortical hypertrophy, or distal pedestals. Stem stability was defined by the absence of progressive migration, progressive radiolucent line around the component, pedestal associated to radiolucent line around the tip of the stem and calcar atrophy associated to one of these signs. Stress shielding was evaluated using the classification of Engh and Bobyn (9). The SPSS statistical software (SPSS, Inc, Chicago, IL) was used to analyze the data (17). The Student's t test was used to analyze the demographic data. The patient self assessments and thigh pain data were compared using chi squared analysis. Harris hip scores, as a whole, were compared using the Mann-Whitney U test. Radiographic data also were submitted to chi squared analysis. The Mann-Whitney U test was used to analyze the stress shielding, the degree of ectopic bone data and the importance of stem subsidence. An alpha level of 0.05 was used to indicate statistical significance in all tests described above.

RESULTS

Fifteen of the proximally hydroxyapatite-coated stems (5.3%) have required revision because of infections in three, persistent thigh pain in two, and mechanical loosening in 10. The mean revision time for persistent thigh pain or stem mechanical loosening was 25 months, ranging from 3 to 48 months. One fully hydroxyapatite-coated stem (0.4%) has required revision at 6 months, as the result of a late femoral fracture. All revision for mechanical loosening occurred for stem failure and none for acetabular failure. The incidence of postoperative complications was similar in the proximal hydroxyapatite and full hydroxyapatite groups including dislocations (3.6% *versus* 2.5%), wound infections (3.2% *versus* 3%), deep vein thrombosis (1.4% *versus* 0.7%), and neurologic injuries (0.4% *versus* 1.1%). The average length of stay in a rehabilitation center was equivalent for the two groups (4.5 weeks *versus* 4.7 weeks). The recovery of full activity either work or day life activity as reported by the patients, took slightly longer for the proximal hydroxyapatite group (90 days) than the full hydroxyapatite group (70 days).

At the most recent follow-ups, there was no significant difference in the Harris hip scores of the patients in the proximal hydroxyapatite group (mean, 93.8 points; range, 27-100; median, 100) and the full hydroxyapatite group (mean, 96.3 points; range, 42-100; median, 100), (p = 0.20). However, there was a statistically significant difference in patient satisfaction when acceptable and unacceptable results were compared. Two hundred fifty seven (91.8%) patients with proximal hydroxyapatite and 270 (97.8%) patients with full hydroxyapatite ranked their outcomes as acceptable. The incidence of thigh pain was statistically significantly higher in the proximal hydroxyapatite group (9.6%) in comparison with the fully coated group (3.3%).

There was no statistically significant difference in orientation of the femoral components in the two groups (p = 0.30). Sixty one percent (172 stems) of proximally hydroxyapatite coated stems and 68% (187) of fully hydroxyapatite coated stems were in neutral. Thirty three percent (92 stems) of proximally hydroxyapatite-coated stems and 24% (66 stems) of fully hydroxyapatite-coated stems were in varus. The full hydroxyapatite group had

statistically less ectopic bone according to Brooker *et al.* (15), than the proximal hydroxyapatite group (p < 0.05) (Table 2). The degree of stress shielding, measured using the classification of Engh and Bobyn (9), was significantly more pronounced in the proximal hydroxyapatite group (p < 0.005) (Table 3). Calcar resorption was seen in 24% of cases in the proximal hydroxyapatite group and 9% of cases in the full hydroxyapatite group, this was statistically significant (p < 0.00001). Table 4

Ectopic bone formation	Proximal hydroxy-apatite	Full hydroxy-apatite
Absent	191 (68.21%)	216 (78.26%)
Class I	56 (20%)	37 (13.41%)
Class II	21 (7.5%)	14 (5.07%)
Class III	11 (3.93%)	9 (3.26%)
Class IV	1 (0.36%)	0

Table 2 – Ectopic bone formation for proximal hydroxyapatite versus full hydroxyapatite.

Stress shielding	Proximal hydroxy-apatite	Full hydroxy-apatite
None	201 (71.78%)	237 (85.9%)
First degree	68 (24.28%)	26 (9%)
Second degree	12 (4.28%)	3 (1.09%)
Third degree	1 (0.4%)	0
Fourth degree	1 (0.4%)	0

Table 3 – Distribution of stress shielding for proximal hydroxyapatite *versus* full hydroxyapatite.

Radiographic analysis	Proximal hydroxyapatite	Full hydroxyapatite	Statistical analysis Chi squared test
Endosteal New Bone			
Gruen Zones 1 and 7	40 (14.3%)	91 (33%)	p < 0.00001
Gruen Zones 2 and 6	252 (90%)	261 (94.5%)	p = 0.46
Gruen Zones 3, 4, and 5	72 (25.7%)	272 (98.1%)	p < 0.00001
Radiolucencies			
Gruen Zones 3, 4, and 5	160 (57.1%)	4 (1.4%)	p < 0.00001
Cortical hypertrophy			
Gruen Zones 2 and 6	130 (46.4%)	68 (22.1%)	p < 0.00001
Calcar atrophy	68 (24.2%)	26 (9%)	p < 0.00001
Pedestals	23 (8.2%)	95 (34.4%)	p < 0.00001

Table 4 – Radiographic fixation analysis for proximal hydroxyapatite *versus* full hydroxyapatite.

compares the incidence of cancellous or cortical hypertrophy and radiolucencies in the two groups. The incidence of radiolucencies in Gruen Zones 3, 4, and 5 was significantly higher in the proximal hydroxyapatite group than in the full hydroxyapatite group (p < 0.00001). A fusiform cortical hypertrophy was observed at the transition between the coated and uncoated regions of the proximally hydroxyapatite-coated stems (fig. 1). The proximal hydroxyapatite group had a greater range of stem migration (mean, 3.2mm; range, 3-4mm; Standard Deviation = 0.5) than the full hydroxyapatite group (mean, 4.8mm; range, 3-10mm; Standard Deviation = 2.6), but this was not statistically significant (p = 0.23). A significantly (p = 0.04) greater number of fully hydroxyapatite-coated stems (271 cases, 98.2%), with none of the four signs of instability as described in the materials and methods section, were considered stable than proximally hydroxyapatite-coated stems (265 cases, 94.6%).

DISCUSSION

The goal of the stem design used in this study was to achieve secure proximal femoral fixation by obtaining intimate bone contact with a coated implant, and avoid thigh pain and stress shielding, by reducing the distal stem diameter. The purpose of this study was to evaluate, for this stem design, the influence of hydroxyapatite coating distribution on the clinical and radiographic outcomes of the hip arthroplasty. This comparative study showed after a mid term follow-up a clear difference in thigh pain, revision rate for aseptic loosening, and radiographic bone remodeling in favor of fully hydroxyapatite-coated stems compared with proximally hydroxyapatite coated stems.

The clinical results observed in this study are consistent with those published concerning hydroxyapatite-coated stems. Geesink and Hoefnagels (2), reported an average Harris hip score of 96 points at 3 years, and Kärrholm et al. (7), an average score of 95 points at 2 years, consistent with the 96 points at 3 years reported in this study. The stems used in these published studies were proximally coated, and associated with a characteristic radiographic remodeling pattern (18). This pattern included a consistent proximal circumferential fixation under the greater and lesser trochanter, as the

80% reported by Ciccotti et al. (6), and the 86% by D'Antonio et al. (19), consistent with the 90% observed in the proximal hydroxyapatite group and the 94% observed in the full hydroxyapatite group. This pattern included also a high prevalence of radiolucent lines around the distal uncoated portion of the stems, as the 68% reported by D'Antonio et al. (19), in a multicenter three year study. This incidence is similar to that observed in the proximal hydroxyapatite group (57.1%), but much higher than that observed in the full hydroxyapatite group (14%). The fusiform cortical hypertrophy observed in the proximal hydroxyapatite group at the transition between the coated and uncoated regions has been reported with proximally coated stems (2, 7, 19). This finding was not present in the full hydroxyapatite group. The distal portion of the proximally hydroxyapatite-coated stems used in the study of Geesink and Hoefnagels (2), or D'Antonio et al. (19), and the one reported by Kärrholm et al. (7), is designed to avoid micromotion by filling the intramedullary canal. Therefore, the radiolucencies around the stem and fusiform cortical hypertrophy may not be clinically important. However, the stem used in this study had a distal portion that was tapered, to reduce stem stiffness that could be associated with thigh pain. Such a stem may be associated with clinically significant motion if it is not well fixed to bone by coating extending to its tip (20). This may explain the significant reduction in thigh pain in the full hydroxyapatite group (3.3%) in comparison with the proximal hydroxyapatite group (9.6%). At a similar follow-up D'Antonio et al. (19), and Kärrholm et al. (7) reported an incidence of thigh pain of approximately 4%. The incidence of ectopic bone formation was comparable with those previously reported (2, 19), but none of them required revision. The reason why this incidence in the less severe form is lower for the fully hydroxyapatite group remained unclear. Similarly no reason was found to explain the greater number of pedestals in the fully hydroxyapatite group, never associated with radiolucencies around the distal portion of the stem. Finally a greater number of stems were found in varus in the proximally coated group, possibly related to a learning curve, but this was not significant.

Theoretical studies have predicted that proximal stress shielding increases when distal bone ingrowth occurs (21). Clinical reports by Engh and Bobyn (9), and finite element analysis (20), indicate that stress shielding of fully porous coated stems is most likely with large, canal filling stems. The stem used in this study is specifically designed not to be canal filling. The fully hydroxyapatite-coated version of this stem was not associated with stress shielding at this relatively short follow-up period. This stem was associated with a significant reduction in osteopenia of the proximal femur relative to the partially hydroxyapatite-coated stem of identical design (fig. 2). The bony response formed at the edge of the hydroxyapatite coating after the insertion of the proximally coated stem may provide excellent load transfer at this location and subsequently much less proximally. Calcar resorption was seen in 9% of cases after 3 years in the full hydroxyapatite group, comparing favorably with the 19% at 2 years observed by Geesink and Hoefnagels (2), and the 61% at 3 years observed by D'Antonio *et al.* (19), with proximally hydroxyapatite-coated and distal filling stems. The radiographic findings observed in this current study with fully hydroxyapatite-coated stems are consistent with those recently published by Trevisan *et al.* (22), using dual energy x-ray absorptiometry. Minimum loss of femoral bone around fully coated stems was seen up to 3 years after surgery. Despite these encouraging results after 3 years, continued monitoring of the patients will be necessary because femoral bone loss still may become a problem after longer follow-up periods. However, in this study the quality of radiographic bone remodeling was more favorable 3 years after

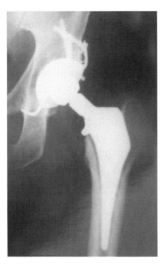

Figure 2 – Solid endofemoral cancellous condensation with minimum proximal osteopenia is seen with a fully hydroxyapatite-coated stem at a 5-year follow-up.

implantation with a full hydroxyapatite coating compared with a proximal hydroxyapatite coating for the same stem design.

Our results show that the fully hydroxyapatite-coated stems migrated less and were more stable than the proximally coated stems. The variations between the two groups are close, and the results may be due to intra-observer variability. Nevertheless, no stem required revision for aseptic loosening in the fully hydroxyapatite group compared with the 10 stems that required revision surgery in the proximal hydroxyapatite group. This is higher than the 0.4% reported by D'Antonio *et al.* (19), in a large number of Omnifit stems after a similar follow-up. However, the Omnifit stems were designed to fill a femur prepared by reaming. In our study, the relatively high rate of mechanical failure found in the proximally-coated group might be related to the total absence of distal canal filling with a very thin distal stem, where fixation is dependent on the cancellous bone compacted by a smooth rasp. The question whether this type of stem coated with a full layer of hydroxyapatite will show less stress shielding than a distal filling stem with no coating, remains open. The early postoperative period after cementless hip arthroplasty is reported to be critical for biological fixation of hydroxyapatite-coated stems (1). Distal extension of hydroxyapatite to the smooth Ti stem in our study suggests that the extended coating leads to superior stem stability in the early postoperative period.

In summary, porous-coated and hydroxyapatite-coated femoral hip stems provide prompt biologic fixation which is associated with encouraging short term clinical results (2, 4, 5, 19). The optimum distribution of a Ti porous coating or hydroxyapatite coating for a given stem design can be determined only by clinical trials in which stems of identical design and different coating distributions are compared. This present comparative study has shown in a large number of patients superior short term results obtained with fully hydroxyapatite-coated stems in term of thigh pain, aseptic loosening, and radiographic bone remodeling compared with proximally hydroxyapatite-coated stems. These data were collected from a stem designed specifically for each individual patient and implanted into compacted femoral bone. Further study is required to extend this comparison into traditional stem systems implanted into a reamed femoral preparation.

The authors are grateful to X. Thirion, MD, PhD, from the Aix-Marseille University Department of Biostatistics for his help.

Reference List

1. Furlong RJ, Osborn JF (1991) Fixation of hip prostheses by hydroxyapatite ceramic coatings. *J. Bone Joint Surg. Br.* 73:741.

2. Geesink RGT, Hoefnagels NHM (1995) Six year results of hydroxyapatite-coated total hip replacement. *J. Bone Joint Surg. Br.* 77:534.

3. Soballe K, Hansen ES, Brockstedt-Rasmussen H *et al.* (1991) Gap healing enhanced by hydroxyapatite coating in dogs. Clin Orthop 272:300.

4. Rothman RH, Hozack WJ, Ranawat A, Moriarty L (1996) Hydroxyapatite-coated femoral stems. A matched pair analysis of coated and uncoated implants. *J. Bone Joint Surg. Am.* 78:319.

5. McPherson EJ, Dorr LD, Gruen TA, Saberi MT (1995) Hydroxyapatite-coated proximal ingrowth femoral stems. A matched pair control study. *Clin. Orthop.* 315:223.

6. Ciccotti MG, Rothman RH, Hozack WJ, Moriarty L (1994) Clinical and roentgenographic evaluation of hydroxyapatite augmented and nonaugmented porous total hip arthroplasty. *J. Arthroplasty* 9:631.

7. Kärrholm J, Malchau H, Snorrason F, Herberts P (1994) Micromotion of femoral stems in total hip arthroplasty. A randomized study of cemented, hydroxyapatite-coated, and porous-coated stems with roentgen stereophotogrammetric analysis. *J. Bone Joint Surg. Am.* 76:1692.

8. Donnelly WJ, Kobayashi A, Freeman MAR *et al.* (1997) Radiological and survival comparison of four methods of fixation of a proximal femoral stem. *J. Bone Joint Surg. Br.* 79:351.

9. Engh CA, Bobyn JD (1988) The influence of stem size and extent of porous coating on femoral bone resorption after primary cementless hip arthroplasty. *Clin. Orthop.* 231:7.

10. Engh CA, Hooten JP, Zettl-Schaffer KF *et al.* (1995) Evaluation of bone ingrowth in proximally and extensively porous-coated anatomic medullary locking prostheses retrieved at autopsy. *J. Bone Joint Surg. Am.* 77:903.

11. Engh CA, Massin P, Suthers KE (1990) Roentgenographic assessment of the biologic fixation of porous surfaced femoral components. *Clin. Orthop.* 257:107.

12. Harris WH (1969) Traumatic arthritis of the hip after dislocation and acetabular fractures: Treatment by mold arthroplasty. *J. Bone Joint Surg. Am.* 51:737.

13. Griffith MJ, Seidenstein MK, Williams D, Charnley J (1978) Socket wear in Charnley low friction arthroplasty of the hip. *Clin. Orthop.* 137:37.

14. Noble PC, Alexander JW, Lindahl LJ *et al.* (1988) The anatomic basis of femoral component design. *Clin. Orthop.* 235:148.

15. Brooker AF, Bowerman JW, Robinson RA, Riley Jr LH (1973) Ectopic ossification following total hip replacement. Incidence and a method of classification. *J. Bone Joint Surg. Am.* 55:1629.

16. Gruen TA, McNiece GM, Amstutz HC (1979) "Modes of failure" of cemented stem-type femoral components : A radiographic analysis of loosening. *Clin. Orthop.* 141:17.

17. SPSS Institute Inc : SPSS 8.01. Chicago, IL, SPSS Inc 1998.

18. Jaffe WL, Scott DF (1996) Total hip arthroplasty with hydroxyapatite-coated prostheses. *J. Bone Joint Surg. Am.* 78:1918.

19. D'Antonio JA, Capello WN, Manley MT (1996) Remodeling of bone around hydroxyapatite coated femoral stems. *J. Bone Joint Surg. Am.* 78:1226.

20. Keaveny TM, Bartel DL (1995) Mechanical consequences of bone ingrowth in a hip prosthesis inserted without cement. *J. Bone Joint Surg. Am.* 77:911.

21. Huiskes R (1990) The various stress patterns of press-fit, ingrown, and cemented femoral stems. *Clin. Orthop.* 261:27.

22. Trevisan C, Bigoni M, Randelli G, *et al.* (1997) Periprosthetic bone density around fully hydroxyapatite coated femoral stem. *Clin. Orthop.* 340:109.

4 The Effect of the Metal Substrate on Biologic Fixation with Hydroxyapatite

William L. Jaffe, MD and Harlan B. Levine, MD

INTRODUCTION

Calcium-phosphate ceramic materials, such as hydroxyapatite, have poor mechanical characteristics that make them unsuitable for load bearing applications (1). Specifically, they are brittle and have both poor tensile strength and poor resistance to impact (2). In order to utilize the osteoconductive properties of calcium-phosphate ceramics in a load bearing application, it is necessary to attach these substances to a material with more favorable mechanical properties. By applying a ceramic to a metal substrate, it is possible to combine the biocompatibility of the ceramic with the strength of the metal. Although implants made entirely of hydroxyapatite have been shown to have very poor mechanical characteristics, HA coatings that have been applied to metal substrates appear to obtain improved mechanical properties, including resistance to fatigue (3, 4, 5, 6). Additionally, although it is possible to place hydroxyapatite on most metal surfaces, most experimental and clinical usage has been with titanium (Ti), a titanium alloy (titanium-aluminum-vanadium, Ti-6Al-4V), and cobalt-chromium alloy (Co-Cr).

This chapter reviews the effect of the metal substrate on the biologic fixation of hydroxyapatite and it evaluates the influence of the metal substrate, surface texture, and HA on biologic fixation. It discusses the results obtained from an implantable bone chamber model used to assess the effects of different metal substrates, varying surface textures, and hydroxyapatite in a canine model of bone-to-prosthesis apposition. It concludes with a brief review of the results of using HA-coated metal substrates in different mechanical environments; the femoral and acetabular components of a total hip arthroplasty are used as a paradigm.

METAL SUBSTRATE

Titanium, Ti-6Al-4V, and cobalt chromium have been used widely in orthopaedic surgery and dentistry, as they have excellent resistance to corrosion from exposure to body fluids and to fatigue from repetitive mechanical loads (7). They have also demonstrated a very good ability to form strong bonds with hydroxyapatite. Titanium-hydroxyapatite interfaces have shown excellent results with mechanical testing in compression (650 megapascals (MPa)), tension (85 MPa), and shear (74 MPa) forces (3, 8). Chemically, titanium is a more reactive metal than cobalt-chromium (9), and it has been demonstrated *in vitro* that titanium is able to form bonds of attachment that are 33% greater than that of cobalt-chromium and hydroxyapatite (5). It has been theorized that this increased bonding strength is secondary to a chemical bond that forms between the titanium metal substrate and the hydroxyapatite in addition to the mechanical interlock between the two materials (3, 8). The suggested mechanism is that, under high temperatures, titanium becomes oxidized and incorporates into the hydroxyapatite lattice.

1. $(n+1) Ca^{10}(PO^4)_6(OH)_2 + nTiO_2 ---\rightarrow nCaTiO_3 + (n-1)Ca10(PO^4)_6(OH)_2 + 3nCa_3(PO4)_2 + nH_2O$
2. $2TiO_2 ---\rightarrow (Ti4+)(TiO4-)$ incorporated into apatite lattice

In a study to evaluate the physical characteristics of hydroxyapatite coatings, Geesink showed that HA coatings on titanium metal substrates have tensile strength and substrate bonding similar to native cortical bone, and that the physical characteristics of HA coatings are at a safe and appropriate level for orthopaedics usage (8). In more recent trials, it has been shown that different surface treatments can enhance the chemical bonding between the metal substrate, bone, and hydroxyapatite or other biologic materials (10, 11, 12). Although the ability of titanium to bond chemically with HA is known, the issue of whether or not this bond influences the tensile strength between HA and titanium has been disputed by some authors. Filiaggi *et al.* were able to show a phosphate diffusion of 25 nm into titanium during plasma spray application of HA, yet through mechanical testing they showed that the bonding between the two substrates could be attributable to primarily to a mechanical interlock, and was possibly dependent upon surface roughness (13). Although titanium is more reactive then cobalt-chromium and is able to form chemical bonds with host tissues, the functional interaction between titanium or CoCr with HA may not be very different.

Titanium and CoCr differ from each other with respect to modulus of elasticity. It is known that CoCr has a modulus of elasticity that is twice that of titanium (220 gigapascals *versus* 110 gigapascals). This makes CoCr the stiffer of the two metals. Due to its lower modulus of elasticity, a titanium femoral stem provides less stress shielding in the proximal femur, and less proximal bone resorption as the load on the proximal femur increases. In comparison, a stiffer CoCr femoral stem transfers loads more distally (14). This has been shown in two dimensional (15) and three dimensional (16) finite element analysis as well as *in vivo* (17).

A consequence of greater stress transfer proximally is the potential for greater motion at the interface between prosthesis and host bone. Huiskes *et al.* (18) compared the effect of stress shielding to proximal interface stresses. They found that as the modulus of elasticity was reduced, proximal stress shielding was diminished, but the proximal interface stresses increased dramatically. The resulting potential for increased motion at the implant-prosthesis interface could lead to decreased bony integration. This has been shown in a canine model, where increased micromotion at the interface site promoted fibrous over osseous ingrowth into an implant (19).

It must be emphasized that, although titanium is less stiff then cobalt-chromium, both of these metals are significantly stiffer than cortical bone, which has a modulus of elasticity of twenty gigapascals. Given that most modern femoral prostheses have generous cross-sections, and that resistance to bending moments decreases proportionally

to the fourth power of the radius of the prosthesis, most prostheses are relatively inelastic when compared to cortical bone. Jaffe *et al.* showed that, although cobalt-chromium has a modulus of elasticity twice that of titanium, the ratio of the structural stiffness of femoral components of identical geometries made from these two materials implanted into femurs was 1.31 to 1.34 (20). Differences in stem stiffness much greater then these values have been shown to not influence bone strain in the proximal femur in a total hip model (21). Although titanium has a modulus of elasticity that is one half that of cobalt-chromium, it is likely that the two metals may transfer loads in a similar fashion when formed into identically shaped prosthesis.

Another factor to consider when comparing titanium and cobalt-chromium with respect to their usage with hydroxyapatite are their coefficients of thermal expansion. Very high temperatures are often utilized during the HA application process. Temperatures as high as 30,000K are reached during plasma spraying (5). To minimize residual stresses at the HA-metal substrate interface that arise from differences in the rate of material expansion/contraction with changes in temperature, it is best to use materials that have similar thermal coefficients. Titanium and hydroxyapatite have a coefficient of 9-10 X 10^{-6}/degree Celcius, *versus* cobalt-chromium and hydroxyapatite, which have a coefficient of 12 X 10^{-6}/degree Celcius (7). The use of titanium with hydroxyapatite will produce less strain at the metal-HA interface than will the use of cobalt-chromium during high temperature HA application.

Surface Texture

The metal substrate can be modified by applying a surface texture in one of three forms: smooth (microtextured), macrotextured, or porous. In preparation for the application of a plasma-sprayed surface coating, the smooth surface is grit-blasted to a surface roughness between four and ten micrometers (μm). The microtextured metal substrate is similar to the microscopic dimensions of hydroxyapatite with respect to surface contour and undulations; it therefore makes an excellent finish on which to apply hydroxyapatite (22). Successful biologic fixation to a bony surface of a grit-blasted metal substrate coated with hydroxyapatite has been demonstrated by several investigators. Failure ultimately occurs at the substrate-coating interface when the construct is subjected to high shear and tensile forces (23, 24). Geesink *et al.* noted a different mode of failure. In a canine model involving transcortical plug push-out testing, they noted ultimate failure either within the hydroxyapatite itself or at the hydroxyapatite-bone interface (3). A metal substrate with a macrotextured surface is better able to resist shear and tensile forces than is a smooth, grit-blasted surface. This may result in increased implant stability and long-term fixation if biodegradation of the HA coating occurs (25). Macrostructuring can take many forms, including grooves, meshes, threads, or deposited metal coatings on the surface of a metal substrate. Grooved surfaces have demonstrated improved fixation *in vivo* both at early follow-up, as well as up to one year following implantation (24, 26). Poser *et al.* conducted a study that demonstrated the sharing of mechanical loads between areas where bone had grown onto the hydroxyapatite surface and where it had grown onto the grooves of the metal substrate. This suggests a "comprehensive" interface between the metal substrate, the grooved macrotexture, the hydroxyapatite surface coating, and the ingrown bone (27).

It is possible to coat a titanium alloy (Ti-6Al-4V) substrate with commercially pure (CP) titanium through an arc-deposition process to form an Arc-dep (AD) macrotextured surface. After first being grit-blasted, this surface can be coated with hydroxyapatite. Although grit blasting the AD surface decreases the surface roughness by 38%, it provides a more suitable surface for the hydroxyapatite coating (28). Despite the decrease in surface roughness, in several animal studies, an arc-deposited substrate coated with hydroxyapatite demonstrated greater biologic fixation than did a similar, uncoated surface (28, 29).

The third type of surface coating is porous coating. Porous coating is a three dimensional structure, commonly beads or wire mesh, that is fixed to the surface of an implant and allows the ingrowth of host bone. This type of surface texture has been used extensively in clinical applications without any surface coating and appears to have an inherent ability to promote the biologic fixation of implant to host bone (30, 31). However, while studies have shown that porous-coated implants are able to maintain clinical stability for many years, retrieval studies have demonstrated mainly fibrous, rather than bony ingrowth into these implants (32,

33, 34). In efforts to improve the osseointegration of host bone into porous surfaces, it was believed the only function of the calcium-phosphate coating was to simply direct the early growth of bone into the pores. For such a limited role, lesser quality calcium phosphate ceramics, including tricalcium-phosphate, have been used. While *in vivo* studies of tricalcium phosphate on a porous surface have shown early improvements in the attachment strength of tissue to implant (35, 36), longer term follow-up has failed to show any long-term advantage of this calcium-phosphate coating (24).

Trials with hydroxyapatite on a porous surface have demonstrated enhanced osseointegration. HA coated surfaces have shown increased tensile strength at the implant-bone interface compared to uncoated porous surfaces (37, 38, 39). Hydroxyapatite coated porous surfaces have also been successful at promoting gap healing between the metal substrate and host bone; in several trials they were shown to bridge gaps of one to two millimeters with bone (8, 40, 41, 42). In a canine model simulating micromotion between an implant and host bone, hydroxyapatite-coated porous implants were compared to porous implants not coated with hydroxyapatite. When compared to the uncoated implants, the hydroxyapatite-coated implants appeared to limit the thickness of the fibrous membrane that formed and induced the formation of fibrocartilage and higher concentrations of collagen (19, 43). After 16 weeks of micromotion, hydroxyapatite possibly induced the formation of bone from fibrocartilage on a porous substrate (44). It is suggested that if, at the time of prosthetic implantation, absolute implant stability or bony contact is not achieved, the addition of HA to a porous-coated implant may promote more bony ingrowth than would an uncoated implant.

Application of Hydroxyapatite Coating

The metal substrate can be covered with hydroxyapatite using several methods. Two of these methods are of significant clinical relevance, plasma spray and solution deposition. Plasma spray has been the most popular method of HA application. In this method, the hydroxyapatite feedstock powder is mixed with a carrier gas and passed through a high temperature electrical arc (30,000 Kelvin). This process melts the surface of the HA and accelerates the particles onto the metal substrate in a "line of sight" pattern (i.e., only those surfaces that are perpendicular to the application beam are coated with HA). Plasma spraying allows a dense, adherent coating of up to 100μm to be applied quickly and accurately to both microtextured and macrotextured metal substrates. As only those surfaces that directly face the application beam get covered with HA, the plasma spraying process results in any three-dimensional surface receiving an uneven pattern of HA coating. Subsequently, "peaks and valleys" form, as the HA is maximally applied to all surfaces perpendicular to the application beam, and not applied to all surfaces either tangent to or hidden from the application beam.

Solution deposition directly addresses this particular limitation of the plasma spray application process. In solution deposition, HA is directly precipitated at low temperature onto the surface of the metal substrate. This produces a pure, highly crystalline, firmly attached HA coating that is evenly distributed over all surfaces. With this method of HA application, the maximum obtainable HA thickness is 2μm (45). Therefore, solution deposition may represent an augmentation to biologic fixation, which would be expected with a thicker coating of HA5n as opposed to providing primary fixation, which would be expected with a thicker coating of HA (5).

Implantable Bone Chamber Model

In our laboratory, we designed an implantable bone chamber to use in an animal model to study the intramedullary bone response to different implant materials, surface textures, and osteoconductive materials in a similar physical environment (46). It was designed to resemble the *in vivo* location of orthopaedic implants in the intramedullary canal. With this implantable chamber, one can reliably measure the affinity of bone for various test materials. The rate at which bone is formed can be measured, as can the quantity and quality of the new bone. This model also allows for the test material-bone interface to be rigorously analyzed.

Implantable bone chambers have been used in previous studies of bone tissues to evaluate physiologic responses and processes, including basic bone function and circulation, normal bone healing, and bone response to different materials and osteogenic factors (47, 48, 49). These early implantable bone chambers were usually made of metal and often consisted of a single large chamber

through which the response of host cortical or cancellous bone could be measured.

In our model, the implantable chamber is constructed of ultra-high-molecular-weight-polyethylene (UHMWPE), which is chosen for several reasons. First, although it is biocompatible, it is relatively inert. Therefore, it will not cause a bony reaction to its presence, thus eliminating the bone response to the chamber itself as a confounding variable to the experimental design. Secondly, it is easily machined and is readily available. It is radiolucent and facilitates the use of high quality radiographs to evaluate ingrown bone in the test chambers. Lastly, as it is nonmetallic and allows for the testing of metallic substances without introducing the confounder of galvanic effects that may result from the interaction between the chamber and test metals.

The implantable bone chamber is a rectangular implant 8mm wide by 25mm long by 10mm deep. It contains a central opening measuring 5mm by 18mm, with eleven slots cut into the floor and ceiling of the central opening to allow the placement of the test substrate in the form of a coupon. Twenty coupons of the various materials to be tested are placed into the slots, thus creating surfaces lining the ingrowth channels. The coupons are placed so that similar materials comprise both sides of the testing channel. Each channel measures 1mm in width between the two testing coupons, 5mm in height, and 8mm in length. A 1mm lip is present at the outer surface of the UHMWPE implant to isolate the intramedullary space from ingrowth of periosteal bone. Additionally, the ingrowth channels are offset 2mm from the outer edge of the implant to ensure they are entirely within the intramedullary space when the chamber is implanted within the intramedullary canal; this effectively discourages bony ingrowth from the endosteal surface. The schematic for the implant chamber model can be seen in Figure 1.

In the canine animal model, the assembled implantable chambers are placed through a cortical window in the lateral distal metaphysis of the distal femur (fig. 2). After implantation, the ingrowth channels are oriented in a perpendicular direction to the long axis of the femur, with the channel openings facing the endosteal surfaces of the intact anterior and posterior cortices.

At the completion of an experiment, the animals are euthanized, and the bone chamber is removed from the distal femur with the use of a diamond

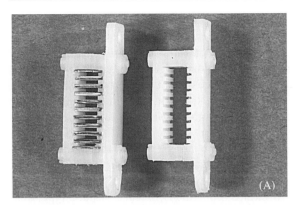

Figure 1 – Implant Chamber Model Schematic. A) Implantable bone chamber without (right) and with (left) metal test coupons. B) Schematic of implantable bone chamber and how coupon "sandwiches" are tested in tension.

(Adapted from Spivak JM, Ricci JL, Blumenthal NC *et al.* "A new canine model to evaluate the biologic response of intramedullary bone to implant materials and surfaces". *J. Biomed. Mater. Res.*, 24:1122-49:1990).

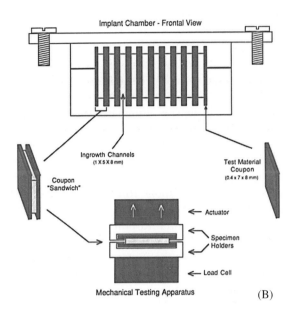

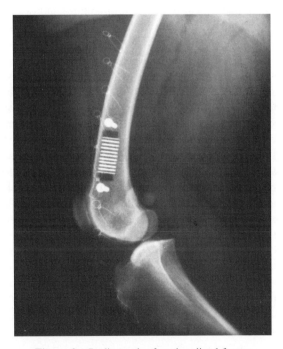

Figure 2 – Radiograph of canine distal femur with implanted bone chamber in distal metaphysis.

wire saw. The contents of the experimental chamber can then be tested as per the experimental design. The bone chambers first undergo Faxitron (high-resolution) radiographs for the quantitative assessment of bone penetration into the channels. The individual units to be evaluated consist of two test coupons with interposed bone and/or soft tissue, which are removed from the bone chamber.

Samples to be evaluated histologically are placed in formalin and embedded in plastic, and the remaining units are prepared for mechanical testing.

The experimental product is a sandwich of two test coupons that have identical opposing surfaces with regard to their metal substrate, surface texture, and coating. They contain the new bone or soft tissue that has grown between them. This "sandwich" readily avails itself to mechanical testing in tension. Mechanical testing in tension is a well validated method of quantifying the interfacial bonding strength between two materials (50, 51). One of the major advantages of tensile testing over other types of mechanical testing is that it eliminates the mechanical interaction between a roughened surface and the surrounding bone and allows a more accurate determination of the bonding, or chemical interaction, between two surfaces.

Others have used the transcortical plug push-out model to evaluate the implant-bone mechanical interactions. This involves implanting the material to be tested directly into cortical bone. Although a popular method of mechanical testing, it has been criticized for its many disadvantages and sources of experimental error (52). The push-out test primarily loads the test subject in shear (38, 24). This allows the surface texture roughness of the test object, as well as the radial stresses of the host bone around the test object, to influence the force required to move the test object rather than isolating the bond between the test samples and bone (52, 53, 54). Secondly, the test results are heavily dependent upon the conformity of the bone-implant interface (55). Any tapering of the implant or cortical window, or any periosteal overgrowth can influence the experimental results. Testing material interactions in tension eliminates many of these variables and allows for a direct determination of the force of adhesion between the experimental coupons and bone.

Although the transcortical plug push-out model may replicate the shear forces exposed to the femoral component of a total hip arthroplasty (THA), the implantable bone chamber model allows for testing in tension, which may more accurately resemble the forces experienced by the acetabular component (56). It is well established that bone growth and remodeling are both heavily influenced by physiologic mechanical forces (57, 58). These forces are both difficult to measure *in vivo* and are virtually impossible to control experimentally in an animal model. By placing the bone chamber in an intramedullary position, we are able to eliminate this variable as a factor in influencing the amount and quality of bone that grows in the experimental chambers. The bone that grows in the chambers is influenced solely by the biological interaction of the native tissues for the material properties, surface texture, and coating of the tested coupon.

Chamber Studies

The implantable bone chamber model has been used to examine the influence on bone formation of different metal substrates, including various metals, surface textures, and osteoconductive coatings. The following three studies are relevant to this chapter.

Study 1: Intramedullary Bone Response to Two Different Surface Textures with and without a Hydroxyapatite Coating (59)

This study utilized the implantable bone chamber to focus on the intramedullary bone response to different titanium and hydroxyapatite implant surfaces. Test coupons were prepared with four different surface coatings: arc-deposited (macrotextured) titanium (AD), hydroxyapatite coated arc-deposited titanium (HA/AD), aluminum grit-blasted (GB) titanium alloy (Ti-6Al-4V), and hydroxyapatite-coated grit-blasted titanium alloy. The hydroxyap-

atite was applied by plasma spray to a thickness of 50μm. The test coupons were placed in the bone chamber and then implanted in the canine animal model. Six animals with chambers in both femora were euthanized at the time periods of 6, 12, and 24 weeks, and a total of 36 bone chambers were retrieved. High resolution radiographs were obtained to assess bone ingrowth. The bone chambers were then disassembled, and the test specimens, which consisted of coupon-tissue-coupon "sandwiches", were mechanically tested in tension to failure. Specimens of each surface type were examined histologically and histomorphometrically for bone ingrowth and bone apposition.

Bone and soft tissue were found to have grown into both ends of all test specimens. At six weeks, the bone was found to be immature, consisting of many thin trabeculae, and a mixture of both poorly organized woven bone and newly remodeled lamellar bone. At 12 and 24 weeks, the bone was found to be progressively more mature and organized, consisting of fewer but thicker trabeculae. Histological examination and high-resolution x-ray showed for all time periods that the arc-deposited surfaces, both with and without hydroxyapatite, showed higher amounts of bone ingrowth into the test chamber and bony apposition to the coupon surface than did grit-blasted surfaces with and without hydroxyapatite. Surfaces with AD/HA showed the highest amounts of bone ingrowth and apposition. In mechanical testing, the uncoated grit-blasted surface failed to show any measurable tensile strength. The arc-deposited surface showed increasing tensile strength with time. The highest tensile strengths were recorded with an AD/HA surface. These samples showed not only the highest tensile strengths for each time period, but also showed increasing tensile strength at each time period. The GB/HA surface showed high tensile strengths at week six (although not as high as AD/HA), but this value decreased with time.

At the three time periods tested, the arc-deposited surfaces, with and without hydroxyapatite, were found to correlate with increasing amounts of bone ingrowth and with greater tensile strengths to failure. In the AD/HA model, the hydroxyapatite appeared to act synergistically with the macrotextured arc-deposited surface to promote the greatest amount of bone ingrowth and the highest tensile strengths. Although the hydroxyapatite coating appeared to increase bone ingrowth and tensile strength on the grit-blasted surface, this effect on tensile strength

	6 weeks	
AD (n = 11)	9.5 ± 7.9	
AD/HA (n = 6)	111.2 ± 59.4*	
GB (n = 10)		0
GB/HA (n = 10)	95.7 ± 57.6*	
	12 weeks	
AD (n = 8)	19.1 ± 13.8	
AD/HA (n = 8)	171.1 ± 43.6*†	
GB (n = 10)		0
GB/HA (n = 7)	82.0 ± 45.6*	
	24 weeks	
AD (n = 11)	49.3 ± 40.0	
AD/HA (n = 6)	207.5 ± 74.0*†	
GB (n = 10)		0
GB/HA (n = 10)	35.4 ± 38.7	

* Significantly greater than AD, $p < 0.05$
† Significantly greater than GB/HA, $p < 0.05$
AD = arc-deposited commercially pure titanium (CPTi). AD/HA = arc-deposited CPTi with plasma sprayed hydroxyapatite. GB = grit blasted commercially pure titanium (CPTi). GB/HA = grit blasted CPTi with plasma sprayed hydroxyapatite.
Adapted from Pereira DS, Ricci JL, Scott D, Casar RS, Jaffe W, Hawkins M, Oh YH, and Alexander H Comprehensive testing of experimental coatings using an implantable chamber model. Transactions Orthopaedic Research Society, 557, 1995 as well as from unpublished data.

Table 1 – Tensile strengths to failure of surface coatings (Newtons, N).

diminished with time. The grit-blasted surface alone showed varying amounts of ingrowth but failed to demonstrate any significant tensile strength at any period. This was attributed to the primarily fibrous rather than bony ingrowth of the coupon-tissue interface in these uncoated GB samples.

The mechanical testing indicated that the degree of roughness of the surface texture is an important determinate of tensile strength. In this experiment, it is believed that the high tensile strength of the arc-deposited samples represents the ability of this surface to interlock with the bone. It also demonstrated that a hydroxyapatite coating can increase the resistance to tensile forces, but that this effect diminishes with time in a microtextured surface (GB) and increases with time in a macrotextured surface (AD).

Study 2: Stimulation of Bone Ingrowth into Porous Beaded Surfaces: Use of Permanent and Resorbable Coatings (60)

The purpose of this study was to compare the intramedullary bone response of a cobalt-chromium porous-coated substrate with various surface enhancements. The three tested substrates included porous cobalt-chrome-molybdenum (PCC), PCC with plasma-sprayed hydroxyapatite (PCC/HA), and PCC infiltrated with resorbable calcium sulfate hemihydrate (PCC/CSH). The interest in testing CSH in this study was prompted by previous trials that indicated this quickly resorbed substance was able to react with body fluids to produce hydroxyapatite-like mineral deposits in surrounding soft tissues. It was found that these deposits could act as a scaffold for ingrowing bone (61).

Test coupons of the three different porous substrates were created. PCC/HA samples were made by plasma spraying a 25-μm layer of hydroxyapatite to a PCC surface. PCC/CSH samples were made by infiltrating a PCC surface with CSH. Using an experimental design similar to the previous study, test coupons were placed into implantable bone chambers which were placed into the distal femora of a canine model. These were retrieved at 3, 6, and 12 weeks. The samples were analyzed by high resolution radiography to measure bone ingrowth, with mechanical testing in tension to assess tensile strengths, and histologically by light microscopy and scanning electron microscopy (SEM) to assess bone ingrowth and apposition.

All specimens at three and six weeks exhibited new bone formation with immature, thin trabeculae comprised of a mixture of disorganized woven bone and newly remodeled lamellar bone. Analysis of high resolution radiographs showed the least amount of bone ingrowth in the PCC sample. The highest quantity of ingrowth was seen with PCC/CSH samples; however, calcium phosphate deposits produced by dissolving CSH are radiopaque and indistinguishable radiographically from bone, and therefore give artificially elevated ingrowth values to these results.

At 3 weeks, SEM analysis showed minimal bone ingrowth or apposition of any of the PCC samples while PCC/CSH samples showed extensive deposits of material resembling bone mineral in the porous matrix. At 6 weeks, there were limited areas of bony ingrowth into the both the PCC and PCC/HA substrates. It was noted that, although there was no demonstrable attachment of bone to the PCC surface, there was direct attachment of new bone to the hydroxyapatite coating in the PCC/HA samples. Although the PCC/CSH samples showed extensive bone ingrowth into the porous surface and bone incorporation of the calcium phosphate deposits, there was no direct attachment of new bone to the PCC surface. By 12 weeks, there was extensive bone ingrowth in both the PCC/HA and PCC/CSH surfaces. Less ingrowth was noted in the PCC samples.

Mechanical testing in tension was then performed to evaluate the substrate-tissue interface. All three samples were found to have increased tensile strength with time. Both PCC/HA and PCC/CSH exhibited a higher tensile strength at all time periods than did PCC alone.

Initial bone contact with the experimental surfaces in this model was minimal. Ultimate fixation was found to depend upon the rate of new bone ingrowth. New bone ingrowth into the uncoated PCC surface was slow and incomplete. The fixation was significantly improved with the addition of an osteoconductive hydroxyapatite coating that provided a surface for direct bone attachment as well as a stimulus for new bone conduction along its surface. PCC/CSH samples had equivalent tensile strengths to PCC/HA samples and were found to stimulate new bone ingrowth into the porous surfaces. The CSH coating was found to resorb within the first 3 weeks, which may limit its clinical usefulness.

Study 3: The effect of alendronate and implant surface on bone integration and remodeling in a canine model (62)

The purpose of this study was to determine the effect of alendronate on bone formation and attachment to metal substrates in a normal and simulated estrogen deficient, calcium deficient canine model. This study was undertaken to determine if alen-

dronate would inhibit bone formation around a metal substrate and limit the potential for osseointegration in a postmenopausal, osteoporotic model. To simulate estrogen and calcium deficiency, the experimental group underwent oophorectomy and was feed a low calcium diet for eight weeks prior to bone chamber implantation. The test coupons were made from the titanium alloy Ti-6Al-4V and were covered with three different surfaces: arc-deposited (AD) commercially pure titanium (CPTi), AD-CPTi with a 50-μm layer of plasma sprayed hydroxyapatite, and chemically textured (microtextured) Ti-6Al-4V with a 50-μm layer of plasma-sprayed hydroxyapatite. Half of the experimental group and half of the control group were administered the drug alendronate at 2.5μm/kg three times per week throughout the study period. The animals were euthanized at 24 weeks post-implantation, and the test bone chambers were retrieved. The samples were analyzed by high resolution radiography to measure bone ingrowth, with mechanical testing in tension to assess tensile strengths. They were also analyzed histologically by light microscopy and scanning electron microscopy (SEM) in order to assess bone ingrowth and apposition.

The results of this study showed that alendronate had no effect on tissue penetration or bone-to-substrate contact. In all cases, the non-hydroxyapatite-coated coupons exhibited largely fibrous ingrowth. In instances where bone was seen, it was not typically in direct contact with the test surface. The mean bone-to-surface contact area was 24.7 ± 1.3%. In contrast, in both of the HA coated surfaces, the amount of bony ingrowth was significantly greater, and there was virtually no fibrous ingrowth. The mean bone to surface contact area

Surface Type	3 weeks	6 weeks	12 weeks
PCC	1.9 ± 3.0 (6)	18.4 ± 16.3 (11)	50.1 ± 20.4 (11)
PCC/HA	12.2 ± 12.7 (7) *	110.0 ± 58.4 (10) *	180.5 ± 69.3 (10) *
PCC/CSH	2.3 ± 3.9 (3) *	164.5 ± 34.0 (4) *	175.5 ± 47.5 (4) *

* Significantly different from PCC groups, $p < 0.05$

PCC = porous cobalt-chrome-molybdenum. PCC/HA = PCC with plasma sprayed hydroxyapatite. PCC/CSH = PCC infiltrated with resorbable calcium sulfate hemihydrate.

Adapted from Ricci JL, Kauffman J, Jaffe WL, Pearlman C, Hawkins M, Alexander H (1997) Stimulation of Bone Ingrowth into Porous Beaded Surfaces: use of permanent and resorbable coatings. Transactions, Orthopaedic Research Society, 759.

Table 2 – Tensile failure strengths of bone-implant interfaces, Newtons (mean ± SD)

was 84.3 ± 3.7%. The quality of the bone seen in these specimens was usually mature and lamellar in nature. As seen both histologically and by SEM, it appeared that bone was attached to and integrated with the HA coating.

Mechanical testing of the samples in tension showed that alendronate had no significant effect on the strength of bony attachment to the different implant surfaces in either the control or oophorectomized animals. This testing did reveal significant differences in quantity and strength of bone that formed on the different surfaces. The strongest bony mechanical construct was found on the AD/HA surface, which showed a trend toward greater attachment strength than did the chemically textured/HA substrate. Both of the HA surfaces had significantly stronger bonds to the host bone than did the AD surface.

Alendronate had no significant influence on bony ingrowth or tensile strength. Mochida, *et al.* similarly found that alendronate has no appreciable effect on the initial fixation of short-term bony

remodeling around HA coated femoral implants (63). The AD/HA surface and the chemically etched/HA surfaces both had a greater percentage of bone ingrowth and formed stronger bony attachments than did the AD surface alone. This was true for both the control and the oophorectomy canine models, and shows that the physiologic response to these substrates coated with hydroxyapatite is equally as robust in a healthy model *versus* one with a deficiency in bone metabolism.

Clinically, hydroxyapatite coated implants are useful in situations where host bone is compromised, such as in the osteoporotic patient or in revision total joint arthroplasty. In the clinical setting, there have been excellent results with HA-coated implants in the osteopenic patient (64, 65, 66). Similarly, HA-coated implants have been successfully utilized in revision surgery, where bone loss is a concern. Looking at the femoral component in revision THA, Geesink (67) found that, although the pattern of bone ingrowth was radiographically more irregular then found in the primary setting, the

Surface Type	Intact Dogs		OVX Dogs	
	Alendronate	No Drug	Alendronate	No Drug
AD	50.7 ± 3.05	48.1 ± 5.25	35.8 ± 2.41	58.2 ± 13.28
AD/HA	84.0 ± 1.05 *	75.9 ± 5.27 *	92.0 ± 3.40 *	69.5 ± 9.01 *
ChemEtch/HA	78.7 ± 3.41 *	81.9 ± 2.08 *	77.7 ± 3.62 *	67.7 ± 5.70 *

* Significantly greater than AD, $p < 0.05$

AD = arc-deposited commercially pure titanium (CPTi). AD/HA = arc-deposited CPTi with plasma-sprayed hydroxyapatite. ChemEtch/HA = chemically textured Ti-6Al-4V with plasma-sprayed hydroxyapatite.

Adapted from Frenkel SR, Jaffe WL, Valle CD, Jazrawi L, Maurer S, Baitner A, Wright K, Sala D, Hawkins M, Di Cesare PE (2001) The effect of alendronate (Fosamax) and implant surface on bone integration and remodeling in a canine model. *Journal of Biomedical Materials Research* 58(6):645-50.

Table 3 – Effect of alendronate treatment on bone penetration,
Percentage bone ingrowth into bone chambers (mean ± SEM).

Surface Type	Intact Dogs		OVX Dogs	
	Alendronate	No Drug	Alendronate	No Drug
AD	89.8 ± 19.7	51.3 ± 12.9	36.2 ± 6.0	105.6 ± 14.8
AD/HA	178.4 ± 14.4 *	153.7 ± 11.8 *	218.2 ± 10.2 *	163.4 ± 26.5 *
ChemEtch/HA	124.5 ± 17.8	95.5 ± 11.3	92.9 ± 29.1	125.2 ± 17.4

* Significantly greater than AD, $p < 0.05$

AD = arc-deposited commercially pure titanium (CPTi). AD/HA = arc-deposited CPTi with plasma-sprayed hydroxyapatite. ChemEtch/HA = chemically textured Ti-6Al-4V with plasma-sprayed hydroxyapatite.

Adapted from Frenkel SR. Jaffe WL. Valle CD. Jazrawi L. Maurer S. Baitner A. Wright K. Sala D. Hawkins M. Di Cesare PE (2001) The effect of alendronate (Fosamax) and implant surface on bone integration and remodeling in a canine model. *Journal of Biomedical Materials Research* 58(6):645-50.

Table 4 – Effect of alendronate treatment on strength of bone attachment:
Tensile testing to failure, Newtons (mean ± SEM).

speed and magnitude of bone ingrowth was remarkable. He found the survival rate of the femoral component to be 93% at 11 years.

Metal Substrate in Clinical Practice: Total Hip Arthroplasty as a Paradigm

Hydroxyapatite on a metal substrate is useful to promote early and more complete osseointegration. It does not, however, guarantee persistent implant fixation and survival. In the long-term, the metal substrate and surface texture play very important roles. This is clearly elucidated in the clinical experiences with HA on femoral and acetabular components in THA.

Radiographically and clinically, there has been great success with HA on femoral prosthesis with different metal substrates. Radiographically, it has been shown that proximally coated HA stems, including smooth, grit-blasted stems, produce a characteristic pattern of remodeling in the femur consistent with excellent biologic fixation. In several studies (68, 69, 70, 71), cortical hypertrophy has been shown consistently at the distal junction between the coated and uncoated regions of the stem. Scott, *et al.* (72) directly compared a porous-coated cobalt-chromium stem on one side and a HA-coated, grit-blasted titanium stem of identical geometry on the other side 5 to 7 years after bilateral total hip arthroplasties in three patients. Radiographically, the HA-coated titanium stems showed substantial cortical hypertrophy immediately distal to the junction between the coated and uncoated zones. The porous-coated stems showed less intense cortical hypertrophy, which was located primarily at the distal tip of the prosthesis. There was no stem subsidence, pedestal formation, or proximal bone loss with either type of stem. Using dual-energy X-ray absorptionmetry (DEXA) analysis, Scott was able to show that there was substantially greater bone mineral density proximally around the HA-coated stem. Of particular note was the increased bone mineral density in the first millimeter of bone directly adjacent to the HA coating as compared to the porous coating. If the degree or mode of fixation was the same between these two stems, then one would not expect to see different patterns of bony remodeling. Scott found that the HA-coated titanium stems had more extensive bone ingrowth in the proximal, coated region of the stem. He hypothesized that this signified greater proximal osseointegration and proximal

load transfer than that which occurred with the porous-coated stem.

Clinically, there has been excellent mid-term and long-term results with HA-coated stems. In a multicenter study of 314 hips (274 patients, average age 51) with a proximally 50µm thick plasma-sprayed, HA-coated, grit-blasted titanium stem, D'Antonio *et al.* (73) showed that, at a minimum of 10 years, HA-coated components did enhance bony ongrowth without significant deterioration of femoral component fixation. Radiographic analysis showed findings of bony remodeling consistent with successful biologic fixation. With a microtextured, fully HA-coated (155-µm thick) stem, Rokkum *et al.* (74) showed excellent results in 100 consecutive THAs at 7-9 years post-operatively. Clinically, the results in this series were excellent. Radiographically, there was evidence of good bony incorporation, and no stem loosening or subsidence was noted. Dorr *et al.* (75) compared bilateral THAs in 15 bilateral patients who were given a porous implant (pore size 750µm) in one hip and an identical porous implant with an HA coating (HA thickness 55µm, pore size 490µm after HA coating) in the other hip. These patients were followed between 5 and 7.9 years. Although there was no difference in Harris Hip Scores between these two different implants, there was radiographic evidence of greater proximal bony remodeling, and there were fewer radiolucent lines with the HA-coated stem. As noted in these clinical studies, there is much evidence that supports the mid-term and long-term success of HA-coated femoral implants with either a microtextured or macrotextured surface on a metal substrate.

The use of hydroxyapatite coating on acetabular components has not initially proven to be as successful as the clinical results of HA-coated femoral stems. In a multicenter study looking at three different cementless acetabular designs in 428 hips (377 patients) at an average follow-up of 7.9 years (range 5.3-9.1 years), Manley *et al.* (76) found that 1% of hydroxyapatite-coated threaded cups, 2% of porous-coated cups, and 11% of hydroxyapatite-coated press-fit cups needed revision because of aseptic loosening. A harbinger of failure of the HA press-fit cups was the appearance of a radiolucency in Charnley acetabular zone III at the implant bone interface. This was typically not seen until two years post-implantation. All HA press-fit implants found to be radiographically loose had been radiographically stable with osseous integration at previous follow-up. Manley concluded that the HA press-fit cups achieved initial stability through peripheral hoop stresses, but ultimately failed because they could not sustain the inferior tensile stress between the implant and the host bone imposed by the activity of the patient. Conversely, porous-coated cups achieved initial stability through hoop stress, but were able to maintain long-term stability by allowing bone or fibrous tissue to grow into the coating. HA-threaded cups achieved immediate fixation by mechanically interlocking the component to the bone and, it is assumed, sustained this fixation because the HA coating directed bone growth into the threads over time.

In a radiographic study comparing 4 year results of an HA grit-blasted cup to an HA-arc deposited cup, Jazrawi *et al.* (77) found a significant reduction in radiolucent lines at, most notably, zone III, the implant-bone interface of the macrostructured HA-AD cup. By contrast, at 4 years, there was no significant decrease in the radiolucent lines around the microstructured HA-coated grit-blasted cup. At an average of 5.1 year follow-up of 105 HA-AD cups, Martell *et al.* reported that no cups had been revised, although three showed evidence of osteolysis in zones I and II (78).

Finite element analysis studies (56) examining the interface stresses around acetabular implants inserted without cement show very high shear or distraction forces in the inferior region of the cup during physiologic loads. If complete bony ingrowth or ongrowth does not occur, then these forces could cause failure at the implant-bone interface. This predicted mechanism of failure may explain the radiolucent lines around the HA grit-

Charnley Zone	GB/HA		AD/HA	
	6 weeks	4 years	6 weeks	4 years
1	28	20	48	8
2	30	32	38	6
3	28	24	32	4

Adapted from Jazrawi LM, Adler EM, Jazrawi AJ, Jaffe WL (2000) Radiographic comparison of grit-blasted hydroxyaptite and arc-deposited hydroxyapatite acetabular components. A four-year follow-up study. *Bulletin of the Hospital for Joint Diseases.* 59(3):144-8.

Table 5 – Percentage of Acetabular Components with Radiolucent Lines in Charnley Zones (Percentage).

blasted cup in zone III in both the Manley and the Jazrawi studies and may help to explain their ultimate failure. The appearance of radiolucent lines, particularly in zone III in a microtextured cup, may signal the loss of mechanical interlock between the implant and host bone, as the relatively smooth metal substrate of the component does not have the surface texture to allow long-term rigid fixation. In contrast, the lack of radiolucent lines adjacent to macrostuctured components, particularly at zone III, may indicate that the mechanical interlock between the macrostructure and the host bone is able to maintain stable fixation, even after the HA coating has been partially or fully resorbed and replaced by host bone. Hydroxyapatite can help incorporate bone onto the metal substrate with both micro and macrostructuring, but the metal substrate must achieve and maintain mechanical interlock with the host bone in order to provide long-term stability of the component. Figure 3 depicts a HA/GB failure at 5 years.

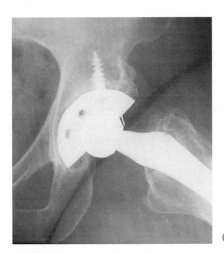

(A)

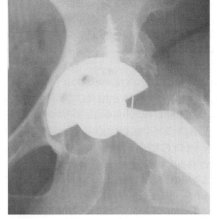

(B)

Figure 3 – HA/GB failure at 5 years. (A) Grit-blasted/hydroxyapatite- coated acetabular implant demonstrating stable fixation 4 years post-operatively. (B) Same component one year later showing loss of fixation with gross displacement.

CONCLUSION

The mechanical properties and biologic potential of a metal substrate determines its ability to both induce formation of new bone and to mechanically or biologically bind to the mineral component of bone or an applied hydroxyapatite surface coating. Although HA can be applied to different metal substrates, it may be able to form a chemical bond with titanium and its alloys. This may improve the mechanical properties and durability of the metal substrate-HA construct and allow increased durability of HA-coated implants.

Surface texture also plays a critical role in influencing the metal substrate-host tissue response. Under equal biological conditions, a microtextured surface causes fibrous tissue growth over its surface with a minimum of bony proliferation or ingrowth. This is the reason for the poor mechanical testing results exhibited by the uncoated, grit-blasted titanium surface in Study 1. An uncoated macrotextured or porous surface, however, has the opposite effect. By nature of its surface characteristics, it is able to promote bony ingrowth and apposition.

Osteoconductive surface coatings strongly influence the deposition of new bone on a metal substrate. This effect, however, may not be permanent and is dependent on the underlying metal substrate and surface coating, as well as on the mechanical forces imposed on the implant. HA-coated macrotextured implants can achieve stable fixation even under tensile forces, while identical HA-coated grit-blasted implants have early failures under similar conditions. It is suggested that this is a result of persistent and enhanced mechanical interlock between a macrotextured implant and bone after the hydroxyapatite is resorbed. An arc-deposited or porous-coated surface allows for strong mechanical interlock between the metal substrate and host bone, while the grit-blasted surface fails to provide sufficient tensile mechanical interlock after the hydroxyapatite has been resorbed or replaced by host bone. Under compression or shear forces, as in femoral fixation, grit-blasted hydroxyapatite has been successful in the long term. However, at the acetabulum where high tensile forces are exhibited, it appears that a macrotextured metal substrate is necessary to provide stable long term fixation.

Reference List

1. Jarcho M (1981) Calcium phosphate ceramics as hard tissue prosthetics. *Clinical Orthopaedics & Related Research* (157):259-78.
2. De Groot K, de Putter C, Sillevis Smitt PAE, Driessen AA (1981) Mechanical failure of artificial teeth made for dense calciumhydroxyapatite. *Science of Ceramics* 11:433-7.
3. Geesink RG. de Groot K. Klein CP (1988) Bonding of bone to apatite-coated implants. *Journal of Bone & Joint Surgery*, British Volume. 70(1):17-22.
4. Kester MA, Manely MT, Taylor SK, Cohen RC (1991) Influence of thickness on the mechanical properties nad bond strength of HA coatings applied to orthopaedic implants. *Trans. Orthop. Res. Soc.* 16:95.
5. Jaffe WL, Scott DF (1996) Total hip arthroplasty with hydroxyapatite-coated prostheses. *Journal of Bone & Joint Surgery* 78(12):1918-34.
6. Manley MT (1993) Calcium Phosphate Biomaterials: A review of the Literature. In: Hydroxylapatite Coatings in Orthopaedic Surgery. Ed RGT Geesink and MT Manley. Raven Press, Ltd, New York, NY: pp 1-23.
7. Sun L, Berndt CC, Gross KA, Kucuk A (2001) Material fundamentals and clinical performance of plasma-sprayed hydroxyapatite coatings: a review. *Journal of Biomedical Materials Research* 58(5):570-92.
8. Geesink RG, De Groot K, Klein CP (1987) Chemical implant fixation using hydroxyl-apatite coatings. The development of a human total hip prosthesis for chemical fixation to bone using hydroxyl-apatite coatings on titanium substrates. *Clinical Orthopaedics & Related Research* (225):147-70.
9. Ducheyne P, Van Raemdonck W, Heughebaert JC, Heughebaert M (1986) Structural analysis of hydroxyapatite coatings on titanium. *Biomaterials* 7(2):97-103.
10. Pham MT, Matz W, Grambole D, Herrmann F, Reuther H, Richter E, Steiner G (2002) Solution deposition of hydroxyapatite on titanium pretreated with a sodium ion implantation. *Journal of Biomedical Materials Research* 59(4):716-24.
11. Kuroda K, Ichino R, Okido M, Takai O (2002) Effects of ion concentration and pH on hydroxyapatite deposition from aqueous solution onto titanium by the thermal substrate method. *J. Biomed. Mater. Res.* 61(3):354-9.
12. Agata De Sena L, Calixto De Andrade M, Malta Rossi A, De Almeida Soares G (2002) Hydroxyapatite deposition by electrophoresis on titanium sheets with different surface finishing. *Journal of Biomedical Materials Research* 60(1):1-7.
13. Filiaggi MJ, Coombs NA, Pilliar RM (1991) Characterization of the interface in the plasma-sprayed HA coating/Ti-6Al-4V implant system. *Journal of Biomedical Materials Research* 25(10):1211-29.
14. Mears DC (1979) Materials and Orthopedic Surgery. Williams and Wilkins. Baltimore, MD.
15. Weinans H, Huiskes R, Grootenboer HJ (1992) Effects of material properties of femoral hip components on

bone remodeling. *Journal of Orthopaedic Research* 10(6):845-53.

16. Cheal EJ, Spector M, Hayes WC (1992) Role of loads and prosthesis material properties on the mechanics of the proximal femur after total hip arthroplasty. *Journal of Orthopaedic Research* 10(3):405-22.

17. Bobyn JD, Mortimer ES, Glassman AH, Engh CA, Miller JE, Brooks CE (1992) Producing and avoiding stress shielding. Laboratory and clinical observations of noncemented total hip arthroplasty. *Clinical Orthopaedics & Related Research* (274):79-96.

18. Huiskes R, Weinans H, Van Rietbergen B (1992) The relationship between stress shielding and bone resorption around total hip stems and the effects of flexible materials. *Clinical Orthopaedics & Related Research.* (274):124-34.

19. Soballe K, Hansen ES, B-Rasmussen H, Jorgensen PH, Bunger C (1992) Tissue ingrowth into titanium and hydroxyapatite-coated implants during stable and unstable mechanical conditions. *Journal of Orthopaedic Research* 10(2):285-99.

20. Scott DF, Jaffe WL (1996) Host-bone response to porous-coated cobalt-chrome and hydroxyapatite-coated titanium femoral components in hip arthroplasty. Dual-energy x-ray absorptiometry analysis of paired bilateral cases at 5 to 7 years. *Journal of Arthroplasty.* 11(4):429-37.

21. Diegel PD. Daniels AU. Dunn HK (1989) Initial effect of collarless stem stiffness on femoral bone strain. *Journal of Arthroplasty* 4(2):173-8.

22. Cook SD, Kay JF, Thomas KA, Haddad RJ Jr (1987) Interface mechanics and histology of titanium and hydroxylapatite-coated titanium for dental implant applications. International *J. Oral and Maxillofac. Implants* 2:15-22.

23. Cook SD, Thomas KA, Kay JF (1991) Experimental coating defects in hydroxylapatite-coated implants. *Clinical Orthopaedics & Related Research* (265):280-90.

24. Thomas KA, Kay JF, Cook SD, Jarcho M (1987) The effect of surface macrotexture and hydroxylapatite coating on the mechanical strengths and histologic profiles of titanium implant materials. *Journal of Biomedical Materials Research* 21(12):1395-414.

25. Svehla M, Morberg P, Bruce W, Zicat B, Walsh WR (2002) The effect of substrate roughness and hydroxyapatite coating thickness on implant shear strength. *Journal of Arthroplasty* 17(3):304-11.

26. Stephenson PK, Freeman MA, Revell PA, Germain J, Tuke M, Pirie CJ (1991) The effect of hydroxyapatite coating on ingrowth of bone into cavities in an implant. *Journal of Arthroplasty* 6(1):51-8.

27. Poser RD, Kay JF, Magee FP, Hadday AK (1993) Preclinical evaluation of the effect of hydroxyapatite on the "comprehensive" bone-implant interface. In: Hydroxyapatite Coatings in Orthopaedic Surgery. pp. 137-149. Edited by RGT Geesink and MT Manley. New York, Raven Press.

28. Hawkins MV, Bauer TW, Friedman RJ, Zimmerman MC, Ricci JL, and Jaffe WL (1995) Evaluation of an arc-deposited CPTI surface with and without hydroxyapatite coating in three *in vivo* studies. Presented as a poster exhibit a the Annual Meeting of The American Academy of Orthopaedic Surgeons, Orlando, Florida, Feb. 17.

29. Periera, DS, Ricci JL, Scott DF, Casar CS, Jafee WL, Hawkins MV, Oh Y, Alexander H (1993) Effects of macroroughness and hydroxyapatite coating on osteointegration and osteoconduction. Read at the Annual Meeting of the Society for Biomaterials, San Francisco, California, March 19.

30. Smith SE, Estok DM 2nd, Harris WH (1998) Average 12-year outcome of a chrome-cobalt, beaded, bony ingrowth acetabular component. *Journal of Arthroplasty* 13(1):50-60.

31. Kronick JL, Barba ML, Paprosky WG (1997) Extensively coated femoral components in young patients. *Clinical Orthopaedics & Related Research* (344):263-74.

32. Bobyn JD, Engh CA, Glassman AH (1987) Histologic analysis of a retrieved microporous-coated femoral prosthesis. A seven-year case report. *Clinical Orthopaedics & Related Research* (224):303-10.

33. Collier JP, Mayor MB, Chae JC, Surprenant VA, Surprenant HP, Dauphinais LA (1988) Macroscopic and microscopic evidence of prosthetic fixation with porous-coated materials. *Clinical Orthopaedics & Related Research* (235):173-80.

34. Cook SD, Thomas KA, Haddad RJ Jr (1988) Histologic analysis of retrieved human porous-coated total joint components. *Clinical Orthopaedics & Related Research* (234):90-101.

35. Berry JL, Geiger JM, Moran JM, Skraba JS, Greenwald AS (1986) Use of tricalcium phosphate or electrical stimulation to enhance the bone-porous implant interface. *Journal of Biomedical Materials Research* 20(1):65-77.

36. Rivero DP, Fox J. Skipor AK. Urban RM. Galante JO (1988) Calcium phosphate-coated porous titanium implants for enhanced skeletal fixation. *Journal of Biomedical Materials Research* 22(3):191-201.

37. Cook SD, Thomas KA, Dalton JE *et al.* (1991) *Trans. Orthop. Res. Soc.* 16:550.

38. Cook SD, Thomas KA, Dalton JE, Volkman TK, Whitecloud TS 3rd, Kay JF (1992) Hydroxylapatite coating of porous implants improves bone ingrowth and interface attachment strength. *Journal of Biomedical Materials Research* 26(8):989-1001.

39. Dalton JE, Cook SD, Thomas KA, Kay JF (1995) The effect of operative fit and hydroxyapatite coating on the mechanical and biological response to porous implants. *Journal of Bone & Joint Surgery.* 77(1):97-110.

40. Cook SD, Thomas KA, Dalton JE, Kay JF (1991) Enhanced bone ingrowth and fixation strength with hydroxyapatite-coated porous implants. *Seminars in Arthroplasty* 2(4):268-79.

41. Søballe K, Hansen ES, Brockstedt-Rasmussen H, Hjortdal VE, Juhl GI, Pedersen CM, Hvid I, Bunger C (1991) Gap healing enhanced by hydroxyapatite coating in dogs. *Clinical Orthopaedics & Related Research* (272):300-7.

42. Søballe K, Hansen ES, Brockstedt-Rasmussen H, Pedersen CM, Bunger C (1990) Hydroxyapatite coating enhances fixation of porous coated implants. A comparison in dogs between press fit and noninterference fit. *Acta Orthop. Scand.* 61(4):299-306.

43. Søballe K, Brockstedt-Rasmussen H, Hansen ES, Bunger C (1992) Hydroxyapatite coating modifies implant membrane formation. Controlled micromotion studied in dogs. *Acta Orthopaedica Scandinavica.* 63(2):128-40.

44. Søballe K, Hansen ES, Brockstedt-Rasmussen H, Bunger C (1993) Hydroxyapatite coating converts fibrous tissue to bone around loaded implants. *Journal of Bone & Joint Surgery*, British Volume. 75(2):270-8.

45. Dumbleton JH (1996) Personal Communication.

46. Spivak JM, Ricci JL, Blumenthal NC *et al.* (1990) "A new canine model to evaluate the biologic response of intramedullary bone to implant materials and surfaces". *J. Biomed. Mater. Res.* 24:1122-49.

47. Albrektsson T (1987) Implantable devices for long-term vital microscopy of bone tissue. *Crit. Rev. Biocompat.* 3:25-51.

48. Winet H. Albrektsson T (1988) Wound healing in the bone chamber 1. Neoosteogenesis during transition from the repair to the regenerative phase in the rabbit tibial cortex. *Journal of Orthopaedic Research* 6(4):531-9.

49. Kalebo P. Jacobsson M (1988) Recurrent bone regeneration in titanium implants. Experimental model for determining the healing capacity of bone using quantitative microradiography. *Biomaterials* 9(4):295-301.

50. Lin H, Xu H, Zhang X, De Groot K (1998) Tensile tests of interface between bone and plasma-sprayed HA coating-titanium implant. *Journal of Biomedical Materials Research* 43(2):113-22.

51. Gross U, Brandes J, Strunz V, Bab I, Sela J (1981) The ultrastructure of the interface between a glass ceramic and bone. *Journal of Biomedical Materials Research* 15(3):291-305.

52. Black J (1989) "Push-out" tests. *Journal of Biomedical Materials Research* 23(11):1243-5.

53. Dhert WJ, Verheyen CC, Braak LH, De Wijn JR, Klein CP, De Groot K, Rozing PM (1992) A finite element analysis of the push-out test: influence of test conditions. *Journal of Biomedical Materials Research* 26(1):119-30.

54. Ricci JL, Spivak JM, Alexander H, Blumenthal NC, Parsons JR (1989) Hydroxyapatite ceramics and the nature of the bone-ceramic interface. *Bulletin of the Hospital for Joint Diseases Orthopaedic Institute* 49(2):178-91.

55. Spivak JM, Ricci JL, Blumenthal NC, Alexander H (1990) A new canine model to evaluate the biological response of intramedullary bone to implant materials and surfaces. *Journal of Biomedical Materials Research* 24(9):1121-49.

56. Rapperport DJ, Carter DR, Schurman DJ (1987) Contact finite element stress analysis of porous ingrowth acetabular cup implantation, ingrowth, and loosening. *Journal of Orthopaedic Research* 5(4):548-61.

57. Wolff J (1892) Das Gaetz der Transformation: Transformation der Knocken. Berlin, Hirschwald.

58. Wolff J (1986) The Law of Remodeling. Maquet P, Furlong R (trans). Berlin, Springer Verlag, (original manuscript 1892).

59. Pereira DS, Ricci JL, Scott D, Casar RS, Jaffe W, Hawkins M, Oh YH, Alexander H (1995) Comprehensive testing of experimental coatings using an implantable chamber model. *Transactions Orthopaedic Research Society*, 557.

60. Ricci J, Kauffman J, Jaffe W, Pearlman C, Hawkins M, Alexander H (1997) Stimulation of Bone Ingrowth into Porous Beaded Surfaces: Use of Permanent and Resorbable Coatings. *Transactions Orthopaedic Research Society*, 759.

61. Ricci JL (1992) *Trans. Soc. Biomater.* 15:49.

62. Frenkel SR, Jaffe WL, Valle CD, Jazrawi L, Maurer S, Baitner A, Wright K, Sala D, Hawkins M, Di Cesare PE (2001) The effect of alendronate (Fosamax) and implant surface on bone integration and remodeling in a canine model. *Journal of Biomedical Materials Research* 58(6):645-50.

63. Mochida Y, Bauer TW, Akisue T, Brown PR (2002) Alendronate does not inhibit early bone apposition to hydroxyapatite-coated total joint implants: a preliminary study. *Journal of Bone & Joint Surgery* 84-A(2):226-35.

64. Kligman M, Kirsh G (2000) Hydroxyapatite-coated total hip arthroplasty in osteoporotic patients. *Bulletin of the Hospital for Joint Diseases* 59(3):136-9.

65. Søballe K, Hansen ES, Brockstedt-Rasmussen H, Hjortdal VE, Juhl GI, Pedersen CM, Hvid I, Bunger C (1991) Fixation of titanium and hydroxyapatite-coated implants in arthritic osteopenic bone. *Journal of Arthroplasty* 6(4):307-16.

66. Søballe K, Gotfredsen K, Brockstedt-Rasmussen H, Nielsen PT, Rechnagel K (1991) Histologic analysis of a retrieved hydroxyapatite-coated femoral prosthesis. *Clinical Orthopaedics & Related Research* (272):255-8.

67. Geesink RG (2002) Osteoconductive coatings for total joint arthroplasty. *Clinical Orthopaedics & Related Research* (395):53-65.

68. D'Antonio JA, Capello WN, Manley MT (1996) Remodeling of bone around hydroxyapatite-coated femoral stems. *Journal of Bone & Joint Surgery* 78(8):1226-34.

69. D'Antonio JA, Capello WN, Crothers OD, Jaffe WL, Manley MT (1992) Early clinical experience with hydroxyapatite-coated femoral implants. *Journal of Bone & Joint Surgery* 74(7):995-1008.

70. D'Antonio JA, Capello WN, Jaffe WL (1992) Hydroxylapatite-coated hip implants. Multicenter three-year clinical and roentgenographic results. *Clinical Orthopaedics & Related Research* (285):102-15.

71.   ⌐, Scott DF (1993) Rationale and clinical application of hydroxyapatite coatings in pressfit total hip arthroplasty. *Seminars in Arthroplasty* 4(3):159-66.

72. Scott DF, Jaffe WL (1996) Host-bone response to porous-coated cobalt-chrome and hydroxyapatite-coated titanium femoral components in hip arthroplasty. Dual-energy x-ray absorptiometry analysis of paired bilateral cases at 5 to 7 years. *Journal of Arthroplasty* 11(4):429-37.

73. D'Antonio JA, Capello WN, Manley MT, Geesink R (2000) Hydroxyapatite femoral stems for total hip arthroplasty: 10- to 13-year followup. *Clinical Orthopaedics & Related Research* (393):101-11.

74. Rokkum M, Brandt M, Bye K, Hetland KR, Waage S, Reigstad A (1999) Polyethylene wear, osteolysis and acetabular loosening with an HA-coated hip prosthesis. A follow-up of 94 consecutive arthroplasties. [see comments.]. *Journal of Bone & Joint Surgery*, British Volume 81(4):582-9.

75. Dorr LD, Wan Z, Song M, Ranawat A (1998) Bilateral total hip arthroplasty comparing hydroxyapatite coating to porous-coated fixation. *Journal of Arthroplasty* 13(7):729-36.

76. Manley MT, Capello WN, D'Antonio JA, Edidin AA, Geesink RG (1998) Fixation of acetabular cups without cement in total hip arthroplasty. A comparison of three different implant surfaces at a minimum duration of follow-up of five years. *Journal of Bone & Joint Surgery* 80(8):1175-85.

77. Jazrawi LM, Adler EM, Jazrawi AJ, Jaffe WL (2000) Radiographic comparison of grit-blasted hydroxyaptite and arc-deposited hydroxyapatite acetabular components. A four-year follow-up study. *Bulletin of the Hospital for Joint Diseases* 59(3):144-8.

78. Martell JM, Mesko JW, Zelicof SB, Avedian R, Whitehurst J, Jaffe WL (2002) The Five-Year Radiographic Performance of an Arc-Deposited and Hydroxyapatite Coated Cementless Titanium Acetabular Design, unpublished data.

5 Proximal Modularity in a Cementless HA-Coated Hip Replacement Assessment of Utility

Michel P. Philippe, MD, Gérard Gacon, MD, André Ray, MD and Alain Dambreville, MD

INTRODUCTION

Cementless fixation of femoral components has made substantial progress, and more than ten years of clinical follow-up data have been accumulated. However, some questions remain unanswered regarding the different modes of fixation for uncemented stems. Therefore, we set out to design an implant that would obtain both primary and secondary fixation in the metaphysis alone, since there was evidence that stress transfer to the rest of the femur takes place in that part of the bone. The lower (diaphyseal) part of the implant was not to be involved in the fixation of the device.

Studies by Noble (1), Rubin (2) and Fessy (3) had shown that there are three femoral morphotypes: the normal pattern, with an intermediate flare index (between 3 and 4.5); the stovepipe pattern, with a wide shaft and a low flare index (< 3); and the champagne-flute pattern, with a wide metaphysis and a narrow shaft, and with a high flare index (> 4.5). In order to obtain primary stability in the metaphysis without wedging the stem in the diaphysis, these different femoral patterns must be borne in mind.

Rather than trying to adjust the bone to the implant by reaming, which might harm the bone, we thought it better to adjust the implant to the bone, by what we have called "monoprogrammation". This has allowed us to design the modular Esop-HA stem.

MATERIAL AND METHODS

The Esop-HA Prosthesis

This device comes in a right and a left version. It has a neck-shaft angle of 135.5° and 10° of ante-version. The implant consists of two pieces, the metaphyseal part and the diaphyseal part. The metaphyseal part is made of a titanium alloy (Ti-6Al-4V), and is shaped in such a way as to fill the metaphysis. It is designed to wedge itself against the side of the greater trochanter as well as against the anterior and posterior aspects of the metaphysis. The horizontal grooves on its surface counteract subsidence. The textured surface of this metaphyseal part is coated with a 70µm layer of hydroxyapatite (HA) to promote secondary fixation. The part comes in ten sizes.

The diaphyseal part is also made of titanium. However, its surface is smooth and does not have an HA coating. It is comparatively short and comes in seven sizes. It serves only as a temporary centralizer until definitive fixation in the metaphysis has been obtained.

As may be inferred from the above, there are 70 possible combinations. This allows the surgeon to cater to the overwhelming majority of cases encountered in hip arthroplasty. The diaphyseal part fits into the metaphyseal part with a cylindrical connection and supplementary screw fixation (fig. 1).

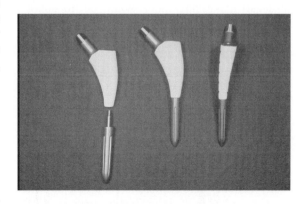

Figure 1 – The modular Esop Stem.

A finite-element study was performed prior to the actual design work, in order to investigate the mechanical behaviour of the connection between the modules. The study was conducted in two stages. The femur was digitized from CT scans, distinguishing between the cortex, the cancellous bone in the metaphysis, and the cancellous bone in the intermediate zone. The prosthesis was then inserted, and the loading conditions were defined using a Pauwels diagram. The load was 2000 N. Calculations were then performed by Cisigraph, to establish deformation, displacements, and stresses. The maximum stress in the connection zone between the two parts was found to be $9.4 daN/mm^2$; this was well below the elastic limit of the material envisaged for the implant.

Concurrently, the French National Test Centre was performing modified fatigue testing, since there were no ISO standards for this type of prosthesis. The implants subjected to these tests were found to withstand 5 million cycles, which proved that the cylindrical connection took most of the stress without transmitting it to the screw thread.

Surgical Technique

At the preoperative planning stage, templates were routinely used. For the metaphyseal part, templating was performed on A/P and on lateral films; for the diaphyseal part, only an A/P film was used. In 71 of our patients, a posterolateral approach was employed, and in 18 cases, the hip was approached through an anterior incision.

At surgery, the diaphyseal diameter was established using specially designed intramedullary "feelers". The diameter of the diaphyseal piece was always one size below that of the last feeler used, so as to make sure there would be no contact between the implant and the inside of the shaft. The metaphysis was prepared with rasps of increasing size, so as to preserve as much cancellous bone as possible. The size of the definitive metaphyseal piece was chosen to match the size of the last rasp found to be stable in both rotation and traction. The neck length was determined using trial heads.

Postoperatively, the patients were managed in identical fashion at all the centres involved in the study. Patients were allowed to get up the day after surgery and to walk immediately, with gradually increased weight-bearing, using two forearm crutches. In all the patients, a suction drain was left in situ for the first 48 hours.

The Study

This was a retrospective multi-centre study involving 89 Esop-HA prostheses implanted between 1991 and 1994 as primary replacements at four centres. The present study could not be considered a consecutive one and will simply serve as a trial clinical series to achieve a better understanding of the proposed design, focusing mainly on the intraoperative selection of implants and technical tips, as well as demographics, complications and radiological findings.

Assessment Protocol

Radiological assessment was performed using a standing A/P film of the pelvis and an A/P and a lateral view of the hip. For the determination of osseointegration and the detection of an radiological changes, the criteria established by Engh *et al.* (4) and by Epinette and Geesink (5) were used. A search was made in the different zones defined by Gruen (6) to detect any reactive lines, spots welds, changes around the stem tip, calcar changes, lucent lines, osteolysis, and migration. Migration was assessed by measuring the distance from the tip of the greater trochanter to the shoulder of the implant. Periprosthetic ossifications were graded using the Brooker system. (7) All the radiographs were digitized and analysed. The radiographs were read by seven independent surgeons. Findings were compared and cross-checked so as to arrive at a homogeneous analysis. Special radiological software (Imagika) and a high-definition radiograph scanner (Vidar System Corporation VXR-8) were used to obtain detailed evidence of any osteolytic lesions and PE wear.

RESULTS

Demographics

Of the 89 implants in the study, 34 were inserted in 32 female patients, and 55 in 48 male patients. The female patients' mean age at surgery was 60 years (range: 45 to 75 years); that of the male patients was 59 years (range: 41 to 78 years).

The most frequent indication was primary osteoarthritis (OA), which accounted for 67% of the cases. OA secondary to acetabular dysplasia accounted for 11%, and essential osteonecrosis for 12%. All the arthroplasties were primary procedures (Table 1).

Diagnosis	N	%
Primary OA	60	67.4
Post-traumatic OA	2	2.3
Rapidly destructive OA	2	2.3
Acetabular dysplasia	10	11.2
Essential osteonecrosis	11	12.4
Fresh femoral neck fracture	1	1.1
Other	3	3.4

Table 1 – Indications for hip replacement.

The mean body mass index (BMI) was 25.4 in the women, and 26.4 in the men; the mean BMI of all the patients was 26.1 (range: 17.58 to 41.02; SD: 4.02). In all, 18% of the prostheses were implanted in markedly obese patients (BMI ≥ 30). For the preoperative anatomical grading, the Fessy index was used. This showed 45 of the femurs to be of the normal pattern, while 17 were stovepipe, and 27 champagne-flute patterns. Analysis of the femoral patterns showed 50.5% of the femurs to have a normal pattern, 19.10% to be stovepipe femurs (a pattern mainly seen in women), and 30.3% to be champagne-flute-shaped.

Complications

The intraoperative complications were confined to three fissures of the femoral neck (3.4%), which were stabilized with an anteroposterior screw in two cases and with cerclage in one case. They did not affect the functional outcome. No fractures of the greater trochanter were observed.

Local complications consisted of three haematomas, of which two required reoperation for drainage. There were three dislocations (3.4%). One occurred immediately postoperatively while the patient was still in hospital and was managed with closed reduction. Two were late dislocations, of which one was trauma-related (road traffic accident) and one was a recurrent dislocation that required reoperation with revision of the cup.

In none of the patients did the stem need revising, and of the implants included in this study, none had the stem removed.

Radiological Results

Implant Positioning

The stem axis was parallel to the femoral shaft axis in 83% of the cases (fig. 2). In 13 cases (15%), it was in varus; however, in only three of these was the angle in relation to the shaft axis > 5°. In three cases, the stem was found to be in valgus; in two of these cases, the angle was < 3°. Any varus angulation seen on the immediately postoperative radiographs remained stable on the films taken during subsequent reviews. By the time of the latest follow-up, there was no evidence of tilting. Varus malalignment was particularly common in young males (mean age: 55 years), who accounted for 12 of the 13 cases seen. Eight of the 13 patients have been followed up for over nine years, and four for between eight and nine years. Their MDA score (mean value: 17.7) was unaffected by this (usually minor) stem varus.

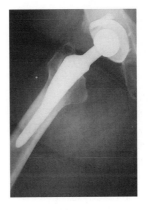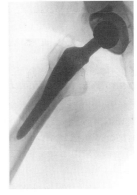

Figure 2 – Typical Esop radiological film at more than 10 years.

This study focused on the bony changes around the implant, specifically, lucent lines, reactive lines, and spot welds.

Lucent lines

Lucent lines are caused by the interposition of fibrous tissue, and are universally considered to be an adverse sign. No such lines were seen in Zones 1 and 7, except for one case that had an abnormal image in these zones, which appeared to be an edge effect.

Reactive Lines

With regard to reactive lines in the entire series, there were 66 cases (74%) without any reactive lines of the kind described above. In the other 23 cases, such lines could be demonstrated in Zones 2, 3, 5, and 6, which correspond to the part of the femoral shaft that houses the smooth, non-HA-coated portion of the stem (fig. 3).

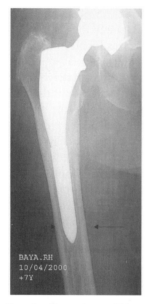

Figure 3 – Reactive line onto non HA-coated zones.

Endosteal densifications

Endosteal densifications, or "spot welds", were found in Zones 2 and 6 in 72% of the cases. They were seen less frequently in Zones 9 and 13 (30% of cases). In five cases (5.6%), there was endosteal ossification at the stem tip associated with thickening in Zone 5. In all of those five cases, the stems were in varus (fig. 4).

Cortical reaction

In three cases, there was thinning of the cortex, observed once each in Zone 5, Zone 3, and Zone 1. Cortical thickening was a feature particularly looked for on the radiographs. It was found once, in Zones 2 and 6, in a patient who had pain seven years post-arthroplasty, with no abnormalities other than cortical thickening. This was the only clinical failure in the series. In five cases, thickening in Zone 5 was associated with an ossification at the stem tip, which was interpreted by us as a response to the varus positioning of the stem detected immediately after implantation.

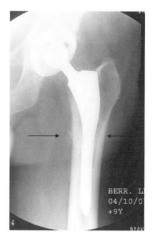

Figure 4 – Typical endosteal new bone formation at the demarcation between coated and non-coated zones.

Calcar changes

In 42 cases (47%) there was calcar atrophy. Five times (6%), this took the form of scalloping. This scalloping was thought to be due to localized osteolysis caused by PE wear debris that had settled at the most dependent part of the articular cavity.

Pedestal formation

The pattern of a pedestal at the stem tip was not seen. However, five stems in varus showed endosteal densification at the level of the stem tip, which was stable and did not have a lucent line separating it from the wall of the shaft (fig. 5).

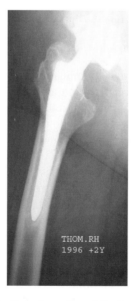

Figure 5 – Bone formation at the tip described as a pedestal.

Femoral osteolysis

Proximal femoral osteolysis in Zone 1A, under the projection of the greater trochanter, was seem four times (4.5%). Distal femoral osteolysis was not, however, observed (fig. 6).

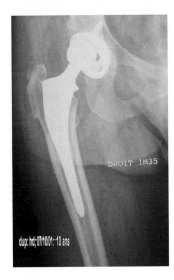

Figure 6 – Major PE wear of the liner without any subsequent osteolysis.

Stem migration

There was only one case of stem migration (8mm). The implant came to rest after the first year. The clinical outcome was not affected, and there was no need for revision surgery. This patient was operated on at the bottom of our learning curve, and the operating surgeon underestimated the size of the metaphyseal piece required. The patient was in pain when he started walking again. Subsequently, however, the implant stabilized and did not subside any further, as shown by the seven-year and ten-year radiographs. No other cases of subsidence were seen.

Periprosthetic ossification

In 62 cases (70%), there were no periprosthetic ossifications. Fifteen patients (17%) had Brooker Class I; seven (8%) had Class II; and 5 (6%) had Class III ossification.

DISCUSSION

Many authors (Delaunay and Kapandji (8), Robinson *et al.* (9)) have reported good results following the insertion of cementless stems with a porous-metal surface and metaphyseal as well as diaphyseal fixation. However, some of the patients in those studies had thigh pain, which remains an adverse effect of non-cemented stems. This problem has been greatly mitigated or eliminated by the introduction of HA coating. It would, however, appear that the nature of the implant surface is not the only relevant factor: the design of the implant may also play a role.

This is why, in the design of our device, we opted for purely metaphyseal fixation. There is wide agreement in the literature (Poss *et al.* (10), Capello, (11), Robertson *et al.* (12), Summer and Turner, (13), Walker *et al.*, (14) Whiteside *et al.* (15), Laine *et al.* (16)) that fixation should be sought in the metapyseal part of the femur.

Load transmission in the metaphysis of an HA-coated femoral component confers two important benefits: no stress shielding, and ease of retrieval without additional bone damage.

No stress-shielding

While it is true that the cortical thinning in the metaphysis and the proximal diaphysis seen with all cementless porous-surfaced stems will not normally lead to loosening, this weakening of the cortex contributes to the deterioration of the periprosthetic bone, which will ultimately result in failure. Preventing this deterioration is, therefore, of considerable importance.

Ease of retrieval without additional bone damage

Since the coating is confined to the upper part of the stem, the device is easier to retrieve. All that is required for detaching the implant from the bone is the insertion of a thin, malleable blade. Retrieval is associated with less bone damage because it involves the separation of a surface bond formed by bone ongrowth. Therefore, it is not necessary to cut through a region of bone ingrowth where bone has grown into the interstices on an implant's surface. With cementless devices fixed in the diaphysis, the main problem used to be implant removal. Cemented devices posed the problem of leaving a thin, devitalized shell once the cement was removed. Both these problems are avoided by the use of a HA-coated device with purely metaphyseal fixation.

Effectiveness of Hydroxyapatite coating

So-called biological fixation is now recognized to be effective (Søballe (17), D'Antonio (18), Onsten (19),

Donnelly (20), Yee (21), Epinette (22)). The HA coating allows rapid and complete bonding to the host bone without an interposed fibrous tissue layer. As a result, there is no need for macrotexturing to allow bone ingrowth, which is a benefit.

Modularity

Several authors (Barrack (23), Bobyn (24), Chmell and Poss (25)) have stressed the disadvantages of modularity. There is a risk of metal particle release and of fretting. The extent to which these potential problems will manifest themselves depends upon the effectiveness of the system used for linking the modular parts together, and on the stress levels to which the system is exposed. It is useful to remember that the maximum stresses (especially torsional stress) will be encountered at the neck-metaphysis junction. Hence, a system that involves linking modules at this junction will entail a major risk of adverse effects after a longer or shorter time in situ. On the other hand, modular head-neck systems have been widely used for a long time, and have proved fairly trouble free, providing there is a good Morse taper lock. The metaphysis-shaft junction is subjected to much lower levels of stress than is the head-neck junction, as shown by studies of systems with proximal modularity (Cameron (26) Andress (27)).

The modular principle adopted in the design of the Esop device allows the surgeon to fit the implant to the morphological pattern of the individual patient's femur. This is a vital point. A CAD study has shown that with a femoral flare of between 25 and 35% (the normal pattern), there are 34 possible combinations of metaphysis and diaphysis provided by the Esop design. For a femoral flare > 35% (champagne-flute pattern), there are 15 different combinations, while for a flare of < 25% (stovepipe pattern), there are 21.

As shown by a recent (June 2001) study (28), surgeons using the Esop stem have made ample use of the facility for implant-to-patient matching provided by this device. The report covered 124 cases followed up for more than nine years. It was seen that the patients with champagne-flute femurs were managed with the largest metaphyseal pieces (13.75, 15, 16.25, 17.5, and 20) together with the smallest diaphyseal pieces (9, 10, 11, and 12). On the other hand, stovepipe patterns were found to have been managed with the smallest metaphyseal components (5, 7.5, 10, 11.25, 12.5) linked to the largest diaphyseal components (12, 13, 14, and 15). We have also studied the manufacturer's data concerning the first 3,433 Esop stems implanted. Each of the seven diaphyseal sizes has been mated with almost all of the ten metaphyseal sizes available, and *vice versa*. Thus, in order to suit the requirements of the individual patient, full use has been made of the mix-and-match potential offered by this modular design.

CONCLUSION

The long-term outcome of any arthroplasty will be governed by a number of factors, all of which must be closely controlled in order to ensure that there will be lasting fixation, as well as the best possible replication of the normal physiological pattern in the host bone. The Esop stem is an original design with three features that, to us, are of fundamental importance: fixation confined to the metaphysis, so as not to interfere with the physiological load transfer pattern; HA coating, to ensure biological "bone-bonding" to give excellent and very long-lasting fixation; and modularity, so as to enable the surgeon to find the combination of implant components that best suits the pattern of the individual patient's femur.

Biomechanical analyses at the R&D stage indicated that this was a valid concept. Mechanical tests then showed that the system was strong enough, and that the use of separate metaphyseal and diaphyseal modules did not harbour any inherent problems. In the judgment of the surgeons who have used the device, modularity – one of the specific features of the Esop stem – has proved a boon. The inherent potential for mix-and-match has been amply utilized to suit the different femoral patterns encountered.

The clinical results obtained so far lead us to anticipate excellent clinical outcomes. Obviously, in order to confirm this impression, all the patients managed with an Esop stem will need to be systematically followed up. Such extended follow-up studies will also need to involve comparisons with other series of HA-coated implants with metaphyseal fixation but without a modular design. From our current viewpoint, however, we can look back upon eleven years of clinical use of the Esop device and note that the clinical and radiological outcomes to date have been promising enough to encourage continuing use (fig. 7).

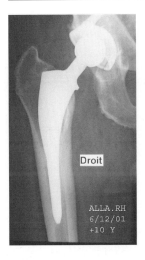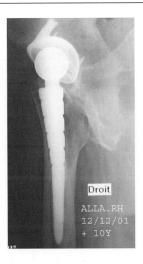

Figure 7 – 10-year radiological evaluation
of a HA-coated Esop: an excellent clinical result.

Reference List

1. Noble PC, Alexander JW, Lindaul LJ, Yew DT, Granberry WM, Tullos HS (1988) The anatomic basis of femoral component design. *Clin. Orthop.* 235:148-65.

2. Rubin PJ, Leyvraz PF, Aubagnac JM, Argenson JN, Esteve P, Roguin B (1992) The morphology of the proximal femur. *J. Bone Joint Surg. Br.* 74:28-32.

3. Fessy MH, Bejui J, Fischer LP, Bouchet A (1995) The upper end of the femur: dimensions of the endosteal canal. *Surg. Radiol. Ann.* 17:155-60.

4. Engh CA, Massin P, Suthers KE (1990) Roentgenographic assessment of the biologic fixation of poroussurfaced femoral components. *Clin. Orthop.* 257:107-28.

5. Epinette JA, Geesink RGT (1995) Radiographic assessment of Cementless Hip Prostheses: ARA, a proposal New Scoring System. Cahiers d'Enseignement de la SOFCOT, 51, Expansion Scientifique. Française, 114-26, English vol, Paris.

6. Gruen TA, Macneice GM, Amstutz HC (1979) Modes of failure of cemented stem type femoral components. A radiographic analysis of loosening. *Clin. Orthop.* 141:17-21.

7. Brooker AF, Bowerman JW, Robinson RA, Riley LH (1973) Ectopic ossification following total hip replacement: incidence and a method of classification. *J. Bone Joint Surg. Am.* 55:1629-32.

8. Delaunay C, Kapandji AI (1998) Survie à 10 ans des prothèses totales de Zweimuller en arthroplastie primaire non cimentée de hanche. *Rev. Chir. Orthop.* 84:412-21.

9. Robinson RP, Deysine GR, Green MT (1996) Uncemented total hip arthroplasty using the CLS stem: a titanium alloy implant with a corundum blast finish. Results at a mean 6 years in a prospective study. *J. Arthrosplasty* 11:286-92.

10. Poss R, Walker P, Spector M, *et al.* (1988) Strategies for improving fixation of femoral components in total hip arthroplasty. *Clin. Orthop.* 235:181-94.

11. Capello WN (1989) Fit the patient to the prosthesis: an argument against the routine use of custom hip implants. *Clin. Orthop.* 249:56-9.

12. Robertson DD, Walker PS, Granholm JW, Nelson PC, Fishman EK Magid D (1987) Design of custom hip stem prostheses using three-dimensional CT modeling. *Journal of Computer Assisted Tomography* 11:804-9.

13. Summer DR, Turner TM (1988) The effects of femoral component design features on femoral modeling. In: Non cemented total hip arthroplasty. 143-155 Edit: Fitzgerald R Raven Press, 1 Vol. New-York.

14. Walker PS, Schneeweis PB, Murphy S, Nelson P (1987) Strain and micromotions of press-fit femoral stem prosthesis. *J. Biomech.* 20:693-702.

15. Whiteside LA, Arima J, White SE, Branam L, Mac Carthy DS (1994) Fixation of the modular total hip femoral component in cementless total hip arthroplasty. *Clin. Orthop.* 298:84-90.

16. Laine HJ, Lehto Muk, Moilanen T (2000) Diversity of proximal femoral medullary canal. *J. Arthroplasty* 1:86-92

17. Søballe K, Hansen ES, Rasmussen HB, Bunger C (1995) Fixation of porous coated *versus* HA coated implants. Cahiers d'Enseignement de la SOFCOT, 51, Expansion Scient. Française, 71-84, Engl vol, Paris.

18. D'Antonio JA, Capello WN, Manley MT (1996) Remodeling of bone around hydroxyapatite-coated femoral stems. *J. Bone Joint Surg. Am.* 78:1226-34.

19. Onsten I, Carlsson AS, Sanzen L , Besjakov J (1996) Migration and wear of a hydroxyapatite-coated hip prosthesis. A controlled roentgen stereophotogrammetric study. *J. Bone Joint Surg. Br.* 78:85-91.

20. Donnely WJ, Kobayashi A, Freeman MA, Chin TW, Yeo H, West M, Scott G (1997) Radiological and survival comparison of four methods of fixation of a proximal femoral stem. *J. Bone Joint Surg. Br.* 79:351-60.

21. Yee AJM , Kreder HK, Bookman I, Davey JR (1999) A randomized trial of hydroxyapatite coated prostheses in total hip arthroplasty. *Clin. Orthop.* 366:120-32.

22. Epinette JA (1995) HA-Coated Omnifit Stems in Primary Hip Replacement: Seven-Year Experience. Cahiers d'Enseignement de la SOFCOT, 51, Expansion Scientifique Française, 215-226, English vol, Paris.

23. Barrack RL, Burke DW, Cook SD, Skinner HB, Harris WH (1993) Complications related to modularity of total hip components. *J. Bone Joint Surg. Br.* 75:688-92.

24. Bobyn JD, Tanzer M, Krigier JJ, Dujovne AR, Brooks CE (1994) Concerns with modularity in total hip arthroplasty. *Clin. Orthop.* 298:27-36.

25. Chmell MJ, Poss R (1995) Avantages et désavantages de la modularité des prothèses totales de hanche. Conférences d'Enseignement de la SOFCOT, 52, Expansion Scient. Française, 1-10, Paris.

26. Cameron HU (1994) The two to six year results with a proximally modular noncemented total hip replacement used in hip revisions. *Clin. Orthop.* 298:47-53.

27. Andress HJ, Lob G, Kahl S, *et al.* (1999) Development of a new modular titanium femoral prosthesis consisting of a head and shaft component. Indications, operation and optimization of the tapered socket connection. *Eur. J. Orthop. Surg. Traumatol.* 9:13-18.

28. Gacon G, Philippe MP, Ray A, Hummer J, Hourlier H, Dambreville A (2001) Modularité métaphyso-diaphysaire et tiges fémorales sans ciment. *Rev. Chir. Orthop.* 87:331-9.

6 Early Clinical Results of an Arc-Deposited Hydroxyapatite-Coated Acetabular Component in Total Hip Arthroplasty

Scott W. Siverhus, MD and Dawanna R. Bryant, CFA

INTRODUCTION

The clinical success of hydroxyapatite (HA)-coated femoral stem components in total hip replacement has been well documented (1). There is conflicting literature support, however, for the use of HA coating on acetabular components. Implant design has been implicated in the variable failure rates reported at early follow up in HA-coated shells (2).

Specifically, the ability of the acetabular shell to provide adequate bone interlock to resist shear forces is considered critical to long-term stability (3, 4). Given the biocompatibility and osteoconductive properties of HA (5), combining it with a macrostructured biocompatible metal surface theoretically presents an appealing combination for acetabular design.

Biologic fixation of implants requires active bone in-growth and remodeling over time to achieve-long term success (6-8). Initial stable fixation and close bone apposition is believed to reduce the occurrence fibrous in-growth and poor clinical function (9-12). Component design, interface biology, and component positioning have each been implicated as contributing to bone in-growth and stress transmission (13-18).

The inferior acetabular sites (i.e., DeLee and Charnley zone III) (19) appear to be particularly susceptible to high local tensile distraction stresses (20, 21). This conclusion from finite element analysis studies correlates well with clinical outcomes studies. Progressive radiolucent lines are frequently identified in zone III in acetabular components that eventually require revision for clinical failure (4). It is postulated that adequate mechanical interlock between the acetabular shell and bone in this area prevents this mechanism of failure.

Previous multi-center experience with HA-coated press-fit cups has yielded results consistent with this failure mechanism (2, 4). Autopsy retrieval studies lend further support to the understanding of the dynamic remodeling process required to maintain continued component stability (22-24). Manley *et al.* (4) compared failure rates of four different acetabular component surfaces at 7.9-year average follow-up. They reported a 6 percent combined failure rate for porous-coated, press-fit Dual Geometry cups. This was consistent with other noncemented series at similar follow-up intervals (25-30). The two HA-coated press-fit cup designs, (Dual Geometry HA and Dual Radius HA) each showed combined failure rates of twenty-two percent. Each of these implants has a 200 micrometer machine-knurled peripheral interface. In contrast, the threaded HA-coated acetabular components in this series (Omnifit Threaded HA cup) showed a combined failure rate of 3 percent. Given our current understanding of the osteoclast removal of the HA coating adjacent to bone, it seems most probable that the press-fit cups failed because of the inability of the machine-knurled fixation interface to resist the tensile stresses over time.

Alternative macro-structured surface finishes were investigated to try to improve the roughness at the bone interface of acetabular shells. Increasing surface roughness improves the resistance to shear forces of the acetabular component (31). The macro-texture selected has to be compatible with application of a uniform overlying HA coating of approximately 50 micrometers thickness (32). Numerous canine implantation studies demonstrated the bone in-growth efficacy of arc-deposited titanium (Ti) macro-structuring which is further enhanced with HA application (33, 34).

In this chapter, we review our early clinical and radiographic results of an arc-deposited titanium (Ti) acetabular component with HA coating (Secur-Fit™, Stryker Howmedica Osteonics, Allendale, NJ) in primary total hip arthroplasty.

MATERIALS AND METHODS

A consecutive series of 78 patients (93 hips) have been prospectively evaluated and followed annually after primary total hip arthroplasty using an arc-deposited HA-coated Ti acetabular component (Secur-fit™, Stryker Howmedica Osteonics ; Allendale NJ). All patients were implanted by a single surgeon (SWS) between March, 1995 and December, 1998. The acetabular shell (fig. 1) has a dual radius external geometry that provides 1.7mm of interference at the peripheral rim. Normalizations increase the offset load transmission to the denser subchondral plate at the acetabular rim. The coarse coating of arc deposited commercially pure titanium (CP Ti) enhances initial cup fixation and improved resistance to shear forces. A 50 micron thick coating of HA (Pure-fix™ HA, Stryker Howmedica Osteonics, Allendale, NJ) is then applied to the arc-deposited surface. This shell is available with or without dome screw holes for additional preliminary fixation. Only patients with ultra high molecular weight polyethylene (UHMWPE) liners are considered.

The decision to use a Secur-Fit™ solid shell or one with clustered screw hole options, was made intraoperatively based on bone quality. Fifty-three hip replacements were preformed using the screwless cup design and thirty using the cluster cup. Additional dome screw fixation was utilized, as needed, based on intraoperative assessment of initial cup stability after impaction.

Of the initial 78 patients, five are deceased from causes unrelated to their surgery and another five are lost to follow-up. This leaves a total of 68 patients with 83 hips still available for annual follow-up evaluation and radiographs for this report.

The femoral components used varied according to patient bone quality and deformities. Of the 83 hips, 30 were performed using a cemented stem, and 53 using a non-cemented stem. All hip replacements were performed using a posterolateral surgical approach. All patients were allowed immediate full weight-bearing as tolerated after surgery. They all participated in an early aggressive range-of-motion and restrengthening program of physical therapy with emphasis on hip dislocation precautions.

Patient demographics (Table 1) reveal an equal male to female ratio (n = 34 males and females) with relatively young average age at the time of surgery (62.5 years old, range = 25 to 85 years old). The most common diagnosis was osteoarthritis (67.8%), and only primary total hip replacements are included. A complete list of diagnoses can be found in Table 2. Six hips required extensive or structural bone grafts at the time of surgery for severe acetabular deficiencies or defects.

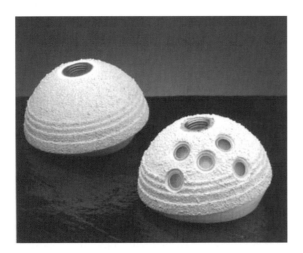

Figure 1 – Secur-fit™ acetabular shells, with and without dome screw holes.

	Females	Male	Total
Patients	34	34	68
Hips	43	40	83
Age (mean)	63.9 yrs	63.5 yrs	62.5 yrs
Age (range)	(28-85)yrs	(25-83)yrs	(25-85)yrs

Table 1 – Patient demographics.

	(Percent)
Osteoarthritis	67.8
Avascular Necrosis	9.7
Rheumatoid arthritis	7.5
Post Traumatic arthritis	6.4
DDH/Protrusio	5.3
Other	3.3

Table 2 – Diagnoses.

The study protocol required preoperative A/P pelvis, A/P hip and Lowenstein lateral radiographs. These were also obtained early postoperatively (two to four weeks) and annually thereafter. All patients completed SF-12 and WOMAC questionnaires, pain and functional analysis at each visit. Global and total Harris hip scores (HHS) and Merle d'Aubigne- Postel (MDA) clinical hip scores were calculated at each interval. All data were collected, compiled and calculated using Orthowave clinical research software (Aria Software, Ltd, Bruay, France).

A three-zone method of evaluation (19) was used for documentation of radiographic changes at each follow-up interval. Any radiolucent lines, osteolytic lesions, radioreactive lines or changes in bone density were recorded. Particular attention was directed to bone remodeling changes in acetabular zone III. Any questionable cases were then digitally copied and further analyzed with color enhancement (Imagika; Clinical Measurement Corporation, Upper Saddle River, New Jersey). Each radiographic detail was then entered into the Orthowave database. Acetabular radiographic scores were calculated at each follow-up interval. Any hip at most recent follow-up that did not have a perfect radiographic score was again reviewed.

The Imagika enhancement process allows detailed visualization of selected areas around the acetabular components. Edge detection algorithms and linear expansion of the gray scale allows the periprosthetic osseous features to be seen more clearly. Radioreactive lines, radiolucent lines and areas of bone-prosthetic spot welding or in-growth are better defined. Component stability was defined as stable with osseous in-growth, stable with fibrous in-growth or unstable as previously described by Manley *et al.* (4).

Eight hips were implanted using ten degree hooded UHMWP liners and seventy-five were implanted with a zero degree hood. Twenty-three hips were implanted using ion-bombarded thirty-two millimeter cobalt-chromium (Co-Cr) femoral heads. Thirty-seven hips were implanted using twenty-eight millimeter ion-bombarded Co-Cr heads, and twenty-three using twenty-eight millimeter zirconia-ceramic heads.

Those patients who received hooded liners and thirty-two millimeter heads tended to be older patients with less clinical concern of long-term polyethylene wear and greater concern for imme-diate hip stability. Those patients who received zirconia-ceramic head components tended to be the youngest patients with greatest clinical concern of long-term polyethylene wear issues.

RESULTS

The mean preoperative Harris Hip score (HHS) was 42.6 (range = 5-68), and at most recent follow-up was 92.0 (range = 62-100). The mean preoperative Merle d'Aubigne-Postel (MDA) score was 8.8 (range 3-12), and at most recent follow-up was 16.5 (range = 11-18). A review of the records revealed that five patients had poor or fair ratings on HHS or MDA scores. Three of these patients had poor functional scores due to other health issues unrelated to their hip replacement surgeries. Another two patients with fair global ratings had low pain scores due to concurrent treatment for trochanteric bursitis. None of these five patients showed any concerning findings on radiographs to suggest acetabular implant loosening.

Two patients underwent an acetabular liner and femoral head revision for early recurrent dislocation, but the acetabular shell and femoral stem components were retained. One patient required removal of a proximal femoral circlage wire that was inserted at the time of replacement for a calcar crack. One patient with developmental dysplasia required femoral stem exchange and bone grafting for nonunion of a femoral osteotomy. No patients have required revision of any of the components for septic loosening, aseptic loosening, mechanical failure, osteolysis, or pain. Figures 2A and 2B show A/P (fig. 2A) and lateral (fig. 2B) radiographs of a cup implanted in a stable position at surgery that remained stable for the next six years of the study.

Eight patients (eleven hips) had less than perfect radiographic acetabular scores and sixty patients (seventy-two hips) had perfect scores. Following Imagika enhancement, only one hip has a confirmed radiolucent line present in zone III which appeared between the fifth and sixth year postoperative follow-up radiographs. A subsequent bone scan showed only increased uptake around the inferior portion of the acetabular prosthesis, suggesting that the component remains stable. Seven of these eleven hips (5 patients) had score reductions due to mild (less than 2mm) asymmetric polyethylene

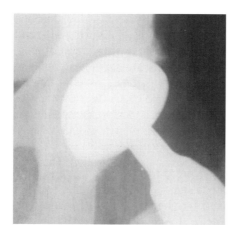 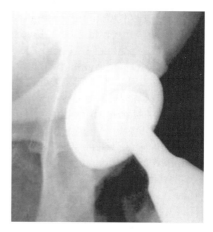

Figure 2A – A/P radiographs at early post-op (left)
and at 6 years follow-up (right).

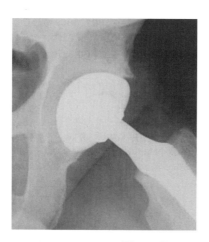 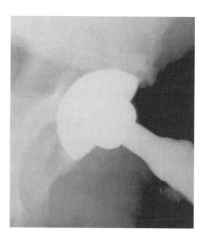

Figure 2B – Lateral radiographs at early post-op (left)
and at 6 years follow-up (right).

liner wear, but showed no evidence of associated acetabular osteolysis or progressive radioreactive/radiolucent lines. One of the eleven hips showed a minimal zone I radiolucency which has actually been filling-in throughout the five year postoperative follow-up. Two hips showed minimal radioreactive lines in zones I and II but demonstrate definite areas of "spot welding" in all zones.

DISCUSSION

Mixed results have previously been reported reguarding the clinical effectiveness of HA-coated acetabular components. Given the consistent suc-

cessful results of press-fit acetabular components and HA-coated femoral components, it is postulated that the variable outcomes of HA-coated acetabular components is design related. Further research into the development of more effective acetabular in-growth surfaces demonstrated the bone in-growth potential of arc-deposited CP-Ti which is further enhanced by fifty micron application of HA. The development of the Secur-fit™ HA acetabular system represents the "second generation" of HA press-fit cup design.

The early clinical results of this second generation HA acetabular component show excellent results in all measures of patient self-reporting scales and radiographically. This is notable in light of the clinical and radiographic findings of the "first generation" press-fit HA acetabular components at similar follow-up interval. The Dual Geometry HA and Dual Radius- HA acetabular components each showed combined failure rates of twenty-two percent at 7.9-year average follow-up. In the cups that failed, radiographs showed a stable interface with osseous in-growth for the first two to three years postoperatively. It was at this time frame, however, that a radiolucent line became evident at acetabular zone III. This radiolucent line then progressed over time as fixation failure to the subchondral bone worsened. This phenomeon of radiolucent line progression was not identified in the more clinically successful Omnifit™ Threaded HA cup or in the porous-coated press-fit Dual Geometry cup. This suggests the importance of achieving a mechanical interlock between the acetabular cup and the underlying subchondral bone in the inferior acetabular zones. It is consistent with the previous predictions of modes of failure from finite element analysis predicting high tensile stresses under physiologic loads at zone III.

In this series of Secur-fit™ HA acetabular components, only one hip showed any concerning radiographic findings to suggest failure of bone in-growth (i.e., radiolucent line). Further image enhancement using Imagika confirmed that only this cup lacks bone in-growth in zone III. This patient remains clinically asymptomatic and is considered to have stable in-growth in zones I and II. No component has required revision for pain, aseptic loosening, septic loosening, mechanical failure or osteolysis. Three hips show radiolucent or radioreactive lines isolated to zones I or II. In each case, these radiographic findings have not developed over the follow-up interval and were seen at the initial post-operative visit. Theses hips will require particularly close follow-up to monitor for clinical and radiographic signs of progression to mechanical failure.

In conclusion, the early (mean = 4.3 year) results with a "second generation" HA-coated press-fit acetabular component are promising. The variable results reported with previous HA cup designs are likely due to differences in implant design. The ability of the surface finish to achieve initial stable fixation, resist local distraction stresses and maintain subchondral fixation over time during bone and HA remodeling seem to be the keys to continued success. These clinical outcome study findings are consistent with predicted modes of failure from numerical modeling (20,

21). They are also consistent with histological findings at autopsy retrieval showing HA and bone apposition most prominent in areas of load transmission (22). Canine studies (7) have demonstrated the most extensive bone in-growth often occurred at the peripheral rim of a press-fit acetabular component. Incomplete apposition between the acetabular dome of the component and native bone often resulted in fibrous interposition, rather than a filling-in with new bone formation. Therefore, lack of radiographic evidence of bone in-growth in Zone II is likely to be less predictive of component failure or loosening then in the peripheral zones, especially zone III.

Reference List

1. D'Antonio JA, Capello WN, Manley MT, Geesink RGT (2001) Hydroxyapatite femoral stems for total hip arthroplasty 10-to13-year followup. *Clin. Orthop.* 1: 101-11.

2. Capello WN, D'Antonio JA, Manley MT, Feinberg JR (1998) Hydroxyapatite in total hip arthroplasty. Clinical results and critical issues. *Clin. Orthop.* 355:200-11.

3. Jazrawi LM, Adler EM, Jazrawi AJ, Jaffe WL (2000) Grit-blasted hydroxyapatite and arc-deposited hydroxyapatite acetabular components. A four year followup study. *Bull. Hosp. Jt. Dis.* 59(3):144-8.

4. Manley MT, Capello WN, D'Antonio JA, Edidin AA, Geesink RGT (1998)Fixation of acetabular cups without cement in total hip arthroplasty. *J. Bone Joint Surg. Am.* 80:1175-85.

5. Jarcho M (1981) Calcium phosphate ceramics as hard tissue prosthetics. *Clin. Orthop.* 157:259-60.

6. Hedley AK, Kabo M, Kim W *et al.* (1983) Bony ingrowth fixation of newly designed acetabular components in a canine model. *Clin. Orthop.* 176:12-23.

7. Harris WH, White RE Jr, McCarthy JC, Walker PS, Weinberg EH (1983) Bony ingrowth fixation of the acetabular components in canine hip joint arthroplasty. *Clin. Orthop.* 176:7-11.

8. Engh CA, Zettl-Schaffer KF, Kukita Y, Sweet D, Jasty M, Bragdon C (1993) Histologic and radiofraphic assessment of well functioning porous-coated acetabular components. J. *Bone Joint Surg. Am.* 77:814-24.

9. Pilliar RM, Lee JM, Maniatopoulos C (1986) Observations on the effect of movement on bone ingrowth into porous-surfaced implants. *Clin. Orthop.* 208:108-13.

10. Sandborn PM, Cook SD, Spires WP, Kester MA (1988) Tissue response to porous-coated implants lacking initial bone apposition. *J. Arthroplasty* 3:337-46.

11. Pilliar RM, Cameron HU, Welsh RP, Binnington AG (1981) Radiographic and morphologic studies of load-bearing porous-surfaced structured implants. *Clin. Orthop.* 156:249-57.

12. Engh CA, Bobyn JD, Glassman AH (1987) Porous-coated hip replacement. The factors governing bone ingrowth, stress shielding, and clinical results. *J. Bone Joint Surg. Br.* 69:45-55.

13. Adler E, Stuchin SA, Kummer FJ (1992) Stability of pressfit acetabular cups. *J. Arthroplasty* 7:295-301.

14. Curtis MJ, Jinnah RH, Wilson VD, Hungerford DS (1992) The initial stability of uncemented acetabular components. *J. Bone Joint Surg. Am.* 74:372.

15. Lachiewicz PF, Suh PB, Gilbert JA (1989) *in vitro* initial fixation of porous coated acetabular total hip components. Biomechanical comparative study. *J. Arthroplasty* 4:201.

16. Morsher E, Bereiter H, Lampert C (1989) Cementless pressfit cup. Principals, experimental data, and three year followup study. *Clin. Orthop.* 249:12.

17. Perona PG, Lawrence J, Paprosky WG *et al.* (1992) Acetabular micromotion as a measure of initial implant stability in primary hip arthroplasty. An *in vitro* comparison of different methods of initial acetabular component fixation. *J. Arthroplasty* 7:537.

18. Won C, Hearn TC, Tile M (1995) Micromotion of cementless hemispherical acetabular components. Does pressfit need adjuctive screw fixation? *J. Bone Joint Surg. Am.* 77:484.

19. DeLee JG, Charnley J (1976) Radiological demarcation of cemented sockets in total hip replacement. *Clin. Orthop.* 121:20-32.

20. Rapperport DJ, Carter DR, Schurman DJ (1987) Contact finite element stress analysis of porous ingrowth acetabular cup implantation, ingrowth and loosening. *J Orthop. Res.* 5(4):548-61.

21. Mann KE (1996) The stress state at the socket/bone interface for well fixed pressfit and threaded HA coated cups. Internal report Osteonics Corp. Allendale, New Jersey.

22. Bauer TW, Stulberg BN, Ming J, Geesink RGT (1993) Uncemented acetabular components. Histologic analysis of retrieved hydroxyapatite-coated and porous implants. *J. Arthroplasty* 8(2):167-77.

23. Bauer TW, Geesink RCT, Zimmerman R, McMahon JT (1991) Hydroxyapatite-coated femoral stems. Histological analysis of components retrieved at autopsy. *J. Bone Joint Surg. Am.* 73(10):1439-52.

24. Tonino A, Oosterbos C, Rahmy A, Therin M, Doyle C (2001) Hydroxyapatite-coated acetabular components. Histological and histomorphometric analysis of six cups retrieved at autopsy between three and seven years after successful implantation. *J Bone Joint Surg Am.* 83(6): 817-25.

25. Cruz-Pardos A, Garcia-Cimbrelo E (2001) The Harris-Galante total hip arthroplasty: a minimum 8 year followup study. *J. Arthroplasty* 16(5):586-97.

26. Taylor AH, Shannon M, Whitehouse SL, Lee MB, Learmonth ID (2001) Harris Galante cementless acetabular replacement in Avascular necrosis. *J. Bone Joint Surg. Am.* 83(2):177-82.

27. Soto MO, Rodriquez JA, Ranawat CS (2000) Clinical and radiographic evaluation of the Harris-Galante cup. Incidence of wear and osteolysis at 7 to 9 years followup. *J. Arthroplasty* 15(2):139-45.

28. Peterson MB, Poulsen IH, Thomsen J, Solgaard S (2000) The hemispherical Harris-Galante acetabular cup, inserted without cement. The results of an eight to eleven-year follow-up of one hundred and sixty-eight hips. *J. Bone Joint Surg. Am.* 82(8):1195-6.

29. Cordero-Ampuero J, Garcia-Cimbrelo E, Munuera L (1994) Fixation of cementless acetabular cups. A radiographic 4-8 year study of 102 porous-coated components. *Acta Orthop. Scand.* 65(3):263-66.

30. Van Flandern G, Bierbaum B, Newberg A, Gomes S, Mattingly D, Karpos PAG (1998) Intermediate clinical follow-up of a dual radius acetabular component. *J. Arthroplasty* 13(7):804-11.

31. Poser RD, Kay JF, Magee FP, Hedley AK (1993) Preclinical evaluation of the effect of hydroxylapatite on the "comprehensive" bone implant interface. In Hydroxlapatite Coatings in Orthopaedic Surgery,137-49. Edited by RGT Geesink, MT Manley. New York, Raven Press.

32. Kester M, Manley MT, Taylor SK, Cohen RC (1991) Influence of thickness on the mechanical properties and bond strength of HA coatings applied to orthopaedic implants. Presented: 37th Annual Meeting, Orthopaedic Research Society, Anaheim, CA, p. 95.

33. Pereira DS, Ricci JL, Scott DF, Casar RS, Jaffe WL, Hawkins MV, Oh YH, Alexander H (1995) Effects of macroroughness and hydroxyapatite coatings on osteointegration and osteoconduction. Presented: Society for Biomaterials, San Francisco, CA: March.

34. Hawkins MV, Bauer TW, Friedman RJ, Zimmerman MC, Ricci JL, Jaffe WL (1995) Evaluation of an arc-deposited CPTi surface with and without hydroxlapatite coatings in three *in vivo* studies. Presented: AAOS Meeting, Orlando, FL: February.

7   Hydroxyapatite-coated Ti6Al4V Implants and Peri-implant Infection

Kees JM. Oosterbos, MD, Charles H. Vogely, MD, PhD, Wouter JA. Dhert, PhD and Alfons J. Tonino, MD, PhD

INTRODUCTION

Replacement of degenerated joints has become one of the most successful surgical procedures in orthopaedics. One of the main reasons for this success was the introduction of polymethylmethacrylate (bone cement), which made long lasting fixation of implant to bone possible. Infections related to the implants have always posed a serious clinical problem leading to an increase in complicated and costly revision arthroplasties with a high mortality (1, 2). Since the introduction of total joint arthroplasties, the infection rate has decreased to less than 1 per cent for a total hip arthroplasty at present (3). The use of antibiotic-impregnated bone cement is considered to be most effective in preventing septic loosening (4). However, the number of patients receiving an arthroplasty is still increasing (5). Therefore, it is obvious that the problem of implant-related infections will further increase in the future in terms of absolute figures.

The most frequently cultured organisms causing such an infection are *Staphylococcus aureus* and *Staphylococcus epidermidis* (6). Other frequently seen micro-organisms are the gram-negative bacilli, such as *Escherichia coli, Proteus, Pseudomonas* and *Klebsiella* (7).

Another problem that became apparent after the introduction of total joint replacement was loosening of the prosthesis without an infection being present (aseptic loosening), especially in younger, and therefore more active, patients. This led to renewed interest in cementless fixation of implants and more research in this area. Noncemented fixation potentially leads to a close and permanent contact between prosthesis and bone (8-17).

One of the most widely used materials for noncemented joint prostheses is titanium, a biocompatible material that permits bone to grow in close proximity to the implant surface (contact osteogenesis) (18, 19). To promote implant-bone contact even more, bioactive materials such as hydroxyapatite, a calcium phosphate ceramic, have been applied to implant surfaces as a coating. Several prosthetic designs using hydroxyapatite coated titanium have proven to be successful after medium term follow-up and are subject of constant evaluation (20-24). Long lasting fixation of these implants will be achieved by functional integration of the prosthesis with the surrounding bone. For the process of bony integration, the early healing phase (days-weeks after implantation) is especially of importance, and is characterised by a cascade of various cellular events at the implant surface (16).

However, the relationship between implant bioactivity and infection susceptibility has not yet been clarified. Therefore we formulated several questions: 1) Will the use of noncemented HA-coated titanium implants influence the rate of postoperative infection?, and 2) Will the use of noncemented HA-coated titanium implants also influence the way in which an infection develops if it does occur?

A study was designed to investigate the infection susceptibility and osseointegration related to peri-implant infection of two commonly used surfaces for noncemented fixation of orthopaedic implants, grit blasted Ti6Al4V as a biocompatible surface, and hydroxyapatite plasma sprayed Ti6Al4V as a bioactive surface. Furthermore, we conducted a postmortem study on a patient who sustained a postoperative infection after total hip replacement. He recovered without removal of the prosthesis and died 6.2 years later from cerebral hemorrage.

MATERIAL AND METHODS

Susceptibility to Infection and Influence of Infection on Osseointegration in Rabbit Tibial Model

The experimental studies are described in detail by Vogely (25) and Oosterbos (26).

Female New Zealand White rabbits were used for the study. Under general anaesthesia and aseptic conditions, titanium cylinders were placed intramedullary in the proximal tibiae of the rabbits. Prior to implantation in the left tibia, a bacterial suspension of *Staphylococcus aureus*, strain Wood-46 (ATCC 10832) (27, 28) was injected into the medullary canal. Different suspensions were used containing either 102, 103, 104 or 105 CFU (colony forming units). The implants were an alloy of titanium, aluminium (6%) and vanadium (4%) (Ti6Al4V) with a cylindrical form (20 × 3.9 mm). The hydroxyapatite (HA) coating had the same characteristics as the coating of clinically used hip implants (24, 29).

Uncoated cylinders were implanted into the contaminated proximal left tibia of 16 rabbits. HA-coated titanium cylinders were implanted into the contaminated tibia of 16 other rabbits. The right tibiae served as control with an identical implant, but without contamination. The animals were monitored clinically and by blood samples (erythrocyte sedimentation rate and white blood-cell counts). After 4 weeks the animals were killed and both tibiae were removed. Postoperatively and after sacrifice X-rays were made. Excision of the proximal tibiae was performed under aseptic conditions. The bone fragments of the anterior half of each tibia were weighed and homogenised. Dilutions from these homogenates were plated on blood agar plates and the following day the bacterial colonies were counted.

For each tibia, the number of viable bacteria per gram of bone was calculated (colony forming units per gram of bone, CFU/g) (25). The implants with the remaining surrounding bone of the posterior half of the tibiae were prepared for histological and histomorphometrical evaluation (26). Proximal and distal sections of each tibia with implant were examined for signs of infection using a light microscope and subsequently scored using a modified scoring system (25) which was based upon the score described by Petty (30). Histomorphometrically the percentage of implant length with direct bone-implant contact (fig. 1) and the percentage of bone area within a radius of 1mm next to the implants (fig. 2) were measured.

RESULTS

The rabbits that received a higher inoculum dose lost more in body weight. In the first week, ESR was more elevated in rabbits that received a HA implant; this difference was no longer noted after 4 weeks. The white blood cell counts were not different for HA and Ti implants. In the left tibia of 8 out of 27 rabbits, radiological signs of infection, such as periosteal reaction, were seen in 6 rabbits that received a HA implant, and in 2 rabbits that received a Ti implant. Six out of these 8 rabbits

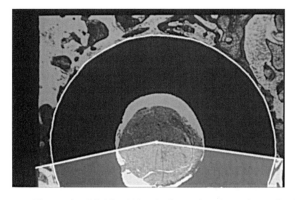
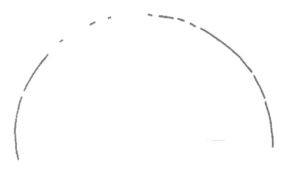

Figure 1 – Digitised histologic section through proximal tibia. In a specific area the part of the implant that was in direct contact with bone (red line) was marked and a percentage was calculated.

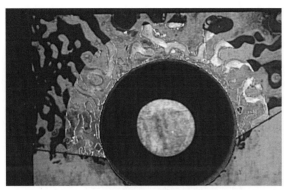
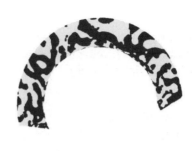

Figure 2 – Digitised histologic section through proximal tibia. Within a radius of 1mm next to the implant the bone was marked (yellow) and a percentage was calculated.

received a 10^4 or 10^5 CFU *Staphylococcus aureus*. No radiological signs of infection were seen in the right tibiae. All animals with radiological signs of infection had a positive culture after 28 days.

Bacteriological cultures from samples of the left tibia were positive in 9 out of 16 rabbits with HA implants, and in 6 out of 16 rabbits with Ti implants. The number of colony forming units per gram (CFU/g) increased with higher inoculum doses, as there was a significant effect of inoculum dosage on bacterial counts ($p \leq 0.025$) (fig. 3). Furthermore, significantly more bacteria were found in the HA group than in the Ti group ($p \leq 0.05$). In two rabbits, positive cultures in the right, control tibia were found (one Ti and one HA implanted rabbit).

Histological evaluation of sections of implants not contaminated with bacteria (right tibiae) showed a normal cortex without periosteal reaction and small Haversian canals. Micro abscesses, granulation tissue, or fibrosis were not seen, and only occasionally a few leukocytes were observed in the medullary canal. Especially in sections from left tibiae, which were contaminated with a high inoculum dosage, severe loss of cortical bone was observed. The remaining cortex showed enlarged Haversian canals and an extensive periosteal reaction. Around the implant in the medulla and the cortex, many leukocytes were found, sometimes accompanied by the formation of micro abscesses and granulation tissue. In some tibiae extensive fibrosis was observed.

With increasing inoculum dosage, both the infected left tibiae with HA and with Ti showed an increase in histopathological semiquantitative scores, as compared to their contralateral control,

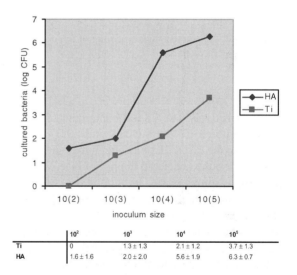

	10^2	10^3	10^4	10^5
Ti	0	1.3 ± 1.3	2.1 ± 1.2	3.7 ± 1.3
HA	1.6 ± 1.6	2.0 ± 2.0	5.6 ± 1.9	6.3 ± 0.7

Figure 3 – Bacteriological cultures from the left tibiae for both implant types as related to inoculum size. On the left axis the mean number of bacteria that were cultured after sacrifice are presented as log colony forming units (CFU) ± standard error.

and for the left contaminated tibiae, there was a significant effect of inoculum dosage on the histopathological scores ($p \leq 0.0005$) (fig. 4). In addition, with increasing inoculum dosage, there was an increasing difference between the HA and Ti implants, which resulted in higher scores for the HA implants ($p \leq 0.05$). This indicates that with increasing inoculum concentration, HA implants developed a more severe infection compared to the Ti implants.

Bone contact measurements for the proximal sections of the right tibiae showed no difference in bone contact between the HA-coated implants and the Ti implants (overall mean percentage 67.0 and

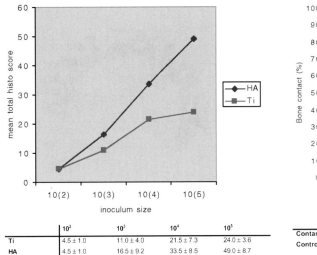

	10^2	10^3	10^4	10^5
Ti	4.5 ± 1.0	11.0 ± 4.0	21.5 ± 7.3	24.0 ± 3.6
HA	4.5 ± 1.0	16.5 ± 9.2	33.5 ± 8.5	49.0 ± 8.7

Figure 4 – Histopathological scoring of the bone from the left tibiae for both implants and various inoculum sizes (mean score ± standard error).

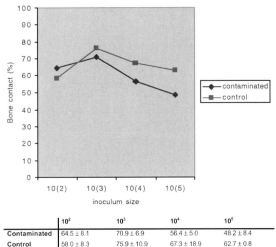

	10^2	10^3	10^4	10^5
Contaminated	64.5 ± 8.1	70.9 ± 6.9	56.4 ± 5.0	48.2 ± 8.4
Control	58.0 ± 8.3	75.9 ± 10.9	67.3 ± 18.9	62.7 ± 0.8

Figure 5b – Bone – Ti-implant contact in the proximal sections. Data are presented as the mean percentage of bone in direct contact with the implant (± standard error) as related to inoculum size.

66.0 respectively). In the left contaminated tibiae, these data were 67.6% for HA and 60.0% for Ti (fig. 5). In the distal sections, the overall mean percentage of bone contact in the right tibiae was 51.6 for the HA implants and 38.8 for Ti (fig. 6). In the left contaminated tibiae, these data were 33.4 per cent and 41.4 per cent, respectively. The bone area measurements for the proximal sections showed the same pattern as the bone contact measurements (fig. 7). The overall mean percentage of bone area

in the right, i.e., not contaminated tibiae was 38.9 for the HA implants and 37.6 for the Ti implants. For the left, contaminated tibiae, these percentages were 42.6 and 35.4, respectively. The inoculum concentration (dosage group) had a significant effect on the bone contact in the distal sections of the HA implants ($p \leq 0.05$) and also on the bone area next to the proximal part of the implant ($p \leq 0.05$). Bone contact and bone area decreased

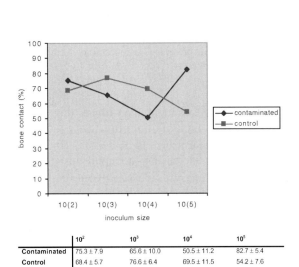

	10^2	10^3	10^4	10^5
Contaminated	75.3 ± 7.9	65.6 ± 10.0	50.5 ± 11.2	82.7 ± 5.4
Control	68.4 ± 5.7	76.6 ± 6.4	69.5 ± 11.5	54.2 ± 7.6

Figure 5a – Bone – HA-implant contact in the proximal sections. Data are presented as the mean percentage of bone in direct contact with the implant (± standard error) as related to inoculum size.

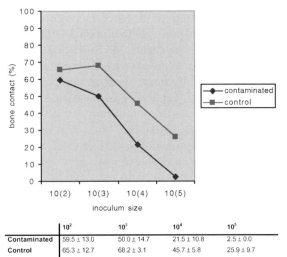

	10^2	10^3	10^4	10^5
Contaminated	59.5 ± 13.0	50.0 ± 14.7	21.5 ± 10.8	2.5 ± 0.0
Control	65.3 ± 12.7	68.2 ± 3.1	45.7 ± 5.8	25.9 ± 9.7

Figure 6a – Bone – HA-implant contact in the distal sections. Data are presented as the mean percentage of bone in direct contact with the implant (± standard error) as related to inoculum size.

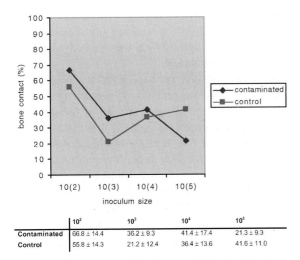

	10^2	10^3	10^4	10^5
Contaminated	66.8 ± 14.4	36.2 ± 9.3	41.4 ± 17.4	21.3 ± 9.3
Control	55.8 ± 14.3	21.2 ± 12.4	36.4 ± 13.6	41.6 ± 11.0

Figure 6b – Bone – Ti-implant contact in the distal sections. Data are presented as the mean percentage of bone in direct contact with the implant (± standard error) as related to inoculum size.

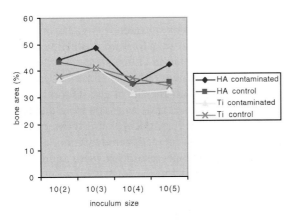

	10^2	10^3	10^4	10^5
HA contam	44.1 ± 2.2	48.7 ± 3.0	35.1 ± 3.3	42.4 ± 3.9
HA control	43.2 ± 9.1	40.6 ± 8.4	35.1 ± 2.1	35.8 ± 7.4
Ti contam	36.2 ± 4.4	41.4 ± 6.3	31.6 ± 7.5	32.4 ± 7.5
Ti control	37.8 ± 8.2	41.4 ± 5.3	37.2 ± 10.7	34.1 ± 8.4

Figure 7 – Bone area in the proximal sections. Data are presented as the mean percentage of bone within a radius of 1mm next to the implant (± standard error) as related to inoculum size.

as a result of increasing inoculum concentration. However, for both the left and right sides separately, there were no significant differences in bone contact or bone area between the two implant types.

When the bone contact and bone area were considered as a function of the presence or absence of infection (i.e., positive or negative culture at sacrifice) we found in the distal sections a difference in bone contact between positive and negative cultures that was significant for the HA implants

($p \leq 0.0001$), but not for the Ti implants, although the effect of infection approached significance ($p = 0.0524$) (fig. 8A). In the proximal sections, there were no significant differences (fig. 8B). With respect to the bone area, we also found no significant differences (fig. 9). Thus, there was a negative

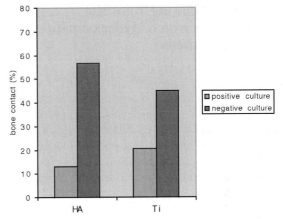

Figure 8a – Bone – implant contact in the distal sections of the left tibiae as related to the results of the cultures.

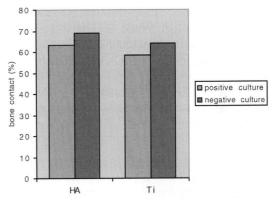

Figure 8b – Bone – implant contact in the proximal sections of the left tibiae as related to the results of the cultures.

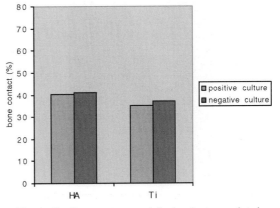

Figure 9 – Bone area around the implants as related to the results of the cultures.

relationship between log CFU and the bone contact in the distal sections (correlation coefficient – 0.69; p ≤ 0.0001), and no significant correlations were found for the bone contact and the bone area data in the proximal sections.

Infection Following Total Hip Arthroplasty with a Hydroxyapatite Coated Prosthesis

Case History

A total hip replacement was performed in the right hip of a 72-year old male (caucasian) because of osteoarthritis and with no history of sepsis in the hip or previous surgery. Just prior to induction of analgesia, the patient received a single dose of prophylactic antibiotics (a second generation cephalosporin). Surgery was uneventful. Thrombosis prophylaxis consisted of administration of subcutaneous heparin from one day preoperatively until 3 days postoperatively, and acenocoumarol, which was started on the day of surgery. There were no problems during the first postoperative days. After 5 days, when the patient started walking, a serious hematoma developed. At the tenth postoperative day, the wound had become swollen, warm, painful, and a fever had developed with a rise of ESR and C-reactive protein (CRP). The operative site was, therefore, opened for extensive debridement, and local antibiotics were left behind (gentamycin beads). An Enterobacter cloacae and a Streptococcus hemolyticus group C were cultured; the infection was treated with vancomycin intravenously.

A second debridement followed at day 21 postoperatively; the second set of gentamycin beads was removed 2 weeks later. Antibiotic therapy was continued intravenously until 2 months after the hip replacement followed by another 2 months of oral antibiotics (ofloxacin and feneticillin). At the time the therapy was discontinued, the infection parameters had been normal (ESR less than 10, CRP less than 5) for more than 4 weeks. Hip movement was restored without difficulty. At 3 months, the Merle d'Aubigné score (31) was 18, which is the maximal score. This remained constant during the entire follow-up period, and the hip performed well until patient death. Radiologically, the hip prosthesis showed no signs of loosening, notwithstanding it was slightly *in varus*. There was a stable position of both components without any change of position or subsidence (fig. 10).

From the second year forward, cancellous densifications were noted in Gruen zones (32) 2 and 6 of the proximal femur, and later in zones 3 and 5. In Gruen zone 4 (at the tip of the femoral prosthesis), an area of sclerosis was seen from the third postoperative year forward, which was interpreted as a sign of distal stem osseointegration. Radiological signs of bone resorption were found initally in Gruen zone 1 at the 5-year follow-up visit.

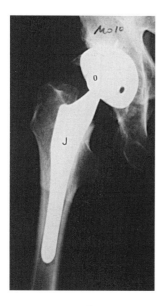

Figure 10a – Postoperative radiograph.

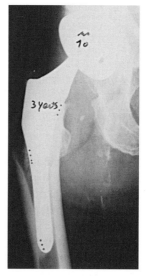

Figure 10b – Radiograph at 3 years postperatively, showing cancellous densification in Gruen zones 2 and 6 as well as in zones 3 and 5. At the tip of the femoral prosthesis an area of sclerosis is seen.

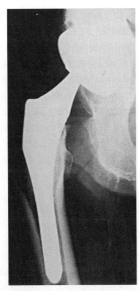

Figure 10c – Radiograph after 6 years.
No migration or subsidence is noted.

The bone around the acetabular component showed a reactive line in DeLee and Charnley (33) zone 1 at the 6 months follow-up visit, which slowly extended into zone 2 at 5 years, but never reached zone 3. No other bone changes were noted in the acetabular region. Technetium scintigraphy was performed at 6 and 12 months after the hip replacement and yearly thereafter. After 6 months, the 3-phase scintigraphy already showed normal blood-flow and bloodpool values indicating that infection was cured. The bone scan demonstrated slightly elevated uptake like in most of the uneventful ABG hip replacements. It was concluded that the scintigraphic pattern at the 5-year follow-up was normal. The patient sustained an intracerebral hemorrage and died 6 years and 6 weeks after the total hip replacement. At the time of the hip operation written consent was given to remove the hip prosthesis after death.

The Implant

An ABG total hip prosthesis was implanted (Anatomique Benoist Gérard, Stryker Howmedica, Newbury, England), a titanium alloy (Ti6Al4V) implant of which the femoral component has a hydroxyapatite coating of the proximal third of the prosthesis and the back of the acetabular component is totally covered with HA (29). The metal acetabular cup has 12 uniform holes through which screws and spikes can be inserted for extra stability. Both components are implanted via press-fit without the use of bone cement. The cup holds a polyethylene insert, the head is of cobalt-chromium with a diameter of 28mm, and several neck lengths are available. The coating was applied by a plasma-spray torch onto a sublayer of titanium in a vacuum. The HA content was more than 90% with a porosity of less than 10% and a Ca:P ratio of 10:6. The crystallinity was 100% before the coating process, and 75% after. The grain size was 20 to 50µm, and the tensile bond strength 62 to 65MPa. The thickness of the HA layer was 60µm ± 30. The roughness of the cup was Ra = 9µm ± 2.5 after sandblasting, 8.5µm ± 2.5 after titan spraying and 5µm ± 1 after HA coating.

Specimen Acquisition and Preparation

The prosthetic components were collected en bloc with the surrounding bone. Unfortunately, the acetabular bone fractured causing the cup to loosen. A reliable assessment of the bone-prosthesis contact in the acetabular area could, therefore, not be made, and these data were discarded. Bone and implant were immersed in buffered formalin for 7 days, subsequently in 70% ethanol for 24 hours. Photographs and radiographs of the specimens were taken. Speciments were then embedded in a PMMA resin. Using a diamond microtome, 20µm thick sections were cut. The sections corresponded to the Gruen zones on the femoral side (fig. 11). They were stained for qualitative histology (paragon staining, a combination of basic

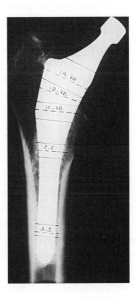

Figure 11 – Radiograph of the proximal femur after explantation, showing good osseointegration of the femoral component and delineating the sections for histology.

fuchsin and toluidine blue) and quantitative histomorphometry. For qualitative analysis, a Polyvar microscope was used; for the quantitative measurements an Axioskop microscope was used which was equipped with a colour-image-analysing system (SAMBA; TITN Alcatel, France).

Bone contact was measured as the percentage of the circumference of the implant that was in direct and close contact with bone. Furthermore, the bone density was measured in several preselected areas around the femoral component and was expressed as a percentage of that specific area that was covered with bone. Residual HA coating was measured as a percentage of the circumference of the implant that was still covered with HA. It must be understood that only fragments of coating of sufficient thickness, i.e., > 5 to 10μm, could be observed, and that the presented values do not take into account very small particles or thin film of HA coating.

RESULTS

The patient's hip prosthesis performed well clinically for more than six years, and the consecutive radiographs of the pelvis taken during the annual follow-up visits did not show any change of position, migration, or subsidence of the components. The stem was well-fixed in the femoral shaft.

Qualitative Histology

Macroscopically, there was a substantial fibronecrotic reaction surrounding the posteromedial half of the proximal part of the femoral prosthesis. Microscopy confirmed the presence of a chronic granuloma. The sections through Gruen zones 1 and 7 showed a large central necrotic cavity that extended up to the interface between prosthesis and surrounding tissue, with an acute and active inflammatory response directly adjacent to it (fig. 12A). Mainly lymphocytes, macrophages and giant cells were present; there were few plasmacells and polymorphonuclear cells. In the granuloma, there were numerous particles from both metallic and polymeric origin. The metallic particles were mainly close to the implant, and the polyethylene debris was in the central necrotic cavity. On the lateral side, there was a high ratio of direct

contact between bone and implant with trabecular bone apposition (fig. 12B).

On the medial side, there was also apposition of bone, but here it did not extend beyond the grooves in the femoral component. The cellularity of the bone marrow was normal without signs of fibroinflammatory infiltrate. Bone density in this area appeared normal. The HA coating was relatively unaffected in the area close to the granuloma, but there was evidence of residual coating all around the prosthesis.

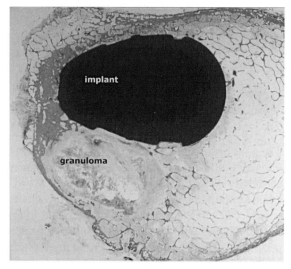

Figure 12a – Histologic section of the proximal femur (Gruen zone 1C-7B) showing the granuloma on the postomedial side of the implant.

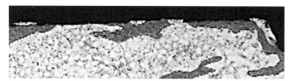

Figure 12b – Detail of section through Gruen zone 1C-7B showing bone apposition (pink) onto the implant (black).

In Gruen zones 2 and 6, the stem was surrounded by a thick fibrous membrane medially and laterally, with a discrete inflammatory reaction. Here, there were no signs of granuloma. On the anterior side there was direct contact between bone and implant (fig. 13a), while on the posterior aspect, there was a thin fibrous layer (fig. 13b). The bone was normal cancellous bone with a low remodelling activity. No more polyethylene or metallic particles were observed in this section.

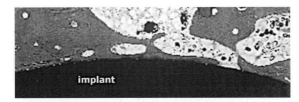

Figure 13a – Section through Gruen zones 2-6 showing direct contact between bone and implant on the anterior side.

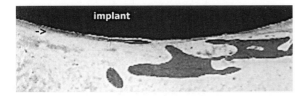

Figure 13b – Section through Gruen zones 2-6 showing a fibrous layer on the posterior side.

More distally, in Gruen zones 3 and 5, there was only a thin fibrous membrane on the anteromedial side. It showed no inflammation. The anterolateral, lateral and posterior sides showed numerous areas of close contact between bone and implant. Bone density appeared normal.

Histomorphometry

In the proximal part of the femur the bone contact values were similar whatever the level of the section (fig. 14); the highest values were seen on the anterior side. The highest percentages of bone contact were measured in the sections through Gruen zones 3 and 5. The bone density gradually increased from proximal to distal (fig. 15). Residual coating (fig. 16) was very limited on all sections except on the posterior side; where the granuloma was located, some 35% of the coating remained. The mean thickness of the observed coating was 23µm.

DISCUSSION

The rather uncomplicated post-infectious clinical course of the patient from the human postmortem study raised questions regarding the influence of the ceramic coating on the infection that occurred, as well as the influence of the infection on the

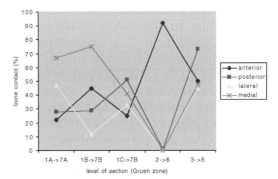

Section level	anterior	posterior	lateral	Medial
1A – 7A	22	28	47	67
1B - 7B	45	29	12	75
1C - 7B	25	51	33	41
2 – 6	92	1	0	0
3 - 5	50	73	45	47

Figure 14 – Bone - implant contact at various levels in the proximal femur presented as the percentage of bone in direct contact with the implant.

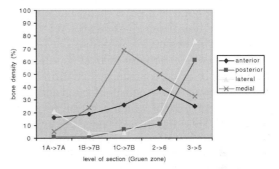

Section level	anterior	posterior	lateral	Medial
1A – 7A	16	1	21	5
1B - 7B	19	1	4	24
1C – 7B	26	7	4	69
2 – 6	39	11	18	50
3 - 5	25	61	76	33

Figure 15 – Bone density around the implant at various levels in the proximal femur.

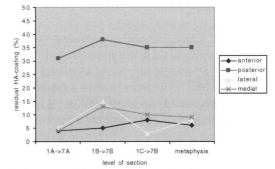

Section level	anterior	posterior	lateral	Medial
1A – 7A	4	31	5	4
1B - 7B	5	38	15	13
1C - 7B	8	35	3	10
metaphysis	6	35	8	9

Figure 16 – Residual HA-coating on the implant at various levels.

osseointegration of the implant. This was, in fact, the reason to design and conduct the animal study.

In the animal study, we demonstrated that infections of biocompatible, noncemented implants can develop after direct contamination of the local implant bed, and that these infections are related to the dose of the original inoculum. We also found that bacteria were more likely to grow onto or next to the HA-coated implants than on non-coated Ti implants, and that the infections that occurred with HA implants were histopathologically more severe. However, the outcome of clinical studies on HA coated implants are quite successful and do not report a higher infection rate (21, 23, 27).

Dhert showed, from histomorphometrical studies on bone contact and bone area, that these parameters can be considered as a representation of implant fixation (34). Inoculum concentration and/or the presence or absence of infection had an effect on the bone contact (at the distal side of the implant) or bone area, particularly for the HA implants. The negative correlation between the number of colony forming units at sacrifice with the amount of distal bone contact confirms a relationship between peri-implant infection and diminished bone ongrowth, which can lead to implant loosening. This diminished bone ongrowth was probably not directly related to the implant type, but more to the severity of infection. Since the HA implants revealed more severe infections, as we demonstrated with the semiquantitative scores, this can explain the histomorphometrical results.

Wilke *et al.* demonstrated for HA-coated implants good osseous ingrowth behaviour, in spite of local infection (35). In our animal study, in case of infection, the percentage of bone contact around the HA implants had decreased in the distal sections only.

Various other groups have studied implant-related infections. Cordero demonstrated that the presence of PMMA bone cement required less bacteria to produce an infection in rabbit femora compared to femora without an implant (36). In another study, he found that PMMA usually appears to be more prone to cause an infection in relation to titanium and cobalt-chromium (37). Hauke described in a rabbit tibial model for titanium, a lower susceptibility to *Staphylococcus aureus* infection as compared with stainless steel (38).

Petty demonstrated in a dog model an early infection of stainless steel and cobalt-chromium alloys, high-density polyethylene, prepolymerised PMMA, and PMMA polymerised *in vivo*. The implants were inserted in the femoral canal after a suspension of bacteria had been injected. Microbiological and histological evaluation demonstrated that all implants were more likely to be associated with infection with Staphylococcus aureus than when surgery was performed without an implant. He concluded that efforts leading to reduction of bacterial contamination in implant surgery are justified (30). However, we have to bear in mind that all these studies are limited by the minimal detectable level of bacteria of ± 1000 CFU/g. This means that a negative culture does not necessarily mean that no bacteria were present. Since we also studied the peri-implant regions histologically, we could correlate negative cultures with histopathological signs of infection. In case of a negative culture, in the majority of cases, the histopathological scores did not indicate a local inflammatory reaction.

In 1987, Gristina described the "race for the surface" theory (39): *"The competition between host tissue cells and bacteria to adhere onto an implanted surface is 'won' by the organisms that arrive first at the implant surface"*. Fast tissue integration of a bioactive material (HA coating) could result in less bacteriological colonisation, as compared to a slower tissue integration of a biocompatible surface (Ti6Al4V). HA coatings are bioactive and well known for their favourable bone-bonding properties, as compared to non-coated Ti6Al4V (9, 10, 11, 40, 41). Biocompatibility could therefore be a determining factor in infection susceptibility or in the development of an infection after contamination of different materials. On the other hand, physical parameters such as surface morphology, porosity, electrical charge, or total surface area could also influence bacterial colonisation.

Since our aim in the animal study was to use the materials as they are applied in the clinical situation, the implant surfaces were not standardised with respect to surface area and porosity. It was previously mentioned that surface roughness may influence bacterial adhesion (42, 43). In addition, according to Naylor *et al.*, the effect of implant surface roughness on infection is also related to differences in colonisation velocity (44). In our experiments, the HA coating had a porosity of less then 10% and there are actual differences in surface architecture between the two implant types. The presence of pores can increase the absolute surface area, despite comparable roughnesses. It can also be hypothesised that bacteria (in a liquid milieu) can more easily migrate into the pores than the tissue cells, and that once the bacteria adhere to the coating surface in the pores, they may be difficult to seize by the host defence system (45). These factors should also be taken into consideration when interpreting the differences that were found between the HA and Ti implants in the animal study.

In the experimental study, we used concentrations of *Staphylococcus aureus*, ranging from very low (10^2) until relatively high (10^5). These unphysiological inoculi were brought in direct contact with the implant. It should be realised that especially the higher concentrations are most likely not to occur perioperatively under uncomplicated, standard circumstances and that, in a clinical situation, contamination will occur in the human tissues rather than on the implant. However, the results from the study do indicate that HA-coated implants can, in the presence of bacteria (e.g., perioperative contamination) more easily develop a more severe infection than uncoated Ti implants. This suggests that precautions to prevent contamination (asepsis) or infection (perioperative antibiotics) are even more important for the highly biocompatible HA-coated implant. This is in particular the case for patients with a higher susceptibility to infection.

In the human postmortem study, there was an overall bone-implant contact of 37%, which is consistent with earlier findings in non-infected THA's with HA-coated hip implants (17). We did note, however, a large cystic granuloma in the metaphysis containing a very large amount of polyethylene and metallic particles along with lymphocytes, macrophages, and giant cells in the metaphysis. There was no bacterial debris, and only a few plasma cells and neutrophils could be identified. We, therefore, concluded that the granuloma formation was mainly due to a foreign body reaction to wear debris.

Osseointegration was circumferential and complete, sealing off the proximal femur and limiting the joint space, since no polyethylene particles were observed distally from the proximal Gruen zones (1 and 7). This is also consistent with earlier findings (17) and confirms that bone ongrowth to the stem followed a normal pattern in this particular patient as well, notwithstanding the infection.

The presence of the granuloma in the proximal femur in the human study showed another interesting phenomenon. The location of the granuloma corresponded exactly with the area of a higher amount (30%) of residual HA coating, while all other proximal surfaces of the stem were covered with less than 10% HA. This can not be explained by lack of dissolution of the coating at lower pH levels as may occur in infection, nor can it be explained by lack of phagocytic activity, as is present in the formation of a PE wear induced granuloma. It can, however, be explained by the lack of bone remodelling activity at the site of the granuloma; in normal bone remodelling osteoclastic-like cells will desintegrate the HA coating with time (41, 46). This observation supports the theory that resorption of HA coating is mainly dependant on the rate of bone remodelling (47).

The human study confirmed that it is possible to eradicate an infection after total hip replacement without the need to remove the prosthesis and that an HA-coated prosthesis may still show a normal pattern of osseointegration.

Reference List

1. Walenkamp GHIM (1990) Infection of orthopaedic prosthesis. Approach to the infected medical device: proceedings of the 5th SB Kurhaus Workshop on antibiotics, Scheveningen, 43-55.
2. Sanderson PJ (1991) Infection in orthopaedic implants. *J. Hosp. Infect.* 18:367-75.
3. Garvin KL, Hanssen AD (1995) Current concepts review. Infection after total hip arthroplasty. Past, present and future. *J. Bone Joint Surg.* 77A:1576-88.
4. Malchau H, Herberts P (1991) Prognosis of total hip replacement. 63rd Annual Meeting of the AAOS, 1996, Atlanta, USA.
5. Okhuijsen SY, Dhert WJA, Faro LMC, Schrijvers AJP, Verbout AJ (1998) De totaleheupprothese in Nederland. *Ned. Tijdschr. Geneeskund* 142:1434-8.
6. Ostendorf M, Malchau H (1998) A report of 302 reoperations for deep infections in THR from the Swedish hip registry. North Sea Biomaterials, 14th European Conference on Biomaterials, The Hague, The Netherlands: ort 8.
7. Maderazo EG, Judson S, Pasternak H (1988) Late infections of total joint prostheses: a review and recommendations for prevention. *Clin. Orth.* 229:131-42.
8. Engh CA, Bobyn JD, Glassman AH (1987) Porous-coated hip replacement. The factors governing bone ingrowth, stress shielding, and clinical results. *J. Bone Joint Surg.* 69-B:45-55.
9. Geesink RG, Groot K de, Klein CP (1987) Chemical implant fixation using hydroxyl-apatite coatings. The development of a human total hip prosthesis for chemical fixation to bone using hydroxyl-apatite coatings on titanium substrates. *Clin. Orthop.* 225:147-70.

10. Geesink RG, Groot K de, Klein CP (1988) Bonding of bone to apatite-coated implants. *J. Bone Joint Surg.* 70-B:17-22.

11. Søballe K, Hansen ES, Brockstedt-Rasmussen H, Pedersen CM, Bunger C (1990) Hydroxyapatite coating enhances fixation of porous coated implants. A comparison in dogs between press fit and noninterference fit. *Acta Orthop. Scand.* 61:299-306.

12. Hardy DC, Frayssinet P, Guilhem A, Lafontaine MA, Delince PE (1991) Bonding of hydroxyapatite-coated femoral prostheses. Histopathology of specimens from four cases. *J. Bone Joint Surg.* 73-B:732-40.

13. Søballe K, Hansen ES, Brockstedt-Rasmussen H, Bunger C (1993) Hydroxyapatite coating converts fibrous tissue to bone around loaded implants. *J. Bone Joint Surg.* 75-B:270-8.

14. Ang KC, Das De S, Goh JC, Low SL, Bose K (1997) Periprosthetic bone remodelling after cementless total hip replacement. A prospective comparison of two different implant designs. *J. Bone Joint Surg.* 79-B: 675-9.

15. Overgaard S, Lind M, Glerup H, Grundvig S, Bunger C, Soballe K (1997) Hydroxyapatite and fluorapatite coatings for fixation of weight loaded implants. *Clin. Orthop.* 336:286-96.

16. Dhert WJA, Thomsen P, Blomgren AK, Esposito M, Ericson LE, Verbout AJ (1998) Integration of press-fit implants in cortical bone: a study on interface kinetics. *J. Biomed. Mater. Res.* 41:574-83.

17. Tonino AJ, Therin M, Doyle C (1999) Hydroxyapatite-coated femoral stems. Histology and histomorphometry around five components retrieved at post mortem. *J. Bone Joint Surg.* 81-B:148-54.

18. Engh CA, Massin P (1989) Cementless total hip arthroplasty using the anatomic medullary locking stem. Results using a survivorship analysis. *Clin. Orthop.* 249:141-58.

19. Mulliken BD, Bourne RB, Rorabeck CH, Nayak N (1996) A tapered titanium femoral stem inserted without cement in a total hip arthroplasty. Radiographic evaluation and stability. *J. Bone Joint Surg.* 78-A:1214-25.

20. D'Antonio JA, Capello WN, Jaffe WL (1992) Hydroxylapatite-coated hip implants. Multicenter three-year clinical and roentgenographic results. *Clin. Orthop.* 285:102-15.

21. Geesink RG, Hoefnagels NH (1995) Six-year results of hydroxyapatite-coated total hip replacement. *J. Bone Joint Surg.* 77-B:534-47.

22. Vedantam R, Ruddlesdin C (1996) The fully hydroxyapatite-coated total hip implant. Clinical and roentgenographic results. *J. Arthroplasty* 11:534-42.

23. Tonino AJ, Rahmy AIA (2000) The International ABG Study Group. The hydroxyapatite-ABG hip system: 5- to 7-year results from an international multicentre study. *J. Arthroplasty* 15:274-82.

24. Oosterbos CJM, Rahmy AIA, Tonino AJ (2001) The ABG hydroxyapatite coated hip prosthesis. Results of 250 hips followed for 5 years. *Int. Orth.* 25:17-21.

25. Vogely HCh, Oosterbos CJM, Nijhof WH, Fleer A, Dhert WJA, Verbout AJ (2000) Effects of hydroxyapatite coating on Ti6Al4V implant site infection in a rabbit model. *J. Orthop. Res.* 18:485-93.

26. Oosterbos CJM, Vogely HCh, Nijhof MW, Fleer A, Dhert WJA, Tonino AJ, Verbout AJ (2002) Osseointegration of hydroxyapatite-coated and non-coated Ti-6Al-4V implants in the presence of infection. A comparative histomorphometrical study in rabbits. *J. Biomed. Mat. Res.* 60: 339-47.

27. Zimmerli W, Waldvogel FA, Vaudaux P, Nydegger UE (1982) Pathogenesis of foreign body infection: description and characteristics of an animal model. *J. Infect. Dis.* 146:487-97.

28. Delmi M, Vaudaux P, Lew DP, Vasey H (1994) Role of fibronectin in staphylococcal adhesion to metallic surfaces used as models of orthopaedic devices. *J. Orthop. Res.* 12:432-8.

29. Tonino AJ, Romanini L, Rossi P *et al.* (1995) Hydroxyapatite-coated hip prostheses. Early results from an international study. *Clin. Orthop.* 312:211-25.

30. Petty W, Spanier S, Shuster JJ, Silverthorne C (1985) The influence of skeletal implants on incidence of infection. Experiments in a canine model. *J. Bone Joint Surg.* 67-A:1236-44.

31. Merle d'Aubigné R, Postel M (1954) Functional results of hip arthroplasty with acrylic prosthesis. *J. Bone Joint Surg.* 36-A:451-75.

32. Gruen TA, McNeice JM, Amstutz HC (1979) Modes of failure of cemented stem type femoral components. A radiographic analysis of loosening. *Clin. Orthop.* 141:17-29.

33. DeLee JG, Charnley J (1976) Radiological demarcation of cemented sockets in total hip replacement. *Clin. Orthop.* 121:20-32.

34. Dhert WJA, Jansen JA (2000) The validity of a single pushout test. In: An YH, Draughn RA, eds. Mechanical testing of bone and the bone-implant interface. Boca Raton, CRC Press : 477-88.

35. Wilke A, Orth J, Kraft M, Griss P (1993) Bone ingrowth behaviour of hydroxyapatite-coated, polyethylene-intruded and uncoated, sandblasted pure titanium implants in an infected implantation site: an experimental study in miniature pigs. *J. Mater. Sci. Mater. Med.* 4:260-5.

36. Cordero J, Munuera L, Folgueira MD (1996) Influence of bacterial strains on bone infection. *J. Orthop. Res.* 14:663-7.

38. Hauke C, Schlegel U, Melcher GA, Printzen G, Perren SM (1997) Local infection in relation to different implant materials. Stainlees steel *versus* titanium intramedullary nails in a rabbit tibia model. 43rd Annual Meeting, Orthopaedic Research Society, San Francisco, California: 301-51.

37. Cordero J, Munuera L, Folgueira MD (1996) The influence of the chemical composition and surface of the implant on infection. *Injury*, 27(Suppl):SC34-7.

39. Gristina AG (1987) Biomaterial-centered infection: microbial adhesion versus tissue integration. *Science* 237:1588-95.

40. Dhert WJA, Klein CP, Wolke JG, Velde A van der, Groot K de, Rozing PM (1991) A mechanical investigation of fluorapatite, magnesiumwhitlockite and hydroxylapatite plasma-sprayed coatings in goats. *J. Biomed. Mater. Res.* 25:1183-200.

41. Dhert WJA, Klein CP, Jansen JA, Velde EA van der, Vriesde RC, Rozing PM, Groot K de (1993) A histological and histomorphometrical investigation of fluorapatite, magnesiumwhitlockite and hydroxylapatite plasma-sprayed coatings in goats. *J. Biomed. Mater. Res.* 27:127-38.

42. McAllister EW, Carey LC, Brady PG, Heller R, Kovacs SG (1993) The role of polymeric surface smoothness of biliary stents in bacterial adherence, biofilm deposition and stent occlusion. *Gastrointest. Endosc.* 39:422-5.

43. Quirynen M, Mei HC van der, Bollen CM, Schotte A, Marechal M, Doornbusch GI, Naert I, Busscher HJ, Steenberghe D van (1993) An *in vivo* study of the influence of the surface roughness of implants on the microbiology of supra- and subgingival plaque. *J. Dent. Res.* 72:1304-9.

44. Naylor PT, Jennings R, Webb LX, Gristina AG (1989) Antibiotic sensitivity of biomaterial-adherent Staphylococcus epidermidis and Staphylococcus aureus. 35rd Annual Meeting, Orthopaedic Research Society, Las Vegas :108.

45. Cordero J, Munuera L, Folgueira MD (1994) Influence of metal implants on infection. An experimental study in rabbits. *J. Bone Joint Surg.* 76-B:717-20.

46. Frayssinet P, Hardy D, Conte P, Delince P, Guilhem A, Bonel G (1993) Histological analysis of the bone-prosthesis interface after implantation in humans of prostheses coated with hydroxyapatite. *J. Orthop. Surg.* 7:246-53.

47. Tonino A, Oosterbos C, Rahmy A, Thèrin M, Doyle C (2001) Hydroxyapatite-coated acetabular components. Histological and histomorphometric analysis of six cups retrieved at autopsy between three and seven years after successful implantation. *J. Bone Joint Surg.* 83-A:817-25.

8   Hydroxyapatite and infection, Results of a Consecutive Series of 49 Infected Total Hip Replacements

Jean-Pierre Vidalain, MD and the ARTRO Group

INTRODUCTION

The biological properties of hydroxyapatite (HA) in the promotion of osseointegration and the achievement of early stabilization have been extensively documented (1, 2, 3, 4). There is reason to believe that the biological fixation provided by HA may also improve the behavior of implant components exposed to infection. Since there is no interposed fibrous tissue, and since living bone is in direct contact with the prosthesis, the resistance of the implant to infection should be enhanced. We have reported (5) our histological findings in tissue samples taken during reoperations for infection where the hip or knee components were either exchanged or left *in situ*. That study showed that HA, while not an anti-infectious agent, could help to control pathogens. At the early stage, the organisms were always seen to be away from the interface, and the septic process looked like a simple acute case of osteomyelitis, which could, therefore, be tackled with appropriate systemic antibiotics (6, 7). It should, therefore, be possible, with the use of HA, to save a larger number of infected prostheses and to obtain a markedly better cure rate in those cases where revision must be performed.

There are, however, very few clinical studies in the literature (8, 9) to show in what way the presence of an HA coating will affect the resistance to infection of the implant components.

We present herein the experience of the ARTRO Group with regard to infective complications which, while rare, may cause a poor functional outcome or worse (10, 11). The investigation was a multi-center retrospective study over a period of more than ten years, beginning in early 1987 and ending in 1998. All the infected devices (whether HA-coated or not) were revised to HA-coated implants.

MATERIALS AND METHODS

There were 49 consecutive cases. The mean time from revision was 72 months (range, 27 to 160 months). These 49 cases had confirmed infections. The criteria for enrollment of a case in the current study was the detection and isolation of bacteria obtained from at least one deep biopsy. We excluded all revised patients in whom bacteria was found by chance during routine intraoperative procurement of tissue samples that were assumed to be uninfected. All the patients were followed up for a minimum of two years. There were no deaths, and none of the patients was lost to follow-up during the time of the study. Over the same period of time, the ARTRO Group performed 7,251 primary hip replacements, of which 0.7% were reoperated for deep infection. In this reoperated group, retrieval or exchange of at least one major component (cup or stem) was performed in two-thirds of the cases (31 out of 49).

There were markedly more men than women (31 males, 18 females). The mean patient age was 62 years. The youngest patient was only 37 years old, the oldest was 86. The general condition of the patients was fairly poor, with only 22 of them rated ASA 1. Only one patient was without any risk factors such as diabetes, steroid medications, cancer, alcohol abuse, or immunodepression. Seventeen patients had one risk factor, while 31 had two or more. Also, many of the patients had undergone surgery before; ten had already been revised before their revision in the present study.

Sixteen of the patients had very early infections, probably acquired at surgery. In 15 cases, there was secondary infection via the bloodstream. In 18 cases, neither the origin nor the time of the infection could be established. Only one patient had a draining sinus. Seventeen patients had obvious signs of local infection. However, in 31 cases, the incision site and the surrounding skin were completely normal. The laboratory results (sed rate, CRP) were almost always suggestive of infection. Scintigraphy was performed in 50% of the cases. Twenty patients underwent a Technetium 99 isotopic scan; three of those 20 patients also underwent Gallium scintigraphy. Whatever the technique used, the result was assessed by the operating surgeon as significant for infection. However, in only 13 cases was the causative agent identified, from swabs or aspirates, prior to revision. In all of the cases, specimens taken at surgery allowed the causative agents to be isolated (Table 1).

	Pathogens	N
Gram + cocci	MSSA	5
	MRSA	14
	MS coag neg staphs	6
	MR coag neg staphs	7
	Streptococci	4
	Enterococci	3
	Others	5
Gram – cocci	E. Coli	3
	Pseudomonas aeruginosa	3
	Others	2
Miscellaneous	Clostridium	1
	Bacterioïdes	1
	Mycobacteria	1
	Others	1

MSSA = methicillin-susceptible *Staphylococcus aureus*; MRSA = methicillin-resistant *S. aureus*; MS coag neg staphs = methicillin-susceptible coagulase-negative staphylococci; MR coag neg staphs = methicillin-resistant coagulase-negative staphylococci.

Table 1 – Causative agents.

Surgical Management

Eighteen patients were managed with irrigation only; in some, the actual bearing components were replaced, but the stem and cup were invariably left *in situ*. In four cases, the implant components were removed, and (for other reasons, usually related to the patients' general condition), the patients were left with a Girdlestone. In seven cases, only one component was exchanged, the reason being that the other component was tight and the radionuclide scan suggested that only one side of the arthroplasty was affected by the infection. In 20 cases, both components were exchanged, either under the same anesthetic (6 cases), or as a staged procedure (14 cases).

All the patients were managed with irrigation, on average for four days; systemic antibiotics (12) were administered for between two months and three years (mean duration, 14 months).

RESULTS

Overall, a definite clinical cure was obtained in 37 patients (no local signs or abnormal laboratory parameters at the latest follow-up) Thus, the definite cure rate was 75%. In 44 patients, improvement of the radiological pattern was consistently seen. Only two patients, neither of whom had a clinical cure, continued to have a typical radiological pattern of infection, with osteolysis, endosteal scalloping, enlargement of the wire tracts, etc. As regards durability of implant fixation, three cups and one stem were revised for what appeared to be mechanical loosening, well away from the site of the septic process and with sterile intraoperative samples.

Functionally, the global MDA score went from 10.7 before surgery to 13.9 at the latest review. These overall results need to be analyzed as a function of the procedure performed (Table 2).

N = 49	Irrigation	Removal	1-component revision	2-component revision
Clinical cure	8/18	2/4	7/7	20/20
Radiological cure	14/18	3/4	7/7	20/20
Loosening	0		0	1
MDA score pre/post	11.6/13.3	7/7.5	12.1/16.6	9.9/15.4
Improvement	+ 1.7	+ 0.5	+ 4.5	+ 5.5

Table 2 – Results as a function of procedure.

Irrigation Only

Eighteen patients were managed in this way. Most of the cases in this subgroup were early infections post-implantation; 15 cases in the first year, and two cases in the second. Most of the infections were acquired at surgery. There was only one case of haematogenous infection, which occurred at ten years.

All the patients had clinical evidence of acute infection and were treated early on. There was local inflammation of the skin, but no sinus tract. The components were found to be tight and were left in place. Irrigation (saline + rifampicin, or saline + betadine) was kept up for a minimum of 48 hours to a maximum of 7 days. Systematic treatment using antibiotics lasted between 3 and 6 months. However, in cases of clinical failure (10 cases), antibiotic treatment lasted until the re-reoperation.

A clinical cure was obtained in only eight cases (44%); the radiographs were considered normal in 14 cases (77%). The MDA score reflects the comparatively low clinical cure rate. The mean global score rose from 11.63 before to 13.29 (range, 6 to 18) at the latest review.

Removal Without Exchange

In four cases, the infected prosthesis was removed but not exchanged. This was either done deliberately, or because a staged procedure that had been planned eventually proved unfeasible.

In all the cases, the patients' general condition was poor. This was not so much because of their age (mean age, 62 years), but because of the association of a number of risk factors, and, above all, because the agents involved (enterococci, salmonellae, and associations of gram-negative agents and anaerobes) were particularly difficult to eradicate. The laboratory parameters never completely returned to normal. While three patients eventually had normal radiographic patterns, only two patients were considered clinically cured. The functional outcome remained poor, with an increase in the MDA score from 7 to only 7.5, following a Girdlestone procedure.

Single-Component Exchange

Seven patients were managed in this somewhat unconventional way. In four cases, only the cup

was exchanged; in three cases, the only component exchanged was the stem. In all the cases, the component left in place was HA-coated. The infection had appeared between 12 months and 36 months postimplantation; in all the cases, onset was sudden and acute. Radionuclide scans consistently showed increased uptake at the site of one of the two components. The causative agent was always isolated at surgery; however, there was no pus in the joint. Since both components were tight, the infected component often proved difficult to remove. In the femur, longitudinal osteotomy had to be performed to facilitate stem retrieval; however, this did not markedly complicate the revision.

Clinical and radiological cure was obtained in all cases, and the MDA score was good (preoperative score: 12.1; postoperative score: 16.6).

Two-Component Exchange

Twenty patients underwent revision of both implant components. In six cases, the exchange was carried out under the same anesthetic; in 14 cases, it was done as a staged procedure, with between one week and a year (mean, nine weeks) between the removal of the infected device and the implantation of the revision prosthesis. The patients were comparatively young (mean age, 60 years); however, many had comorbid conditions: six were rated ASA 3, and 13 had more than two risk factors. Many of the patients had undergone prior surgery: 15 had been operated on more than twice, while nine had undergone at least one previous revision.

In the majority of cases, the implant had become secondarily infected. The mean time to the appearance of signs of infection was 15 months (range, three weeks to five years). Few of the patients received early treatment; on average, there had been three months between the first signs and symptoms and the institution of treatment. While there was strong laboratory evidence of infection (sed rate on average 50 mm; mean CRP 87 mg/L), the local condition was perfectly normal in 15 cases (only one draining sinus), and in three-quarters of the patients, the causative agent was identified only in the samples taken at surgery. The bacterial flora was fairly standard (3 × MSSA, 3 × MRSA, 5 × *S. epidermidis*, *etc.*). Only one patient had an association of *S. aureus* and an enterococcus. Systemic antibiotics were given for a mean of 21 weeks (range, two months to 14 months).

Radiologically apparent lesions were comparatively limited on the acetabular side, and always allowed the use of a threaded or a press-fit hemispherical cup, without the need for a reinforcement ring or for structural grafts. On the femoral side, in more than 50% of the cases, the lesions were SOFCOT (13) Stages II and III. All of these infected stems were revised to non-screw-locked, long, entirely HA-coated stems In some of the cases, a Wagner osteotomy was used to facilitate the removal of a perfectly integrated cementless stem. This allowed ready debridement of the infected tissues, and reconstruction with a screw-locked long-stem implant (14) was straightforward (Table 3).

N=20	Stage I	Stage II	Stage III	Stage IV
Cup	6	9	4	1
Stem	12	4	3	1

Table 3 – Radiological lesions-SOFCOT severity scale.

A clinical cure was obtained in all the cases. Throughout the study, there was no instance of renewed flare-up of the infection. The radiological images were consistently rated normal (disappearance of signs of bone resorption; return to a healthy pattern of the host bone at the implant sites) (fig. 1 and 2).

There were no mechanical failures (migration or loosening) on the femoral side. On the acetabular side, one cup had to be revised after more than ten years, because of a large PE wear debris granuloma, in a case of severe wear of the insert. In terms of the functional outcome, the MDA score improved by almost five points, from 9.9 preoperatively to 14.7 at the latest review.

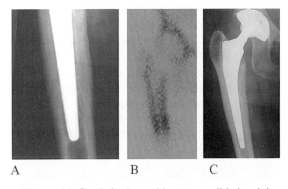

Figure 1A-C – Infection, with osteomyelitis involving the entire shaft, and loosening of an HA-coated stem (A and B). Radiological result at 5 years from one-stage revision to another HA-coated stem (C).

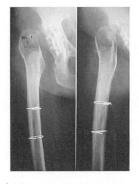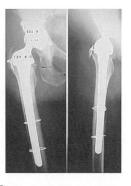

A   B

Figure 2A-B – Two-component staged revision to an HA-coated long-stem device (A). Radiological result at nine years (B).

DISCUSSION

The overall clinical cure rate in the patients managed with HA-coated implants was 75%. This is in line with the mean rates reported for cemented implants, especially for those using antibiotic-laden cement (1, 15, 16, 2, 17). However, the observation that the different treatment modalities in the study produced different cure rates may be useful in deciding how to treat infected implants.

Leaving aside the Girlestone procedures (which would be resorted to only where the patient's condition or the infection are particularly severe, and whose functional outcome is bound to be poor), "irrigation only" gave the poorest results. The decision to treat with irrigation only is often taken purely on the local appearance of the hip (local infection; perfectly stable components). The presence of an HA coating does not appear to substantially increase the resistance to infection, even if the site is accessible to systemic antibiotics. In four of our 18 cases managed with irrigation only, there was persistent or newly emergent radiological evidence of chronic infection, necessitating revision surgery. We therefore feel that "irrigation only" cannot be recommended as a treatment strategy. It tends to underestimate the severity of the situation, and since these patients are in good condition, they should be able to stand more aggressive management (16).

Single-component exchange is not a very logical strategy, and is not an established treatment modality. We were surprised to find that, overall, the clinical and radiological results were excellent. In fact, the patients managed in this way had the best functional scores at the latest review.

Notwithstanding the results obtained with single-component exchange, revision of both implant components is required in order to obtain a complete and lasting cure of the infection. We did not find any difference in outcome following one-stage and two-stage revisions. In order to spare the patient a second operation, it would therefore justifiable to consider revision for infection in one sitting. Where the femoral components to be removed are tight, a transfemoral approach may have to be used. However, we have never found this to be associated with any problems at reconstruction, and have not witnessed any particular complications. As a rule, the radiological pattern will return to normal.

CONCLUSION

The present study was not performed to show that the risk of infection is less with HA-coated than with conventional prostheses. Septic complications are generally not very frequent following total hip replacement. What we wanted to show, in the light of our ten-year experience at many centers, was the utility of HA coatings in revision arthroplasty for infection. Histological studies of some retrieved hips (5) had shown that, at least in the presuppurative phase, the implant-bone interface had remained uninfected and was still tight, and that the pattern of the adjoining bone marrow was that of a simple acute osteomyelitis. Under these conditions, conservative management with appropriate systemic antibiotics could be envisaged. However, a more aggressive approach, with single-component or, preferably perhaps, two-component exchange, would appear to hold greater promise in terms of cure rates. In this respect, HA should be seen as an effective means of controlling infection; however, it cannot be relied upon in isolation, and must be combined with medical treatment and sound technique (16). Hydroxyapatite is at least a credible alternative to the use of antibiotic-laden cement.

Reference List

1. Capello WN, D'Antonio JA, Feinberg JR, Manley MT (1997) Hydroxyapatite coated total hip femoral components in patients less than 50 years old. Clinical and radiographic results after five to eight years of follow-up. *J. Bone Joint Surg. Am.* 79:1023-9.

2. Tsukayama DT, Estrada R, Guistilo RB (1996) Infection after Total Hip Arthroplasty. A study of the treatment of one hundred and six infections. *J. Bone Joint Surg. Am.* 78A, 512-23.

3. Vidalain JP (2001) Long Term Results with a Fully-HA coated Prosthesis (15-year Experience). *Key Engeneering Materials.* Vols 192-195:1021-4.

4. Vidalain JP (2001) Minimum 10-year results of a fully HA-coated Hip System. *J. Bone Joint Surg. Br.* 83B, Sup II, 116.

5. Vidalain JP, Frayssinet P (2000) Prothèses Articulaires à revêtement HA et Complications Septiques. Analyse histologique des tissus péri prothétiques provenant de 10 ablations d'implants. AOLF 2000. *Rev. Chir. Orthop. Reparatrice Appar. Mot.* 86:210-1.

6. Itokazu M, Matsunaga T, Kumazawa S, Oka M (1994) Treatment of osteomyelitis by antibiotic impregnated porous hydroxyapatite block. *Clin. Mater.* 17 (4):173-9.

7. Kawanabe K, Okada Y, Matsusue Y, Iida H, Nakamura T (1998) Treatment of osteomyelitis with antibiotic-soaked porous glass ceramic. *J. Bone Joint Surg. Br.* 80: 527-30.

8. Lecuire F, Collodel M, Basso M, Rubini J, Gontier D, Carrere J (1999) Revision of infected total hip prostheses by ablation reimplantation of an uncemented prosthesis. 57 case reports. *Rev. Chir. Orthop.* 85:337-48.

9. Oosterbos CJ, Rahmy AI, Tonino AJ (2001) Hydroxyapatite coated hip prosthesis followed up for 5 years. *Int. Orthop.* 25(1):17-21.

10. Havelin LI, Engesaeter LB, Espehaug B, Furnes O, Lie SA, Vollset SE (2000) The Norvegian Arthroplasty Register: 11 years and 73,000 arthroplasties. *Acta Orthop. Scand.* 71(4):337-53.

11. Vielpeau C (1986) Sauvetage des Prothèses Totales Infectées. Cahiers d'enseignement de la Sofcot. Conférences d'Enseignement 1986. *Expansion Scientifique Française,* 26:161-84.

12. Desplaces N (1998) Antibiothérapie curative chez l'adulte en chirurgie orthopédique et traumatologique. Cahiers d'enseignement de la Sofcot. Conférences d'Enseignement 1998. *Expansion Scientifique Française.* 66:235-47.

13. Migaud H (2000) Reprises fémorales dans les arthroplasties de la hanche ; classification des pertes de substance. Symposium Sofcot 1999. *Rev. Chir. Orthop. Reparatrice Appar. Mot.* 86:38-40.

14. Laffargue Ph, Delalande JL, Meyer E, Decoulx J (1996) Voie transfémorale *versus* endo-fémorale dans les reconstructions prothétiques des prothèses totales descéllées. *Rev. Chir. Orthop.* 87, II, 91.

15. Lortat-Jacob A (1998) Prothèses de Hanche Infectées. Cahiers d'enseignement de la Sofcot. Conférences d'Enseignement 1998. *Expansion Scientifique Française* 66:61-81.

16. Symposium Sofcot (2001) Les Reprises de Prothèses Totales de Hanche Infectée. *Rev. Chir. Orthop. Reparatrice Appar. Mot.* 88.2002 (Suppl. 5), p. 159-216.

17. Van Hoye M, De Cuyper A, Naert P, Brabants K (1997) The HA-coated ABG socket in revision arthroplasty. *Acta Orthop. Belg.* 63 (Sup I):103-5.

9   The 13 Year Experience of a Novel Cementing Technique Using HA Granules: Interface Bioactive Bone Cement (IBBC)

Hironobu Oonishi, MD, PhD, Seok Cheol Kim, MD, PhD and Hiroshi Fujita, MD, PhD

INTRODUCTION

Since Sir John Charnley first used doughy acrylic cement to secure total hip components, cemented total hip replacements (THRs) have been one of the most successful procedures in orthopaedic surgery (1). Improvements in cementing techniques soon followed, such as usage of cement guns and low viscosity cements. Additionally, distal cement plugs were inserted in order to pressurize the femoral canal and create a more effective bone-cement interface (2-4).

Even with contemporary cementing techniques, cement pressurization is often imperfect, especially in the fixation of acetabular components. This contributes to the high failure rate and aseptic loosening observed with cemented acetabular components (5-7). Even when using the best surgical techniques, there is a limit to what can be achieved with pressurized cement. The use of bioactive materials interposed at the bone-cement interface, with the hope of achieving further interdigitation, may be an attractive option. Using a rabbit model, we found that the integrity of the bone-cement interface was significantly improved when hydroxyapatite (HA) granules were interposed at the bone-cement interface (8-9).

Based on this observation, the process of interposing HA granules at the bone-cement interface has been used since 1983 on markedly sclerotic bone, as well as at bone graft sites in total hip revision cases (8-10). HA granules of varying sizes have been combined and used as grafting material in massive acetabular defects. Having obtained satisfactory results in all those cases with no apparent radiolucent lines at the interface (8-10), we have been using HA granules at the bone-cement interface of THR components since 1987.

MATERIALS & METHODS

This method involves placing less than two layers of fine, porous HA granules 100 to 500μm in diameter with a porosity of 35% to 48% (average 42%) between the bone and cement. Although HA granules of 300 to 500μm in diameter were used initially, they were later reduced to 100 to 300μm, as it was found those sizes adhere to bone more easily. HA of 100 to 300μm must be used on the surface of completely hemostatic bone. On the areas with slight bleeding, the use of larger 300 to 500μm HA granules is more appropriate, as granules smaller than 300μm will blend into the blood. As a result, blood will be present between the HA and bone cement. Additionally, low viscosity bone cements should not be used with HA granules, because the HA granules will sink into it. We used CMW-Type I as the PMMA bone cement.

The senior author (HO) refers to this procedure as the interface bioactive bone cementation technique (IBBC). IBBC fixes the bone cement and HA granules mechanically and, after several days, chemically bonds the HA granules to the bone. Bony tissue then enters the spaces between HA granules. Strong, reliable fixation can be anticipated, as the many small surface irregularities of the HA granules serve as micro anchors for the cement. Fixation of the component to bone via IBBC can be considered as full contact cementless fixation using HA coating.

EXPERIMENTAL STUDIES

Histological Studies

Holes 6mm in diameter and 10mm in depth were made in both femoral condyles of mature rabbits, and IBBC was carried out (fig. 1). In groups of three, rabbits were sacrificed at 2, 3, 4, 6, 12 and 24 weeks, and at 3 years after implantation. Nondecalcified hard tissue specimens were prepared and examined by optical microscopy, scanning electron microscopy (SEM), and back-scattered electron image.

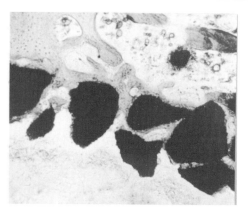

Figure 3 – Two weeks after surgery of IBBC. Nondicalcified hard tissue specimens were stained by Toluidine blue and observed by optical microscopy. New bone had entered a majority of the spaces among the HA granules in the first layer.

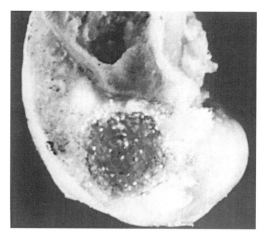

Figure 1 – Cut surface of the femoral condyle six weeks after surgery.

Holes 6mm in diameter were made in both femoral condyles of mature rabbits. HA granules of 100-300μm in diameter were smeared in less than two layers over the bone surface of the hole, and the hole was filled with bone cement.

One week after surgery, new bone began entering the first layer and adhering to the HA granules (fig. 2). At two to three weeks after surgery, new bone had entered a majority of the spaces surrounding the first layer of HA granules (fig. 3), and at 4 weeks, entered a majority of the spaces in the second layer. At 6 weeks, all spaces were filled with new bone, thus forming a unified body (fig. 4). Three years after surgery, bone ingrowth into the spaces of HA granules was the same as that seen at 6 weeks. The HA granules and bone cement bonded mechanically (8-10).

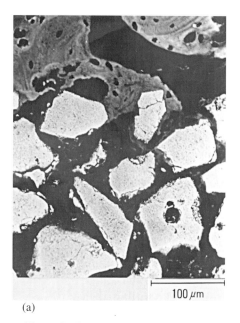

(a)

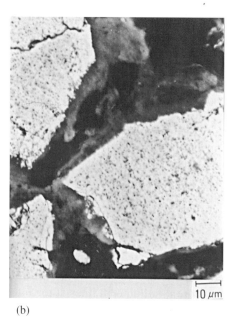

(b)

Figure 2a, b – One week after surgery using the interface bioactive bone cement technique (IBBC).
New bone ingrowth into the spaces of the first layer of HA granules began and the new bone surrounded the HA granules.

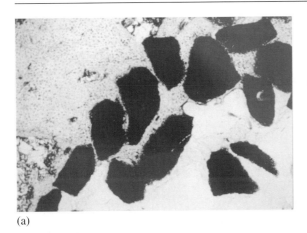

(a)

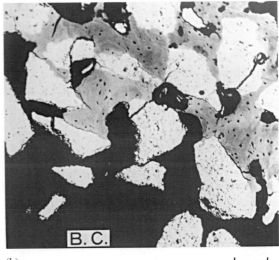

(b)

Figure 4a, b – Six weeks after surgery of IBB. Hard tissue specimens stained by Toluidin blue was observed by optical microscopy (a) and grinded hard tissue specimens were observed by a back-scattered electron image (b).

Bonding Strength Tests

The bonding strength of interface bioactive bone cementation (IBBC) has two important aspects: the adhesive strength of the cement to HA, and that of the HA granule layer to bone.

Bonding Strength of Bone Cement to Square HA Blocks

This surgical procedure is performed in wet areas. Therefore, a square HA block ($7 \times 9 \times 15$mm) was placed in physiological saline solution to absorb water. Bone cement was then applied to the wet HA block, and the adhesive strength was compared to that between cement and a square block of dry titanium (Ti). Titanium and HA with varying degrees of roughness were used, and the Instron Universal tester was employed at a push-out rate of 0.1mm/min crosshead speed.

It was estimated that the adhesive strength between wet HA and bone cement was roughly three to seven times greater than that between dry titanium and bone cement (Table 1) (8-10).

	Surface Roughness (Ra)	Shear Strength (MPa)
Ti	0.31 μm	0
	0.62	1.3
	5.68	7.0
HA	0.88	3.6
	1.04	7.1

Table 1 – Bond (shear)-strengths of bone cement to square HA block or Ti block with the various degrees of surface roughness.

Bonding Strength of the HA Granules Layer to Bone

The interface bioactive bone cementation technique (IBBC) was tested on mature rabbits. Holes with a 6mm diameter and a depth of 10mm were made in both femoral condyles (fig. 1). The rabbits were sacrificed in groups of three at 2, 4, 6, 12 and 24 weeks after implantation, and a push out test was performed. HA coating applied to a smooth titanium surface was used as a control. Figure 5 shows the

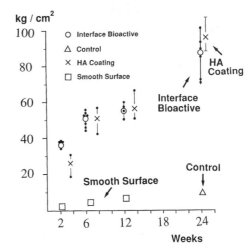

Figure 5 – Push-out test results.
Interface bioactive : IBBC technique.
Control : only cementing.
HA coating : HA coating on the smooth Ti surface.
Smooth surface : smooth surface.

results of the push out tests. The mean adhesive strength at 2, 4, 6, 12 and 24 weeks after implantation was 15, 27, 35, 55 and 35kg/cm^2, respectively.

A relatively strong initial fixation was obtained immediately after implantation using the IBBC technique. Two weeks after implantation, the bonding strength of IBBC was higher than that of the HA coating on the smooth titanium surface, but at six weeks after implantation, the bonding strength of IBBC became similar to that of HA coating. Figure 6 shows the section of the fracture site after the push-out test, which was conducted 6 weeks after implantation.

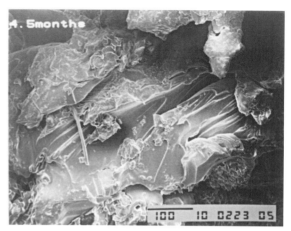

Figure 7 – Fracture surface resulting from the push-out test, five weeks after IBBC operation.

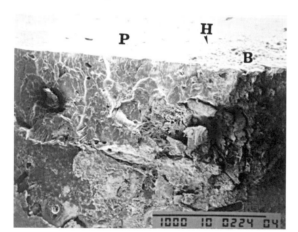

Figure 6 – The section of the fracture site after push-out test six weeks after IBBC operation.
P : PMMA bone cement.
H : HA granule layer.
B : Bone.

The surfaces of the test pieces were observed by SEM after the push out test in order to investigate the fracture zone that was created when the test pieces were pushed out. The fractures resulting from the push out test occurred in the HA granules layer from 2 to 6 weeks after implantation, and occurred in both the HA granules layer and the surrounding bone layer after 12 weeks (fig. 7).

These results indicated that the strength of the HA granule layer gradually increased after surgery and reached almost the same level as the bone around the HA granule layer after 12 weeks. In these experiments, the bonding strength of bone cement to bone by interposing HA granules was found to be adequate.

In subsequent clinical cases, stress shielding was not found. When cement fixation using PMMA bone cement is performed, excellent initial fixation can be obtained. However, after a period of time, a connective tissue membrane may form between the bone and bone cement, particularly in the acetabulum. This may lead to component loosening.

When cementless fixation with a HA-coated component is performed, micromotion of the component may occur if the initial fixation is insufficient. Therefore, we are confident that IBBC combines the fixation advantages of both conventional PMMA bone cement and HA (8-10).

CLINICAL STUDIES

In 1984, we began using the IBBC technique in selected THR revision surgery cases. Good results were obtained, and no radiolucent lines were visible in the IBBC area. Since 1987, the IBBC has been performed in more than 2500 joints.

Materials

A modified Charnley-type prosthesis (KC®, Kyocera Co. Ltd., Kyoto, Japan) was used in combination with a 28mm alumina ceramic head. The femoral component was grit-blasted, collared, cobalt-chromium. All-polyethylene acetabular components with a thickness of more than 10mm were used. The largest stem sizes feasible for each case were used. All the operations were performed by the senior author (HO) using the lateral or anterolateral approach with the patients in supine position.

HA granules were manufactured by sintering at 1200°C after which they were sieved to obtain granules of several sizes (Bioceram P®. Sumitomo Cement Co. Ltd. Tokyo, Japan).

CMW®-type I bone cement (CMW, Laboratories Ltd, Blackpool, UK) was used for both acetabular and femoral component fixation.

Surgical Procedures

For the IBBC technique to be effective, good hemostasis must be present before cementing. For complete hemostasis, blood pressure must be kept under 90mm Hg.

The acetabulum must be pressurized by fine bone reamed in the acetabulum to achieve hemostasis. After five minutes of pressurization, good hemostasis can be obtained, even after reamed bone is removed by a water rinse. If bleeding areas are found after a water rinse, reamed bone may be used to fill the bleeding areas only. Complete hemostasis in the acetabulum can be obtained by using these procedures. After good hemostasis is achieved, HA granules (100 to 300µm or 300 to 500µm) of 2 to 3g are smeared (using fingers) in less than 2 layers along the entire bone surface. Bone cement is then inserted, followed by insertion of the acetabular component.

After the bone plug is inserted into the femoral canal, gauze is used for several minutes to compress the femoral canal, then a hydrogen peroxide rinse is applied. Immediately after wiping away the hydrogen peroxide, 2 to 4g of HA granules are smeared on the inner surface of the femoral canal with a special instrument holding at the tip of the long clamp a longitudinal, halved silicon tube 7 to 8mm in diameter and 30mm in length. This enables HA granules to be smeared throughout the entire femoral cavity.

Immediately after smearing the HA granules, bone cement is inserted quickly using a cement gun via a so-called second-generation cementing technique. Cement pressurization was obtained because the largest stem size possible was used. Because the patient is in a supine position, sometimes a small amount of blood occasionally flows out to the greater trochanter area. Therefore, bone cement is inserted at the same time the blood is being aspirated from the greater trochanter by an aspirator. When bleeding is found in an extensive area after smearing the HA, the whole area of the femoral canal should be pressed and wiped with gauze. Even when gauze is pressed into the after the HA is smeared, the HA granules are rarely removed. Because HA is porous, it adheres well to wet bone.

In order to gauge the effectiveness of smearing the HA granules with our original instrument, experimental studies were performed using cadaveric bone. As a result, it was found that after smearing the HA granules using our special instrument, the HA was smeared extensively and rather evenly throughout the femoral canal (fig. 8).

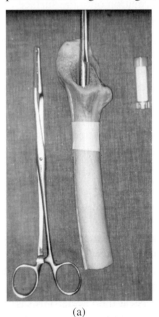 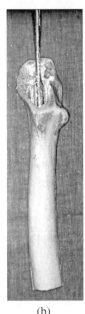 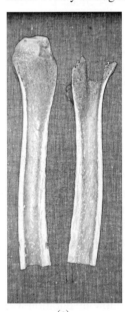 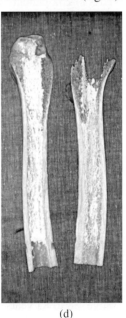

    (a)   (b)   (c)   (d)

Figure 8 – IBBC technique was performed by using a cadaveric femoral bone.
a) Before smearing HA granules on the inner surface of the femur.
b) After smearing HA granules.
c) Longitudinal section of the femur before smearing HA granules.
d) Longitudinal section of the femur after smearing HA granules.

When complete hemostasis cannot be obtained, it is preferable to use HA granules of larger sizes (300 to 500µm) both the acetabulum and femur, as smaller sizes (100-300µm) may sink into the blood, resulting in a space between the HA and cement (8-10).

Post-operative Weight Bearing Time

Permitting full weight bearing at 4 to 6 weeks after surgery is considered the safest, earliest time if an initial fixation is insufficient. The following results were obtained from our animal experiment: (1) new bone sufficiently entered into spaces among HA granules, and (2) bone adhesive strength reached 50% of the final strength. However, as found in the acetabulum, numerous micro anchor holes were made, and in the femur full contact was completely achieved compared to the cementless stem. With good initial fixation, full weight bearing can be allowed before 2 weeks.

Clinical Cases

Patients and Evaluation Method

This cementing technique was used between 1987 and 1989. The patient group was comprised of 268 THRs in 232 patients (Male: 11, Female: 221). The diagnosis was degenerative osteoarthritis due to congenital dysplasia in 231 hips (199 patients), rheumatoid arthritis in 15 hips (12 patients), avascular necrosis of the femoral head in 12 hips (11 patients), femoral neck fracture in 10 hips (10 patients). Structural, autogenous bone graft was used in 215 dysplastic hips. At the beginning of 1987, HA granules were smeared only in zones 3 and 4 or, in some cases, only in zone 4; a good hemostasis was not obtained in some cases. Five patients died (5 hips) and 30 patients (45 hips) were lost to follow-up. Most patients lost to follow-up lived too far away or were too old to visit our hospital, or they moved and did not inform us of their new address. Thus, 218 THRs (197 patients Male:11, Female:186) comprised the study group and were followed-up radiologically and clinically. The average patient age at the time of the index operation was 58.2 years (range, 38 to 82 years). The follow-up duration was 11 to 13 years. The patients were followed-up at regular intervals, and clinical evaluation was performed using (Charnley's modification of) Merle d'Aubigné's criteria. Evaluation of the radiography was performed by one of the authors (NK) inde-

pendently, without the knowledge of the patient clinical status. The presence of radiolucent lines (RLL) was evaluated, and their location was identified according to the three zones described by DeLee and Charnley for acetabular components (11) and the seven zones described by Gruen *et al.* for femoral components (12). The presence of osteolysis in the pelvis and the femur was carefully assessed. Osteolysis was defined as a focal area of balloon-shaped lucency, and not linear lucency.

Clinical & Radiological Findings

The average preoperative clinical score was 3.11 points. At the time of the most recent follow-up, the average score was 5.85 points. One hip was revised due to aseptic loosening of the acetabular component, because microanchor holes were not made. Two hips were revised due to infection. Another two hips dislocated and were managed with closed reduction. One patient sustained a femoral shaft fracture, which was fixed with a plate and screws.

General radiological appearance

The bone-cement interface in this study group was more clearly defined as compared to that seen with other methods of cemented THR. This was probably due to new bone formation onto the surface of the HA granules (fig. 9, 10).

The RLL in the study groups could potentially appear at two interfaces, namely, cement-HA and HA or cement-bone. The RLL between HA and cement occurs when the cementing is performed in the bleeding area. The RLL between HA and cement was identified in 5 patients (4 acetabular component and 1 femoral component). The lines did not progress after three years, and they did not influence clinical outcome (fig. 11). Thus, we focused on the RLL between HA-bone interface.

The RLL Around the Acetabular Component

Six acetabular components were defined as radiologically loose, and one hip was revised seven years after the operation. RLLs more than 2mm thick were seen in zone 3 in one patient after six years and progressed to a 4mm thickness at nine years. The other eight acetabular components were associated with a RLL of less than two mm (zone 3: 6 cups, zone 1: 2 cups) at the latest follow-up. Twelve components were associated with a RLL of less than one mm (zone 1: 8 cups, zone 2: 1 cup, zone 3: 3 cups).

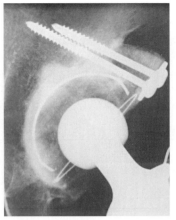
(a)

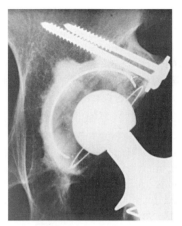
(b)

Figure 9 – IBBC technique was performed on the dysplasic acetabulum.
Acetabular bone graftings were performed from anterior to posterior margin.
a) three months after surgery.
b) 13 years after surgery.

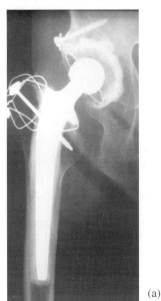
(a)

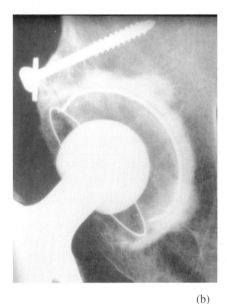
(b)

Figure 10 – IBBC technique
was performed
on the dysplasic acetabulum.
a, b) 13 years after surgery.

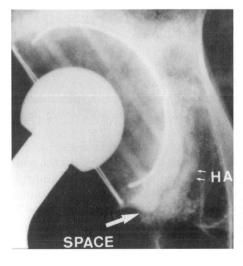

A RLL in zone 1 appeared in a case of with no bone grafting on the dysplasic acetabulum. This is because the bone at zone 1 was sclerotic, and it is difficult for HA or cement to adhere to sclerotic bone.

As at the beginning of 1987, HA granules were smeared only at zone 3 and 4 or only zone 4 in some cases, and a good hemostasis was not obtained in some cases. Radiologically loose acetabular components were observed in these cases.

Overall, the radiological loosening rate for the acetabular component was 2.8%.

Figure 11 – 13 years after surgery.
IBBC technique was performed on the bleeding area.
The spaces (RLL) appeared between HA and bone cement at Zone 3.
The spaces never progressed.

The RLL Around Femoral Components

No femoral component was defined as radiologically loose (fig. 12). Two components were associated with RLLs of 2mm in zones 1 and 2. Osteolysis was observed in zones 4 and 5 in 2 hips, 5 and 9 years after surgery, respectively.

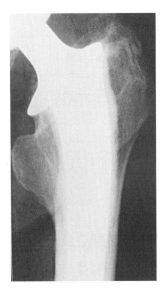

Figure 12 – IBBC technique was performed on the femur. Radiograph at 13 years after surgery.

Histological Studies of Clinical Cases

Histological studies were performed in three clinical cases, a fractured femur, a late infection, and movement of the metal backed socket from cement.

On the dense bone, such as a cortical bone and subchondral bone, new dense bone grew readily into the spaces of HA granules smeared on the dense bone, and new dense bone layers were formed by new bone and HA granules (fig. 13).

On the cancellous bone, new cancellous bone grew into the spaces of HA granules with the same density of cancellous bone.

These clinical histological results corresponded to those of animal experiments.

Pros and Cons in IBBC and HA Coating

The pros and cons of IBBC and HA coatings were compared. From the viewpoint of HA materials, with IBBC neither peeling off nor absorption of HA occurs.

From the viewpoint of the prosthesis, if the IBBC coating area is completely covered, but distribution of HA is not even, the strength of the fix-

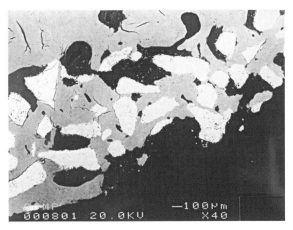

Figure 13 – Materials were retrieved due to movement of the metal backed socket from the cement ten years after surgery. IBBC was performed on the subchondral bone region of the acetabulum. Non decalcified hard tissue specimen was observed by back scattered scanning electron microscopy imaging.

ation is merely adequate. When an entire surface is coated with HA, the fixation strength may be too strong, and stress shielding may occur. With IBBC, when complete contact is obtained immediately after surgery, initial fixation is certain. With HA coating, complete total contact may or may not be obtained; therefore, initial fixation is uncertain. With IBBC, the size variation of prostheses can be limited. With an HA coating, many sizes of prostheses must be prepared. With IBBC, a metal backed socket is unnecessary. HA-coated acetabular components are associated with reduced thickness of polyethylene because of the need for metal backing of the acetabular shell; the thinner polyethylene potentially poses the problem of increased wear. Furthermore, initial stability is not always obtained with so-called press fit components, and additional screw fixation, which may cause fretting and corrosion, may be necessary. In IBBC, the cost of the prostheses is not expensive.

From the viewpoint of surgical technique, with IBBC, good hemostasis is indispensable, and the technique of smearing the HA is important. However, stem positioning in CDH with severe anteversion is easy.

From the viewpoint of clinical results, stress shielding rarely occurs with IBBC, but occurs quite often with a HA coating. Adequate fixation is always obtained with IBBC, but not always with a HA coating. Removal of the component is not difficult with IBBC, but is often difficult with a HA coating. With IBBC, when the component is inserted into a bleeding area, RLL appear between HA. However, with IBBC, the probability of an occurrence of micro-motion and thigh pain is very low.

From the viewpoint of material and prosthesis, IBBC is supposed to be superior to HA coating. However, from a viewpoint of surgical technique and conditions, IBBC is rather difficult.

DISCUSSION

As HA granules are porous, they adhere easily to the wet bone. Complete hemostasis is very important while cementing, because smaller HA granules will sink in the bleeding area and spaces, or RLL may appear between HA and cement. When good hemostasis is difficult to obtain, it is better to use larger HA granule sizes of 300 to 600μm.

Several long-term follow-up cases of IBBC total hip replacement have demonstrated excellent longevity of the femoral component, exceeding that of the acetabular components (3-4). The failure rate seen with acetabular components has not been reduced by the use of so-called second generation cementing techniques. Mulroy *et al.* reported that the total rate of radiological loosening was 9% for the femoral component and 49% for the all-polyethylene cemented acetabular component at a mean follow-up of 11.2 years (3). Madey *et al.* also reported that the total rate of radiological loosening was 3% for the femoral component and 22% for the acetabular component at minimum follow-up of 15 years (4). Hybrid fixation was then introduced in response to this disparity between the longevity of cemented femoral and acetabular components, and it has demonstrated low complication rate after a minimum of 10 years follow-up (13). This fixation method, however, is associated with reduced thickness of polyethylene because of the need for metal backing, and this potentially poses the problem of increased wear. Furthermore, initial stability is not always obtained with so-called press fit components, and additional screw fixation, which might cause the fretting and corrosion, may be necessary.

Hydroxyapatite (HA) has been used as a coating on implants because of its ability to conduct new bone across the gap between the bone-implant interface, thus enhancing component stability (14-16). The HA coating has been shown to be effective in the fixation of femoral components (17),

but the cost-effectiveness of the acetabular components is still controversial (17-18). Although the cement fixation of the acetabular components provides good initial stability, "biological mode" of failure due to foreign body reaction at the bone-implant interface has been suggested (19). The cementing technique used in this study could be regarded as a coated implant stabilized with cement at the time of implantation.

The reduced incidence of RLL around the femoral and acetabular components might be, in some part, due to the radiodensity of the HA granules present in the interface. However, we histologically demonstrated that the majority of interposed HA granules were incorporated into host bone, after which they underwent remodeling, forming a convoluted, dense bone-cement interface (20). Thus we believe that the reduced incidence of RLL is attributable to the continued bone formation and remodeling adjacent to HA granules. This effect is of particular importance in view of the fact that bone formation and remodeling have been shown to be universally present in well-fixed total joint prostheses (21-23). Another important effect of this well-integrated bone-implant interface is that the migration of particles and subsequent osteolysis was prevented by its sealing effect. In fact, we found a very low prevalence of osteolysis, in spite of the fact that we used relatively large head sizes in this study group.

HA coating on the prostheses has been reported to undergo resorption (24, 25) and some inflammatory reactions (26), and third body effects (27) of fragmented HA have been reported. Another concern is that the roughness of the HA granules might cause the degradation of the bone cement. There were, however, no untoward clinical complications attributable to the use of HA granules at a mean follow up of 13 years. We histologically confirmed negligible foreign body reactions in the specimens retrieved after 10 years service *in vivo* (20). This is probably because the particle size of HA granules used was relatively large (ø =100 to 300μm or 300 to 600μm) and the majority of them were incorporated into trabeculae without a macrophage reaction.

When the pros and cons of IBBC and HA coating are compared with IBBC, neither peeling off nor absorption of HA occur. As the coating area can be controlled and distribution of HA is uneven, fixation strength is adequate and stress shielding does not occur. If full contact is completely obtained, initial fixation is certain. The large variety of prosthetic sizes is not needed. A metal-backed acetabular shell is unnecessary. The cost of the prosthesis is not expensive. The removal technique of the component and the cement is not difficult. However, good hemostasis is very important.

From a viewpoint of material and prosthesis, IBBC is superior to HA coating. However, from viewpoint of surgical technique, IBBC is rather difficult.

In conclusion, the cementing technique with HA granules was associated with very low incidence of loosening, osteolysis and RLLs, especially with the acetabular components. There were no untoward clinical complications attributable to the use of HA granules. Based on these results, we are confident in the continuous use of this cementing technique and we anticipate more favorable long-term clinical results.

Reference List

1. Wroblewski BM (1986) Charnley low friction arthroplasty of the hip: Review of the past, present status, and prospect of the future. *Clin. Orthop.* 210:37-42.

2. Oh I, Carlson CE, Tomford WW *et al.* (1978) Implant fixation of the femoral component after total hip replacement using a methylmethacrylate plug. *J. Bone Joint Surg.* 60A:608.

3. Mulroy RD, Harris WH (1990) The effect of improved cementing techniques on component loosening in total hip replacement. *J. Bone Joint Surg.* 72B:757-60.

4. Madey SM, Callaghan JJ, Olejniczak JP, Goetz DD, Jonston RC (1997) Charnley total hip arthroplasty with use of improved techniques of cementing. *J. Bone Joint Surg.* 79A:53-64.

5. Shulte KR, Callaghan JJ, Kelly SS, Jhonston RC (1993) The outcome of Charnley total hip arthroplasty with cement after a minimum twenty-year follow-up. *J. Bone Joint Surg.* 75A:961-4.

6. Sochart DH, Porter MI (1997) The long term results of Charnley low-friction arthroplasty in young patients who have congenital dislocation, degenerative osteoarthritis, or rheumatoid arthritis. *J. Bone Joint Surg.* 79A:1509-617.

7. Callaghan JJ, Forest EE, Olejniczak JP, Goets DD, Johnston RC (1998) Charnley total hip arthroplasty in patients less than fifty years old. *J. Bone Joint Surg.* 80A:704-14.

8. Oonishi H, Kushitani S, Aono M, Maeda E, Tsuji E, Ishimaru H (1989) Interface bioactive bone cement by using PMMA and hydroxyapatite granules. Bioceramics vol. 1 Ishiyaku-Euro America; p. 102-7.

9. Oonishi H (1991) Interfacial reactions to bioactive and non-bioactive bone cement. The Bone Biomaterial Interface Davies JE, editors. University of Toronto Press, Toronto, p. 321-33.

10. Oonishi H, Kushitani S, Yasukawa E (1998) Clinical results with interface bioactive bone cement. Hip Surgery; Material and Developments, Edited by Sedel L. and Cabannela M., p. 65-74, Martin Dunitz (UK).

11. DeLee JG, Charnley J (1976) Radiological demarcation of cemented sockets in total hip replacement *Clin. Orthop.* 121:20-32.

12. Gruen TA, McNiece GM, Amstutz HC (1979) "Modes of failure" of cemented stem type femoral components. A radiological analysis of loosening. *Clin. Orthop.* 141:17-27.

13. Smith EM, Harris WH (1997) Total hip arthroplasty performed with insertion of the femoral component with cement and the acetabular components without cement. *J. Bone Joint Surg.* 79A:1827-33.

14. Oonishi H, Yamamoto M, Ishimaru H, Tsuji E, Aono M, Ukon Y (1993) The effect of hydroxyapatite coating on bone growth into porous titanium alloy implants. *J. Bone Joint Surg.* 71B:213-6.

15. Maisterelli GL, Mahomed M, Fornasier V, Antonelli L, Li Y, Binnington A (1993) Functional osseointegration of hydroxyapatite-coated implants in a weight-bearing canine model. *J. Arthroplasty* 8:549-54.

16. Søballe K, Hansen ES, Brockstedt-Rasmussen H, Bünger C (1993) Hydroxyapatite coating converts fibrous tissue to bone around loaded implants. *J. Bone Joint Surg.* 75B:270-8.

17. Donnely WJ, Kobayashi A, Freeman MAR, Chin TW, Yeo H, West M (1997) Radiological and survival comparison of four different methods of fixation of a proximal femoral stem. *J. Bone Joint Surg.* 79B:351-9.

18. Thanner J, Kärrholm J, Harberts P, Malchau H (1999) Porous cup with and without hydroxyapatite-tricalcium phosphate coating. 23 matched pairs evaluated with radiostereometry. *J. Arthroplasty* 14:266-71.

19. Schmalzried TP, Kwong LM, Jasty M, Sedlacek RC, Haire TC, O'Connor DO, Bragdon CR, Kabo JM, Malclom AJ, Harris WH (1992) The mechanism of loosening of cemented acetabular components in total hip arthroplasty: Analysis of specimens retrieved at autopsy. *Clin. Orthop.* 274:60-78.

20. Oonishi H, Kadoya Y, Iwaki H, Kim N (2000) Hydroxyapatite granules interposed at bone-cement interface in total hip replacements. Histological Study on Retrieved Specimens. *J. Applied Biomat.* 53:174-80.

21. Linder L (1994) Implant stability, histology, RSA and wear-more critical questions are needed. *Acta Orthop. Scand.* 65:654-8.

22. Freeman MAR, Plante-Bordeneuve P (1994) Early migration and late aseptic failure of proximal femoral prostheses. *J. Bone Joint Surg.* 76B:432-8.

23. Kärrholm J, Borssén B, Löwenhielm G, Snorrason F (1994) Does early micromotion of femoral stem prostheses matter? *J. Bone Joint Surg.* 76B:912-7.

24. Linder F, Böhn G, Huber M, Acholz R (1994) Histology of tissue adjacent to an HAC-coated femoral prosthesis. A case report. *J. Bone Joint Surg.* 76B:824-9.

25. Overgaard S, Lind M, Josephsen K, Maunsbach AB, Bünger C, Søballe K (1998) Resorption of hydorxyapatite and fluorapatite ceramic coatings on weight-bearing implant: A quantitative and morphological study in dogs. *J. Biomed. Mater Res.* 39(1):141-52.

26. Grimm D, Schwartz E, Ukata S, Hicks D, Hsu J, Puzas J, Rosier R, O'keefe R (1999) Hydroxyapatite particles induce monocyte production of TNF-Alfa and bone resorption. Trand ORS, 24(1)-243.

27. Morscher EW, Hefti A, Aebi U (1998) Severe osteolysis after third-body wear due to hydroxyapatite particles from acetabular cup coating. *J. Bone Joint Surg.* 80B:267-72.

CLINICAL EXPERIENCES
IN PRIMARY HIPS
AT A MINIMUM OF 10 YEARS

1 Two Decades of Hydroxyapatite Coatings in Total Hip Replacement

Marc George, FRCS, Marion Mueller, FRCS and John Shepperd, FRCS

INTRODUCTION

Approximately 850,000 total hip replacements (THRs) are performed worldwide each year (1). This number will continue to rise due to an aging population, longer life expectancies, and the continuing need for hip replacement in younger patients. Therefore, long term results are of the utmost importance. Aseptic loosening is the major long-term concern, followed by component wear. Despite improved cementing techniques (2), disappointing long-term results with cemented prostheses, especially in the young (3) led to the introduction of uncemented porous coated implants in the hope of achieving long-term stability via bony ingrowth. Results of these long-term prostheses have been variable, with subsidence and thigh pain being particularly problematic (4).

The introduction of hydroxyapatite-coated prostheses in the 1980's yielded excellent initial results that are now being backed up by long-term studies. Hydroxyapatite (HA) ceramic is a bioactive material that promotes bony fixation into the implant surface coating. In hip surgery, it is believed that hydroxyapatite was first utilised in revision hip replacement. Pelvic underpinning was developed for major acetabular floor defects by Shepperd (5). This procedure has been used in 113 cases performed since 1981. HA-coated tubes have subsequently been used at femoral revision to bypass badly damaged bone. Ideally, the results of these procedures should be compared to alternative procedures, such as impaction bone grafting, by using randomised, controlled trials. The first HA-coated primary hip prosthesis in humans was implanted in 1985 by Furlong.

Titanium has proved to be the most suitable implant substrate material for hydroxyapatite coatings (6), which are usually applied by plasma spraying techniques. Despite strongly voiced anecdotal claims, it is unclear what thickness is optimal. Layers thinner than 30mm may be ineffective due to excessively rapid resorption. Conversely, the risk of fractures occurring in the ceramic coating may increase with thicker layers (7). Most hip replacement coatings are at least 50mm. There is, however, no consensus regarding either the importance of coating thickness, or whether full or partial coating is preferable. The bonding that occurs between implant and bone in hydroxyapatite implants allows equal transfer of mechanical forces and prevents micromotion, which is believed to be a key factor failure in failure of implant fixation.

THE HASTINGS EXPERIENCE OF HYDROXYAPATITE-COATED (HA) TOTAL HIP REPLACEMENTS

Interest in hydroxyapatite coatings in hip replacement began in Hastings, England, in 1981, with the first orthopaedic use in revision hip surgery outlined supra. In 1986, a series of JRI-Furlong hip replacements began. During a sixteen year period beginning in 1986, we evaluated five different stem designs and six different cup designs (Tables 1A and 1B). Our longest experience is with the JRI hip replacement.

Between 1986 and 1991, 346 HA-coated total hip replacements were performed in 301 patients (mean age 67 years, range 45-85). Thirty-eight patients had sequential bilateral replacement performed under one anaesthetic, and an additional 7 patients had contralateral replacement after an interval. Surgery was performed via a Watson-

Year	Stem
In use since 1986	JRI Furlong stem
1986-89	JRI Furlong stem - Used with cemented all poly cup
1989-93	JRI Furlong stem - Used with HA coated screw cup
1992	JRI Furlong stem - Used with present CSF press fit cup
1989	ABG stem and cup
1989	Panatomic uncoated stem
1994	Panatomic partially coated stem
1995	Trial: Osteonic partial coated *vs* JRI fully coated stem
1996	Panatomic fully coated stem
2001	Anca-Fit Modular HA Hip replacement

Table 1A – Primary Hydroxyapatite Hips Used in Hastings.

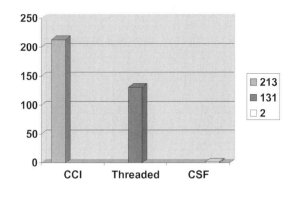

Table 1B – Types of HA Cup.

Jones approach by or under the supervision of one surgeon (JANS). Three doses of perioperative antibiotics were used. Patients were mobilised fully weight-bearing immediately, with the exception of intraoperative fracture, where only partial weight-bearing was allowed for the first six weeks.

Patients were evaluated at six, twelve, twenty-six and fifty-two weeks, and at annual intervals thereafter in dedicated joint replacement clinics with all cases logged in a hip register. Clinical evaluation was with the modified Merle D'Aubigne and Postel hip score8. Radiological assessment of anteroposterior pelvic and lateral hip radiographs was carried out at each visit. Femoral bonding was assessed by the presence of cancellous densification and spot welds. Femoral and acetabular lucencies were noted according to the classifications of Gruen9 and De Lee and Charnley (10). At ten to sixteen years mean follow up, 171 patients (202 hips) were still alive with no deaths related to surgery. Merle D'Aubigne & Postel score averaged 5.8 for pain, 5.7 for movement and 5.2 for function.

FEMORAL COMPONENT

The same femoral component was used in all cases (Furlong HAC, JRI Instrumentation Ltd., London UK), which is manufactured from titanium alloy, has a cylindrical stem, and consists of a cone with a vestigial fin for primary mechanical fixation. It is fully coated with a 200mm thickness of hydroxyapatite (fig. 1). A 32mm ceramic head was used in all cases (Furlong). Sixteen intraoperative technical fractures of the femur occurred, but fifteen were minor and required only a protected period of weight-bearing. One underwent cerclage wiring. All fractures united without detriment to the anchorage or further complications.

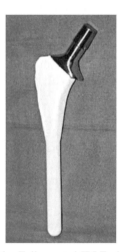

Figure 1 – Fully coated JRI Furlong Stem.

Intraoperative fractures are well documented during uncemented hip replacement (11, 12) but need to be taken into context. Although minor cracks are not uncommon, these do not affect outcome, and significant fractures requiring operative intervention are rare. A higher fracture rate was described in the first 100 Hastings JRI hips (13).

This was most likely due to the learning curve phenomenon of a new stem design (14). There were three late femoral shaft fractures, all of which occurred after significant trauma. One patient was revised for traumatic loosening of the femoral component following polytrauma from a road traffic accident eleven years following surgery. This was the only aseptic case of femoral revision. In one further case, both components were removed for presumed sepsis from an ipsilateral retrograde femoral nail. Infection was never proven, and the patient subsequently had a second stage hydroxyapatite hip replacement with an excellent outcome. Two further cases required revision of infected prostheses, one after revision for a trunnion fracture, and another following revision of a loose cemented prosthesis to a HA-coated stem with pelvic underpinning acetabular reconstruction. Indications for all revisions are shown (Table 2). No other femoral component is awaiting revision, and all HA coated components are well bonded, with complete absence of periprosthetic lucent lines.

We have not had problems with stem subsidence. Although common, is within the limitations of measurements on routine x-rays. However, from studies performed with radiostereometric analysis (RSA), the subsidence encountered in some uncemented series does not appear to be a problem in HA cases. Less subsidence is seen with HA-coated stems as compared to either porous coated or cemented (15).

All the stems used in this series were fully hydroxyapatite-coated. We orignally intended to randomise against a series of uncoated identical stems, but the second cohort encountered two early postoperative fractures and was subsequently abandoned. Although fully coated stems provide a greater surface area for interface bonding, it has been suggested that proximal coating may reduce stress shielding. At present, this is an unresolved controversy, with excellent long-term results also seen with partially coated stems (16). No difference in outcome has been seen in the short to medium term in a randomised-controlled trial comparing partial and fully coated prostheses (17). Functional adaptation is to be expected, but the distinction between this accepted phenomenon and dysfunctional adaptation remains unclear.

CUP DESIGN

Although the excellent results of HA-coated stems have been reproduced in other studies (16), the choice of cup is evidently more critical. Results of threaded cups without HA coating have been disappointing, but coating appears to dramatically improve these results. Manley *et al.* reported poorer results with the HA-coated press fit cup than porous-coated or threaded cups18. In our series, the sequential change of cups has allowed us to compare different patterns of failure between cup designs. Initially, a cemented acetabular component was used in all cases (Furlong CCI, fig. 2) with a HA-coated threaded cup (Furlong, fig. 3) introduced in 1989. The press-fit HA-coated cup (Furlong CSF, fig. 4) was introduced in 1991. Two cases using this cup are included at the end of this series. We continued using the threaded cup until 1993. No intraoperative acetabular fractures have been encountered, but we have had one late acetabular fracture following significant trauma.

Of the original cemented cups five have been revised. Although this is a similar proportion to the four revisions for aseptic loosening with fibrous interposition between the component and bone in the threaded cup group, a further 25% of the

Acetabular	No	Femoral	No
Wear (cemented)	0	Traumatic Loosening	1
Wear (threaded)	4	Aseptic Loosening	0
Aseptic Loosening(cemented)	5	Deep Infection	3*
Aseptic Loosening(threaded)	4	Trunion fracture	1
Deep Infection	3*		

* 3 patients had both components removed for deep infection.

Table 2 – Revisions.

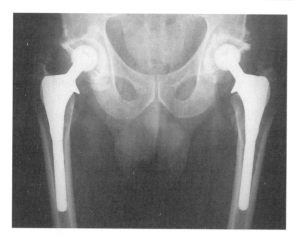

Figure 2 – Bilateral JRI hips with cemented cups 14 years postoperatively.

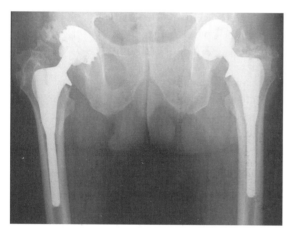

Figure 3 – Bilateral JRI hips with threaded cups 11 years postoperatively. Note the increased wear on the left-hand side, which is in a suboptimal position.

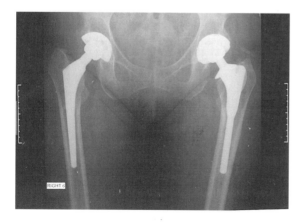

Figure 4 – Left hip JRI with CSF cup. Right hip Osteonics.

cemented cups show radiological signs of loosening, but none requires revision on clinical grounds. Although the cemented cups have shown evidence of loosening and osteolysis in the long term, they have shown less wear than the threaded cups. Four revisions have been due to worn liners, and many more show marked signs of eccentric polyethylene wear. No other component is awaiting revision, and all HA-coated components are well bonded.

We suspect the increased wear seen in the threaded cup group may be due in part to the design of the parallel threaded cup, which makes insertion and correct cup positioning difficult, and risks stripping the HA coating at the tip of the threads during implantation. The 32mm head is also known to increase polyethylene wear (19), although this was constant in both groups. Other authors have suggested that an absence of pain following total hip arthroplasty using HA-coated implants may cause greater polyethylene wear as a result of greater activity (14).

Since 1993, we have routinely used a press fit CSF cup. Although it is beyond the scope of this chapter to discuss cases at less than ten years, we have not experienced the early failures described in other studies. We have also not encountered the phenomenon of "backside wear" with these cups. At 5-9 years, we have had no cases of aseptic loosening, which suggests the failure described by Manley *et al.* (18) is due to prosthesis design rather than failure of HA coatings to withstand the tensile stresses between the bone and the cup. In fact, in the majority of cases, we have not found it necessary to augment the press-fit cups with screws. This allows minor adjustments of the cup in order to achieve the most congruent position.

Hydroxyapatite is an osteotrophic material that encourages both endosteal and implant ossification. Formation of bridging trabeculae between the stem and the bone via mechanical and chemical bonding is widely seen and described (20). This ensures mineralised continuity between implant and bone, with subsequent absorption of micromovement by the trabeculae. Two thirds of the HA coating is absorbed, and twenty five percent of this is replaced by bone with the absence of a fibrous membrane at the interface, which results in less micromotion and subsequently, less loosening (21). This biological fixation is far stronger than cemented or any other uncemented technique and approaches the strength of cortical bone (22). This correlates well with the long-term results above, where no atraumatic aseptic loosening of the stem has occurred within 16 years.

The issue of HA debris has been raised, with possible concern about HA degradation products causing third body wear. Results are controversial and have depended on whether specimens are retrieved at autopsy or revision (23, 24). HA dissolution and delamination has been found in revision cases. The same is not true of autopsy cases, where bone formation is seen without a fibrous interface. It may be that damage at retrieval led to the findings in the revision cases. Particle separation and abrasive wear in hot pressed implants with thick coarse coatings has been described (25). It is arguable that third body wear may be less in HA hips as compared to porous-coated and cemented ones (26). Although many of our cases showed bony resorption at the calcar, this was not seen elsewhere. Unlike other forms of fixation, the intimate bone-prosthesis bond prevents passage of particulate debris at the bone implant interface.

CONCLUSION

A previously published study on the first 100 cases (13) showed no cases of aseptic loosening at 9-12 years. With results now at up to 16 years, the only case of femoral loosening followed major trauma. Clinical results remain excellent. We place no lifestyle limitations on our patients. HA-coated hip replacements show exceptionally reliable bonding with a wide range of different designs of implant, regardless of shape, size or extent of coating. This is in contrast to cemented hip replacements, in which strikingly different results have been observed with minor modifications in design or cementing technique. The behaviour and results of HA-coated implants are quite different to uncoated ones and should not be placed together in an "uncemented" bracket. In our series, the long-term results are outstanding, and we would challenge the best of cemented replacements to approach within 5% or our long-term survival rate. With the use of HA-coated hip implants, the problem of aseptic loosening appears to be nearing resolution.

Reference List

1. Trends & Dynamics in Global Orthopaedics: US & European Hip Implants. Ref SZME0011. Datamonitor, April 2000.

2. Oishi CS, Walker RH, Colwell CW (1994) The femoral component in total hip arthroplasty: six to eight year follow up of one hundred consecutive patients after use of third generation cementing technique. *JBJS* 76-A (7):1330-6.

3. Collis DK (1984) Cemented total hip replacement in patients who are less than fifty years old. *JBJS* 66-A (3):353-9.

4. Engh CA, Culpepper WJ, Engh CA (1997) Long term results of use of the anatomic medullary locking prosthesis in total hip arthroplasty. *JBJS* 79-A (2):177-84.

5. Butler-Manuel PA, James SE, Shepperd JA (1992) Pelvic underpinning: eight years' experience. *JBJS* 74-B(1):74-7.

6. Geesink R (2002) Osteoconductive Coatings for Total Joint Arthroplasty. *CORR* 395:53-65.

7. De Groot K, Geesink R, Klein CP (1987) Plasma sprayed coatings of hydroxylapatite. *J. Biomed. Mater. Res.* 21:1375-81.

8. D'Aubigne RM, Postel M (1954) Functional results of hip arthroplasty with acrylic prosthesis. *JBJS* 36-A (3): 451-75.

9. Gruen TA, McNeice GM, Amstutz HC (1979) "Modes of Failure" of cemented stem-type femoral components. *CORR* 141:17-27.

10. DeLee JG, Charnley J (1976) Radiological demarcation of cemented sockets in total hip replacement. *CORR* 121:20-32.

11. Mont MA, Maar DC, Krackow KA (1992) Hoop stress fractures of the proximal femur during hip arthroplasty. *JBJS* 74-B:257-60.

12. Schwartz JT, Mayer JG, Engh CA (1989) Femoral fracture during non-cemented total hip arthroplasty. *JBJS* 71-A (8):1135-42.

13. McNally SA, Shepperd JA, Mann CV (2000) The results at nine to twelve years of the use of a hydroxyapatite coated femoral stem. *JBJS* 82-B (3):378-82.

14. Geesink RGT, Hoefnagels NH (1995) Six-year result of hydroxyapatite-coated hip replacement. *JBJS* 77-B (4): 534-47.

15. Karrholm J, Malchau H, Snorrason F et al. (1994) Micromotion of femoral stems in total hip arthroplasty. A randomized study of cemented, hydroxyapatite-coated, and porous-coated stems with roentgen stereophotogrammetric analysis. *JBJS* 76-A:1692-705.

16. D'Antonio J et al. (2001) Hydroxyapatite Femoral Stems for Total Hip Arthroplasty. *CORR* 393:101-11.

17. Santori FS, Ghera S, Moriconi A et al. (2000) Results of the anatomic cementless prosthesis with different types of hydroxyapatite coating. *Orthopedics* 24(12): 1147-50.

18. Manley MT, Capello WN, D'Antonio JA *et al.* (1999) Fixation of Acetabular cups without cement in total hip arthroplasty. *JBJS* 80-A (8): 1175-85.

19. Livermore J, Ilstrup D, Morrey B *et al.* (1990) Effect of femoral head size on wear of the polyethylene acetabular component. *JBJS* 72-B(4):518-28.

20. Engh CA, Bobyn JD: Porous-coated hip replacement: The factors governing bone ingrowth, stress shielding, and clinical results. *J. Bone Joint Surg. Br.* 69:45-55.

21. Søballe K, Hansen ES, Brockstedt-Rasmussen H *et al.* (1993) Hydroxyapatite coating converts fibrous tissue to bone around loaded implants. *JBJS* 75-B (2):270-8.

22. Geesink RGT, DeGroot K, Klein CP (1988) Bonding of bone to apatite-coated implants. *JBJS* 70-B(1):17-22.

23. Bloebaum RD, Beeks D, Dorr LD *et al* (1994) Complications with hydroxyapatite particulate separation in total hip arthroplasty. *CORR* 298:19-26.

24. Jaffe WL, Scott DF (1996) Total Hip Arthroplasty with hydroxyapatite-coated prostheses. *JBJS* 78-A(12): 1918-34.

25. Morscher EW, Hefti A, Aebi U (1998) Severe osteolysis after third body wear due to hydroxyapatite particles from acetabular cup coating. *JBJS* 80-B(2):267-72.

26. Bauer T, Taylor SK, Jiang M *et al.* (1994) An indirect comparison of third-body wear in retrieved hydroxyapatite-coated, porous, and cemented femoral components. *Clin. Orthop.* 298:11-8.

2 Corail Stem Long Term Results Based upon the 15-Year Artro Group Experience

Jean-Pierre Vidalain, MD

INTRODUCTION

It has been 15 years since Corail prostheses were first implanted. The early clinical and radiographic results provided convincing evidence of the value of the HA-induced bond between living host bone and the inert device (1). During that period, we have performed 2,956 primary total hip arthroplasties using HA-coated components.

This large series provides valuable information and instruction (2, 3, 4). First, we shall present statistical and demographic data, followed by our clinical and radiological results, with particular emphasis on the most prominent facts. Lastly, survivorship curves will be presented, leading to the conclusion that Corail is a highly dependable hip system.

MATERIALS AND METHODS

Components

On the femoral side, the standard Corail stem has been used in all cases (2,956).

The Corail stem is made of forged titanium alloy (TiAl6V4). It is straight, with a quadrangular cross-section. The proximal part is flared in the sagittal and the coronal planes to provide three-dimensional stabilization in the metaphyseal area. The distal portion has a taper in order to produce a stiffness gradient and to avoid medullary canal blocking. Macrotextural features (horizontal and vertical grooves) enhance primary mechanical stability, which may be further augmented by the use of an optional collar. The HA coating is applied to the entire stem in order to prevent the release of

metal ions, to provide for maximum osseointegration at the interface, and to prevent the interposition of a fibrous membrane around the distal portion of the stem. The coating parameters are the same for all the different prosthetic components. Hydroxyapatite powder is applied according to an atmospheric plasma spray process. The thickness of the ceramic layer is 150 microns.

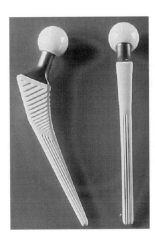

Figure 1 – The standard CORAIL stem.

On the acetabular side, operators have chosen HA-coated components (2,308) for the large majority of patients (Table 1). The titanium alloy Tropic cup is hemispherical. Primary stability is ensured by a self-tapping equatorial thread. For additional fixation, radial screws may be inserted. A polar hole allows in-situ grafting. In the hemispherical Atoll cup stability comes from impacting the over-sized shell into the acetabulum to achieve a press-fit. The two cups are fully HA-coated, and take concentric PE liners with or without an extended lip around half the liner circumference.

Femur	Standard Corail Stem		2,956
Acetabulum (Cementless)	HA-coated Press-Fit : Atoll Screwed : Tropic	256 2,052	
			2,308
	NON HA-coated Press-Fit : Screwed : Others :	70 105 23	
			198
Acetabulum (Cemented)		388	
NR		62	
			450

Table 1 – Implanted Prosthetic components.

Patients

We implanted 2,956 CORAIL prostheses (2,580 patients) between September 1986 and December 2000. Excluding patients deceased (116 = 3.9%) or lost to follow-up (65 = 2.1%), this leaves over 2,775 cases available for analysis (mean follow-up, 54 months). Two hundred forty-three cases have more than 10-year follow-up.

As far as demographics is concerned, the age distribution of patients shows a perfect Gauss curve, indicating the wide range of options offered by the Corail femoral stem, which can be used in very young to very old patients (mean age 66.7 years, range 17-101).

Sex distribution (male, 49.8%) or operated side prevalence (right, 65%) do not need to be commented on. In our activity, over 70% of implanted patients are operated on for primary osteoarthritis of the hip; however, HA-coated stems also give very good results in fractures of the femoral neck in the elderly (7%) in whom rapid and minimally aggressive surgery is desirable. Other diagnosis (necrosis 7%, dysplasia 4%, CDH 1%, RA 1%) represent a marginal section.

All the patients were examined at the third and twelfth month, then every 2 years. All clinical and radiological data were stored and analyzed through our computerized hip database DPS (DePuy Hip Soft).

RESULTS

Clinical Findings (Global Series N = 2,775)

The complication rate is not very high (7.3%) and complications (202) are not specific to hydroxyapatite coating (intra-operative complications 1.2%, early complications, 3.1%, late complications, 3.0%) (Table 2).

Intra-operative complications n : 34 = 1.2%	
Cracks	21 = 0.7%
Fractures	11 = 0.4%
Perforations	2 = 0.1%
Early complications n : 86 = 3.1%	
DVT	17 = 0.6%
PE	2 = 0.1%
Hematoma	15 = 0.5%
Sepsis	4 = 0.2%
Dislocations	42 = 1.4%
Nerve palsy	6 = 0.3%
Late complications n : 82 = 3.0%	
Ectopic bone	25 = 0.9%
Pain	9 = 0.3%
Revisions	48 = 1.8%

Table 2 – Distribution of the different complications.

It is interesting to note the low rate of ectopic ossifications, and we do point out the absence of interface failure, either mechanical or biological. We have had no aseptic loosening to this date.

Finally, we shall refer to 48 implant removals, 16 stems and 32 cups for different reasons, none of them being related neither to a failure of the biological fixation nor to a HA induced problem. Among the 16 Corail stems revised (0.5%), a femoral shaft fracture destabilized the prosthetic component in 9 cases, 5 deep infections needed a one stage re-implantation, and 2 head breakages damaged the Morse cone of the stem. On the acetabular side, 32 cups (1%) were revised, 24 non HA-coated components, where the migration occurred very soon during the first post-operative years. Only 8 HA-coated shells (2 Tropic cups and 6 Atoll cups), have been changed for excessive wear (7 cases) and major lysis (14 cases).

Functional Results

Functional results have been rated as excellent using the Postel Merle d'Aubigné or Harris hip scores. According to the PMA hip scale, the mean pre-op score was 11.29. It was 17.20 at the last control (Table 3). 86.3% of the arthroplasties were totally pain-free, and 56.4% of the hips were considered as strictly normal (PMA score 18), no pain, no limp, normal range of motion (Table 4).

	PRE-OP%			Last Control%	
	PMA	HHS	PMA	HHS	PMA	HHS
Excellent	18	>=98	0	1	56	59
Good	>= 15	>=80	2	3	34	30
Fair	>= 12	>=60	13	11	9	10
Poor	<12	<60	85	85	1	1
Mean			11.29	59.3	7.2	95.7

Table 3 – Functional results PMA/HHS score.

PMA score	%
Pain = 6	86
Motion = 6	90
Activity = 6	65
Global = 18	56.4

Table 4 – Functional evaluation.

In 371 cases (13.7%), patients complained of very slight uncharacteristic hip pain unrelated to walking. We report 9 patients suffering from groin pain related to a psoas tendinopathy. No patients experienced thigh pain.

Radiological Findings (More than 10-y FU Series : N = 243)

The radiological analysis, especially of the oldest series with a follow-up over 10 years, provides some certainties for short term and intermediate term. However, the discussion is still open concerning long term questions. All the radiological files of this series were evaluated by two independent surgeons.

HA advantages for the early post-operative period are now well established. 70.4% of the patients show radiological evidences of bone-ingrowth. The different aspects of this new-bone formation have been described in a previous publication (5); however, we can recall the X-ray criteria of implant osteointegration, such as, newly formed trabecular bone connecting the endosteal bone to the implant, orientation of bone along strength distribution lines (tensile and compression strengths), organization of the neo-osteogenesis along the length of the implant depending on the prosthetic surrounding (cancellous or cortical) and on the distance between the endosteal bone and the implant, and lack of periprosthetic radiolucent lines.

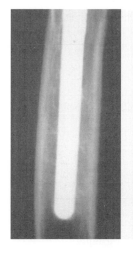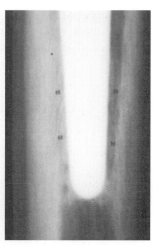

Figure 2 – Osteointegration of a fully HA-coated stem. Note bone bridges and the trabecular newly formed bone at the tip of the prosthesis.

With regard to the lack of periprosthetic radiolucent lines, with a Corail stem, these signs are slightly seen in the metaphyseal area, but neo-osteogenesis is clearly evident in zones 3, 4 (89%; 4A = 82%,4B = 77%) and 5, coming from one or two cortices, but the distal tip of the implant remains free in the medullary canal. New-bone formation in this zone never takes on the radiological aspect of the pedestal described by Engh. In fact, this new bone is never dense, but always trabecular, looking like the sails of a sail boat.

On the pelvic side the absence of any radiolucent lines is the proof of close bone-bonding. This phenomenon must be considered a healing process (such as fracture consolidation). Several scintiscans confirm the physiological and non-evolutive character of bonding osteogenesis on both sides:

the femoral site is vital immediately after surgery, and scintigraphic activity is intense as early as the 8th day. This activity is seen on all implant zones but is concentrated in zone 1 (greater trochanter) and zone 4 (distal part). Finally, the process decreases quickly, as scintigraphies become old by the end of the first year. Five-year images are purely physiological.

During the intermediate period, the mechanical features of the implants most likely play the main role. The overall design has already provided primary stability which is needed for a successful osteointegration. Macro and microstructures must secure secondary and final stability even in case of more or less coating resorption.

In the series (243 cases) which has a follow-up over the tenth year, we can note that the rate of subsidence of the femoral component is very low (Table 5).

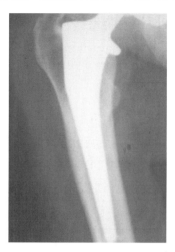

Figure 3 – Femoral remodeling 10 years after implantation of a CORAIL stem : aside from slight resorption of the calcar, note the physiological remodeling of the surrounding bone.

Migration	Collar	Collarless	N:243	%
0mm	136	88	224	92.1
< 2mm	0	12	12	4.9
> 2mm-< 5mm	2	4	6	2.5
> 5mm	0	1	1	0.4
Total	2	17	19	7.8%

Table 5 – Corail stem stability.

All the implants that migrated (19/243 = 7.8%) did so during the first 3 months, then stabilized (migration < 2mm in 4.9% of the cases, > 5mm in 0.4%). The prostheses incorporating a collar appear to be more stable (2/19).

On the acetabular side, using a traditional radiological method, we were not able to establish a significant difference in terms of stability between the screwed cup Tropic and the press-fit component Atoll.

Bone remodeling seems to be contained within physiological limits, and conventional X -Ray is the usual technique used to estimate structural modifications of the recipient site.

There were no lucencies in any of the zones. This finding was remarkable, especially in zone 1, which is subject to tensile stress. While this absence of lucencies does not mean that the HA coating will last forever, it certainly differs from the pattern observed with all the other cementless

implants that do not have a HA coating. However, reactive lines were noticed in few cases in zone 1. The meaning of such reaction is not well understood.

There were virtually no cases of isolated cortical hypertrophy, even where the stem was in varus with cortical impingement at the stem tip. Calcar reshaping is very common (45% at 10 years). The pattern was cortical thinning and blunting of bone edges. Trochanteric osteopenia can be seen in very few files, so far.

In all our series, we have only 0.4% cases of major stress-shielding (Table 6) according to Ch. Engh's criteria (6). Females are involved in 90% of these cases due to several risk factors: femoral neck fracture, pre-op osteopenia, wide femoral canal, *etc.*

N = 243 > 10-Y FU		
Isolated calcar remodeling	109	44.8%
Stress-shielding		
Grade I	17	6.9%
Grade II	6	2.4%
Grade III	1	0.4%

Table 6 – Mechanical bone remodeling.

However, it is now well known that after arthroplasty, early modifications of bone structure are infraradiological. Among the different techniques currently used to quantify the variations of bone, biphotonic absorptiometry is today the most simple and reproducible.

We started in 1990 a remodeling DEXA evaluation of the surrounding bone after THA (7).

Nowadays, there is a general agreement on the reality of a significant bone loss after THA. This loss occurs early (third month), and is more important proximally, mainly in zone 7. This phenomenon is intense during the first year, then slows down. An equilibrium seems to be reached beyond the 5th year (Table 7).

	3 months	1 year	2 years	3 years	5 years
Zone 1	–11.04%	–12.37%	–12.64%	–13.22%	–12.37%
Zone 4	+ 6.45%	–3.04%	–1.94%	+2.97%	–8.66%
Zone 7	–21.90%	–40.76%	–42.46%	–42.99%	–49.49%

Table 7 – Average bone mineral density variation in a series of 42 patients.

We tried to establish a correlation with different factors: age, sex, implant size and femur morphology. In terms of sex, bone loss is always more important in the female group. This fact seems to suggest that osteoporosis might have a great influence in terms of remodeling.

We did not observe any significant variation according to the patient ages during the first years after implantation. However at the 5th year evaluation, we noticed, notably in area 7, a bone loss in proportion of the patient age (Table 8).

Age	Zone 1	Zone 4	Zone 7
40-50	– 0.25	+ 0.25	– 0.35
50-60	– 0.12	+ 0.05	– 1.40
60-70	– 0.20	– 0.05	– 1.71
70-80	– 0.30	– 0.02	– 2.10
80-90	– 0.32	+ 0.27	– 2.45

Table 8 – 5th year bone loss (g/cm^2) according to patient ages.

We were not able to appreciate the preventive role of the collar support in the remodeling of the calcar region. Bone loss was more or less identical in both groups (collar or collarless) without any statistical signification.

The mechanical features of the implant, and femoral morphology, seem to play a major role. Stiffness depends on the material and on the size of the implant. With such a device, stiffness is mainly important at the metaphyseal level. In the upper part of the femur, when the filling index is important, bone loss is constant and increases in proportion with the implant size (Table 9).

Stem size	10	11	12	13	14	15	16
Zone 1	–5%	–6%	–22%	–23%	–25%	–30%	–29%
Zone 7	–24%	–36%	–41%	–60%	–52%	–65%	–61%

Table 9 – Bone loss (%) in the metaphyseal area.

Aseptic loosening is probably the main question concerning the future of HA-coated implants. No revision has been performed on the femoral side for such a complication. However, PE wear is a reality (8, 9, 10, 11) and osteolysis a potential risk of destabilization (12, 13). In our oldest series, using the Livermore method (20), the mean linear wear is 1.2 mm at the 10th year, but we can note an abnormal wear (between 2 and 3 mm) in 13% of the cases.

Linear osteolysis, and limited granuloma have been observed in 20 cases in zones 1 and 7, and in 12 cases in zones 2 and 6. There is no sign of osteolysis in any zone in all the cases of regular wear. On the acetabular side, granuloma are rather extensive, especially in zone 2 (15 cases = 0.5%)

The original bone-implant link, without fibrous interposition, is probably a seal reducing fluid circulation, and therefore, preventing PE debris migration. We have never seen extensive osteolysis along the mid and distal parts of the stem. In cases of premature wear, we were not able to establish a correlation with different factors such as weight, patient activity, acetabular component orientation (4).

All in all, in this series we have never encountered any aseptic loosening of the femoral component. If we take as "end point" any failure of the biological fixation, the survival probability of the Corail prosthesis is 100% all along the follow-up. Usually, the end point reference is the exchange of the stem for any reason. Therefore, the overall survivorship rate is 98.3% (95% CI 97.2 to 99.5) at 10 years for the Corail stem, and 96.3% (95% CI 94.7 to 97.9) for the whole arthroplasty.

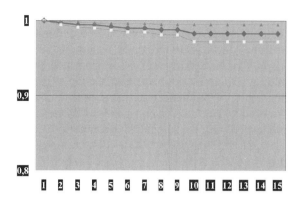

Figure 4 – Survival probability of the standard Corail stem (Confidence interval 95%) Patients "on file" at 10 y: 243 ; 11 y : 194 ; 12 y : 159 ; 13 y : 87 ; 14 y : 37.

DISCUSSION

It is now well established that hydroxyapatite is not toxic, does not produce inflammatory or allergic reactions, and is not carcinogenic (14, 15, 16, 17). Still, four problems remain unsolved: HA resorption and long-term stability, osteolysis that is occasionally observed, polyethylene wear and potential risk of granuloma, and difficulty removing an HA-coated stem, particularly when it is well ingrown.

Resorption of hydroxyapatite is more or less inescapable due to both chemical dissolution and cell degradation. However, the kinetics of this degradation process is influenced by a number of factors which are still not clearly understood, and consequently, are not well known (18, 19).

Cell degradation is followed by a bone formation process identical to the creeping substitution process that is seen in graft incorporation, and with time, sporadically, where hydroxyapatite coating has disappeared, the new bone is directly in contact with the metal of the implant, without any interposition of fibrous tissue (20). It is not established that the degradation scenario described through different post-mortem explanta occurs in the same way in younger patients. We can report that in all the revisions concerning traumatic periprosthetic fractures, the coating was still intact on the two-third distal parts. In cases of partial resorption, the degradation only concerned the metaphyseal area of the prosthesis. Today, we strongly believe that HA is not a temporary go-between, useful only in the initial period, but also that it encourages long

term fixation (20), and that the thickness of the coating (150μ) probably plays a significant role. We have never seen lucent lines that could suggest disruption between implant and bone (21, 22).

Osteolysis has been discussed in some outstanding publications (23, 24) which, in our opinion, are just anecdotal, as there is no evidence that these lytic phenomena are strictly associated with hydroxyapatite (10). As a matter of fact, granulomas observed include both hydroxyapatite crystals, and metal and polyethylene wear debris. On the contrary, we have had a number of cases where grains of hydroxyapatite were neither free nor responsible for lytic phenomena. Most of the time, these debris are being recycled and gradually incorporated into new bone. All our major cases of osteolysis are strictly correlated to excessive or/and accelerated PE wear. All linear osteolysis was confined to the proximal one-third of the stem ; no diaphyseal endosteal lysis was found. The quality of the bonding interface is now generally confirmed ; bioactive fixation is more an advantage than a drawback. The extensive HA coating of the stem seals the whole interface and blocks the migration of wear debris (25).

Are there free hydroxyapatite particles in the articular cavity that may cause third-body wear ? First, it should be remembered that delamination of an HA coating is essentially a technological problem that only occurs with very thick coatings (the thickness of our coating is well under critical values) or with coatings applied to inappropriate substrates, particularly PE.

With a highly reliable technology, this phenomenon is virtually non-existent (26). Polyethylene wear is not more significant with HA-coated implants than with any other type of replacement (27). The average annual wear curve of polyethylene cups that we presented during a SOFCOT meeting does not show that HA-coated implants are associated with significantly more rapid wear. In literature (9, 10, 13) reporting excessive wear with HA-coated components, we can always note other parameters playing a more significant role, *eg*, ball size (32mm), material (stainless steel), cup size (< 50mm) diameter.

In any case, crystals of calcium phosphate are, indeed, occasionally found within the surface of polyethylene liners. In some cases, we clearly see the incorporation of calcium phosphate in the bearing surface of the polyethylene liner. But, as Patrick Frayssinet pointed it out in his presentation during an EORS meeting, there is no evidence that these calcium phosphates are hydroxyapatite and that they originate from implant coatings. As a matter of fact, calcium phosphate inlays are found in the surface of almost all polyethylene liners, whether cups are cemented or cementless without hydroxyapatite.

What about revisions? Sixteen femoral stems have been revised. In most cases, the implant was loose as a result of a septic process or a fracture which had destabilized the interface. In 7 cases only did we revise a well ingrown implant, more particularly for breakage of a ceramic component with a badly damaged Morse cone. The eventual difficulties in removing a well-integrated, fully-coated implant are often a great source of concern. Extraction of the stem is always possible through a transfemoral approach. This is a well planned option that minimizes additional bone sacrifice and makes reconstruction of the femoral shaft around the new stem an easy procedure and almost routine.

The relationship between the extent of the coating, the extent of fixation, and the modifications of the femoral bone pattern after implantation is very controversial. However, we can recall that Huiskes (28) has shown, in a finite element model, that relative to a fully bonded stem, coating on the proximal one-third of the stem reduces the amount of resorption from 54% to 50% only. In addition, there is not a graduated load transfer, and stress concentration occurs at the edge of the coating. Material, shape and size of the femoral component are much more relevant factors than the percentage of the coated surface in term of remodeling (29). With the standard Corail stem, the periprosthetic bone metabolism seems to be contained within physiological limits.

CONCLUSIONS

In conclusion, this study continues to demonstrate that the benefits of HA should not be confined to an early but temporary role. Bioactive coatings may contribute to the durability of stability by significantly reducing osteolysis and the risk of delayed aseptic loosening.

In the short run, hydroxyapatite improves clinical results significantly in providing superior stability thanks to osseointegration. In the interme-

diate term, the mechanical characteristics of the implant will likely play a critical role, although it becomes more and more evident that the quality of load transfer is also dependent on the nature of the bond between the implant and the host site. In addition, a full coating does not increase the rate of proximal bone resorption in so far as the shape of the stem prevents distal blockages and harmonizes strain distribution on the bone with a progressive rigidity gradient.

One can assume in the long run that preservation of long-term stability and excellent bone trophicity will further increase the durability of the implant. Let us hope that the 98.3% survival rate of the Corail femoral stem will be maintained during the next decade.

Reference List

1. Vidalain JP *et al.* (1993) The Corail Prosthesis. 5-year experience of the Artro Group. *Acta Orthop. Belg.* 59:165-9.

2. Vidalain JP *et al.* (1997) HA Coating : Ten-year experience with the Corail system in primary THA. *Acta Orthop. Belg.* 63:93-5.

3. Vidalain JP *et al.* (1999) The Corail system in primary THA: results, lessons and comments from the series performed by the ARTRO Group (12-year experience). *Eur. J. Orthop. Surg. Traumatol.* Vol 9, No. 2:87-90.

4. Vidalain JP *et al.* (2001) Long Term Results with a Fully-HA-coated Prosthesis (15-year Experience). Key Engeneering Materials. Vols 192-195:1021-4.

5. Vidalain JP *et al.* (1994) The Corail THR System in Primary Hip Arthroplasty. Seven-year Experience of the Artro Group. Cahiers d'Enseignement de la SOFCOT, No. 51, Hydroxyapatite Coated Hip and Knee Arthroplasty.

6. Engh CA, Bobyn JD (1988) The influence of stem size and Extent of Porous Coating on Femoral Bone Resorption after Primary Cementless Hip Arthroplasty. *Clin. Orthop.* 231:7-28.

7. Vidalain JP *et al.* (1994) Densitometry in the analysis of Femoral Remodeling Following the Implantation of an HA-Coated Prosthesis. Cahiers d'Enseignement de la SOFCOT, No. 51, Hydroxyapatite Coated Hip and Knee Arthroplasty.

8. Charnley J, Halley DK (1975) Rate of wear in total Hip Replacement. *Clin. Orthop.* 112:170-9.

9. Fisher J (1994) Wear of UHMWPE in Total Artificial Joints. *Current Orthopaedics* 8:164-5.

10. Howling GI, Barnett PI, Tipper JL, Stone MH, Fisher J, Ingham E (2001) Quantitative characterization of polyethylene debris isolated from periprosthetic tissue in early failure knee implants and early and late failure Charnley hip implants. *J. Biomed. Mater. Res.* 58:415-20.

11. Livermore J, Ilstrup D, Morrey B (1990) Effect of Femoral Head Size on Wear of the Polyethylene Acetabular Component. *J. Bone Joint Surg. Am.* 72A:518-28.

12. Rokkum M, Reigstad A. Total Hip Replacement With an Entirely Hydroxyapatite-Coated Prosthesis. *J. Arthroplasty* Vol. 14, No. 6, 199.

13. Rokkum M, Brandt M, Bye K, Hetland KR, Waage S, Reigstad A (1999) Polyethylene wear, osteolysis and acetabular loosening with an HA-coated hip prosthesis. A follow-up of 94 consecutive arthroplasties. *J. Bone Joint Surg. Br.* 81 B:582-9.

14. Casas J, Cots M, Rodriguez J (1999) Hyroxyapatite coated Femoral Component. Surgical Technology International VII. 369-376. Universal Medical Press Inc.

15. Donnely WJ, Freeman MAR, Scott G (1998) Hydroxyapatite Coating. The Adult Hip:1041-1046. Lippincott-Raven.

16. Frayssinet P, Machenaud A, Vidalain JP, Cartillier JC, Conte P, Bonnevialle P (1994) Interface Membranes: Intersest of Orthopaedic Materials which do not Provoke their Formation. Cahiers d'Enseignement de la SOFCOT, No. 51, Hydroxyapatite Coated Hip and Knee Arthroplasty.

17. Geesink RGT (2002) Osteoconductive Coatings for Total Joint Arthroplasty. *Clin. Orthop.* 395:53-65.

18. Frayssinet P, Hardy D, Hanker JS, Giammara BL (1995) Natural history of bone response to hydroxyapatite coated hip prostheses implanted in human. *Cells and Materials,* Vol. 5, No. 2.

19. Hardy D, Frayssinet P, Bonel G *et al.* (1994) Two-year outcome of hydroxyapatite-coated prostheses: two femoral prostheses retrieved at autopsy. *Acta Orthop. Scand.* 65:253-7.

20. Søballe K, Hansen S, Rasmussen HB, Jorgensen PH, Bünger C (1992) Tissue ingrowth into Titanium and Hydroxyapatie-Coated Implants during Stable and Unstable Mechanical Conditions. *J. Orthop. Res.* Vol. 10, No. 2.

21. Havelin L, Espehaug B, Vollset S, Engesaeter L (1995) Early aseptic loosening of uncemented femoral component in primary total hip replacement. A review based on the Norvegian Arthroplasty Register. *J. Bone Joint Surg. Br.* 77B:11-7.

22. Havelin L, Engesaeter L (1997) Results of 2054 primary uncemented hydroxyapatite coated hip prostheses. *J. Bone Joint Surg. Br.* 79B:Supp II.

23. Bloebaum RD, Beeks D, Dorr LD *et al.* (1994) Complications with hydroxyapatite particulate separation in total hip arthroplasty. *Clin. Orthop.* 298:19-26.

24. Bloebaum RD, Dupont JA (1993) Osteolysis from a press-fit hydroxy-apatite-coated implant: a case study. *J. Arthroplasty* No. 8.

25. Frayssinet P, Hardy D, Tourenne F, Rouquet N, Delincé P, Bonel G (1994) Osseointegration of Plasma Sprayed HA-coated Hip Implants In Humans. Cahiers d'Enseignement de la SOFCOT, No. 51, Hydroxyapatite Coated Hip and Knee Arthroplasty.

26. Bonel G, Tourenne F, Rouquet N, Frayssinet P (1994) Hydroxyapatite and Plasma Spraying. Cahiers d'Enseignement de la SOFCOT, No. 51, Hydroxyapatite Coated Hip and Knee Arthroplasty.

27. McKellop H, Shen FW, Lu B, Cambell P, Salovey R (2000) Effect of sterelization method and other modifications on the wear resistance of acetabular cups made of UHMWPE. A hip-simulator study. *J. Bone Joint Surg. Am.* 82-A:1708-25.

28. Huiskes R, Weinans H (1994) Biomechanical Aspects of Hydroxyapatite Coatings on Femoral Hip Prostheses. Cahiers d'Enseignement de la SOFCOT, No. 51, Hydroxyapatite Coated Hip and Knee Arthroplasty.

29. Head WC, Bauk DJ, Emerson RH (1995) Titanium as the material of choice for cementless femoral components in Total Hip Arthroplasty. *Clin. Orthop.* 311:85-90.

3 Long-term Survivorship Analysis of Hydroxyapatite-Coated Hips

Based upon a 15-Year Clinical Experience with Three Different Models of HA-Coated Omnifit Stems

Jean-Alain Epinette, MD and Michael T. Manley, PhD

"The question today is not whether THR is working. The question of today is how various THRs compare with each other."

Henrik Malchau

INTRODUCTION

Survivorship analysis has become one of the most reliable tools as far as long term outcome of implants is concerned (1-3). With reference to the works of the Scandinavian registers (4-6), the main goals of this method of analysis are first to report an updated epidemiological analysis of hip replacement, second to identify risk factors for failures leading to revision procedures, and finally, to describe the importance of continual improvement of surgical technique by independent risk factor analysis.

As a contribution to the evaluation of the long-term outcome of hydroxyapatite (HA)-coated hips, the present study reports on a series of 2,199 cases where HA stems were used in primary surgery and that were followed up from 1987 to 2002. The HA stems used were the Omnifit-HA stem, and two slightly modified HA Omnifit stems, the Omniflex-HA, and the HA Omnifit FC. All femoral stems were manufactured by Osteonics Corp., Allendale, NJ.

The overall cumulative survival rates of the HA stems were collected, and the results of the different designs were compared. The analysis of modes of failures according to various "end points" relating to the different models proved interesting, as did the comparative results from specific cohorts with respect to different parameters and patient-related variables.

MATERIALS & METHODS

The HA-coated Stems

The three stems used were successively the HA-Omnifit (fig. 1a), then the HA Omniflex, and the HA Omnifit FC (Stryker-Osteonics, Allendale, USA) (fig. 1b).

The Omnifit femoral prosthesis used had a dense, 50-micron thick surface treatment of HA, with the pure, highly crystalline HA applied circumferentially to the proximal one-third of the stem. The surface of the implant was a grit-blasted, roughened, collarless straight titanium alloy implant with normalization steps on the anterior and posterior surfaces. The proximal third is coated with HA applied by a plasma-spray technique. The HA coating was 50 microns thick (range 45-65 microns) and fully dense (porosity < 20%). The content of HA after spraying was greater than or equal to 95%, the crystalline phase of HA after spraying was greater than or equal to 70%, the tensile bond strength was greater than or equal to 65MPa, and the fatigue life was greater than 10^7 cycles at 8.3MPa.

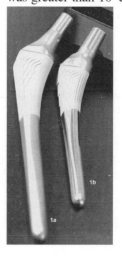

Figure 1 – a) HA Omnifit Stem; b) HA Omnifit FC.

The HA Omniflex stem has an identical proximal HA coating with similar characteristics, and differs from the Omnifit by the distal geometry of the stem (fig. 2). Distally the stem has a tip ranging between 10mm and 22mm that can be trimmed to the exact shape of the bone shaft in order to fill it completely, but without producing a stable bond with the host bone at this level.

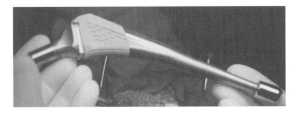

Figure 2 – HA Omniflex.

The HA Omnifit FC stem was approximately 2.5 cm shorter than the other stem designs, was non modular, and was expected to allow for increased flexibility over the current Omnifit design due to the incorporation of distal flutes. In general, this stem had the same proximal geometry as the others, but offered enhanced augmentations on the lateral and medial surfaces (grooves). The HA Omnifit FC stem incorporated a plasma-sprayed coating on a grit-blasted titanium substrate; this was similar to the current Omnifit design. The stem was distally polished to discourage distal bone ingrowth and/or fixation.

The Series

From June 1987 to February 2001, 2,199 primary hip replacements in 1,821 patients were performed as a consecutive series by one of us (JAE) at the Bruay Clinic in France. With respect to the type of stem, HA Omnifit stems (48.5%) were the predominantly implanted stem from 1987 until 1995 (1,066); 114 HA Omniflex stems (5.2%) were used during two years, 1991 and 1992. Use of the Omnifit FC stem began in 1992 and became a routine procedure from 1994 until 2001, with 1,019 cases implanted (46.3%). From 1987 until 1989, all stems were matched with the titanium, plasma-sprayed Arc 2f acetabular cup, then the HA-coated Arc 2f from was used from 1990 to date in almost all cases (98.8%) with the exception of 26 cups from various designs, including 4 bipolar implants and 10 HA press-fit cups. Poly-

ethylene (PE) bearings were used in 1,640 cases (74.6%), ceramic on ceramic (C/C) bearings (also referred to as alumina/alumina) in 544 hips (24.7%), and Crossfire PE bearings were used in the remaining 15 cases (0.7%). A head diameter of 32 mm was used in the very first cases in 1987 and 1988, then later on when C/C bearings were used. All other hips received a 28mm head. The choice for the various implants of the current study was dictated solely by an expected improvement in the design of the devices, and the broad indications for the use of HA-coated implants (no limitation due to age, aetiology, or shape of the medullary canal). Only poor bone quality with unacceptable primary fixation at the time of the trial led to implantation of a cemented component; this occurred in less than 5% of the cases.

Methods

The clinical course of each patient was evaluated preoperatively, early postoperatively (five to ten weeks), at six months, one year, and yearly thereafter. The entire study was carried out at the CRDA (Center of Research and Documentation of Arthroplasty) located in Bruay, France. At the various post-implantation follow-up periods, those patients able to travel to the clinic received clinical and radiographic review. Those unable to attend because of advanced age or a disability unrelated to the operated hip were evaluated by telephone interview for pain, function, and the retention of their implants. All clinical data and radiological images were stored for both retrieval and analysis in a computerized hip database, (OrthoWave, ARIA, Bruay, France). Any visible change of the component was measured on sequential radiographs.

Using Kaplan-Meier methodology (7) to evaluate survivorship, we calculated the cumulative survivorship rate for the HA-coated stems at 15 years follow-up using both revision for aseptic loosening and revision for any cause as the two survivorship endpoints. The survivorship study analysis started with a total number of 2,199 hips and stopped at 12 years with 66 patients "at risk" at that follow-up time; after that point in time, the number of cases under 30 did not allow for statistically significant tests. On all survival diagrams, the 95% confidence interval is indicated, and upper/lower survival rates corresponding to the confidence interval of 0.05 were calculated. The standard error increases with a decreasing number of prostheses at risk. None of the curves are depicted when there are less than 30 hips remaining at risk.

The StatWave statistical module of OrthoWave allows a comparison of survival rates between two cohorts based upon the same type of endpoint. In such a case, statistical tests could be displayed for addressing this comparison, including p value, through two tests, Mantel-Haenszel and Log rank (chi square). Naturally, isolated acetabular failures with retention of the stem at reoperation were excluded from the current study.

According to the Kaplan and Meier statistical procedures, material patient-related factors and implant-related factors were analyzed by estimation of the survival function for the implants depending on age, gender, aetiology and type of implant (7). Specific interest was paid to reoperations and revisions. We followed the policy described by the authors of the Swedish register, *reoperation* describes "any new hip operation on a patient who has previously undergone total hip replacement", while *revision* involves "exchange or removal of one or both components. Exchange of line or head component is not considered as a revision (4)".

RESULTS

Demographics

With respect to demographics, the average age was 67 years (18-91 years). Four cohorts were defined according to age: less than 40 years in 79 hips (3.6%), between 40 and 59 years in 490 hips (22.3%), between 60 and 79 years in 1446 hips (65.8%), and over 80 years in 184 hips (8.4%). Of the total population receiving implants, 730 were male (875 hips, 39.9%) and 1,091 were female (1,320 hips, 60.1%). The median value for BMI was 26.6 (SD: 4.84). Only 35% of patients were considered to be normal weight, while mild obesity was recorded in 43% of the patients, medium obesity in 21%, and severe obesity in the remaining 1%. Aetiology was mainly osteoarthritis in 84.8% of hips, followed by avascular necrosis of the femoral head in 11.7%, and rheumatoid arthritis in less than 2%. CDH was 1.1%, while no fresh fracture or revision cases were enrolled in the study.

As expected, cross correlation between age and aetiology demonstrated a significant difference, with an average age of 49.9 years for necrosis, *versus* 63 years for inflammatory lesions, and 67.4 years for osteoarthritis; this difference was significant for both ANOVA (p = .05) and Kruskal & Wallis test (p = .001). Similarly, osteoarthritis was found mainly in females, and necrosis in males (Chi square test, p = .001).

Of the 2,199 primary hips in the current study, 1,892 hips (86.04%) in 1,570 patients remained "on file" at a maximum follow-up, while 14 hips (0.64%) in 13 patients were lost to follow-up, and 203 patients (241 hips, 10.96%) died for reasons unrelated to the operated hip(s). Regarding revisions and failures, there were 3 retrievals in 3 patients for infection (0.14%), and 17 retrievals in 17 patients (0.77%) for secondary fractures; these were classified as revisions due to non hip-related reasons.

One patient experiencing a clinical failure did not undergo any revision due to poor health. Implant failure with retrieval of the two components occurred in 3 cases (in 3 patients; 0.14%), while in 11 cases (in 11 patients, 0.50%), femoral failure was isolated with retrieval of the stem. In 17 cases (in 17 patients; 0.77%), retrieval involved only the acetabular cup or bipolar with retention of the stem. These 17 cases were excluded from the stem survivorship analysis, which enrolled all retrievals for any cause (hip-related failure, infection and traumatic fracture) with "revision" as endpoint following the "Scandinavian register" policy, and all "failures" as endpoint, i.e., all hip related failures, having been reoperated or not.

Overall Results

When taking into account revision for any reason as endpoint, the overall cumulative survival rate, starting with 2,182 cases (i.e., 2,199 primaries less the 17 isolated acetabular failures that were excluded from the series) reaches at 5 years 98.10% ± 0.0067, then falls to 96.27% ± 0.0135 at 10 years, and finally, is 95.32% ±0.0135 at 12 years, with 66 hips remaining "at risk" at this follow-up period (fig. 3). Interestingly, when selecting only hip related failures as endpoint, revised or not, these cumulative rates were 98.98% ±0.0043 at 5 years, then 98.47% ±0.0080 at 10 years, and finally, 98.15 ±0.0080 at 12 years (fig. 4).

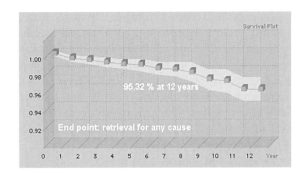

Figure 3 – Survival curve at 12-year follow-up period in primary arthroplasty of HA stems with "retrieval any cause" as endpoint. Confidence intervals are at 0.05.

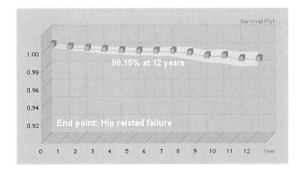

Figure 4 – Survival curve at 12-year follow-up period in primary arthroplasty of HA stems with "hip-related failure" as endpoint . Confidence intervals are at 0.05.

Of the 2,182 operated cases, 35 hips (1.60%) underwent revision for any cause. Of these retrievals, 15 revisions were assessed as hip-related failures, which represents a failure rate of 0.69%. These revision cases are as follows, and are also shown in Table 1.

There were three infected hips in three patients at 1, 2, and 6 years, with one infection per type of stem (Omnifit, Omniflex, and Omnifit FC). There were seventeen non hip related fractures in 17 patients, with 4 fractures before the second year, 6 between the third and fifth year, 4 between the sixth and ninth year and the remaining 3 fractures at the tenth year. Seven cases were HA Omnifit, nine were Omnifit FC and one was Omniflex. Four hips in four patients underwent revision for hip failure involving the two components, in two HA Omnifit stems, one Omniflex stem and one Omnifit FC. The reasons for revision were neurological disease leading to recurrent dislocations in two cases, a painful hip at 3 years, and a loosening at 7 years. These two latter cases were reoperated on in another clinic. Eleven hips in eleven patients were revised, with isolated retrieval of the stem in 5 HA Omnifit stems, 1 Omniflex, and 5 Omnifit FC. Follow-up periods were less than 2 years in 7 hips, 2 cases at 8 year, and 2 cases at 10 years. Interestingly, the five failures of the Omnifit FC stems were due to a fracture of the lesser trochanter that occurred in the early postoperative period for no apparent cause. Fracture leading to reoperation occurred similarly in one HA Omnifit and one HA Omniflex stem. The four remaining failure cases, all of the four being HA Omnifit, were due to recurrent dislocations in one case ; one subsidence at 3 years, one typical loosening at 5 years, and 1 painful hip in one patient treated for Paget lesions.

In summarizing the complications that led to revision, we noticed some interesting features. The infection rate leading to retrieval is low (0.14%). Non hip related fractures due to falls are commonly observed in older patients with generally poor health. In this particular group, the revision rate is 0.78% and is similar for each stem design. Recurrent dislocations were found in 0.14% of cases, and again can be seen as a common adverse effect

Reason for Revision	Whole series	Omnifit	Omniflex	Omnifit FC
Infection 3	(0.14%)	1 (0.09%)	1 (0.88%)	1 (0.10%)
Accidental fracture	17 (0.78%)	7 (0.66%)	1 (0.88%)	9 (0.89%)
Dislocation	3 (0.14%)	2 (0.19%)	0	1 (0.10%)
Loosening	2 (0.09%)	2 (0.19%)	0	0
Painful Hip	2 (0.09%)	1 (0.09%)	1 (0.88%)	0
Subsidence	1 (0.05%)	1 (0.09%)	0	0
Crack/Fracture	7 (0.32%)	1 (0.09%)	1 (0.88%)	5 (0.49%)
No. of retrievals	35 (1.60%)	15 (1.41%)	4 (3.54%)	16 (1.58%)

Table 1 – Types, numbers and percentages of reasons for revision of retrieved stems (isolated femoral or global revision), in the whole series (N:2182) and in each of type of stem: HA Omnifit (N:1066), HA Omniflex (N:113) and HA Omnifit FC (N:1013).

in the elderly, especially when neurological lesions are observed. There was no correlation with the type of stem used. Conversely, loosening, unexpected painful hips, or subsidence can be related to poor fixation and, finally, a failure of the HA interface. The overall failure rate of the HA fixation was 0.23% in 5 cases out of 2,182 hips. Interestingly, however, these complications occurred with the HA Omnifit stem in four cases, *versus* one case with the Omniflex (painful hip), and no fixation failures with the short stem HA Omnifit FC. The rate of fixation failure is then 0.36% in HA Omnifit (1,066 cases), 0.88% in Omniflex (113 cases), and 0% in Omnifit FC (1,013 cases).

However, the rate of unexpected fractures (0.32%) could be viewed as significant and involved mainly the Omnifit FC stem, with 5 cases of the 7 fractures of the overall series, leading to a rate of 0.45% for the FC stem, *versus* 0.09% for the HA Omnifit. (The low number of Omniflex stems yields a non significant percentage and cannot be taken into account.) Furthermore, a comparative survivorship analysis between the HA Omnifit and the Omnifit FC, while selecting any unexpected fracture that was not recorded as accidental, demonstrated a significant difference at p: 0.02, according to both Mantel-Haenszel and Logrank tests.

Finally, the overall rates of retrievals were different for the three models of HA stems, from 1.4% with the HA Omnifit up to 1.6% with the HA Omnifit FC, and 3.5% with the HA Omniflex stem. However, if we take into account the rate of aseptic loosening, i.e., loosening, pains or subsidence, the best results were provided by the Omnifit FC, with a 0% failure rate, up to 0.4% with the HA Omnifit stem, and 0.9% with the HA Omniflex. Conversely, poor results were recorded for the FC Stem with regard to non accidental fractures occurring early after the operation, reaching a high percentage of 0.5%, *versus* 0.1% with the HA Omnifit stem, and demonstrating a significant difference through the different tests at the expense of the FC stem.

The specific assessment of the various modes of failure allows a particular study enrolling all failures that would be related to a lack of fixation over years, such as painful hip, subsidence or radiological loosening (Table 2). These failures might define a specific analysis with "aseptic loosening" as endpoint.

As we recorded 5 aseptic loosening cases in the series, at 2,3,7,8 and 10 years, thus the cumulative

FU period	N "at risk"	Retrieval any cause	Hip-related failures	Aseptic loosening
0	2,182	11	5	0
1	1,631	3	2	0
2	1,368	3	2	1
3	1,110	2	1	1
4	969	1	1	0
5	871	3	0	0
6	754	1	0	0
7	678	2	1	1
8	608	5	2	1
9	539	1	0	0
10	491	3	1	1
11	110	0	0	0
12	66	0	0	0
Total		35	15	5

Table 2 – Breakdown of revisions according to follow-up periods postoperatively, due to any cause for retrievals, the related numbers including hip-related failures, which include aseptic loosenings.

survival rates were 99.82% ± 0.0023 at 5 years, down to 99.49% ± 0.0063 at 10 years and, finally, 99.16% ± 0.0063 at 12 years, with 66 hips remaining "at risk" at this follow-up period (fig. 5).

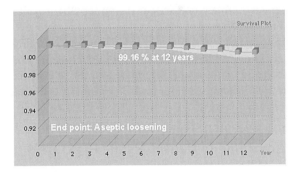

Figure 5 – Survival curve at 12-year follow-up period in primary arthroplasty of HA stems with "aseptic loosening" as endpoint. Confidence intervals are at 0.05.

Comparative Survivorship Analyses According to the Various Models

"Hip Related Failure" as Endpoint

The cumulative survivorship analyses with hip-related failure as endpoint for each of the three models demonstrated at the latest follow-up period the following rates: 98.57% ± 0.0089 at 12 years for the HA Omnifit, 97.29% ± 0.0255 at 10 years for the HA Omniflex, and 98.23% ±0.0128 at 6 years for the Omnifit FC. Interestingly, statistical tests carried out for the Omniflex and Omnifit FC *versus* HA Omnifit did not demonstrate any significant difference at 0.05, according to both Mantel-Haenszel and Log rank tests.

"Aseptic Loosening" as Endpoint

It may be of interest to focus on this particular breakdown according to various models, since the HA-coating was the same onto each of the models. Thus, the different designs would have a direct relationship with successes or failures. The cumulative survivorship analyses with aseptic loosening as endpoint for each of the three models demonstrated at the various follow-up periods the following rates:

At 6-years, 99.97% ± 0.0025 for the HA Omnifit, 99.04% ± 0.0186 for the HA Omniflex, and 100% ± 0.0000 for the Omnifit FC. At 10-years, 99.48% ± 0.0074 for the HA Omnifit, and 99.04% ±0.0186 for the HA Omniflex, and at 12-years, 99.10% ± 0.0074 for the HA Omnifit.

The FC stem reaches at present 10 years of maximum follow-up and, to date, zero aseptic loosening has been recorded. Despite the fact that a survival curve cannot be drawn over 6 years due to an insufficient number of cases (i.e., under 30), results might be considered as the best of the three models. However, statistical tests carried out for Omniflex and Omnifit FC *versus* HA Omnifit did not demonstrate any significant difference at 0.05, according to both Mantel-Haenszel and Log rank tests.

Comparative Survivorship Analyses According to Patient-Related Factors in HA-Coated Stems with Hip-Related Failures as Endpoint

Several parameters related to patients, such as age, gender or aetiology, would likely affect changes in the outcome of the arthroplasty. In order to obtain consistent statistical tests, we selected homogenous cohorts enrolling a significant number of cases. The maximum follow-up will be dictated by the number of cases remaining "at risk", which must not fall below 30 cases.

Age

The use of HA-coated implants might be questionable in the elderly; conversely, it seems rea-sonable to use hydroxyapatite for younger patients, as this population places greater physical challenges on an implant. Thus, it was interesting to draw the different cumulative survival curves for three cohorts, according to age.

Results at the 10-year follow-up are as follows: 99.31% ± 0.0128 for patients under 50, 98.13% ± 0.0098 for patients between 50 and 74 years of age, and 98.04% ± 0.0141 for patients over 75 years of age.

The results were unexpectedly similar in the three cohorts. This was confirmed by statistical tests carried out for the youngest and oldest patients *versus* patients between 50 and 74 years of age. These tests did not demonstrate any significant difference at 0.05, according to both Mantel-Haenszel and Log rank tests.

Gender

Comparative analysis was carried out for males and females. Results obtained at the 11-year follow-up are as follows: 99.25% ± 0.0068 for males, and 97.47% ±0.0122 for females. Despite the supposed better results recorded in the male population, statistical analysis did not confirm any significant difference at 0.05.

Aetiology

Due to the low number of other types of diagnoses, such as rheumatoid arthritis, we could assess only the results of osteoarthritis and necrosis. Results at 11-years are as follows: 98.41% ± 0.0085 for osteoarthritis, and 100% ± 0.0000 for avascular necrosis.

Despite the supposed better results recorded in the patients operated on for avascular necrosis, as no failure had been reported, tests did not confirm any significant difference at 0.05 for both the Mantel-Haenszel and the Log-rank.

Weight

Being overweight is sometimes assessed as a significant predictor for failures. A study by Schurman *et al.* (8) identified 75 kilograms as a limit that led to higher failure rate when exceeded. Our results with any femoral failure as endpoint with 1,018 hips in patients over 75 kilograms in weight *versus* 1,283 cases under this weight demonstrated survival rates at 12 years of 95.79% ± 0.0183 in the former group *versus* 97.80% ± 0.0104 in the latter, with no statistical difference at 0.05, according to both Mantel-Haenszel and Log rank tests. In addition, although these authors assessed that age was significant in overweight patients up to 75 years in age, we could not find any significant difference, especially when the given limit was 75 years old and 75 kilograms of weight.

DISCUSSION

The estimation of the survival function for the implants as described by Kaplan and Meier in 1958 has become a tremendous tool for any long lasting outcome studies in arthroplasty, since computerized databases have taken advantage of the newest developments and techniques over the years. This cumulative survivorship analysis helps answer fundamental questions, such as the success of failure of arthroplasty on the whole, the real benefit afforded by some innovative techniques regarding designs and mode of fixation of implants, or patient-related factors. Comparisons between different survival rates would be reliable, provided that 1) the compared cohorts are statistically significant, 2) the computerized database that collects, stores, and analyzes the data is relevant and, finally, 3) that the appropriate questions are asked based on an appropriate selection of cohorts along with judicious checking of "end points" (9-10).

The current study reports on a homogenous series of over 2,000 cases of hydroxyapatite-coated hips used in primary arthroplasty followed-up as a prospective continuous study for fifteen years. Data were collected and analyzed by the OrthoWave program, which comprises a statistical module (StatWave) that allows all kinds of descriptive analyses, cumulative survival rate calculations, and the related statistical tests. Three different HA-coated stems were analyzed. These stems belonged to the same family of Omnifit implants and had an identical grit-blasted substrate, an identical plasma-sprayed coating, and a similar design overall. Differences between the three stems were minor, such as stem length, augmentation structures at the upper aspect, and anticipated differences in terms of the elasticity of the metallic device.

These features certainly allowed us to provide consistent answers to specific questions about various outcomes of HA-stems in hip arthroplasty.

How can we consider the overall results of HA-coated stems regarding the arthroplasty itself, then the implant on the whole and, finally, the success or failure of the fixation afforded by the HA interface?

The appropriate choice of the selected "endpoint" allows a precise assessment of results regarding the arthroplasty, the implant, or the interface, as summed up in Table 3. Results of the arthroplasty itself take into consideration the final status of the operated patient, and record the fact of whether or not the implant was retrieved, whatever the cause for revision. Thus, we select "retrieval due to any cause" as endpoint. The over 95% final rate of "surviving" stems at 12 years can be considered as agreeable in a non selected series at an average age of 67-years, with respect to the high rate of accidental fractures reaching almost 1% and, naturally, jeopardizing the overall outcome.

On the whole, the results afforded by the implanted stem can evaluate the success or the failure of the implant type chosen by a surgeon. Failures can be analyzed and involve several factors. Dislocations or unexpected cracks might involve the design of the implant and the instruments, the method of the surgeon, or any acrobatic feats of the patients, while late loosening, pain, or subsidence are directly related to both the mechanical and biological fixation of the HA-coated stem. Endpoint will be "hip-related failures" in order to assess the result of the implant on the whole. Results were over 98% at the 12-year period.

While selecting as endpoint the failures due to a lack of fixation leading to subsidence, radiological loosening, or unexpected pain, one might directly assess the success or failure of the HA-coatings as means of "biological" long lasting fixation. This study could point out the survival rate of these HA-coated stems, and according to "aseptic loosening" as endpoint, the final rate of 99.16% at 12 years of follow-up period allows us to confirm the excellent clinical results previously reported.

Survival of...	Endpoint	Survival rate	"Worst case scenario"
"arthroplasty"	Retrieval any cause	95.32%	0.9397
"implant"	Hip-related failure	98.15%	0.9735
"HA fixation"	Aseptic loosening	99.16%	0.9853

Table 3 – Cumulative survivorship analysis as an assessment of long lasting success of the arthroplasty, the implant, and the HA fixation. The "worst case scenario" is computed as each survival rate minus the confidence interval at 0.05.

When affording innovative changes in terms of prostheses design, engineers' proposals are based upon lab tests, mathematics, and saw bone based conclusions. Were they beneficial regarding the distal tip of the Omniflex or the normalization steps and flutes of the short stem Omnifit FC ?

A paper presented by Manley *et al.* at the New Orleans AAOS in 1990 summed up some laboratory tests about "effects of stem design parameters, stem fit and bone quality on the torsional stability of femoral stems". Interestingly, the Omniflex geometry was superior to any other design, since "to manage the natural distal torsional and axial motion occurring with stems that achieve proximal load transfer, the surface finish characteristics of the distal tip are paramount. A cylindrical geometry is the only one that allows distal pistoning and rotation while presenting a consistent, biocompatible area of contact to the endosteal surface of the femur". On the other hand, with respect to the expected improvement afforded by the shortened Omnifit FC stem, "fluted and conical", conclusions were as follows: "Biomechanical testing has shown the superiority of distal flutes in providing increased flexibility while maintaining torsional stability over designs employing windowed, tapered, or hollow distal geometries…"

At the end of the day, surgeons and engineers would consider the comparative results of long term clinical experience with humility, provided that serious prospective studies were carried out and carefully analyzed. In fact, a decade later, no significant difference arose with respect to survivorship analyses between both the "distal tipped" Omniflex, and the "shorter and fluted" Omnifit FC stem, as compared to the original HA Omnifit stem, while considering either any "hip-related failure" or "aseptic loosening" as endpoint.

However, some additional details of the analyses pointed out some interesting conclusions about the different designs, especially between HA Omnifit and the short stem Omnifit FC. Despite the fact that statistical tests did not confirm any superiority of this shorter geometry when compared to the longer original stem, zero aseptic loosening was never reported with this FC stem, even after 10 years of clinical use. Additionally, the Ortho-Wave program allows computation of clinical scores, and rises up comparisons between the different brands according to various clinical assessment, mainly, the Harris Hip Score. Interestingly, the average values of this HHS score, based upon the patients of the current study, were the same (96.6) for both the Omnifit and the Omniflex stems, with no statistical difference at 0.05 (test of ER, Student-Fisher, Mann & Whitney). This confirmed the lack of any significant benefit afforded by the new features of the Omniflex.

Conversely, the mean values of the HHS for respectively the HA Omnifit (HHS: 96.6) and the shorter FC stem (HHS: 98.9) demonstrated a significant difference according to the various tests: $p < 0.001$ at both the test of ER and at the Mann & Whitney test. This should be critical for confirming proven better results with this FC stem. Unfortunately, the high incidence of fractures reported with that stem was a concern. This was confirmed by the statistical tests when selecting any "non accidental fracture" as endpoint. We suspect the increased fracture rate with the FC stem may be related to the medial grooves in the proximal stem body, which led to cracks and fractures induced by high torsional loads in weak bones. Again, clinical long term expertise is critical to confirm or invalidate the real benefit of innovative features.

Currently, HA-coated implants are widely used, especially in hip replacement. Should we restrict the indications, with respect to age or aetiology, due to different results in the long run for any kind of cohort ?

For years, we used hydroxyapatite coated implants for the vast majority of our cases, without any formal limitation due to age or aetiology. The only limitation for a stem with this "bioactive" fixation has been the lack of primary mechanical stability at the time of the operation.

The current study confirmed two previous assessments in terms of HA-coated stems. HA implants provided excellent survival rates at the 10-year follow-up period in any subgroup of population, in the youngest patients as well as the elderly, being said that young patients achieved the best survival rate at 99.31%, which is considered very encouraging in this "challenging" group. Interestingly, we computed the average HHS scores for patients with 10 year of minimum follow-up, who were under age 50 *versus* patients between ages 51 and 70. The average HHS was slightly better for the younger patients at 99.08 points, *versus* 98.48 points for the older patients, while statistical tests (Mann & Whitney and Wilcoxson) did not demonstrate any significant difference.

Similarly, the breakdown according to gender, weight, or aetiology did not demonstrate any significant statistical differences in terms of survivorship analysis, despite the better results that seemed to be obtained by males and avascular necrosis (AVN) cases, most likely due to the majority of AVN in young males.

All survival rates provided by all subgroups with hip-related failure as endpoint were between 97.47% and 100% at 10 years, which certainly would confirm the interest of these HA-coated stems in almost all of the primary indications, considering that only clinical concerns, not economic ones, have been taken into account for the patient selection.

Normally, the estimation of the survival function of implants follows the same rules in all survivorship analyses, which allows some comparisons through some National registers, mainly the Scandinavian ones, between HA-coated implants and cemented ones, at similar and consistent follow-up period of time. Is the Charnley cemented stem still the gold standard in terms of long term outcome in hip arthroplasty ?

The current book sums up the 10- to 15-year experience with HA implants. It seemed of interest to check all survival rates reported by all the authors of the current book with regard to HA stem results in primaries at 10 years of follow-up. Interestingly, the list of these survival rates, listed in Table 4, confirms that all these survival rates were between 96% up to 100%.

Scandinavian National Registers certainly represent the worldwide reference in terms of Hip register and survivorship analysis. We would like to refer to both the Swedish "Update and Validation of results from the Swedish National Hip Arthroplasty Registry – 1979 to 1998", presented by Henrik Malchau *et al.* at the 67th Orlando AAOS in 2000 (4) and the "prospective studies of hip prostheses and cements – A presentation of the Norwegian Arthroplasty Register – 1987 to 1999" by Leif I. Havelin and Lars B. Engesaeter (6).

Author	Femoral Implant	Survival rate
Tonino	ABG 1	99.34%
D'Antonio-Capello	HA Omnifit	99.6%
Vidalain	Corail	100%
Nourissat	ABG 1	97.62%
Toni	Anca fit	96%
Argenson	Symbios HA	96.7
Petit	PRA	98.75%
Epinette-Manley	HA Omnifit/flex/FC	99.16%

Table 4 – Survival rates at 10 years of Follow-up with aseptic loosening as endpoint, reported by all the authors of the current book (see table of contents for related details).

Based upon a global number of cases of 73,244 cases between 1988 and 1998, the Swedish Register states that "using modern cementing technique, a 94.6% 10-year survival is obtained for hip replacement with index diagnosis osteoarthosis and revised due to aseptic loosening". With respect to the different models of cemented hips, "…the improvement during the second period for cemented implants is obvious, and the 10-year survival for most cemented implants in Sweden is now between 93 and almost 97%". In particular, the 10 year survival rate for the Charnley hip was 92.8%, in which "the failures are predominately related to the femoral component. Conversely, "the Exeter polished implant has performed as well as the best implants" with 96.1% at 10 years.

The Norwegian register carried out a comparative study between HA-coated, porous-coated, cemented, and uncoated stems. Considering aseptic loosening as endpoint, HA-coated stems performed better. With a risk ratio of 1 for HA-coated stems, this risk increased to 2.1 (p-value of 0.01) for porous stems and 6.8 (p-value < 0.001) for cemented hips. Thus, based upon this study, "…compared to HA-coated stems (n=4,648), both the porous-coated (n=1,264) and cemented (n=2,839) stems had increased risks for revision, both for revisions due to any cause and for revisions due to aseptic stem loosening". According to the summary of this register study, "uncemented HA stems had better results than cemented stems at 10 years of follow-up… Cemented hip prostheses with high viscosity Palacos or Simplex cement had generally good results, with a 10-year survival of 95% or better".

Despite the differences between the 10-year cemented survival rates and the results provided by HA-coated stems from both these registers and chapters from this book, it leads one to infer that HA survival rates are clearly better. However, all these figures should be interpreted cautiously.

Nonetheless, now that survivorship analyses for HA-coated implants can be reported at 10 years and more, results from all studies demonstrate survival rates at least as good as the best cemented implants, and often significantly better.

CONCLUSIONS

Provided that prospective series can be adequately collected, stored, and analyzed through a dedicated computer program, survivorship analyses could be seen as the best outcome study tool in order to compute the long term results of a given implant, and to compare survival rates of different sub series according to any implant related or patient related parameter (1-3, 8-9).

The OrthoWave software allowed us to carry out a survival study of 2,199 primary hips, based upon a 15-year experience with three quite similar HA-coated femoral implants, the HA Omnifit, the HA Omniflex, and the HA Omnifit FC, which differ from each only slightly. Results with 66 patients remaining "at risk" at the 12-year follow-up period demonstrated extremely encouraging cumulative survival rates. Various endpoints led to assessment of three types of "survival". The survival of the arthroplasty itself, with any retrieval due to any cause as endpoint was 95.32% (worst case scenario at CI of 0.05: 0.9397). The results afforded by the implant itself, grouping all hip-related failures as endpoint, gave a survival rate of 98.15% (worst case scenario at CI of 0.05: 0.9735). The particular study of failures and causes for retrieval allowed us to check all failures related to lack of fixation and aseptic loosening, such as pain, radiological loosening and subsidence. Thus, the survival rate with aseptic loosening as endpoint reached 99.16%, with a "worst case scenario" at 0.9853.

The three Omnifit stems that were successively used had the same type of coating and almost the same proximal geometry. Differences regarded mainly the distal portion of the stem, with a "distal tip" for the Omniflex, and a shorter, fluted and conical stem for the Omnifit FC. These modifications did not lead to significant differences in term of survival rates. Similarly, no statistical difference

arose from comparative survivorship analyses according to age, gender, and aetiology.

Furthermore, survival rates provided by the HA Omnifit stems through the current study compare favorably with all the survivorship analyses reported by all the authors of this book. Survivorship for all HA stems at 10 years ranged from at least 96% up to 100% for the best records. Conversely, the survival rates provided by the cemented stems, as published in the Scandinavian registers, seem to reach a ceiling at 97% at the 10-year follow-up period, including a survival rate of 92.8% with the cemented Charnley hip.

For years, hydroxyapatite-coated implants were often considered a passing fancy and a "here today, gone tomorrow" attempt to improve the classic and well regarded cemented prostheses. Publications at present begin to report excellent long lasting HA results at 15-years of clinical experience, and this makes all the difference. The cemented Charnley hip no longer need be considered the "gold standard". Clearly, hydroxyapatite-coated implants are here to stay.

Reference List

1. Dorey F, Amstutz HC (1986) Survivorship analysis in the evaluation of joint replacement. *J. Arthroplasty* 1(1):63-9.
2. Dorey F, Amstutz HC (1989) The validity of survivorship analysis in total joint arthroplasty. *J. Bone Joint Surg. Am.* 71(4):544-8.
3. Laupacis A (1989) The validity of survivorship analysis in total joint arthroplasty. *J. Bone Joint Surg. Am.* 71(7):1111-2.
4. Herberts P, Ahnfelt L, Malchau H, Strömberg C, Andersson GBJ (1989) Multicenter clinical trials and their value in assessing Total Joint Arthroplasty, *Clin. Orthop.* 249; 48-55.
5. http://www.jru.orthop.gu.se.
6. http://info.haukeland.no/nrl.
7. Kaplan EL, Meier P (1958) Non parametric estimation from incomplete observations. *J. Am. Stat. Assoc.* 457-81.
8. Schurman DJ, Bloch DA, Segal MR, Tanner CM (1989) Conventional cemented total hip arthroplasty. Assessment of clinical factors associated with revision for mechanical failure. *Clin. Orthop. Mar.* (240):173-80.
9. Garellick G, Malchau H, Herberts P (2000) Survival of hip replacements. A comparison of a randomized trial and a registry. *Clin. Orthop.* (375):157-67.
10. Nardi D, Terzi S, Toni A (1998) The importance of statistics in documentation on hip prostheses. *Chir. Organi Mov.* Jul-Sep; 83(3):221-30.

4 Hydroxyapatite Femoral Stems for Total Hip Arthroplasty: 10-14 Year Follow-up

James A. D'Antonio, MD, William N. Capello, MD, Michael T. Manley, PhD, Rudolph G.T. Geesink, MD, PhD, William L. Jaffe, MD

INTRODUCTION

The current report details the performance of hydroxyapatite-coated femoral implants implanted in patients at five centers. The patients were followed up prospectively for as long as 14 years. The primary objectives were to evaluate long-term stem fixation, functional results, and radiographic bony response to the implant. Long-term fixation of the femoral stem, particularly in the young and active patient, remains a challenge because of aseptic loosening and progressive osteolysis. Failure of first generation cemented systems and techniques (1-6) stimulated the search for new designs, new cement techniques, and cementless fixation. The use of second and third generation cement techniques, and the use of porous ingrowth implants, has improved the ability to achieve long-term fixation of the femoral stem (7-16). However, aseptic loosening, osteolysis and/or thigh pain continue to be a problem with some designs (9, 14, 17-22).

During the past fifteen years, the authors studied the use of hydroxyapatite coatings for the fixation of orthopaedic implants to bone. Early work conducted in canine models showed that in the presence of a hydroxyapatite coating, bone filled gaps around cortical plugs, intramedullary rods, and hip implants, and a bone seam proliferated on these devices (23-27). Coated implants were tightly fixed to bone at follow-up, whereas uncoated control implants were not. With hydroxyapatite-coated implants, bone was conducted onto surface features (normalization steps) by the coating, whereas with uncoated implants, these features remained unfilled by bone. Additional studies have demonstrated that a coating of hydroxyapatite increases the speed, strength, and amount of bony attachment to an implant without an intervening fibrous tissue membrane (19, 28-34).

During the past 14 years, the authors have used a hydroxyapatite-coated tapered titanium femoral stem without a porous coating, and results at 2-, 5-, and 10-year minimum follow-up have been published (35-39). These reports showed excellent early and midterm clinical results with very low failure rates and minimal thigh pain.

The intent of the current study was to measure the efficacy of fixation provided by the hydroxyapatite coatings in total hip replacement and to compare the results with controls provided by the contemporary literature.

MATERIALS & METHODS

From 1987 to 1990, fifteen surgeons implanted 380 Omnifit-HA stems in eight centers. Five surgeons in four centers continue to follow these patients beyond ten years.

At present, 199 patients (232 hips) have a minimum ten-year and maximum 14-year (average 12.1 year) follow-up for review. Twelve patients (14 hips, 5.2%) died before the 10-year follow-up, and one patient died after the 10-year evaluation. Ten patients (11 hips, 4.2%) have less than ten year follow-up. Ten patients (10 hips, 3.7%) have had femoral revisions.

All of the patients received the same hydroxyapatite-coated Ti alloy femoral stem (fig. 1, Stryker Howmedica Osteonics, Allendale, New Jersey). The stem is grit-blasted, is straight but tapered, and has a double wedge proximal configuration with normalization steps. Stem surface roughness was 3 to 4.3mm before the application of hydroxyapatite coating and 4.3 to 8.1 after. A dense 50mm thick layer of hydroxyapatite was applied circumferentially to the proximal 1/3 of the stem by plasma spray technique. This proximal hydroxyapatite coating was more than 90% hydroxyapatite by weight, and has been previously described (24-26). Combined with the femoral stem, 143 hydroxyapatite threaded sockets were implanted, 74 hydroxyapatite press-fit sockets were implanted, 47 porous press-fit sockets were implanted, and three patients (three hips) received a bipolar prosthesis.

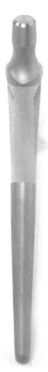

Figure 1 – The Omnifit-HA femoral stem.

Fifty-two percent (106 hips) of patients were men. The mean age of the patients at the time of the operation was 51.3 years (range, 18-73 years), and 35% of these patients (81 hips) were under the age of 50 years at the time of implantation with average age of 39 years (range, 18-49 years). The mean weight was 77 kilograms (range, 36-122 kilograms). The principle diagnoses were: osteoarthritis (159 hips, 68.5%), avascular necrosis (27 hips, 11.6%), previously failed implant (13 hips, 5.6%), rheumatoid arthritis (11 hips, 4.7%), posttraumatic arthritis (8 hips, 3.4%), congenital hip dysplasia (11 hips, 4.7%), femoral fracture (one hip, 0.9%), and other (two hips, 0.9%; one synovial chondromatosis and one acetabular fracture) (Table 1).

Twelve patients (14 hips) died before the ten-year follow-up. One patient died at 10.5 years postoperatively; this patient's data are included with the minimum 10-year follow-up. Ten patients with eleven hips have not yet returned for their minimum ten-year visit.

The level of pain as well as functional parameters such as the distance the patient could walk, stair climbing ability, the need for external support, sitting ability, limp, and participation in recreational activities were evaluated at each visit, and a composite Harris Hip Score was calculated (40). A score of 90 to 100 points was considered an excellent result; 80-89 points was considered a good result, 70-79 points was considered a fair result; and 69 points or less was considered a poor result. Anteroposterior (AP) and lateral radiographs of the hip were made preoperatively and at all postoperative visits. The radiographs obtained postoperatively were evaluated for radiolucency, periosteal cortical hypertrophy, and cancellous condensation in the zones described by Gruen *et al.* (41). In addition, subsidence of the implant and erosion of cortical bone (osteolysis). Zones 1 and 7 on the AP radiographs and Zones 8 and 14 on the lateral radiographs represented the proximal hydroxyapatite coated areas of the femoral stem. The definitions of radiolucency, periosteal cortical hypertrophy, and cancellous condensation have been previously described (37).

The performance of the femoral stem implant was evaluated in three ways. The rate of mechanical failure was defined as the number of stems revised for aseptic loosening and the number that were determined to be loose by the radiographic criteria of Engh *et al.* (42). The rate of clinical failure was defined as the number of stems revised because of osteolysis or pain plus those stems associated with pain that limited activities of daily living. Finally, the combined failure rate was defined as the sum of the mechanical failures and the clinical failures. Survivorship analysis based on mechanical failure and combined failure as the end point was calculated.

RESULTS

One hundred ninety-nine patients (232 hips) with a minimum 10-years follow-up (mean 12.1 years) were evaluated. Forty-six hips have incomplete evaluations (one or more fields incomplete or have responded to phone questionnaires and mailings, or both), and 206 hips have complete radiographic evaluations. A complete evaluation (a calculable Total Harris Hip Score) is available at latest follow-up for 186 hips evaluated between 10 and 14 years. Of these 186 hips, 139 (75%) had good to excellent results, and 10.8% (25 hips) had a Harris Hip Score below 70 points.

The preoperative Harris Hip Score for the patients with complete data was 43.1 points, and the Harris Hip Score at last evaluation averaged 87.9. Five patients (2.2%) complained of mild (4 patients) to marked (1 patient) thigh pain. Twenty-five patients had Harris Hip scores below 70 points. These scores are attributed to acetabular failure (8 patients) and other non-hip related problems (17 patients). Of the 17 patients with other non-hip related problems, investigators reported 4 cases with medical problems, 7 with multiple joint/back problems, 4 with bursitis, 1 with ectopic bone, and 1 etiology unknown.

Radiographic evaluation revealed that 100% of the non-revised stems evaluated at minimum ten-years (206 stems) were bony stable. Nine of the revised femoral stems also were read as bony stable before they were revised for reasons other than mechanical failure. Reactive line formation was found around the uncoated distal tip in 102 hips (50%), and seven hips (3.4%) had a radiodense line formation in the hydroxyapatite-coated proximal zones. An additional seven hips (3.4%) had a non-progressive rounded reactive line in the trochanter and proximal portion of Zone 1. Where radiolucent lines were present, they were always parallel, never divergent, and they were never associated with the formation of a so-called pedestal. Cancellous condensation was seen about the mid and distal stem in 100% of cases, most commonly seen in Zones 6 and 2 at the distal end of the hydroxyapatite coating, and was present in 94% (190 stems) and 96% (196 stems) of those two zones, respectively. Cortical hypertrophy was seen in 64% of cases (128 stems), most commonly in Zone 5, where it was present in 50% of all hips (103 stems). Atraumatic subsidence of more than 3mm occurred in four hips during the first year; none of those hips became unstable, and none have additional subsidence thereafter. Traumatic subsidence of 10mm occurred at 10 years postoperatively and was related to periprosthetic fracture requiring revision of one stem. No hip had endosteal osteolysis, but 41% had some evidence of osteolysis in the proximal most areas of Zones 1, 7, 8, or 14 (fig. 2), and in 13% (23 hips) pelvic osteolysis was

observed. The radiographic changes as previously reported progressed and changed from Years 1 through 5 but thereafter remained stable without change (fig. 3). In this group of patients with a minimum 10-years and maximum of 14-years follow-up, there were 33 socket revisions. One porous press-fit socket was revised for loosening. Nineteen hydroxyapatite press-fit sockets were revised: 16 for loosening, and three for polyethylene wear. Thirteen hydroxyapatite-threaded sockets were revised: one for dislocation, seven for polyethylene wear, and five for loosening. Two femoral stems in this group were revised, one for the previously mentioned traumatic

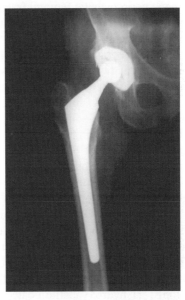

Figure 2 – Forty-one percent of the hips had some form of osteolysis in the proximal most areas of zones 1, 7, 8, or 14.

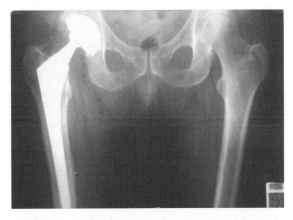

Figure 3 – Radiographic changes were observed during the first five years, after which the hips remained stable without change. Predictable and consistent remodeling occurred around the stems.

subsidence, and one revised with the acetabular component for polyethylene wear in order to implant a ceramic-on-ceramic hip system in a young patient.

Two hundred fifty-five of the 267 stems (96%) have not been revised. For the total population of 230 patients (267 hips) initially enrolled in the multicenter study, revisions include isolated femoral revisions in four patients, femoral revisions combined with acetabular revisions in eight patients, and an additional 36 isolated acetabular revisions. There were four isolated femoral revisions; one for aseptic loosening; two for repair of post traumatic periprosthetic femoral fracture; and one discretionary stem revision for excessive anteversion, neck/socket impingement. Eight patients (8 hips) had both components revised: three for deep joint infection; two well-fixed stems for pain of unknown etiology; and three discretionary revisions at the time of revision of the acetabulum where the stems were well-fixed. The one femoral revision for aseptic loosening was revised 9.5 years postoperatively because of polyethylene wear and progressive proximal femoral osteolysis. The two patients who had revision surgery for pain of unknown etiology in the lower extremities had surgery by two surgeons who were not part of the multicenter study group. Both stems were well fixed at the time of revision, and difficult to revise. The 36 isolated acetabular revisions occurred for the following reasons: one porous press-fit socket for loosening; 21 hydroxyapatite coated press-fit sockets with 19 revised for loosening and 2 for polyethylene wear and osteolysis; and 14 hydroxyapatite threaded sockets revised, one for dislocation, six for aseptic loosening, and seven for polyethylene wear and/or osteolysis.

At 10 to 14 years, the survivorship of the femoral stem based on mechanical failure was 99.6%; based on the combined failure rate, it was 98.9%. The mechanical failure rate of the femoral stems included only the one for aseptic loosening (0.4%). No stems were radiographically loose. Two potential clinical failures occurred. Both were for pain of unknown etiology in two patients who had revision surgery. Adding the clinical failures to the mechanical failures gives a device-related combined failure rate on the femoral side of three hips (1.1%). The acetabular mechanical failure rate was 10.6%, and the combined failure rate was 14.4%. The individual socket types had a mechanical and combined failure rate as follows: porous press-fit sockets 2.1% and 2.1%; hydroxyapatite press-fit sockets 25.7% and 28.4%; and hydroxyapatite threaded sockets 5.6% and 11.2%.

DISCUSSION

The intent of the current study was to follow the clinical course of a series of patients receiving hydroxyapatite-coated total hip replacements. Measurements of the study outcome included clinical and radiographic analyses and measurements of implant survival rates. The contemporary literature was designed as a control. In comparing the findings from a recent literature search (Table 2), the authors assumed that a radiographic analysis was done blinded and data collection was done on a prospective basis.

The results from animal studies indicated that, even when implants were loosely placed or subjected to interface motion, a stable bone fixation interface could be obtained with the specific hydroxyapatite coating that we evaluated (9, 25-26, 43-44). Other authors have now shown similar results (16, 29, 32-34, 45-47). In several animal studies conducted before the current clinical investigation, cortical plugs and intramedullary rods implanted in hips in canines all were fixed tightly to bone when harvested (26, 44). Where uncoated control implants were used, they were loose and surrounded by fibrous tissue at sacrifice. Histologic evaluation of specimens confirmed the closed apposition between the hydroxyapatite coated implants and bone. The adaptation of the bone interface into implant surface contours (normalization steps) seen with, but not without, the hydroxyapatite coating in the canine hip study further suggest the potential utility of this coating for fixation of orthopaedic devices. This finding of bone growth into implant steps was later confirmed for human implants in an early clinical femoral stem retrieval at autopsy (43, 48). Other autopsy retrievals have shown the presence of extensive circumferential bone apposition to a hydroxyapatite-coated titanium femoral stem (49). In addition, clinical trials have shown with roentgen stereophotogrammetric analysis techniques that less micromotion and subsidence occurs with hydroxyapatite-coated implants compared with porous coated or cemented implants of the same design (33, 46).

The current clinical study began in the Netherlands in 1987 and at eight sites in the United States in 1988 within a clinical trial regulated by the Food and Drug Administration. Earlier reports evaluated the populations of European and the United States separately (35-37, 39, 50) although the current study combines the series. The authors have followed the patients prospectively since their inception for up to 14 years and measured a femoral mechanical failure rate of 0.4%. Additionally, when the data from the patients under 50 years of age in our study were isolated from the entire study cohort, it was found that the femoral mechanical failure rate for 90 hips implanted in patients under 50 years of age was 1.1%. This result compares very favorably with reported failure rates for hip arthroplasty that frequently have reached double digits at moderate periods of follow-up in young and active patients (1-6, 10, 18). Additionally, the mean Harris Hip Score for this patient population at latest follow-up was 87.9 points (range, 32.5-100 points). The success achieved with the hydroxyapatite femoral stem used in our study has now been confirmed with other hydroxyapatite coated stem designs (33, 47, 51-55).

Predictable and consistent remodeling occurred around the hydroxyapatite femoral stems (fig. 3). During the first 5 years postoperative, progressive cancellous condensation fills in about the stem where the stem does not initially contact the endosteal surface. Reactive lines are seen frequently around the uncoated distal tip but rarely in the hydroxyapatite coated zones. Cortical hypertrophy progresses throughout the middle to distal stem zones. The authors think that these remodeling changes are a secondary stabilization of the stem. Osteolysis has been confined to the most proximal Gruen zones indicating an excellent seal against polyethylene debris migration. Only one patient has had femoral fixation threatened by osteoylyis, and that patient had surgery revision at 9.5 years. Acetabular osteolysis was seen in 13% of the patients. Although no evidence of hydroxyapatite was found as a cause of osteolysis, the authors recognize that osteolysis is a problem with cementless fixation.

As reported previously, the overall success rate with the acetabular components has not matched that of the hydroxyapatite coated femoral stem (27). Although the porous press-fit sockets and hydroxyapatite-threaded sockets have had satisfactory results with mechanical failure rates of 2.1% and 5.6% respectively, the hydroxyapatite press-fit sockets had a mechanical failure rate of 25.7%. The analysis of these components led the authors to the conclusion that the fixation interface for the hydroxyapatite-coated press-fit sockets failed because the fixation interfaces could not withstand the tensile stresses between the bone and cup that occur at the interface beneath the implant during patient activity. By comparison, the hydroxyapatite-coated threaded cups and porous coated cups remain interlocked with bone to resist the tensile stresses and have similar, acceptable mechanical failure rates of 2.1% to 5.6%.

Because of the different results achieved with cups and stem, it is the authors' belief that while a hydroxyapatite coating may produce short-term interface fixation and favorable bone remodeling at fixation interfaces, long-term stability of the implant is dependant on the inherent stability provided by the device design. Thus, early success with the press-fit hydroxyapatite-coated cups turned to mid-term failure because of the inability of the smooth fixation interfaces to withstand the applied loading in the acetabulum. By comparison, the hydroxyapatite-coated threaded cups were interlocked with bone and maintained long term stability. Similarly, the femoral stem now has demonstrated long term success, in the short-term because of the favorable remodeling provided by the coating and now in the long term because of the inherently stable stem design.

CONCLUSION

The clinical results of this multicenter study evaluating the use of a hydroxyapatite-coated femoral titanium stem support the experimental findings that hydroxyapatite increases the speed, strength, and amount of bony attachment to a titanium prosthesis. The femoral stem with a hydroxyapatite proximal coating has performed exceedingly well in a young and active patient population and in the hands of a variety of surgeons. Its implantation has resulted in progressive remodeling of the femur about the implant and permitted patients to return to a high level of activity with a low risk of activity related thigh pain. The circumferential hydroxyapatite coating has prevented the migration of polyethylene wear debris distal to the femoral neck resection level. The current results at more than

10-years follow-up compare favorably with any published results in total hip arthroplasty.

Acknowledgments

The authors thank the surgeons in the United States who were part of the Investigational Device Exemption study of these implants: B. Bierbaum MD, Boston, MA ; D. Mattingly MD, Boston, MA.

Reference List

1. Chandler HP, Reineck FT, Wixson RL, McCarthy JC (1981) Total hip replacement in patients younger than thirty years old. *J. Bone Joint Surgery* 63A:1426-34.

2. Collis DK (1984) Cemented total hip arthroplasty in patients who are less then fifty years old. *J. Bone Joint Surgery* 66A:353-9.

3. Collis DK (1991) Long term (twelve to eighteen year) follow-up of cemented total hip arthroplasty in patients who are less than fifty years old: A follow-up note. *J. Bone Joint Surgery* 73A:593-7.

4. Devitt A, O'Sullivan T, Quinlan W (1997) 16- to 25-year follow-up study of cemented arthroplasty of the hip in patients aged 50 years or younger. *J. Arthroplasty* 12:479-89.

5. Dorr LD, Kane III TJ, Conaty JP (1994) Long-term results of cemented total hip arthroplasty in patients 45 years old or younger. *J. Arthroplasty* 9:453-6.

6. Dorr LD, Luckett M, Conaty JP (1996) Total hip arthroplasty in patients younger than 45 years: A nine-to-ten year follow-up study. *Clin. Orthop.* 260:1226-34.

7. Ballard WT, Callahan JJ, Sullivan PM, Johnston RC (1994) The results of improved cementing techniques for total hip arthroplasty in patients less than 50 years old. *J. Bone Joint Surgery* 76A:959-64.

8. Barrack RL, Mulroy Jr RD, Harris WH (1992) Improved cementing techniques and femoral component loosening in young patients with hip arthroplasty: A 12-year radiographic review. *J. Bone Joint Surgery* 74B:385-9.

9. Engh Jr CA, Culpepper WJ, Engh CA (1997) Long-term results of use of the anatomic medullary locking prosthesis in total hip arthroplasty. *J. Bone Joint Surgery* 79A:177-84.

10. Glassman AH, Engh CA, Culpepper Jr WJ (1996) Cementless total hip replacement in patients fifty years of age or younger: A five year minimum follow-up study. *Ortho. Trans.* 20:139.

11. Hellman EJ, Capello WN Feinberg JR (1999) Omnifit cementless total hip arthroplasty: A 10-year average follow-up. *CORR* 364: 164-74.

12. Malchau H, Wang YX, Karrholm J, Herberts P (1997) Scandinavian multicenter porous coated anatomic total hip arthroplasty study. Clinical and radiographic results with 7 to 10 year follow-up evaluation. *J. Arthroplasty* 2:133-48.

13. McLaughlin JR, Lee KR (2000) Total hip arthroplasty in young patients: 8-13 year results using an Uncemented stem. *CORR* 373:153-63.

14. Oishi CS, Walker RH, Colwell Jr CW (1994) The femoral component in total hip arthroplasty. Six to eight year follow-up of one hundred consecutive patients after use of third generation cementing technique. *J. Bone Joint Surgery* 76A:1330-6.

15. Sakalkale DP, Eng K, Hozack WJ, Rothman RH (2000) Minimum 10-year results of a tapered cementless hip replacement. *CORR* 362:138-44.

16. Smith SE, Harris WH (1997) Total hip arthroplasty performed with insertion of the femoral component with cement and the acetabular component without cement: Ten to thirteen year results. *J. Bone Joint Surg.* 79A: 827-33.

17. Callaghan JJ, Forest EE, Sporer SM, Goetz DD, Johnston RC (1997) Total hip arthroplasty in the young adult. *CORR* 344:257-62.

18. Heekin RD, Callaghan JJ, Hopkins WJ, Savory CG, Xenos JS (1993) The porous-coated anatomic total hip prosthesis inserted without cement: Results after five-to-seven years in a prospective study. *J. Bone Joint Surgery* 75A:77-91.

19. Kim YH, Kim JS, Cho SH (1999) Primary total hip arthroplasty with a cementless porous-coated anatomic total hip prosthesis: 10- to 12- year results of a prospective and consecutive series. *J. Arthroplasty* 14: 538-48.

20. Smith SE, Estok II DM, Harris WH (2000) 20-year experience with cemented primary and conversion total hip arthroplasty using so-called second generation cementing techniques in patients aged 50 years or younger. *J. Arthroplasty* 15:263-73.

21. Sporer SM, Callaghan JJ, Olejniczak JPO, Goetz DD, Johnston RC (1998) Hybrid total hip arthroplasty in patients under the age of fifty: A five to ten year follow-up. *J. Arthroplasty* 13:485-91.

22. Xenos JS, Callaghan JJ, Heekin RD *et al.* (1999) The porous coated anatomic total hip prosthesis, inserted without cement. *J. Bone Joint Surg.* 81A:74-82.

23. DeGroot K, Geesink RGT, Klein CPAT, Serekian P (1987) Plasma sprayed coating of HA. *J. Biomed. Mater. Res.* 21:1375-81.

24. Geesink RGT (1989) Experimental and clinical experience with hydroxyapatite-coated hip implants. *Orthopedics* 12:1239-42.

25. Geesink RGT, deGroot K, Klein CPAT (1988) Bonding of bone to apatite-coated implants. *J. Bone Joint Surgery* 70B:17-22.

26. Geesink RGT, Manley MT ed (1993) Hydroxyapatite Coatings in Orthopaedic Surgery, New York, Raven Press.

27. Manley, MT, Capello WN, D'Antonio JA, Ediden AA, Geesink R (1997) Revision rates and radiographic changes associated with different socket interface technologies. *J. Bone Joint Surgery*.

28. Cook SD, Thomas KA, Dalton JE *et al.* (1992) Hydroxyapatite coating of porous implants improves bone

ingrowth and interface attachment strength. *J. Biomed. Mater. Res.* 26:989-1001.

29. Dalton JE, Cook SD, Thomas KA, Kay JF (1995) The effect of operative fit and hydroxyapatite coating on the mechanical and biological response to porous implants. *J. Bone Joint Surgery* 77A:97-110.

30. Søballe K, Hansen ES, Brockstedt-Rasmussen H, Nielson PT, Rechnagel K (1991) Histologic analysis of a retrieved hydroxyapatite-coated femoral prosthesis. *Clin. Orthop.* 272:255-8.

31. Søballe K, Hansen ES, Brockstedt-Rasmussen H *et al.* (1991) Fixation of titanium and hydroxyapatite-coated implants in osteopenic bone. *J. Arthroplasty* 6:307-16.

32. Søballe K, Hansen ES, Brockstedt-Rasmussen H, Pedersen CM, Bunger C (1990) Hydroxyapatite coating enhances fixation of porous coated implants. A comparison in dogs between press-fit and noninterference fit. *Acta Orthop. Scand.* 61:299-306.

33. Søballe K, Toksgiv-Larsen S, Gelineck J *et al.* (1993) Migration of hydroxyapatite-coated femoral prostheses. A roentgen sterophotogrammetric study. *J. Bone Joint Study* 75B:681-7.

34. Tisdal CL, Goldberg VM, Parr JA *et al.* (1994) The influence of a hydroxyapatite and tricalcium-phosphate coating on bone ingrowth into titanium fiber-metal implants. *J. Bone Joint Surgery* 76A:159-71.

35. Capello WN, D'Antonio JA, Feinberg JR, Manley MT (1997) Hydroxyapatite coated femoral components in patients less than fifty years old. *J. Bone Joint Surgery* 79A:1023-9.

36. D'Antonio JA, Capello WN, Crothers OD, Jaffe WL, Manley MT (1992) Early clinical experience with hydroxyapatite-coated femoral implants. *J. Bone Joint Surgery* 74A:995-1008.

37. D'Antonio JA, Capello WN, Manley MT (1996) Remodeling of bone around hydroxyapatite-coated femoral stems. *J. Bone Joint Surgery* 78A:1226-34.

38. D'Antonio JA, Capello WN, Manley MT, Geesink, R (2001) Hydroxyapatite femoral stems for total hip arthroplasty: 10-13-year followup. *CORR* 393:101-11.

39. Geesink RGT, Hoefnagels NHM (1995) Six-year results of hydroxyapatite-coated total hip replacements. *J. Bone Joint Surgery* 77B:534-47.

40. Harris WH (1969) Traumatic arthritis of the hip after dislocation and acetabular fracture: Treatment by mold arthroplasty. An end-result study using a new method of result evaluation. *J. Bone Joint Surgery* 51A:737-55.

41. Gruen TA, McNeice GM, Amstutz HC (1979) "Modes of failure" of cemented stem-type femoral components: A radiographic analysis of loosening. *Clin. Orthop.* 141:17-27.

42. Engh CA, Massin P, Suthers KE (1990) Roentgenographic assessment of the biologic fixation of porous-surfaced femoral components. *Clin. Orthop.* 257:107-28.

43. Bauer TW (1993) The histology of HA-coated implants. In Geesink RGT, Manley MT (eds). Hydroxyapatite coatings in Orthopaedic Surgery, New York, Raven Press, 305-18.

44. Manley MT, Kay JF, Yoshiya S, Stern LS, Stulberg BN (1987) Accelerated fixation of weight bearing implants by hydroxyapatite coatings. *Orthop. Res. Soc.* 33 Annual Meeting.

45. Burr DB, Mori S, Boyd RD *et al.* (1993) Histomorphometric assessment of the mechanism for rapid ingrowth of bone to HA/TCP coated implants. *J. Biomed. Mat. Res.* 27:645-53.

46. Kroon P-O, Freeman MAR (1992) Hydroxyapatite coating of hip prostheses. Effect on migration into the femur. *J. Bone Joint Surgery* 74B:518-22.

47. Søballe K, Hansen ES, Brockstedt-Rasmussen H, Bunger C (1993) Hydroxyapatite coating converts fibrous tissue to bone around loaded implants. *J. Bone Joint Surgery* 75B:270-8.

48. Bauer TW, Geesink RG, Zimmerman R, McMahon JT (1997) Hydroxyapatite-coated femoral stems. Histological analysis of components retrieved at autopsy. *J. Bone Joint Surgery* 73A:1439-52.

49. Tonino AJ, Therin M, Doyle C (1999) Hydroxyapatite-coated femoral stems. Histology and histomorphometry around five components retrieved at post mortem. *J. Bone Joint Surgery* 81B:148-54.

50. Jaffe WL, Scott DF (1996) Total hip arthroplasty with hydroxyapatite-coated prostheses. *J. Bone Joint Surgery* 78A:1918-34.

51. Araujo CA, Gonzalez JF, Tonino AJ and the International ABG study group (1998) Rheumatoid arthritis and hydroxyapatite-coated hip prostheses. Five-year results. *J. Arthroplasty* 6:660-7.

52. Furlong RJ, Osborn JF (1991) Fixation of hip prostheses by hydroxyapatite ceramic coatings. *J. Bone Joint Surgery* 73B:741-5.

53. Karrholm J, Malchau H, Snorrason F, et al. (1994) Micromotion of femoral stems in total hip arthroplasty. *J. Bone Joint Surgery* 76A:1692-705.

54. Overgaard S, Lind M, Glerup H *et al.* (1996) Hydroxyapatite and fluorapatite coatings on loaded implants. *Acta Orthop. Scand.* 67(Suppl 267):59.

55. Tonino AJ, Rahmy AIA and the International ABG Study Group (1998) The hydroxyapatite-ABG hip system. 5-7 year results from an international multicenter study. *J. Arthroplasty* 15:274-82.

5   Clinical Experience
with the ABG Total Hip Arthroplasty

Christian Nourissat, MD, José Adrey, MD, Daniel Berteaux, MD and Christian Goalard, MD

INTRODUCTION

The ABG Cement-Free Hip prosthesis is a cementless implant made from $TiAl_6V_4$ titanium alloy proximally coated with a thin Hydroxyapatite (HA) coating. From a series of 294 prostheses implanted in 282 patients who had a primary hip replacement between February 1989 and March 1990, we report the outcome at 10 years (mean follow-up period = 124 months). The cumulative survival rate of all 294 prostheses was 97.62% for the stem, 95.92% for the cup (confidence interval = 95%).

Of the 177 surviving hips with original prostheses, the mean pre-operative Merle D'Aubigne (MDA) score (1) was 8.94/18, compared with a mean post-operative score of 17.63/18. Radiological results showed good adaptation of the bone around the implant, with the osseointegration remaining constant without lucent or reactive lines (2) in the areas with hydroxyapatite (HA) coating. However, we observed some polyethylene wear and osteolysis, which will be discussed in this chapter.

MATERIALS AND METHODS

Between February 1989 and March 1990, 294 ABG total hip prostheses, with cementless cups and cementless stems, were implanted by the authors in a continuous series. The operations, all primary surgical interventions, were performed by 4 orthopaedic surgeons at three different centers. All cases have been followed up at 10 years. The patients (117 female, 165 male, 282 patients and 294 hips) had a mean age at the time of primary THR of 64.66 (28.33 to 86.58) years. Indications for hip replacement are listed in Table 1

Primary osteoarthritis	170 (57.82%)
Dysplasia	63 (21.4%3)
Protusio & osteoarthritis	23 (7.82%)
Primary necrosis	16 (5.45%)
Secondary necrosis	3 (1.02%)
Rapid destruction osteoarthritis	7 (2.38%)
Rheumatoid arthritis	5 (1.70%)
Post-traumatic osteoarthritis	4 (1.36%)
Other mechanical complications	3 (1.02%)

Table 1 – Indications.

Statistical analysis was performed using the Kaplan-Meier method (3) to evaluate survival of the implant with regard to the rate of revision 10 years post implantation. Survival curves with corresponding confidence intervals (95%) were generated with failure defined according to the following 3 endpoints: the revision of any component; the revision of the acetabular component; and the revision of the femoral component.

Patients were evaluated both clinically and radiologically with the original prosthesis *in situ*. For the clinical examination, the Merle D'Aubigné (MDA) functional grading system was used (1). The radiological examination consisted of 3 X-rays: 1 anterior/posterior view of the femoral stem, 1 lateral view of the femoral stem, and 1 lateral view of the cup. A detailed analysis was performed to analyze the position and stability of the stem and cup and the reaction of the bone in contact with, and at distance from, the implant. The femoral stem was assessed using the 7 A/P Gruen zones (4), and the cup was assessed using the 3 DeLee-Charnley zones (5). Ossification of the femoral stem was graded according to the Brooker Ectopic Ossification Grading system (6), and the cup was assessed for wear according to the procedure as described by Livermore (7).

The presence of cyclic osteolysis was looked for on X-rays in the anterior and lateral view at the level of the femur and acetabulum, and a multifactorial analysis was performed to assess whether the following factors favored its occurrence: age and activity of the patients, gender, and polyethylene wear. Additionally, progression of femoral and acetabular osteolysis was compared.

Surgical Procedure

Pre-operative planning with the use of templates is essential to determine implant sizing. In the choice of the implant to be inserted, the main criterion is optimal metaphyseal fill. As much of the cancellous bone in the metaphysis as possible must be preserved in order to prevent contact between the implant and cortex. The stem must be centered in the medullary cavity of the diaphysis without any *varus* or *valgus* deviation.

We recommend an exact-fit implantation of the cup into the subchondral bone. This was performed in 94% of the cases in this series. Before implanting the final cup, it is essential to achieve excellent stability of the trial cup by hollowing out the acetabulum. Size 52mm was most commonly used (series range 46mm to 60mm). Eighty-seven percent of the cups were fixed solely with the spikes; most often, two spikes were used. In 13% of cases where the primary stability appeared to be inadequate, stability was achieved by replacing one spike with a screw.

In 54% of cases, a standard insert was used, and a flanged insert was used in 46% of cases. A head with a diameter of 22.22mm in cobalt chrome was implanted in only a single case (0.34%). In the other 293 cases (99.66%), a head with a diameter of 28mm was used. Eighty-two percent of the heads used were zirconia oxide.

The posterior approach was used in 74% of cases, and the anterior approach in 26%.

Due to a high performance instrumentation, peri-operative complications were rare: 5 cases of the femoral calcar splitting (1.7%), and 1 fracture of the greater trochanter (0.3%) were noticed and corrected during the operation.

Post-Operative Management

Patients got out of bed 24-48 hours after surgery and were weight-bearing with the use of crutches for the first month. Medical complications were observed in 6.8% of cases, of which 1.7% were thrombo-embolic complications. Post-operative surgical complications occurred in 4% of the cases: 1 femoral fracture (0.3%) on day 10 due to a fall, was corrected with a cemented prosthesis and reconstruction of the femur, 11 dislocations (3.7%) required orthopaedic reduction, but 3 of the 11 dislocations were reduced surgically. These dislocations correlate with the learning curve. Now that we no longer perform a capsulectomy and suture the capsular plane very carefully during the operation, the rate of post-operative dislocations is less than 1%.

10-Year Results

In June 2000, 10 years after implantation, 177 of the original 294 prostheses were recorded as functioning. Fifty-two cases were classified as deceased, 42 were lost to follow-up, and 23 were revised. Most of the time, the revisions were partial and were excluded from the 10 years analysis. We observed 2 infections. Other re-interventions during the first five years were linked to mechanical complications. After five years, problems linked to bearing surface, wear, and osteolysis, were responsible for re-interventions, as listed in Table 2.

More than half of the original 294 prostheses were recorded as functioning. Taking all 294 primary interventions into consideration, results showed that the ABG-HA prosthesis has a 92.18% survival rate at 10 years post implantation, if the change of the implant or only a part of the implant is a criteria of failure (Figure 1). The femoral component has a 97.62% survival rate (Figure 2), and the acetabular component has a survival rate of 95.92% (Figure 3).

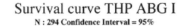

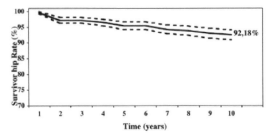

Figure 1 – Survival curve: revision of any component for prosthesis in primary THA : 92,18% at 10 years post implantation.

Cause and year of hips	Resulting of occurrence	Number change
Dislocation:		
1st	H, I	2
1st	C, H, I	1
Thigh pain:		
2nd	H, I, S	1
4th	H, I, S	1
Acetabular		
5th	C, H, I	1
7th	C, H, I	1
Acetabular		
7th	C, H, I	1
9th	C, H, I	1
10th	C, H, I	2
Femoral osteolysis		
6th	H, I	1
9th	H, I	2
Polyethylene wear:		
8th	C, H, I	1
Acetabular fracture:		
9th	C, H, I	1
Femoral fracture:		
1st	H, I, S	1
Femoral fracture:		
4th	H, I, S	1
Zirconia head		
2nd	H I	1
5th	H, I, S	1
Loosening		
2nd	C, H, I, S	1
Infection*		
2nd	C, H, I	1
Haemategenus		
5th	C, H, I, S	1
Total number of revisions		23

*Methicillin-resistant *Staphylococcus aureus*.
** E. Coli.

Table 2 – Cause, year and resulting change to prosthesis 10 years post implantation (C: Change of cup; H: Change of head; I: Change of insert; S: Change of stem).

RESULTS

Clinical Results

Clinical results were analyzed using the Postel Merle d'Aubigné (PMA) score. Ninety-five percent of the cases had very good results (PMA score > or = 17) and an average score increasing from 8.94 in the preoperative stage to 17.63 after 10 years (13 to 18) with 80% of the hips at 18. The same observation can be made for the pain score, which increased from 2.52 at the preoperative stage to 5.96 after 10 years. Ninety-six percent of the hips are at D6 (Table 3).

MDA	Average Scores	
(n=177 prostheses)		
	Before implantation	After implantation
Total/18	8.94	17.63
Pain/6	2.52	5.96
Mobility/6	3.02	5.86
Function/6	3.40	5.82

Table 3 – MDA (Postel-Merle d'Aubigne) scores before implantation and at 10 years post implantation.

This retrospective analysis of the clinical results demonstrates very high stability and the absence of early thigh pain conventionally observed with cementless implants without bioactive coating. These results correspond to the results generally published on bio-active coated hip prostheses.

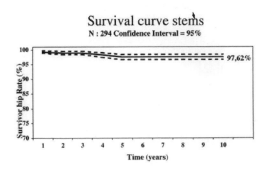

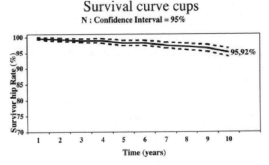

Figures 2 and 3 – Survivorship analysis for ABG Hip Prosthesis in primary THA at 10 years with regard to ABG stem (Fig.2) at 97.62%, and ABG cups (fig. 3) at 95.92%

Radiological Results

All the patients were re-examined after 3 months and every two years thereafter.

An standing position X-ray of the pelvis was taken as was an X-ray centered on a frontal view of the femur as well as a view displaying the entire stem and cup (Figure 4).

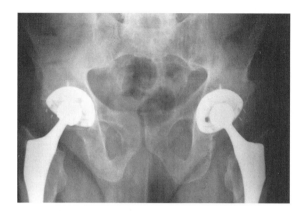

Figure 4 – ABG I THA: 10-year results on the left-ABG II THA: 5-year results on the right.

In the acetabulum, analysis of the cup position showed 80.55% with an angle of less than 45°, 15.28% with an angle of 45° to 50°, and 4.17% with an angle of more than 50°. Examination of the reaction of the bone in contact with the cup revealed an excellent bone-implant interface. We observed radiological silence in all three De Lee-Charnley zones (5). This radiological silence was observed after 3 months and remained unchanged at 10 years. Lucent lines, classically found in zone 3 with cementless cups without HA, were not observed with the ABG cups. There was no evidence of fracture or lucent lines around the spikes or the screws, indicating an absence of micro-movement in those areas (Figure 5).

In the femoral anterior/posterior view, 92.6% of the hips were centered: 7.4% were in varus and 0% in valgus. On the lateral views, no stems showed any cortical contact. Structural changes of femoral bone became evident at 3-6 months, with cancellous bone densification evident in the upper Gruen zones (1c, 2, 6, 7a and 7b). This densification remains stable at 10 years and relates to the prosthesis requirement of metaphyseal anchorage. Cortical thickening was observed in 9 cases (6%), in zones 3 and 5. Lucent lines often found in the

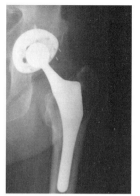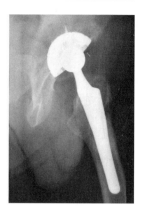

Figures 5a and 5b – ABG THA 10-year results A/P view (a) and lateral view (b).

metaphyseal zone 1 with cementless prosthesis without biological coating are rarely seen with the ABG prosthesis. In five percent (5%) of cases, a small lucent line is observed in zone 1A where the stem is not coated with HA. Similarly, reactive lines were observed from the first year onward in zones 3, 4, 5, all of which are zones without HA coating.

This radiological analysis confirms the osteointegration of the implants. Osteointegration is observed from the third month and remains constant, due to the initial stability of the implant. It is not correlated to age, sex, weight, or aetiology and remains stable over time, with no change during the 9-10 years of follow up, and seems to be directly related to the bioactive coating.

Polyethylene Wear

From the fifth year, a radiological measurement of the wear based on the Livermore procedure using a template (7), was included in the radiological files. At 10 years, the average wear is 0.79mm, which corresponds to an average annual wear of 0.08mm. Twenty-five percent of hips had no measurable wear, 75% showed measurable wear, of which 15% had an excessive wear (>0.12mm/y) of 1.3 to 3mm. This excessive wear is sometimes observed early. We could not find a significant correlation between wear, weight, aetiology or inclination of the cup. However, this wear seems to be correlated with the age and therefore the activity of the patient: The average age at the time of the intervention for patients with no measurable wear was 65 years (48-81), the average age at the time of the intervention for patients with measurable wear was

61 years (29-77), and the average age at the time of the intervention for patients with excessive wear was 58 years (33-76). However, excessive wear was more frequently observed in young men. Wear factors seem to be related to age, PE thickness (small cup) and quality, and to zirconia heads. However, in a retrieval study, we demonstrated that there was no third body wear related to HA resorption.

Osteolysis

The presence of osteolysis was detected on the femur and on the acetabulum.

Between 5 and 10 years, we observed 55 cases, 34 on the femur, 21 on the acetabulum, and 9 at both sites. Three cases of femoral osteolysis were reoperated with change of the insert and of the head, but without changing the stem or the cup. Six cases of acetabular osteolysis were reoperated with change of the cup, insert, and head but without changing the stem. We also grafted the cysts.

At 10 years, the incidence of osteolysis is twenty three percent (23%), and is more frequent at the femoral level (18.29%) than at the acetabular level (8.23%). A multifactorial analysis demonstrates three important risk factors, age, polyethylene wear, and individual factors. The level of physical activity can be related to age. The average age at the time of the hip intervention for patients with osteolysis at 10 years was 57.98 years, but for patients with acetabular osteolysis it was 47.46 years, with a very clear female predominance (72%). The average wear of hips with osteolysis after 10 years is 1.12mm (0-3mm) while the average wear of hips with no osteolysis is 0.69mm (0-2.8mm). Out of the 38 hips with osteolysis, 3 hips have no wear, 35 have measurable wear, of which 11 have excessive wear (>0.12mm/year). This wear was particularly seen in patients with small acetabula or in patients that were implanted with zirconia heads. The analysis of these explanted heads revealed a high percentage of grains in monoclinical phase. Individual factors clearly play a role, as some patients present early osteolysis without excessive wear; in bilateral cases, osteolysis is sometimes seen in both operated hips.

In our series, as far as prognosis is concerned, it seems important to differentiate acetabular osteolysis from femoral osteolysis. Acetabular osteolysis is more frequent in younger women, especially if they were implanted with a small cup and a zir-conia head. Acetabular osteolysis is mainly cyclical and located in the 3 Charnley zones. Femoral osteolysis is more frequent in men; it is always metaphyseal, never diaphyseal, and in 45% of cases is localized in Gruen zone 7a.

Osteolysis can occur when debris such as polyethylene particles induce bone damage by a chemical phenomenon involving the action of cytokines. In the femur, osteolysis occurs only at the metaphyseal level, providing strong evidence that HA is an excellent barrier to particle migration. At the acetabular level, particles migrate through the holes of the cup by a fluid pumping effect.

DISCUSSION

The specifications of the ABG-HA prosthesis are based on the primary stability of the implant associated with its shape. This is the necessary condition to achieve secondary fixation, due to the osteoconductive properties of HA. The retrospective clinical and radiological analyses of our series confirm that these specifications were fulfilled.

Clinical Results

In clinical terms, the results are excellent and are achieved from the third month after surgery onward. They were maintained in the various cases followed up to the tenth year after implantation as 86% of the hips were given a score of 18 on the MDA (1) scale. If moderate thigh pain was observed at 3 months, it disappeared at 1 year. Only 2 patients had to be revised for mechanical pain. Their pain was related to stems that were too big, with diaphyseal radiological contact and scintigraphic hot spots at the tip of the stem.

Radiological results

The reactions of the bone after implantation of an ABG hip prosthesis with hydroxyapatite are worthy of examination from the third month onward, in particular at a distance from the implant on account of their potentially evolutive nature.

Bone in contact with the implant

The reactions of the bone in contact with the implant provide a measure of osseointegration and therefore of the osteoconductive role of the hydroxyapatite (8, 9). In the acetabulum, the important feature is the radiological "silence" which is observed in all cases, with the acetabular bone seating perfectly maintained. This radiological silence appears at an early stage and is maintained over the 10-year follow-up. In the femur, densification of the cancellous bone in the metaphyseal zone appears from the third month in the anterior and lateral views, in accordance with the specifications. This densification becomes more pronounced as the years pass, spreading to zones 2 and 6. It remains stable at the 10-year follow-up with no alteration. The reactive lines were only observed around the zones 3, 4, and 5 of the stem, areas that have no HA coating. This occurs at an early stage, is seen from the third month onward, and can be confirmed histologically by the analysis of an explant removed because of poor positioning.

Bone at distance from the implant

At distance from the implant, the reaction of the bone is evidence of biomechanical disturbance caused by the placement of the implant; this disturbance is related to the surgical technique and the design of the implant. For the cup, the rationale requires the concept of "exact fit" with subchondral implantation. This was achieved in 94% of cases in our series. The bone seating is perfectly uniform in direct contact with the cup, without reactive or lucent lines. With regard to the impacted hemispherical shape, the forces must be transmitted uniformly to the subchondral bone, avoiding peak forces, especially in the area of primary fixation.

For the stem, the specifications require the concept of metaphyseal anchoring with undersizing in the diaphysis. As elastometric studies have shown, the transmission of forces into the diaphysis is more uniform when the implant is fixed in the upper metaphysis. Radiological analysis confirmed this with a low incidence of rounding of the calcar (16% at 10 years) and the rarity of cortical thickening in zones 2 and 6 (< 5%). This is why it appears essential to maintain a small safety triangle of cancellous bone in the lower exterior zone of the greater trochanter, in order to improve the transmission of forces to the femoral cortical bone. Oversizing in the metaphysis must be avoided. This was responsible for one case of pain lasting 2 years with appearance of cortical thickening in zones 2 and 6 in the second year after the operation.

Similarly, oversizing in the diaphysis must be avoided. This calls for flexible reaming. If not, there is a risk of radiological cortical thickening in zones 3 and 5 and excessive distal fixation as shown on CT scan analysis. The implant must be positioned with neither a varus nor a valgus deviation; varus alignment can give rise to pain at an early stage, which disappears over time, but may be associated with cortical thickening in zone 3. All this emphasizes the importance of pre-operative planning and close respect of the surgical technique. Even when the prosthesis is well positioned and correctly sized, the concept of the implant and therefore its design may give rise to changes in bone seating.

Wear and osteolysis

The remaining problem is that of the bearing surface between head and insert, with polyethylene wear, and in consequence, osteolysis in the medium term. However, Southwell (10) showed that the incidence of acetabular osteolysis is underestimated and requires complementary views.

Polyethylene wear has been the subject of many publications (11-14). Its occurrence has been blamed on the diameter and the material of the head, the thickness of the polyethylene, and the method of fixation of the cup and the design of the cup (cemented cup or metal-backed cup). The mean annual wear reported in the literature is between 0.1 and 0.2mm. The mean wear at ten years in our series is 0.79mm (0.08mm/year). However, whereas 25% of the hips had no measurable wear, 75% had measurable wear among which 22% had excessive wear (>0.12mm/year). This excessive wear was occasionally observed at an early stage; at the 5-year follow-up, it was seen in 8.3% of cases.

We have not seen any influence of gender, weight, aetiology, head diameter (32mm heads were not used), cup diameter, or angle on wear. Wear appears to be affected by age and therefore how active the patient is; the mean wear in patients under the age of 60 at the time of the operation is 0.98mm (0mm-3mm) at 10 years, whereas in the case of patients over the age of 70 at the time of the operation, it is 0.41mm (0mm-1.4mm). The analysis of explants originating from revisions on account of wear or osteolysis revealed no third body wear associated with resorption of HA coating. The problem of insert thickness and polyethylene quality remains; wear was blamed on sterilization procedures (irradiation).

WH Harris considers that osteolysis is the number one problem with hip prosthesis in 2000. Its frequency varies and has been reported in a number of publications; however, it appears to be observed more frequently with cementless prostheses than with cemented prostheses. Osteolysis may be discovered when clinically evident loosening occurs, but it is most commonly clinically silent and is discovered in the course of routine assessments. It may be located on the acetabulum, on the femur, or both on the femur and the acetabulum. It is undoubtedly underestimated in radiological examinations, especially in the acetabulum, and this may have the effect of increasing its incidence, especially in the acetabulum (hence the value of 3/4 views as demonstrated by Southwell). Out of the 294 hips, osteolysis was observed in 55 cases at the various follow-up examinations between 5 to 10 years; 34 were located in the femur and 21 in the acetabulum. In 9 cases, it was present both in the femur and the acetabulum. Nine hips were re-operated because of osteolysis; three cases of femoral osteolysis (2 men, 1 woman) required the insert and the head to be changed without changing either the cup or the stem and involved an allograft of cancellous bone in the femoral metaphysis. Six cases of acetabular osteolysis (5 women, 1 man) required change of cup, insert and head, with no change of stem; in 5 cases an ABGII-HA cup of a larger size had to be re-implanted with autograft and in 1 case a cemented cup had to be implanted. At 10 years, when including patients who died and patients lost to follow-up, the incidence of osteolysis is 23%; 18% for the femur, and 8% for the acetabulum.

Osteolysis is occasionally detected early, from the fifth year in our series. Its incidence increases with time (5% at 5 years, 23% at ten years). We felt that it was appropriate to compare femoral and acetabular osteolysis in terms of progression.

Femoral osteolysis, which is most frequent, is most readily encountered in men with a mean age of 60 years. It was observed solely in the metaphyseal zone and never in the diaphyseal zone. Most often lesions are confined to Gruen zones 7A or 1A (47%) and are usually clinically silent. Three of the 34 cases of femoral osteolysis observed were re-operated on (8.8%).

Acetabular osteolysis is less common, and predominantly observed in young, active women with a mean age of 47 years. It is often discovered on account of pain of mechanical origin with presence of cysts revealed by X-ray analysis. Lesions are occasionally multiple and located in one or more DeLee-Charnley zones. They often necessitate revision surgery because 6 hips (28.5%) out of the 21 with acetabular osteolysis were re-operated on, two of them in the same patient.

A multifactorial analysis enabled us to demonstrate several factors which favor the occurrence of osteolysis – age, gender, and polyethylene wear – being said that this rate of osteolytic lesion may be sometimes difficult to address (15). Age is usually related to the activity level of the patient. The mean age at the time of the arthroplasty in the series was 65 years. Mean age of patients with femoral osteolysis was 58 years, but it was 47 years for patients with acetabular osteolysis. Even though patients with femoral osteolysis were predominantly male, there was a very distinct predominance of women in cases of acetabular osteolysis (72%). At 10 years, the mean polyethylene wear of hips with osteolysis is 1.12mm, whereas the mean wear of hips without osteolysis is 0.69mm. Of the 38 hips with osteolysis, 3 hips had no wear, 35 had measurable wear, and of these 11 had excessive wear. This degree of wear was encountered mainly in small cups (< 54mm) and with zirconia heads, as pointed out by Kim *et al.* (16). The analysis of explants revealed a high percentage of grains in the monoclinical phase.

As for the mechanism of osteolysis, it is clear that the role of polyethylene particles must be borne in mind, as their accumulation has a cytotoxic effect on the bone (17). Individual factors arise because in five patients (10 hips) the osteolysis was bilateral, with an acetabular location in 9 cases out of ten. Two female patients had both hips re-operated on. The predominance of women among the cases of acetabular osteolysis raises the problem of the quality of the cancellous bone associated with the bone remodeling classically observed during menopause. However, the implant must share part of the blame. As a number of authors have stressed, the thickness and in particular the quality of the polyethylene must undoubtedly be taken into account. We were impressed, during revision surgery for wear or osteolysis, by the yellowish and delaminated appearance of the inserts. In several explants with minimal wear, we found that particles had entered by impingement between the neck and the flange of the insert when a hooded insert was used. In addition, particles migrate into the acetabulum via the holes of the cup by means of a pumping effect, and then accumulate in the cancellous bone of the acetabulum (hence a modified design of the ABG II cup without holes). At the femoral level, hydroxyapatite appears to form an excellent barrier to particle migration, as we have encountered only cases of metaphyseal osteolysis, and never diaphyseal osteolysis.

CONCLUSION

At follow-up after 10 years, the clinical results with the ABG HA prosthesis are comparable to those in the best series of hip replacement operations published in the literature. To achieve such results the surgical technique must be adhered to strictly. Radiology reveals that osseointegration is stable and durable with no sign of loosening of the cup or of the stem. However, we are worried by the problems associated with the bearing surfaces, occasionally with excessive polyethylene wear or osteolysis, the incidence of which is 23.17% at 10 years. This prompts us to make use of ceramic-ceramic bearing surfaces in young and active subjects.

Reference List

1. Merle D'Aubigne R (1990) Numerical classification of the function of the hip. *Rev. Chir. Orthop. Reparatrice Appar. Mot.* 76(6):371-4.

2. Epinette JA, Geesink RGT (1995) Radiographic assessment of cementless hip prostheses: ARA, a proposed new scoring scoring system – in Cahiers d'Enseignement de la SOFCOT: "Hydroxyapatite Coated Hip and Knee Arthroplasty", L'Expansion scientifique Ed. Paris, France, n° 51:114-26.

3. Kaplan EL, Meier P (1958) Non parametric estimation from incomplete observations. *J. Am. Stat. Assoc.* 457-81.

4. Gruen TA, McNeice GM, Amstutz HC (1979) "Modes of failure" of Cemented Stem type femoral components. A Radiographic Analysis of Loosening. *Clinical Orthopaedics* 141:17-27.

5. DeLee JG, Charnley J (1976) Radiological demarcation of cemented sockets in total hip replacement. *Clin. Orthop.* (121):20-32.

6. Brooker AF, Bowerman JW, Robinson RA, Riley RH (1973) Ectopic ossification following total hip replacement: incidence and a method of classification. *J. Bone Joint Surgery* 55-A: 1629-31.

7. Livermore J, Ilstrup D, Morrey B (1990) Effect of femoral head size on wear of the polyethylene acetabular component. *J. Bone Joint Surg. Am. Apr.* 72(4):518-28

8. Geesink RG (2002) Osteoconductive coatings for total joint arthroplasty. *Clin. Orthop.* (395):53-65.

9. D'Antonio JA, Capello WN, Manley MT, Geesink R (2001) Hydroxyapatite femoral stems for total hip arthroplasty: 10- to 13-year follow-up. *Clin. Orthop.* (393):101-11.

10. Southwell DG, Bechtold JE, Lew WD, Schmidt AH (1999) Improving the detection of acetabular osteolysis using oblique radiographs. *J. Bone Joint Surg. Br.* 81(2):289-95.

11. Pollock D, Sychterz CJ, Engh CA (2001) A clinically practical method of manually assessing polyethylene liner thickness. *J. Bone Joint Surg. Am..* 83-A(12):1803-9.

12. Dumbleton JH, Manley MT, Edidin AA (2002) A literature review of the association between wear rate and osteolysis in total hip arthroplasty. *J. Arthroplasty.* 17(5):649-61.

13. Terefenko KM, Sychterz CJ, Orishimo K, Engh CA Sr (2002) Polyethylene liner exchange for excessive wear and osteolysis. *J. Arthroplasty* 17(6):798-804.

14. Bragdon CR, Malchau H, Yuan X, Perinchief R, Karrholm J, Borlin N, Estok DM, Harris WH (2002) Experimental assessment of precision and accuracy of radiostereometric analysis for the determination of polyethylene wear in a total hip replacement model. *J. Orthop. Res.* 20(4):688-95.

15. Engh CA Jr, Sychterz CJ, Young AM, Pollock DC, Toomey SD, Engh CA Sr (2002) Interobserver and intraobserver variability in radiographic assessment of osteolysis. *J. Arthroplasty* 17(6):752-9.

16. Kim YH, Kim JS, Cho SH (2001) A comparison of polyethylene wear in hips with cobalt-chrome or zirconia heads. A prospective, randomised study. *J. Bone Joint Surg. Br.* 83(5):742-50.

17. Akisue T, Bauer TW, Farver CF, Mochida Y (2002) The effect of particle wear debris on NFkappaB activation and pro-inflammatory cytokine release in differentiated THP-1 cells. *J. Biomed. Mater. Res.* 59(3):507-15.

6   The ABG Hydroxyapatite-Coated Hip Prosthesis Followed-up for 9-11 Years

Alfons J. Tonino, MD, PhD, Kees J.M. Oosterbos, MD, Ali I.A. Rahmy, MD
and Wendy D. Witpeerd

INTRODUCTION

When John Charnley pioneered total hip arthroplasty (THA) more than 30 years ago, fixation and wear of the components were the two major challenges he faced; these two problems have still not been totally resolved. To achieve permanent fixation, the surfaces of uncemented prostheses are textured with, for example, a metal porous coating or a hydroxyapatite (HA) coating, to allow direct bone ingrowth or ongrowth.

Animal and postmortem studies indicate that HA-coated implants have osteoconductive properties by enhancing direct bone formation at the interface without the formation of an intermediate layer of fibrous tissue (1-7), thus forming a secure, strong bond with living bone over a relatively short period of time even under loaded conditions (1-10). Extensively porous-coated cementless implants also have good results with biologic fixation (11). However, with these extensively coated stems, there were concerns regarding thigh pain and the development of proximal bone atrophy through stress shielding (11-14).

As it is certain that the occurrence and severity of thigh pain are not related to patient factors, or even to the presence or absence of osseointegration, it was thought that proximal offloading at the femoral metaphysis could potentially decrease the incidence of thigh pain and at the same time preserve bone stock in this area. Therefore, new stems were designed for proximal offloading by way of proximal osseointegration only. Indeed, early and medium clinical results with proximally HA-coated prostheses have shown reliable proximal osseointegration (15-20) with negligible mid-thigh pain.

It became clear that a mismatch between the elastic modulus of these uncemented stems and the femoral diaphysis must be one of the decisive factors for the origin of thigh pain, but the issue of proximal stress shielding in the long term still needed to be determined. We know that augmented proximal stress shielding-induced bone resorption can theoretically start a failure scenario (26). Therefore, the long-term success of most prostheses is directly influenced by the distribution of stress transfer, which mainly depends on prosthetic design and bonding characteristics (21-25). Extensively porous-coated cementless stems are designed for total stem osseointegration and will therefore produce even more stress shielding (21, 22, 26).

The hip prosthesis described in this article is designed for only proximal osseointegration and, therefore, only proximal off loading. To enhance further proximal offloading and to inhibit distal off loading, the stem had an anatomic shape, which permitted distal overreaming. This prospective one-center study presents the clinical and radiographic results of 151 consecutive primary total hip arthroplasties (THA) with a cementless HA coated prosthesis designed for proximal stem osseointegration. The first goal was to evaluate, through clinical and radiographic assessment, whether or not the prosthesis did fulfill the design criteria. The second goal of the study was to confirm that proximal circumferential osseointegration reduces or eliminates femoral diaphyseal osteolysis.

PATIENTS AND METHODS

Between May 1990 and August 1992, 151 consecutive primary THA's were performed in 134 patients in our teaching hospital using a cementless

HA-coated prosthesis. The average age of the patients at the time of surgery was 68 years (range 34-84 years). Forty hips were implanted in men and 111 in women; the mean body weight of the patients was 72kg (range 37-110kg), and their mean height was 1.65cm (range 1.25-1.95cm). The left hip was replaced in 66 cases, the right hip in 85. Primary osteoarthritis was the most common diagnosis (126 cases), followed by rheumatoid arthritis (13 cases), avascular necrosis (5 cases), femoral neck fracture (3 cases) and 4 cases for other reasons.

The Anatomique Benoist Girard (ABG, Stryker Newbury, England) hip prosthesis (fig. 1) was used. The stem is available in 9 sizes and is made of a titanium alloy (Ti6Al4V). The proximal third is HA-coated and has a macrorelief scaled surface. The scales on the anterior, posterior, and medial surfaces were designed to transform any shear forces into compression forces. There is an area of transition between the coated metaphysis and the non coated diaphysis of the stem to avoid chipping of the HA during insertion.

To accommodate the proximal anatomic press-fit, there is a bend of 7° starting 1cm distal of this transition point, whereas the neck shows an extra 5° antetorsion giving a total of 12° of anteversion to the coronal plane. This accommodation is important to obtain proximal rotational stability, regardless of diaphyseal fill. The stem is not polished distally but has a grit-blasted surface texture (roughness 2.59µm) and incorporates a slight distal taper. The acetabular component is a hemispherical, totally HA-coated press-fit cup available in 14 sizes. We used 28mm cobalt-chromium (CoCr) heads for all cases, including hips with a diameter less than 50mm.

The HA coating was applied with a vacuum plasma-spray torch on a sublayer of pure titanium, to improve the tensile adhesion of the HA of the implant. This vacuum treatment maximized the quality and homogeneity of the coating. The HA coating of the implant had the following characteristics: a chemical purity of 100% crystallinity before coating as determined by X-ray diffraction at low speed and > 75% crystallinity post-coating. The porosity was < 10%. The tensile bond strength was 62 to 65MPa, and the thickness was 60mm (±20). The roughness of the HA-coated parts was 3 to 4mm. Each batch was tested to ensure that the specifications were achieved.

The surgery was performed in a standard operating theatre, and 3 different consultants operated. Systemic prophylactic antibiotics and oral anticoagulation were administered routinely. The approach was lateral (Hardinge approach) in 98 cases and anterolateral (Watson-Jones) in 53; no trochanteric osteotomies were made. The distal femur was reamed to a diameter slightly greater (1-1.5mm) than the diameter of the stem that was to be inserted. Full weight bearing with crutches was allowed immediately postoperatively.

All patients were included in a prospective follow-up study using the Merle d'Aubigné functional scoring system (27). They were reviewed again clinically and radiographically at 3, 6, and 12 months after surgery, and yearly thereafter. All changes were described using the Gruen zones (28) for the proximal femur and the De Lee and Charnley zones (29) for the acetabulum. Augmented wear was defined as a linear wear rate of > 0.1mm/year. Osteolysis was defined as a scalloped erosion of greater than 2mm in diameter at the bone-prosthesis interface. Resorption or densification of bone was not quantified but was graded as present or absent when compared with the previous set of radiographs. The position of the stem was considered to be in varus or valgus when it showed a deviation of ≥ 3° from the neutral. Likewise, using a radiographic template, both cranial and medial

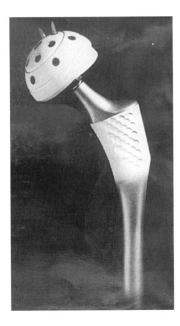

Figure 1 – The ABG hip prosthesis.

migration of the socket and the head were measured on standing AP radiographs. The stem was qualified as completely filling the medullary canal when less than 1mm was measured on both sides between the stem and the cortex on the AP radiograph. The components were defined as being fixed by osseointegration when there was no subsidence or migration and no formation of radiolucent or radiodense lines along the HA-coated portions of the prosthesis.

Statistical analysis of the results was performed, and the influences of clinical and radiographic variables were studied using the chi-square tests, the two-tailed Student's t test or logical regression, depending on group characteristics. Statistical significance was set at P < 0.05. Survival was calculated using revision or pending revision due to aseptic loosening as the definition of failure.

RESULTS

Forty-four patients (46 hips) died during the first 9 to 11 years from causes unrelated to the hip. None of them had a revision, and their clinical notes at the last annual assessment recorded similar outcomes to those of the living patients. None of the patients were lost to follow-up; 105 hips were available for evaluation, and 101 original stems and 100 original cups were still *in situ*.

Perioperatively, 5 fissures of the proximal femur occurred. Two perioperative fractures of the greater trochanter were displaced over time, and one needed internal fixation. There were 5 wound hematomas, one superficial infection, and 3 deep infections. Two cured completely, but the third one ended with a Girdlestone in a patient who had had an infected but healed osteosynthesis for a lateral femoral neck fracture. This patient did not want to be reoperated. Two transient lesions of the femoral nerve were seen, while one sciatic lesion recovered only partially. This last patient was reoperated elsewhere two years later to shorten the leg. Both components were fully osseointegrated at revision. There were two early dislocations. None developed into a recurrent dislocation. There were three late stem revisions; one after a periprosthetic fracture 5 years after the index THA, one for unexplained thigh pain and one in the patient with the ischiatic nerve lesion. All four patients without the original stem had been operated on by the same consultant.

The clinical results are summarized in Table I and show a marked improvement in pain and total scores from pre-operative (MdA = 8) to the 3-month visit onward (MdA = 15) up to 10 years (MdA = 17). There was a low incidence of early (10%) and late thigh pain (6%). The inclination of the metal acetabular component as measured on standing AP radiogram was between 40° and 55° in 68% of the hips. In 32% of the hips, the angle was 55° or more. All acetabular components showed good osseointegration without any migration. In 13 hips, osteolytic changes appeared in the pelvic bone around the acetabular component (fig. 2). Signs of augmented polyethylene wear were noted in 43 cases at 10 years. Cups that were inserted with an inclination of 55° or more showed significantly augmented wear (P < 0.001). Five cups had to be revised after a mean of 9.2 years (range 7.7-10.7) because of augmented PE-wear induced acetabular osteolysis. All five patients had positive Technetium uptake after earlier normal scintigraphic patterns were observed. Two of these five cups showed aseptic loosening and migration, while the other three were still firmly fixed at revision. No cup revisions were pending at the last date of follow-up.

	Pre-operation (N=151)	3 months (N=150)	10 years (N=105)
Pain	1.9	5.5	5.8
Mobility	3.7	5.6	5.9
Ability to walk	2.7	4.6	5.7
Total	8.3	15,7	17.4

Table 1 – Clinical results: Merle D'Aubigné Functional Grading (mean scores)

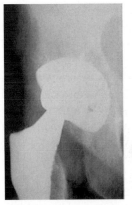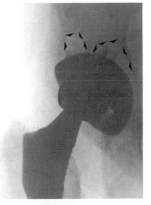

Figure 2 – Case 17. There is progressive osteolysis of the acetabulum after 9 years, necessitating cup revision.

On the first postoperative radiograph, 20 femoral stems were in varus and 1 was in valgus. The positions did not change significantly during the follow up. Slight distal migration of the stem (< 5 mm) was observed in 3 patients at 3 months, but had stopped at 6 months. Late subsidence occurred in only one patient who sustained a periprosthetic fracture of the proximal femur after a fall; the stem became loose and was revised.

Structural changes of the femoral bone became apparent between 3 and 6 months after THA. Densifications of cancellous bone were seen along the femoral stem at the point of transition between the coated and non-coated parts of the stem in Gruen zones 2 and 6, from 3 months onward. These endosteal bone densifications were progressive in frequency and appeared in 63% of cases in Gruen zones 2 and in 69% of cases in Gruen zone 6 at 5 years. At 10 years, it appeared in Gruen zone 2 in 81% of the cases and in Gruen zone 6 in 86% of the cases. From 1 year onward, these areas of bone apposition slowly expanded distally into the upper parts of Gruen zones 3 (45%) and 5 (44%) at 5 years and were noted in Gruen zone 3 in 84% of the cases and in Gruen zone 5 in 86% of cases at 10 years.

Between the first and second year postoperatively, endosteal reactive lines became visible on radiographs in Gruen zone 4. The incidence increased strongly between the second and third year, after which its incidence decreased to the level at one year follow-up. At 1 year, it was 47%, at 3 years 80%, at 5 years 63%, and at 9 years 45%.

Resorption of bone was mainly observed in Gruen zone 7A; it was observed with progressive frequency particularly after the second year. Later, it also became prominent in Gruen zone 1. At 5 years, it was present in Gruen zone 7 in 43% of the hips. Thereafter, it progressed slowly to 48% in this area at 9 years. In Gruen zone 1, it was present in 50% of the hips at 5 years, and by 9 years it had progressed to 74%.

Densification of cortical bone was observed in Gruen zones 2, 3, 5, and 6 from 3 years onward and measured 12%, 3%, 3%, and 15%, respectively, at the 5-year visit. There was only progression in Gruen zones 3 and 5 because at 10 years the percentages for cortical bone densification were 14%, 19%, 34%, and 14% for Gruen zones 2, 3, 5, and 6 respectively.

The pattern of peripheral thickening of the femoral cortex followed that of cortical bone densification. Observed from the third postoperative year

onward, it was noted in 10%, 7%, 5%, and 7% of the hips in Gruen zones 2, 3, 5, and 6, respectively, at the 5-year visit. At the last follow-up, these figures were 14%, 13%, 30%, and 17%, respectively.

Small cyst formation (< 5mm in diameter) as a sign of polyethylene-wear induced osteolysis was observed in Gruen zone 7A in 3 cases at 9 years and in Gruen zone 1 in 8 cases at 9 years. However, no radiolucent lines around any femoral component were noted, and there were no signs of impending failure of any stem or cup.

Periarticular ossifications were recorded using the Brooker grading system (5). At the last visit, 44% of the hips had grade I ossifications, 6% had grade II, 2% had grade III, and 0% had grade IV.

The cumulative survival at 10 years was 98.78% (fig. 3) for the acetabular component (95% confi-

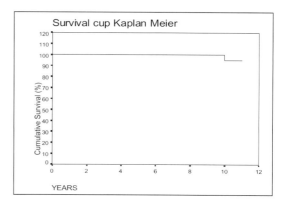

Figure 3.

dence interval between 0.97 and 0.99) and 100% (fig. 4) for the femoral stem (95% confidence interval between 0.99) and 1.00 taking aseptic loosening as an endpoint. For the worst case scenario,

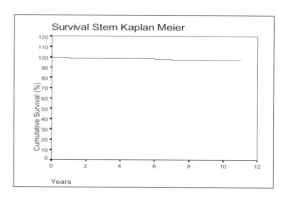

Figure 4.

this figure was 95.85% (3 extra cup revisions), (95% confidence interval between 0.921 and 0.985) for the acetabular cup and 96.70% (3 extra stem failures), (95% confidence interval between 0.959 and 0.996) for the stem. The combined cumulative survival rate for both cups and stems is given in figure 5.

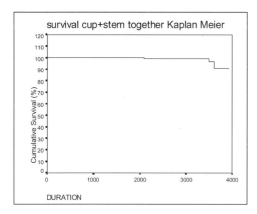

Figure 5.

DISCUSSION

With a mean follow-up period of 10.1 years, the clinical results of this prosthesis may now be compared with the 10-years results of several other non-cemented prostheses (30-36). Since the patients were considerably older (mean age 68 years) than patients in most other studies, one might assume that the present study contained more patients with poorer quality bone stock. Although only 50% had a good bone stock score when evaluated using the modified Singh index, this did not compromise clinical success and osseointegration.

Survival rates of cemented stems have increased through time together with improvement of cementing techniques (37, 38, 39). The same can now be observed with cementless stems, where improvements of the coating have resulted in even slightly better long term survival rates, with figures for aseptic loosening smaller than 1% after 10 years of follow up (35-36). This means that the concept of bone ongrowth to proximal, HA-coated and proximal porous-coated stems is a valid concept for long term fixation of this component.

While for cemented stems survival rates are mainly determined by cement properties and

cementing techniques rather than prosthetic design, the large differences of survival rates for different uncemented stems are more a reflection of the large differences in design and surface structure rather than surgical technique. Nevertheless, also from our series it became obvious that one surgeon (with a stem failure rate of 4/18 THA or 22%) can be a key variable for surgical outcome.

This concept of bone ongrowth and persistent osseointegration is also acknowledged by histology and histomorphometry from cadaver retrieved specimens after years of successful hip function (6, 7). However it was also noted from these studies that the HA layer was nearly resorbed after 7-8 years of implantation, and that ongoing fixation of the components in the long term was rather more dependent of the quality and roughness of the underlying surface texture of the substrate.

Although the survival rate of this acetabular cup was also very high (98,78%) at ten years, taking aseptic loosening as endpoint, the survival rate dropped to 96.70% when taking revision as endpoint; this is also seen in many other studies (40-43). The poor performance of press-fit cups in these studies has been the success limiting factor of the procedure. However, also in screwed cups like the Harris-Galante cup, augmented polyethylene wear induced osteolysis (24%), was noted after a mean of 7 years follow-up (44). Although from the patients view it is irrelevant to separate the survival of the acetabular and the femoral component, from the investigators point of view and for further research it matters quite a lot.

Therefore, there is reason for concern about the relatively high percentage of polyethylene induced acetabular osteolysis in these kind of press-fit metal-backed cups with open screw holes. From our series, we can indicate three reasons for this elevated level of PE-wear. First, the decision we made when using 28mm heads instead of 22mm heads in cups under 50mm size. This decision had directly negative consequences for the thickness of the polyethylene liner, and as is clear from literature, a certain amount of thickness of the polyethylene liner is mandatory for preventing accelerated wear (45.46). Second, the wrong placement of the cup in too steep a position (> 55°) had negative consequences. In four of the five cup revisions, the cup showed a lateral opening between 55° and 73°. Although technical faults of surgical technique are a rather constant factor in hip surgery (47), this factor should and could be minimized by continuous attention to surgical detail. We do suggest a much larger place for surgical technique in re-education programs, apart from the further development of navigation techniques, which surely will become standard procedure in the future.

Last but not least, we think that the 10 of 12 holes of this cup which were not used for a spike or screw also form an important risk factor by allowing ingress of polyethylene wear particles into the open, reamed acetabular bone. While it has been shown that short periods of oscillating fluid pressure directed at an osseointegrated titanium-bone interface may lead to osteolysis (48-50) and debonding, it is also obvious that the pressure gradient through a large hole is much less than through a small hole. Manley *et al.* (51) observed the highest frequency of osteolysis in DeLee-Charnley zone I for cups with small holes, while the threaded cup with only one larger central hole showed osteolysis in zone II only. Also, our observations from the radiographs, and our experiences during cup revision, do confirm that the noted osteolysis starts from the empty screw holes and is predominantly in DeLee-Charnley zone I. Therefore, we do believe that the fluid pressure theory is one of the most important causes for the rapid spread of polyethylene wear particle debris into the acetabular bone.

In contrast to the noted acetabular osteolysis, no distal or linear osteolysis around the stem was observed in any case after 9 to 11 years of follow up. Also, in the cases that augmented acetabular osteolysis, where the extended joint space surely also had extended to the femoral side, only very moderate local cystic osteolysis was noted in 8 cases. This can only be explained by a complete proximal sealing of the medullary cavity by circumferential bone ongrowth. Histology of retrieved autopsy specimens have acknowledged this circumferential sealing through circumferential osseointegration (6).

The radiographic bone remodelling is characterized by a specific pattern of bony features in the proximal femur. Positive bone remodelling during the first 3 years in the form of endosteal bone apposition in Gruen zones 2 and 6 suggests that the load transfer from stem to femoral bone starts to occur mainly in this area, and that the prosthesis is securely bonded there. Somewhat later during the follow-up, between the third and fifth year, a slow process of bone resorption (negative bone remodeling) in the region of the lesser and greater

trochanter starts. The concomitant formation of a reactive line around the distal part of the stem in Gruen zones 3, 4, and 5 is thought to be consistent with the presence of a local fibrous interface as a result of micromotion in this area without distal offloading.

These three characteristic radiographic features did at first confirm the design goal for the femoral stem – that osseointegration should occur mainly proximally. In fact, after 5 years, most of the bone apposition occurs adjacent to that part of the femoral stem where the HA coating ends, the so-called transitional zone. We would have expected the apposition to occur more proximally, since the coating was present only on the proximal one third of the stem. Instead, we found that the region in which the most prominent cancellous and cortical densifications were observed gradually shifted from proximally in Gruen zones 2 and 6 to more distally in these same zones, or even more distally into Gruen zones 3 and 5. Formation of new bone in the area near the lower edge of HA coatings was predicted by Huiskes *et al.* (21) using finite element analysis. The explanation was that particularly in this area endosteal stress concentrations are caused by the abrupt transition from a bonded to a loose interface.

However, concomitant with the decrease in incidence of the reactive line after the 5 year follow up, the incidence of cortical thickening, and especially of cortical densification, is clearly augmented, especially for Gruen zone 3 and 5. This also indicates a shift from proximal offloading to distal offloading. Other authors already observed more cortical thickening around HA-coated stems in a much earlier stage. D'Antonio *et al.* (18) observed 47% cortical thickening in Gruen zone 5 along with 63% calcar resorption after 6 years with a proximally coated stem. Geesink and Hoefnagels (16) using the same design of prosthesis reported nearly the same figures. Vedantam and Ruddlesdin (52), inserting a completely HA coated stem, reported 26-46% cortical hypertrophy in Gruen zones 3 and 5 after only 2 years with femoral neck resorption in more than 57% of cases.

The phenomenon of cortical hypertrophy was also noted with cementless, non-HA coated stems. Mulliken *et al.* (53) reported this cortical hypertrophy in 35% of their patients, especially in Gruen zones 3 and 5. In non-cemented, porous-coated hips, it was observed that poorly fitting stems were less likely to become fixed by bony ingrowth. Therefore, in order to achieve predictable fixation, it was advised to implant the stem with a tight fit at the isthmus and to fill the medullary canal completely. These authors advised inserting the largest stem that the femoral canal will allow. But in a former article (20), we already showed that the concept of transitional load transfer from proximal to distal is morphologically dependent on the way the stem fills the medullary canal. Mulliken *et al.*, in their study of 416 non-cemented THAs (53), could not explain this finding, but Whiteside (54), in his study on the effect of stem fit on bone hypertrophy, observed that 24 of the 67 patients in the tight distal stem group showed distal cortical hypertrophy, while none of the 38 patients with a loose distal fit, did. Therefore, diaphyseal fill is not pursued with the ABG prosthesis, and this may be the explanation for the less than 30% distal cortical thickening observed in Gruen zone 5 after 10 years of follow-up.

Therefore, anatomical shape, distal overreaming and a proximal coating have proven to be all three determining factors for reducing distal offloading.

CONCLUSION

Our results confirm that fixation by means of bone ongrowth of this proximally HA-coated hip prosthesis is very reliable and a valid concept for enduring component fixation, irrespective of factors such as age, sex, weight, activity or quality of bone stock and diagnosis.

Secondly, radiographic follow-up showed that bone remodelling around the stem was an ongoing process with most of the positive bone remodelling (bone formation) preceding the negative bone remodelling (bone resorption). As distal cortical densifications and distal peripheral cortical thickening were augmented primarily between 5 and 9 years, this sign of augmented distal offloading does challenge the original concept of this prosthesis. It was in reconsidering the starting concept of this proximal HA-coated stem intended for only proximal stress transfer and proximal off loading that the ABG II stem was developed. This ABG II stem is shorter and is distally polished to prevent distal bone ongrowth in order to prevent distal off loading.

Thirdly, because of the observed augmented polyethylene wear induced acetabular osteolysis behind the empty screw holes, a no-holes metal backed cup was developed along with the development of other bearings like crosslinked, stabilized polyethylene and ceramic bearings. Our findings do suggest that this hydroxyapatite coating provides an excellent, stable prosthesis-bone interface and is preferable to any other fixation method.

References List

1. Overgaard S, Lind M, Glerup H *et al.* (1995) Hydroxyapatite and fluorapatite coatings for fixation of weight loaded implants. *Clin. Orthop.* 336:286.

2. Søballe K, Hansen ES, Brockstedt-Rasmussen H, Bunger C (1993) Hydroxyapatite coating converts fibrous tissue to bone around loaded implants. *J. Bone Joint Surg.* 75-B:270.

3. Bauer JD, Geesink RCT, Zimmermaan R, McMackon JT (1991) Hydroxyapatite coated femoral stems. *J. Bone Joint Surg.* 74-A:1439.

4. Frayssinet P, Hardy D, Conte P *et al.* (1993) Histological analysis of the bone-prosthesis interface after implantation in humans of prostheses coated with hydroxyapatite. *J. Orthop. Surg.* 7:246.

5. Hardy DCR, Frayssinet P, Guilhem A *et al.* (1991) Bonding of hydroxyapatite coated femoral prostheses: histopathology of speciments from four cases. *J. Bone Joint Surg.* 73-B:732.

6. Tonino AJ, Therin M, Doyle C (1999) Hydroxyapatite coated femoral stems: histology and histomorphometry around five components retrieved at autopsy. *J. Bone Joint Surg.* B 81-B:148.

7. Tonino AJ, Oosterbos C, Rahmy A, Therin M, Doyle C (2001) Hydroxyapatite-coated Acetabular Components. *J. Bone Joint Surg.* 83-A:817.

8. Donnelly WJ, Kobayashi A, Freeman MAR *et al.* (1997) Radiological and survival comparison of four methods of fixation of a proximal femoral stem. *J. Bone Joint Surg. Br.* 79:351.

9. Søballe K, Hansen ES, Brockstedt-Rasmussen H *et al.* (1991) Gap healing enhanced by hydroxyapatite coatings in dogs. *Clin. Ortop.* 272:300.

10. Geesink RGT, de Groot K, Klein CPAT (1988) Bonding of bone to apatite coated implants. *J. Bone Joint Surg.* 70-B:17.

11. McAuley JP, William J, Culpepper MA, Charles A. Engh (1998) Total hip arthroplasty. Concerns with extensively porous coated femoral components. *Clin. Orthop.* 355:182-8.

12. McAuley JP, Moreau GM, Ostrowski J, Desjardins DR (1998) Proximal versus extensively coated femoral components in total hip arthroplasty : Clinical and radiographic comparison. *Orthop. Trans.* 21:1131.

13. Campbell AC, Rorabeck CH, Bourne RB, Chess D, Nott L (1992) Thigh pain after cementless arthroplasty: Annoyance or ill omen? *J. Bone Joint Surg.* 74-B:63-66.

14. Engh CA, Bobyn JD (1988) The influence of stem size extent of porous coating on femoral bone remodeling after primary cementless hip arthroplasty. *Clin. Orthop.* 231:7-28.

15. Geesink RGT, Hoefnagels NHM (1995). Six-year results of hydroxyapatite coated hip replacement. *J. Bone Joint Surg.* 77-B:534.

16. Tonino AJ, Romanini L, Rossi P *et al.* (1995) Hydroxyapatite coated hip protheses. *Clin. Orthop.* 312:211.

17. D'Antonio JA, Capello WN, Manley MT (1996) Remodeling of bone around Hydroxyapatite coated femoral stems; *J. Bone Joint Surg.* 78-A:1226.

18. Garcia Araujo C, Gonzalez FJ, Tonino AJ, International ABG Study Group (1998) Rheumatoid arthritis and hydroxyapatite coated hip prosthese: five year results. *J. Arthroplasty* 6:660.

19. Tonino AJ, MD, AIA Rahmy and the International ABG Study Group: (2000) 5- to 7- Year results from an international multicentre study. *J. Arthroplasty* 15:274.

20. Oosterbos C, Rahmy A, Tonino AJ (2001) Hydroxyapatite coated hip prosthesis. Int. Orthopaedics.

21. Huiskes R, Weinans H, Dalstra M (1989) Adaptive bone remodeling and biomechanical design considerations. *Orthopaedics* 12:1255.

22. Huiskes R (1990) Various stress patterns of press-fit, ingrowth and cemented femoral stems. *Clin. Orthop.* 261:27.

23. Skinner HB, Curlin FJ (1990) Decreased pain with lower flexural rigidity of uncemented femoral prostheses. *Orthopaedics* 13:1223.

24. Franks E, Mont MA, Maar DC *et al.* (1992) Thigh pain as related to bending rigidity of the femoral prostheses and bone. *Trans. Orthop. Res. Soc.* 38:296.

25. Mont MA, Hungerford DS (1997) Proximally coated ingrowth prostheses: a review. *Clin. Orthop.* 344:139.

26. Huiskes R (1993) Failed innovation in total hip replacement: diagnosis and proposals for a cure. *Acta Orthop. Scand.* 64:699.

27. Merle d'Aubignee R, Postel M (1954) Functional results of hip arthroplasty with acrylic prosthesis. *J. Bone Joint Surg.* 36-A:451.

28. Gruen TA, McNeice JM, Amstutz HC (1979) Modes of failure of cemented stem type femoral components: a radiographic analysis of loosening. *Clin. Orthop.* 141:17.

29. DeLee JH, Charnley J (1979) Radiological demarcation of cemented sockets in total hip replacement. *Clin. Orthop.* 121:20.

30. Engh CA, Culpepper WJ and Ch. A Engh (1997) Long-term results of use of the anatomic medullary locking prosthesis in total hip arthroplasty. *J. Bone Joint Surg.* 79-A:177.

31. Malchau H, Herberts P, Xing Wang Y, Karrholm J, Romanus B (1996) Long-term clinical and radiological results of the Lord total hip prosthesis. *J. Bone Joint Surg.* 78-B:884.

32. McLaughlin, Kyla R Lee (1997) Total hip arthroplasty with an uncemented femoral component. *J. Bone Joint Surg.* 79-A:900.

33. Eingartner C, Volkmann R, Winter E, Maurer F, Sauer G, Weller S, Weise K (2000) Results of an uncemented straight femoral shaft prosthesis after 9 years of follow-up. *J. Arthroplasty* 440:447.

34. Hellman EJ, William N, Capello, Feinberg JR (1999) Omnifit cementless total hip arthroplasty; a 10-year average follow-up. *Clin. Orthop.* 164:174.

35. McNally, SA, Shepperd JAN, Mann CV, Walczak JP (2000) The results at nine to twelve years of the use of a hydroxyapatite coated femoral stem. *J. Bone Joint Surg.* 82-B:378.

36. Delaunay C and Kapandji AI (2001) Survival analysis of cementless grit-blasted titaniom total hip arthroplasties. *J. Bone Joint Surg.* 83-B:408.

37. Britton AR, Murray DW, Bulstrode CJ, McPherson K, Denham RA (1996) Long-term comparison of Charnley and Stanmore design total hip replacements. *J. Bone Joint Surg.* 78-B:802.

38. Schulte, Callaghan JJ., Kelley SS, Johnston RC (1993) The outcome of Charnley total hip arthroplasty with cement after a minimum twenty-four follow-up. *J. Bone Joint Surg.* 75A:961.

39. Kale AA, Della Valle CJ, Frankel VH, Stuchin SA, Zuckerman JD, Di Cesare PE (2000) Hip arthroplasty with a collared straight cobalt-chrome femoral stem using second-generation cementing technique. *J. Arthroplasty* 2:187.

40. Bono JV, Sangord L, Toussaint JT (1994) Severe polyethylene wear in total hip arhtroplasty. *J. Arthroplasty* 9(2):119-25.

41. Barrack RB, Folgueras A, Munn B, Tvetden D, Sharkey P (1997) Pelvic lysis and polyethylene wear at 5-8 years in a uncemented total hip. *Clin. orthop.* 335: 211-7.

42. Hozack WJ, Rothman RH, Eng K, Mesa J (1996) Primary cementless hip arthroplasty with a titanium plasmasprayed prosthesis. *Clin. Orthop.* 333:217-25.

43. Owen TD, Moran CG, Smith SR, Pinder IM (1994) Results of uncemented porous-coated anatomic total hip replacement. *J. Bone Joint Surg.* 76:258-62.

44. Soto MO, Rodriquez JA, Ranawat CS (2000) Clinical and radiographic evaluation of the Harris-Galante Cup. *J. Arhtroplasty* 2:139.

45. Livermore J, Ilstrup D, Morrey B (1990) Effect of femoral head size on wear of the polyethylene acetabular component. *J. Bone Joint Surg.* 72A:518.

46. Devane PA, Robinson EJ, Bourne RB, Rorabeck CH, Nayak NN, Horne JG (1997) Measurement of ployethylene wear in acetabular components inserted with and without cement. *J. Bone Joint Surg.* 79A:682.

47. Herberts P, Malchau H (2000) Long-term registration has improved the quality of hip replacement; *Acta Orthop. Scand.* 71 (2):111-121.

48. Vis van der HM, Aspenberg P, Kleine de R, Tighelaar W, Noorden van CJF (1998) Short periods of oscillating fluid pressure directed at a titanium-bone interface in rabbits lead to bone lysis. *Acta Scand. Orthop.* 69:5-10.

49. Vis van der HM, Aspenberg P, Marti RK, Tighelaar W, Noorden van CJF (1998) Fluid pressure causes bone resorption in a rabbit model of prosthetic loosening. *Clin. Orthop.* 350:201.

50. Aspenberg P, Vis van der H (1998) Migration, particles and fluid pressure. A Discussion of causes of prosthetic loosening. *Clin. Orthop.* 352:75.

51. Manley MT, Capello WN, D'Antonio JA, Edidin AA, Geesink RGT (1998) Fixation of acetabular cups without cement in total hip arthroplasty. A comparison of three different implant surfaces at a minimum duration of follow-up of five years: *J. Bone Joint Surg.* 80A:1175.

52. Vendantam R, Ruddlesdin C (1996) The fully hydroxyapatite coated total hip implant. *J. Arthroplasty* 11:534-42.

53. Mulliken BD, Bourne RB, Rorabeck CH, Nayak N (1996) A tapered titanium femoral stem inserted without cement in a total hip arthroplasty: *J. Bone Joint Surg.* 78:1214-25.

54. Whiteside LA (1989) The effect of stem fit on bone hypertrophy and pain relief in cementless total hip arthroplasty. *Clin. Orthop.* 247:138-47.

7 Ten-Year Follow-Up Experience with an Hydroxyapatite-Coated Hip Arthroplasty

Aldo Toni MD, PhD, Francesco Traina MD, Susanna Stea BSCi., Barbara Bordini, BSCi., Enrico Guerra, MD, Alessandra Sudanese, MD and Armando Giunti, MD

INTRODUCTION

Total hip arthroplasty (THA) is one of the most commonly performed orthopaedic procedures. Despite the fact that it is widely investigated, there is a deficiency of long-term follow-up studies (27, 30) and none, to our knowledge, of cementless fully hydroxyapatite-coated arthroplasties with a ceramic on ceramic coupling. Independently from the fixation technique employed for the stem, wear debris produced in polyethylene-metal couplings were described as a possible cause of cortical osteolysis (5, 8, 15, 36). In our series, the ceramic bearing removes the confounding presence on outcomes of polyethylene wear. We report the ten year results of 151 prosthesis with a collarless hydroxyapatite-coated femoral stem and ceramic on ceramic coupling.

PATIENTS AND METHODS

Between June 1990 and December 1991, 147 consecutive patients underwent primary total hip arthroplasty (THA) with hydoxyapatite-coated femoral stems and ceramic-ceramic bearing surfaces (AnCA Cremascoli, Milan, Italy). All were primary surgeries, there were no specific exclusions; fifty-nine patients were male and 92 female, with a mean age of 58 years (male 59.6 ± 10.4, female 57.0 ± 9.0). Among these 147 patients, 4 underwent a bilateral replacement, for a total of 151 implants (Table 1). Charnley classification of patients (6) and preoperative diagnosis are shown respectively in Table 1 and 2. Ten died for causes unrelated to the surgery, still having their stem in place at the time of the last intermediate inquiry.

Variable	Patients	Prosthesis	Male	Female	Percent
Gender					
Male	57	59			39%
Female	90	92			61%
Total number	147	151			100%
Age*					
0-40	8	8	3	5	
41-69	131	135	49	82	
70 or more	8	8	5	3	
Total	147	151	57	90	
Charnley class**					
A Unilateral, healthy		84			56.8%
B Bilateral, healthy		45			30.4%
C Uni/bilateral, medical problems		19			12.8%
Bone graft					
No		135			89.4%
Femoral		6			4.0%
Acetabular		10			6.6%
Antibiotic prophylaxis					
Cefazolina		118			78.1%
Cefotaxime		33			21.9%
Thromboembolic prophylaxis					
Heparin		50			33.1%
Indobufene		96			63.6%
Heparin and Indobufene		5			3.3%
Body mass index§					
≤ 30		116			82.9%
≥ 30		24			17.1%

Table 1 – *mean age: male 59.6 ± 10.4, female 57.0±9.0; ** 3 lack values; § 11 lack values.

One died from postoperative complications; thirty nine of the surviving patients were lost to follow up.

All patients underwent a preoperative antibiotic prophylaxis, 78% with Cefazolina and 22% with

Diagnosis	Patients	Percent
Primary osteoarthritis	100	66.2%
Dysplastic osteoarthritis	25	16.5%
Rheumatic disease	8	5.3%
Post traumatic arthritis	6	4.0%
Post traumatic necrosis	5	3.3%
Idiopathic head necrosis	5	3.3%
Post infective arthritis	1	0.7%
Neck fracture	1	0.7%
Total	151	100%

Table 2 – Preoperative diagnosis of 151 implants.

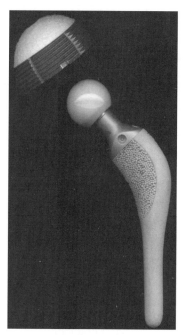

Figure 1 – AnCA Anatomical HA-coated hip prosthesis.

Cefotaxime. Local or general anaesthesia was uniformly employed; all surgeries were performed with the patients in a supine position and using the lateral surgical approach, according to the Charnley technique, without trochanteric osteotomy. A bone graft was used only in a few cases when the acetabular or femoral bone stock was judged inadequate to hold a cementless prosthesis.

The AnCA hip arthroplasty uses a cobalt-chrome alloy stem, 13 cm long, anatomically shaped, proximally porous-coated in the medial, anterior, and posterior faces, and fully-coated with plasma-sprayed hydroxyapatite (HA). The HA coating has an average thickness of 130 m with a porosity of 5%. The Ca/P ratio is 1.72, with 50% of amorphous content, and a crystalline phase after spraying of 47%. The tensile bond strength is > 36 MPa.

The tapered neck is matched with a dense alumina 32mm ball of three different insertion depths, – 4/0/+ 4 mm (Biolox®, Cerasiv, Stuttgart, D). The socket, made of dense alumina, is contoured by a threaded titanium alloy (Ti-6Al-4V) ring 18mm high, and has a 3-D porous alumina bead coating (Poral®) in the remaining dome outer surface (fig. 1).

Routine management included a peri- and post-operative prophylaxis for deep venous thrombosis until full weight bearing (Table 1). Patients were allowed to begin immediate rehabilitation exercises at bed on first postoperative day, and to a minimum weight bearing with two crutches on fourth postoperative day. Full weight bearing was usually achieved after 45 days.

The Merle D'Aubigné and Postel score (28) for pain, range of motion and ability to walk was recorded before and after surgery at each review. The Quetelet ratio (22) or body mass index (BMI) was calculated to evaluate the relative obesity of patients, obesity was recorded for an index of 30 or higher (Table 1).

An anteroposterior view of the pelvis and a frog-lateral view of the involved hip was taken at 45 days, 3 and 6 months, 1 year and afterwards annually.

The bone-prosthesis interface was evaluated according to Gruen's regions of interest (ROI) for the stem (16), looking for bone bridges, contact and radiolucent lines smaller, equal or grater than 2mm. Definitive radiographic fixation and stability was evaluated using Engh's score (12) for uncemented implants. Heterotopic bone formation was recorded by Brooker's criteria (4).

The results were analysed by the Kaplan-Meier product-limit method to estimate the cumulative probability of revision; the survival analysis has been performed since at least 20% of the sample was still reviewed in order to have steady statistical results, and a 95% confidence intervals were chosen. Furthermore, to calculate the survival analysis, those lost to follow up were considered with the same survivorship trend of the controlled group as also supported by Dorey and Amstutz (10, 34). The Wilcoxon and the log-rank tests were employed to compare the survivorship curves of patients younger or older than 60 years and male *versus* female.

RESULTS

Complications

Among the 147 patients, one died because of post-operative complications, while 10 died for reasons unrelated to the hip a long time after the hip operation. During surgery 2 patients had had a fissure fracture of the calcar, but recovered perfectly, postponing the full weight bearing for 2 weeks; one case was a fracture of the great trochanter that was successfully circle wired. During hospitalisation, 11 local and 10 systemic complications were recorded with no consequence, among these were two embolisms and a cardiac infarction (Table 3). In one case, one month far from the surgery, the prosthesis was completely removed with Girdlestone's procedure because of septic loosening. Among the others, 6 cups required revision surgery for aseptic loosening, and 6 stems were revised for thigh pain. Four dislocations occurred in the first two weeks after surgery. They were treated with a cast; revision surgery for recurrent dislocation was never performed.

	Number of cases
During surgery	
Calcar fissure fracture	2
Great trochanter fracture	1
Local	
Deep joint infection	1
Deep venous thrombosis	2
Sciatic nerve palsy	1
Hematoma	4
Dislocation	3
Systemic	
Died during hospitalization	1
Pulmonary embolism	2
Infarct	1

Table 3 – Early complications.

Evaluation of the Retrieved Stems

At revision surgery, the stems were firmly fixed to the bone. The cortical bone was thin, and caution was required at the removal to avoid major damage to the femur. A whitish powder mould surrounded the stems retrieved; the HA coating loss was macroscopically evident, since the metallic stem surface was largely exposed.

In one case, a histological evaluation was performed; the stem was removed 23 months after the first surgery for thigh pain without signs of radiological and scintigraphic loosening. Microscopically, the HA coating was randomly lost, while at the outer boarder of the beads it mostly appeared to be of normal thickness. Elsewhere, it was detached in gross blocks or tiny crystals, but the crystals were never smaller than 2-3μ. Bone trabeculae contacted directly either residual HA or metallic surface, and sometimes were ingrown to the outer surface of the detached HA blocks, lacking continuity between bone and stem (fig. 2). Metallic debris were also detached, but without a histiocytic or giant cell reaction.

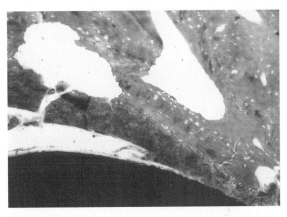

Figure 2 – The arrow show the bone tissue contacting the fragmented parts of the hydroxyapatite coating, which act as a "reef", preventing contact bone apposition to the metallic surface.

Clinical and Radiological Results

The mean Merle D'Aubigné rating improved from 10 before operation to 16.2 at the latest follow up (from a mean of 3, 3.7, 3.2 to 5.5, 5.4, 5.4). A leg length discrepancy was present before surgery in 89 patients of our series (mean 1.7 cm); in 63 patients an equal leg length was restored, in 14 cases it was improved, and in 6 cases it was unchanged. In 16 cases (among these were ten cases with an equal leg length before surgery) it worsened; after surgery a leg length discrepancy was present in 36 patients.

On the first postoperative radiograph, 18 femoral stems were in valgus and 5 in varus. The radiological results of the stem are shown in Tables 4 and 5. Radiolucent lines were seen more frequently in Zone 1, even if spot welds of endosteal bone for-

Gruen zone	Endosteal spot welds	Contact	Radiolucency < 2mm	Radiolucency > 2mm	Total
I	57.1%	38.8%	2.05%	2.05%	100%
II	57.1%	41.8%	0.0%	1.1%	100%
III	43.8%	55.1%	1.1%	0.0%	100%
V	29.6%	70.4%	0.0%	0.0%	100%
VI	50.0%	48.9%	1.1%	0.0%	100%
VII	26.5%	72.4%	0.0%	1.1%	100%

Table 4 – Radiological interface evaluation of the stem in 98 patients (percentage of cases).

Gruen zone	Normal bone	Hypertrophy < 50%	Hypertrophy > 50%	Bone reabsorp	Cortical thinning	Total
I	55.1%	0.0%	0.0%	43.8%	1.1%	100%
II	70.4%	4.0%	3.1%	21.4%	1.1%	100%
III	56.1%	30.6%	4.1%	9.2%	0.0%	100%
V	51.0%	39.8%	6.1%	3.1%	0.0%	100%
VI	66.3%	9.2%	5.1%	19.4%	0.0%	100%
VII	23.4%	2.1%	0.0%	73.4%	1.1%	100%

Table 5 – Radiological bone remodeling evaluation of the stem in 98 patients (percentage of cases).

mation were mainly present in the proximal third of the stem. A high rate of stress shielding, grades 3-4 according to Engh and Bobyn's criteria (11), was evaluated in the 17.3% of the cases, while stress concentration was present in the 49% of the cases (7.1% of high grade). In Zone 4, an abundant pedestal formation was present in 15.3% of the cases, but radiolucent lines thicker than 2mm were never seen (Table 6).

According to the Engh's roentgenographic fixation and stability score for cementless implants (12) bone stability was recorded in all cases but two in which there was a pain free fibrous stability. A calcar resorption was recorded in any case greater than 10mm, and a late subsidence of the femoral stem was never seen. In 18 cases a high grade of heterotopic bone formation (Brooker 3 or 4) was present; however, an excision of the periprosthetic ossification was never required.

Statistical Results

The Kaplan-Meier cumulative probability of 150 prosthesis not having revision for loosening at 10 years predicted a rate of survival for the prosthesis of 92.5% (95% CI 88 to 96), and for the stem of 96% (95% CI 92.5 to 99) as shown in Figure 3 and 4 and related Tables 7 and 8. In this series, considering the survival analyses at ten years follow up, any statistically significant influence of factors as age and gender was seen, while for the numerical paucity of the subgroups, the C Charnley patients and the high BMI patients were not investigated.

Apex (zone IV)

	Unchanged	Small pedestal formation	Radiolucency < 2mm	Abundant pedestal formation	Radiolucency > 2mm
Interface	27.6%	53.0%	4.1%	15.3%	0.0%
	Normal bone	Hypertrophy < 50%	Hypertrophy > 50%	Bone reabsorption	Cortical thinning
Bone remodelling	68.3%	25.5%	5.1%	1.1%	0.0%

Table 6 – Radiological evaluation of the stem tip in 98 patients (percentage of cases).

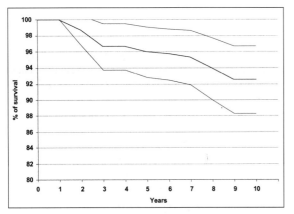

Figure 3 – Kaplan-Meier cumulative probability of 150 prosthesis not having revision for loosening at 10 years. The thinner lines indicate 95% confidence intervals.

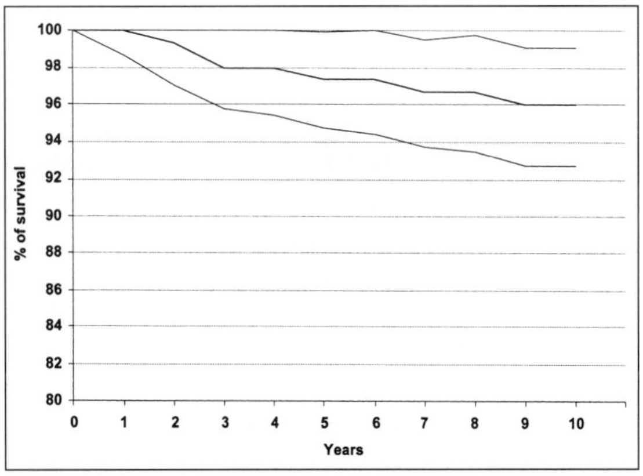

Figure 4 – Kaplan-Meier cumulative probability of 150 stems not having revision for loosening at 10 years. The thinner lines indicate 95% confidence intervals.

Year	% of survival	CI of 95%	
0-1	100.00	100.00	100.00
1-2	98.66	96.82	100.50
2-3	96.64	93.74	99.54
3-4	96.64	93.74	99.54
4-5	95.97	92.81	99.13
5-6	95.67	92.51	98.83
6-7	95.28	91.87	98.69
7-8	93.89	90.03	97.75
8-9	92.51	88.26	96.76
9-10	92.51	88.26	96.76

Table 7 – Cumulative survival rate of the prosthesis at 10 years.

Year	% of survival	CI of 95%	
0-1	100.00	98.69	100.00
1-2	99.33	97.08	100.00
2-3	97.99	95.74	100.00
3-4	97.99	95.38	100.00
4-5	97.31	94.70	99.92
5-6	97.31	94.41	100.00
6-7	96.63	93.73	99.53
7-8	96.63	93.45	99.81
8-9	95.94	92.76	99.12
9-10	95.94	92.76	99.12

Table 8 – Cumulative survival rate of the isolated stem at 10 years.

DISCUSSION

The aim of this study was to evaluate the ten year survival rate of a cementless HA-coated stem. The 92.5% survival rate of the AnCA prosthesis at 10 years follow up does not differ from the 93% rates of other prostheses followed by The Swedish National Total Hip Arthroplasty Register. Even though Soderman and Colleagues (33) analysing the Register data, found clinical failure rates between 13% and 20% for all implants after 10 years, our surviving population had better clinical outcomes. Moreover, the survival analysis of AnCA prosthesis is mainly subject to the poor survival rate of a non hydroxyapatite-coated threaded cup as also observed by Yahiro *et al.* (39). The 96% survival rate of our HA-coated stem is comparable to that of other published series at 10 year follow-up (5, 18, 19, 24, 25, 27).

The fragmentation into the surrounding tissues of HA coating found at histological analysis, also reported by Collier *et al.* (7) and by Morscher *et al.* (29), did not impair the osteointegration; nevertheless, the "reef" effect of bone trabeculae bonded to gross blocks of coating may have jeopardized the integration of the stem, leading to a mechanical failure. This delamination was not detected in other histological studies (1-3, 13, 14, 17, 32, 35, 37) and as suggested by Tonino *et al.* (36) and by Geesink *et al.* (15) it probably depends on the quality of the HA coating; the 130μ thick, 50% pure HA coating of our series likely has weak mechanical properties and a high chance of delamination and abrasion.

The clinical results of our series are satisfactory, especially for pain. At the latest follow up, 91% of the patients have a Merle D'Aubigné score for pain of 5 or 6, and 65% are pain free; even better results were obtained in the majority of cases where we were able to restore an equal leg length.

During the radiological evaluation, we have seen a high endosteal bone condensation on the proximal part of the stem, probably due to the combined activity of the HA coating and the anatomical shape of the stem (Zone I, II, VI). Tonino *et al.* (36) with a 5 to 7 years follow up using an anatomical HA-coated stem documented similar findings (Zone II and VI), while Vedantam and Ruddlesdin (38) in a medium follow up study and McNally *et al.* (27) at a mean 10 year follow up reported, with a fully HA-coated prosthesis, a distal incidence of subcortical bone spot welds. We have also frequently seen an abundant pedestal formation in Zone 4 (15.3%), but this finding had not impaired the stability of the prosthesis.

In our series, the high symmetrical cortical bone remodelling about the distal part of stem had not implicated a high rate of proximal cortical thinning (1.1% in Zone I, II and VII), but we have found proximal bone resorption due to possible stress shielding (43.8% and 73.4% respectively in Zone I and VII). However, this finding of a distal load transfer represents a subject of dispute in the international literature.

Huiskes (21) suggests a proximal coating to prevent stress shielding, even if he emphasizes the role of the rigidity of the stem alloy and believes that a full coating enhances the holding power of the stem in the pre- and post-ongrowth phases. He also quotes the outcomes of Skinner *et al.* (31) and Keaveny and Bartel (23) who predicted, using finite-element analyses, a less bone resorption with proximal coatings.

Nonetheless D'Antonio *et al.* (8) and Geesink *et al.* (15) using a proximal coated prosthesis observed, in a 6 years follow up, a high incidence of cortical thickening in Zone 5 (47% and 44%) and atrophy of the calcar (63% and 69%).

Our 10 years of follow up has shown that a HA-coated stem has an overall good outcome, the HA coating has not shown particular contraindications, and its mechanical properties are related to the thickness and the amorphous content.

Reference List

1. McNally SA, Shepperd JA, Mann CV, Walczak JP (2000) The results at nine to twelve years of the use of a hydroxyapatite-coated femoral stem. *J. Bone Joint Surg. Br.* 82B:378.

2. Murray DW, Carr AJ, Bulstrode CJ (1995) Which primary total hip replacement? *J. Bone Joint Surg. Br.* 77B:520.

3. Capello WN, D'Antonio JA, Manley MT, Feinberg JR (1998) Hydroxyapatite in total hip arthroplasty. Clinical results and critical issues. *Clin. Orthop.* 355:200.

4. D'Antonio JA, Capello WN, Manley MT (1996) Remodelling of bone around hydroxyapatite-coated femoral stems. *J. Bone Joint Surg. Am.* 78A:1226.

5. Geesink RG, Hoefnagels NH (1995) Six-year results of hydroxyapatite-coated total hip replacement. *J. Bone Joint Surg. Br.* 77B:534.

6. Tonino AJ, Rahmy AI (2000) The hydroxyapatite-ABG hip system: 5- to 7-year results from an international multicentre study. The International ABG Study Group. *J. Arthroplasty* 15:274.

7. Charnley J (1972) The long-term results of low-friction arthroplasty of the hip performed as primary intervention. *J. Bone Joint Surg. Br.* 54B:61.

8. Merle D'Aubigné R, Postel M (1954) Functional results of hip arthroplasty with acrylic prosthesis. *J. Bone Joint Surg. Am.* 36A:451.

9. Jellife DB, Jelliefe EF (1979) Underappreciated pioneers: Quetelet: man and index. *Am. J. Clin. Nutr.* 32:2519.

10. Gruen TA, McNeice GM, Amstutz HC (1979) Modes of failure of cemented stem-type femoral components: a radiographic analysis of loosening. *Clin. Orthop.* 141:17.

11. Engh CA, Massin P and Suther KE (1990) Roentgenographic assessment of the biologic fixation of porous surfaced femoral components. *Clin. Orthop.* 257:107.

12. Brooker AF, Bowerman JW, Robinson RA, Riley LH Jr (1973) Ectopic ossification following total hip replacement: incidence and a method of classification. *J. Bone Joint Surg. Am.* 55A:1629.

13. Dorey F, Amstutz HC (1989) The validity of survivorship analysis in total joint arthroplasty. *J. Bone Joint Surg. Am.* 71A:544.

14. Toni A, Stea S, Bordini B, Traina F: Lost to follow up in hip prosthesis register: experience of RIPO. *Acta Orthop. Scan. Suppl.* 73(305S):49.

15. Engh CA and Bobyn JD (1985) Biological fixation in total hip arthroplasty. Edited by Thorofare, New Jersey, Slack.

16. Soderman P, Malchau H, Herberts P, Zugner R, Regner H, Garellick G (2001) Outcome after total hip arthroplasty: Part II. Disease-specific follow-up and the Swedish National Total Hip Arthroplasty Register. *Acta Orthop. Scand.* 72:113.

17. Yahiro MA, Gantenberg JB, Nelson R, Lu HT, Mishra NK (1995) Comparison of the results of cemented, porous-ingrowth, and threaded acetabular cup fixation. A meta-analysis of ye orthopaedic literature. *J. Arthroplasty* 10:339.

18. Havinga ME, Spruit M, Anderson PG, van Dijk-van Dam MS, Pavlov PW, van Limbeek J (2001) Results with the M. E. Muller cemented, straight-stem total hip prosthesis: a 10-year historical cohort study in 180 women. *J. Arthroplasty* 16:33.

19. Hellman EJ, Capello WN, Feinberg JR (1999) Omnifit cementless total hip arthroplasty. A 10-year average follow-up. *Clin. Orthop.* 364:164.

20. Keisu KS, Mathiesen EB, Lindgren JU (2001) The uncemented fully textured Lord hip prosthesis: a 10- to 15-year follow up study. *Clin. Orthop.* 382:133.

21. Paprosky WG, Greidanus NV, Antoniou J (1999) Minimum 10-year-results of extensively porous-coated stems in revision hip arthroplasty. *Clin. Orthop.* 369:230.

22. Collier JP, Surprenant VA, Mayor MB, Wrona M, Jensen RE, and Suprenant HP (1993) Loss of hydroxyapatite coating on retrieved, total hip components. *J. Arthroplasty* 8:389.

23. Morscher EW, Hefti A, Aebi U (1998) Severe osteolysis after third body wear due to hydroxyapatite particles from acetabular cup coating. *J. Bone Joint Surg. Br.* 80A:267.

24. Bauer TW, Geesink RC, Zimmerman R, McMahon JT (1991) Hydroxyapatite-coated femoral stems: histological analysis of components retrieved at autopsy. *J. Bone Joint Surg. Am.* 73A:1439.

25. Bloebaum RD and Dupont JA (1993) Osteolysis from a press-fit hydroxyapatite coated implant: a case study. *J. Arthroplasty* 8:195.

26. Bloebaum RD, Beeks D, Dorr LD, Savory CG, DuPont JA and Hofmann AA (1994) Complications with hydroxyapatite particulate separation in total hip arthroplasty. *Clin. Orthop.* 29:19.

27. Frayssinet P, Hardy D, Rouquet N, Giammara B, Guilhelm B and Hanker J (1992) New observations on middle term hydroxyapatite-coated titanium alloy prostheses. *Biomaterials* 13:668.

28. Furlong RJ and Osborn JF (1991) Hydroxyapatite ceramic coatings. *J. Bone Joint Surg. Br.* 73B:741.

29. Hardy DCR, Frayssinet P, Guilhelm A, Lafontaine MA, Delince PE (1991) Bonding of hydroxyapatite-coated femoral prostheses: histhopatology of specimens from four cases. *J. Bone Joint Surg. Br.* 73B:732.

30. Søballe K, Gotfredsen K, Brockstedt-Rasmussen H, Nielsen PT, Rechnagel K (1991) Histologic analysis of a retrieved hydroxyapatite-coated femoral prosthesis. *Clin. Orthop.* 272:255.

31. Tonino AJ, Oosterbos C, Rahmy A, Therin M, Doyle C (2001) Hydroxyapatite-coated acetabular components: histological and histomorphometric analysis of six cups retrieved at autopsy between three and seven years after successful implantation. *J. Bone Joint Surg. Am.* 83A:817.

32. Tonino AJ, Therin M, Doyle C (1999) Hydroxyapatite-coated femoral stems: histology and histomorphometry around five components retrieved at post mortem. *J. Bone Joint Surg. Br.* 81B:148.

33. Vedantam R, Ruddlesdin C (1996) The fully hydroxyapatite-coated total hip implant: clinical and roentgenographic results. *J. Arthroplasty* 11:534.

34. Huiskes R (1996) Biomechanics of non cemented total hip arthroplasty. *Curr. Opin. Orthop.* 7:32.

35. Skinner HB, Kim AS, Keyak JH, Mote CD Jr. (1994) Femoral prosthesis implantation induces changes in bone stress that depend on the extent of porous coating. *J. Orthop. Res.* 12:553.

36. Keaveny TM, Bartel DL (1995) Mechanical consequences of bone ingrowth in a hip prosthesi inserted without cement. *J. Bone Joint Surg. Am.* 77A:911.

37. De Groot K (1987) HA coatings for implants in surgery. In High Tech Ceramic, pp. 381-386. Edited by P. Vincencini. Amsterdam, Elsevier Science.

38. Herberts P, Malchau H (1997) How outcome studies have change total hip arthroplasty practices in Sweden. *Clin. Orthop.* 344:44.

39. Kester MA, Manley MT, Taylor SK and Cohen RC (1991) Influence of thickness on the mechanical properties and bond strength of HA coatings applied to orthopaedic implants. *Trans. Orthop. Res. Soc.* 16:95.

8   The Symbios Hydroxyapatite Custom Stem at 10 Years

Jean-Noël Argenson, MD and Jean-Manuel Aubaniac, MD

INTRODUCTION

The custom made hip prostheses is now integrated into the whole concept of computer assisted hip arthroplasty, which includes computer assisted preoperative planning, computer assisted designing of custom hip prostheses, and computer assisted hip surgery. This paper will focus on custom made hip prostheses and will describe the elements leading to the design and clinical use of custom stems. It will also discuss the fabrication and biomechanical evaluation of custom made hip prostheses.

The Rationale for A Custom Stem and A Custom Neck

Why custom ?

The loosening rate of conventional cemented stems reported in the literature ranges from 2% to 56% (1, 2, 3, 4, 5, 6, 7, 8). For young age patients in a large group of 8,406 cases collected from the national Swedish register, the failure rate was 30% at eleven years (9) for patients younger than 55 years old. The high level of activity in such patients increases significantly the stresses applied on the component and may explain higher failure rates (1, 2, 6, 10, 11).

Since Judet in 1978 (12), cementless fixation of femoral stem has been proposed as an alternative to cemented fixation. The results of uncemented stems reported from the Swedish register in 1998 were not encouraging (9). This was for a number of reasons, which largely included use of old types of designs. Nevertheless, cementless fixation for femoral stem prostheses has its own requirements, which include proximal adaptation and avoidance of micromovements in order to obtain an optimal load transmission to the bone (13). These princi-

ples are advocated in order to avoid stress shielding and thigh pain, the two complications most often reported with cementless stems (14, 15).

The specific issue with young age patients is not only the level of activity, but also the wide range of proximal femoral anatomies (16). The femoral anatomy can consist of a high canal flare index with a champagne fluted femur, described by Noble (17). However, for congenital or traumatic reasons, it can also lead to a narrow, curved, and excessively ante or retroverted proximal femur. These anatomical issues lead some authors to avoid using cementless fixation in young patients because of the difficulty of meeting the requirements of proximal femoral adaptation in such cases (2, 11).

When considering these two conflicting goals, cementless fixation and adaptation to all types of proximal femoral anatomy, it seems a logical response obtain a custom stem for each case of differing femoral anatomy.

Why a custom stem and a custom neck ?

For many clinicians, a custom device is designed to completely fill the femoral cavity, but it still uses a conventional prosthetic neck. However, the clinical experience of these types of designs showed us that the extramedullary part of the stem, i.e., the prostheses neck, was at least of equal importance in order to restore the correct hip function.

The design of a three-dimensional custom neck allows for correction in length, lever arm, and anteversion. The clinical consequence of such design is the restoration of leg length, abductor function, and proper lower limb rotation. The appropriate anteversion of the neck may also contribute toward reducing the dislocation rate. The mechanical goal of such a neck design is also to optimize load transmission to the bone stem interface. Finite element analysis has shown the influence of the extramedullary parameters on the stem stability and stress transfer (18).

If the intramedullary stem design is based on the reconstruction of the proximal femoral anatomy, the design itself does not match the whole internal femoral anatomy. Contact in the proximal area is imperative when trying to obtain stability in rotation. The distal diameter of the stem is reduced to avoid any cortical impingement distally – a possible source of thigh pain with maximally canal filling stems. It is thus extremely important to preserve all cancellous bone around the entire stem, top to bottom, by the use of a smooth compactor that is shaped identically to the final prostheses.

This whole concept, addressed by Aubaniac and Essinger in 1987, led to the development of software for cancellous bone density evaluation and three-dimensional custom neck design. This is the rationale behind the Symbios® custom concept (Symbios Inc., Yverdon, Switzerland). The concept and the first results were published for the first time in 1992 (19), and the use of this technology for solving the problems faced in osteoarthritis following high congenital dislocation of the hip was presented at the American Academy of Orthopaedic Surgeons in 1993 (20). The preoperative radiological data requires information from both X-rays and a CT-Scan. Based on that information, the preoperative planning relocates the new center of rotation and the new position of the greater trochanter in both the craniopodal and mediolateral planes (21).

The Design And Fabrication of Custom Made Hip Stem Prostheses

Preoperative Data

X-ray data

The radiographic analysis is based on several x-ray views. A full view of the two limbs using scanography is needed to assess the overall anatomical status of the pelvis and limbs and to evaluate the extent of pelvic imbalance by assessing bilaterally the position of the hip rotation centers in the vertical axis. A frontal pelvis view is used to determine the extent of lever arms between the rotation centers and the corresponding femoral axes. Discrepancies are recorded and are used later in the pre-operative planning to correct the anatomy of the diseased joint so that full restoration of the

pelvic balance can be achieved. Eventually, frontal and lateral x-ray views of the diseased joint are needed to complete the x-ray data set (fig. 1).

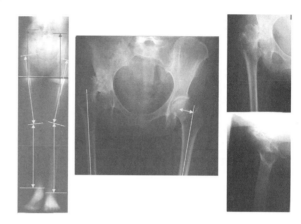

Figure 1 – Typical set of pre-operative X-ray data including scanography, frontal pelvic, and hip frontal and lateral views.

CT Data

Data obtained from a computerized tomography scanner are necessary for the design of the intramedullary femoral stem and for the planning of the extramedullary part of the joint reconstruction. Except in special cases, the CT data acquisition must follow an established protocol detailed by Symbios. However, in special cases, such as very severe congenital dislocations, the radiologist may have to select a modified protocol based on the x-ray status.

The intramedullary femoral anatomy is assessed by CT views taken every 5 mm from the acetabular summit down to the bottom of the lesser trochanter, then every 10 mm to the femoral isthmus.

The extramedullary planning requires CT views taken at three different levels. The first view is at the base of the femoral neck (assessment of helitorsion axis), the second is at the knee level, across the femoral condyles (assessment of posterior bicondylar axis), and the third is at the foot level, by the second metatarsus axis (assessment of foot axis) (fig. 2).

Pre-operative Planning

Acetabular Cup

If the contralateral hip is healthy, planning the rotation center of the replaced joint and the socket size

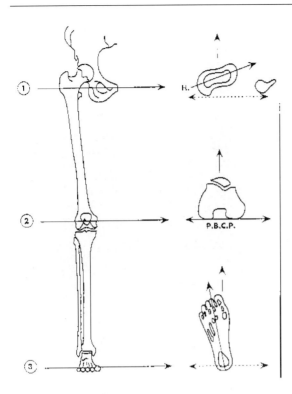

Figure 2 – CT views required for the extramedullary planning 1) above the lesser trochanter, 2) knee, 3) foot.

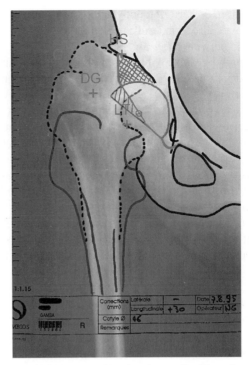

Figure 3 – Pre-operative planning on the X-ray frontal view with (a) anatomical landmark registration (in red), planning of the acetabular socket, and positioning of the greater trochanter.

is performed by reproducing the contralateral geometry on the x-ray frontal pelvis view (fig. 3). In presence of a bilateral lesion, and in most high dislocation cases, the position of the rotation center and the size of the acetabular socket are determined by the surgeon. In certain cases, the size is determined using the CT view passing through the center of the true acetabulum, which allows further assessment of bone stock (fig. 4). Results are then reported on the x-ray pelvic view.

New Position of the Femur

The future position of the femur as determined, for instance, by the location of the greater trochanter, is determined on the frontal view based on the position of the acetabular socket, on the desired lengthening as determined from the scanogram, and on the neck lever arm (fig. 3). This position will determine the level of the femoral cut and will determine the correct neck lever arm on the frontal view. However, osteotomy of the greater trochanter may be necessary in cases where extensive lengthening is required due to an inappropriate anteroposterior position of the greater trochanter due to excessive anteversion.

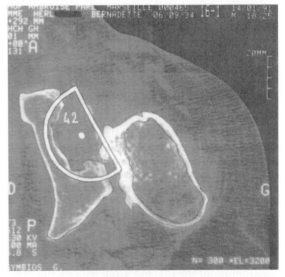

Figure 4 – Planning of the acetabular socket using CT image.

Neck Anteversion

The anteversion angle of the prosthesis neck must be set such that normal gait anatomy can be restored. The normal gait anatomy requires three conditions: foot axis showing 10°-20° of external rotation, posterior bicondylar axis perpendicular to the gait direction, and anteversion of the femoral neck between 15° and 20° with respect to the bicondylar axis. It has been shown that in most cases of congenital dysmorphism, the upper femur axis (also called the helitorsion axis and defined as the axis passing across the longer diameter at the level of osteotomy) is not aligned with the neck axis (22). This phenomenon is usually not taken into account in standard prostheses. In such cases, this often results in an over or under correction of the prosthetic anteversion angle, thus preventing full restoration of the normal gait.

By superimposing the three CT views of the osteotomy level (usually above the lesser trochanter), and of the knee and foot levels, it is possible to calculate the correction angle to add (or subtract) to the helitorsion angle in such a way that a final prosthetic anteversion angle of 15°-20° is achieved.

Design of the Intramedullary Section

Contouring

Raw CT data is processed by numerical thresholding in order to exclude non bony structures from the images. Following this "image filtering" step, the design engineer runs an image analysis program to select both the internal and external contours of the bone section on each femoral CT slice. This contouring process is usually fully automatic, except in the area of the femoral neck and in cases where significant artifacts seen the CT images indicate that manual intervention is needed.

Matching CT and X-ray Data

First, anatomical landmarks on the diseased joint must be registered. These landmarks will be used later for the definition of the osteotomy. The summits of the greater and lesser trochanters (GT and LT), the digital gap (DG) and the femoral head summit (HS) are localized and indicated on the x-ray frontal view (fig. 3).

The next step in the design process consists of superimposing the CT and x-ray data on the same image file. For this step, frontal and lateral radiographic views of the diseased hip are first digitalized using an x-ray compatible image scanner. The contouring data obtained during the previous step is numerically added to the digitalized x-ray views. A manual fitting of the two types of images is then performed independently on the frontal and lateral view (fig. 5).

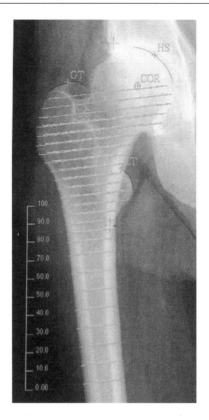

Figure 5 – Matching of CT and X-ray data in the frontal plane.

Definition of Osteotomy Geometry

Once merging of CT and x-ray data is completed, osteotomy directions are calculated and added to the image file. The level of the osteotomy is defined by taking into account such issues such as neck length, optimized stability in rotation, and optimized bone stock preservation.

Generation of the Initial Stem and Extraction

Based on the internal contouring data, the design software uses numerical interpolation procedures to generate the first draft of a stem shape, which is limited to the intramedullary zone. However, the very precise reproduction of the femoral internal contour on this first draft makes it often of little use unless it is modified, as local protrusions and depressions at the bone surface would prevent any movement of the stem within the femur (fig. 6a). Therefore, it is necessary to simulate numerically the extraction of the stem from the femur. This is done in successive steps during which the stem is extracted incrementally by rotations and translations in the three main orthogonal axes.

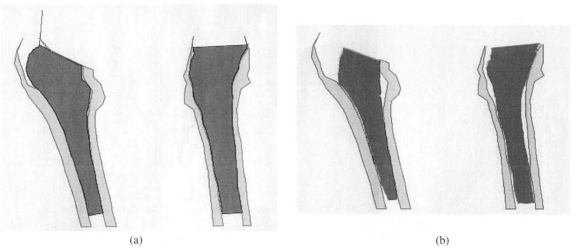

(a)   (b)

Figure 6 – a) Generation of initial stem with protrusions preventing insertion,
b) Modified stem after the extraction process.

During each repeated step, incremental stem shape modifications are performed by the software in order to allow the extraction while maintaining the contact zones necessary for optimized mechanical support of the stem in the femur. Optimized support is sought in medial, lateral, and anterior metaphyseal areas. At the end of the simulation, a new, modified version of the stem is obtained that can be implanted into the femur with a very restricted degree of freedom for the insertion path (fig. 6b).

Final Corrections

At the end of the extraction process, the numerical data from the new stem shape is integrated into the CT data. This enables the design engineer to view each CT section together with the corresponding stem section. By switching to the editor mode of the software, the engineer can also perform a final design "tune up", during which he can still implement slight modifications on each stem section to further optimize the bone-prosthesis fit.

Stem Validation

The final step in the design of the intramedullary part of the femoral stem involves simulating subsidence of the stem in the femoral canal in order to be sure the stem is in contact with the cortical bone even in the worst case scenario. A numerical 3-point bending simulation test is then performed to validate the mechanical resistance of the stem.

Design of the Extramedullary Section

The design of the extramedullary part of the stem is performed the same way in the frontal and lat-eral planes as it is in the sagittal plane. The determination of the anteversion angle of the prosthesis neck, taking into account the correction for heli-torsion, was explained earlier. With the intramedullary stem integrated in the x-ray frontal view, the design engineer calculates the optimized combination of CCD angle, neck length, and head offset, while taking into account the planned rotation center and lever arm.

Planning and Prosthesis Validation

Together, the surgeon and the design engineer at Symbios conduct the pre-operative planning of a custom made prosthesis. Following the planning, the design of the stem is done entirely by the design engineer. Therefore, the final design must be validated by the surgeon before the actual fabrication of the prosthesis. For this, Symbios provides the surgeon with a patient file including the CT composite view, the normal gait restoration scheme, the x-ray frontal (with osteotomy parameters, fig. 7), and lateral view with the designed stem.

Fabrication

Stem Machining

Upon validation of the stem design and pre-operative planning by the surgeon, the fabrication of the prosthesis can proceed. For this, the stem CAD data is transferred into a CAM software program that pilots a 5-axis milling machine. At the same time, a compactor with a smooth surface is machined with the same design as the stem itself.

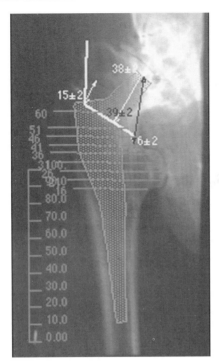

Figure 7 – Composite X-ray frontal view with integration of intra- and extramedullary stem sections.

It is used for compaction of the cancellous bone before the stem itself is introduced (fig. 8).

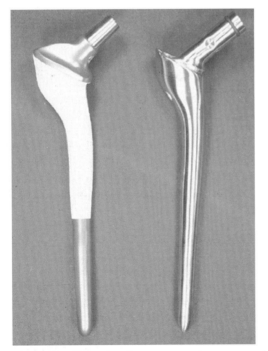

Figure 8 – Example of porous coated custom made prosthesis together with the corresponding "rasp" for compaction of cancellous bone and implant preparation.

Materials and Coatings

Wrought Ti6Al4V titanium alloy is used most of the time for the fabrication of the stem; in a very few cases, stainless steel stems are produced upon request of the surgeon. The rasp itself is made out of wrought stainless steel. After machining, the prosthesis stem undergoes a surface plasma spray coating procedure, which can vary from one stem to the other, depending again on the surgeon's request. In most cases, an initial ~300 mm thick layer of porous titanium is applied to the stem on the intramedullary section of the stem, from the osteotomy level down to the distal level at which the transition from an elliptic to a circular section takes place. A ~80 mm thick layer coating of porous hydroxyapatite (HA) is then applied over the porous titanium coated area.

Sterilization and Packaging

The final steps in the production of the prosthesis are the gamma sterilization and the final packaging procedure, which is performed in clean room conditions.

All in all, the surgeon planning a custom made hip stem prostheses can expect the entire design process to take about five weeks. This time period begins with the delivery of patient's x-ray and CT data to the designer, and ends with delivery of the final prostheses and ancillary implements to the surgeon.

THE CLINICAL EXPERIENCE

Surgical Consideration

The extramedullary custom neck has been able to solve many of the surgical difficulties faced in the cases of excessively anteverted upper femurs often found in dysmorphic or dysplastic hips. Using CT-Scan measurements, we found extreme values up to 85° in some etiologies (23). In those cases, the retroversion included in the custom neck offset was able to restore an appropriate anteversion of 15 to 20° on the knee condylar plane (24). In such cases, some authors have described the association of a derotational osteotomy to a conventional stem (14), but the restriction in postoperative weight bearing and the incidence of non union of the osteotomy may increase the morbidity of the procedure. Another solution would be the use of a modular neck; however, in cases of great anteversion, the possibilities for correction are limited by the risk of fretting.

The intramedullary custom stem aims to preserve the dense cancellous bone compacted towards the inner cortical femur by the use of the smooth compactor. This compactor, of identical intra- and extramedullary shape to the final prosthesis, is used as a trial prosthesis during surgery. The preservation of this cancellous bone is of great importance for secondary biologic fixation to the hydroxyapatite (HA) coating on the final prosthesis. Our clinical and radiological experience prompted us to move from using proximally coated HA stems to using fully coated HA stems (25).

Clinical Indications

Conditions where normal hip anatomy cannot be restored with a standard neck and a standard stem is often encountered in dysmorphic and dysplastic hips (fig. 9a, 9b, 9c). Younger patients often place high, long-term demands on an implant and require full and quick recovery of function. The significant change in the results reported in the Swedish register seems to be at approximately 65 years of age, with a high failure rate of conventional implants under that age (9). Average life expectancy has been increasing. This means a 65 year old patient may, on average, expect to live for another twenty years (26). Therefore, it is important to provide implants that have extended functional lives.

Clinical Results

The clinical implantation of this Symbios custom concept (Symbios, Yverdon, Switzerland) began in our department in January, 1990. Between January, 1990 and January 2000, 1,156 cementless custom stems have been implanted. Focusing only on patients 65 years old or less, and excluding revisions of another prostheses, the series consists of 726 hips. The mean age of the patients was 52 years (range 17-65 years), and the mean weight was 72 kg (range 49-147). The etiologies included osteoarthritis in 273 cases (38%), avascular necrosis in 101 cases (14%), congenital dislocation of the hip in 200 (18%) and dysmorphy in 152 hips (20%). After 1 to 10 years follow-up, eight patients were dead, 28 were lost to follow-up (3.8%), and 11 were excluded because they had less than one year of follow-up. This left 680 hips to study at an average of 5.6 years of follow-up. The clinical Harris hip score averaged 99 points (range 84 – 100) for the 387 extremely satisfied patients and averaged 95 points (range 83 – 100) for the 279 satisfied patients. At the time of follow-up, 98% of the patients ranked their result as excellent or good, eight patients (1.2%) found no change, and six patients were disappointed (0.8%) with a mean Harris score of 80 points.

Seven hips were revised for sepsis (1%), and eleven were revised for aseptic failure (1.6%). These revisions for aseptic failure consisted of nine cases of loosening, one fracture, and one case of persistent pain. Nine of these eleven aseptic fail-

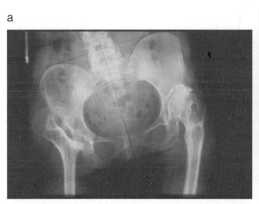
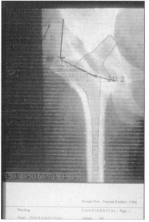
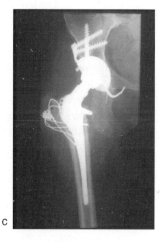

Figure 9 – a) Preoperative pelvis A/P view of bilateral CDH, with high dislocation on the right hip.
b) Custom stem planning. c) Postoperative A/P view of the right hip after 5 year follow-up of the prosthesis.

ures occurred with the proximal HA coating used originally. Considering stem revision for aseptic failure as an end point, the Kaplan-Meier survivorship analysis showed a 96.7% survival rate at 10 years, with a 95% confidence interval. The dislocation rate for all etiologies was 1.7% (12 cases) and considering only patients with primary osteoarthritis, 0.04% (3 cases).

DISCUSSION

These clinical results at 10 years are encouraging. They are at least as good as or better than clinical reports previously reported results in young age groups using modern cementing techniques with conventional cemented implants (3, 7, 11, 27, 28, 29, 30, 31, 32, 33), or using standard cementless prostheses (14, 15). The goals set in 1990 seem to have been reached in 2000, with an increased stem longevity for patients under 65 years old, a reduced dislocation rate regarding the 0.6% to 15% rate reported in the literature (34), and a return to full social and sport activities.

The remaining problems for the current use of custom stems are the higher price, the delay for conception, and surgeon adaptation. The price difference between conventional and custom implants has moved from a factor to five to a factor to two during the ten last years, and this process is expected to continue in the coming years. With the regular use of teleradiology, the 5 week delay for stem fabrication may soon be reduced to 3 weeks.

Finally, with the custom concept, the orthopaedic surgeon no longer needs to have a large number of implant sizes in the operating room ; only one compactor and one final prosthesis are needed. Use of custom implants has a learning curve, but it is quickly achieved by the full computerized preoperative planning, which is helpful during surgery. Once this adaptation is achieved, this custom concept may be able to solve a number of surgical difficulties previously encountered with conventional implants.

CONCLUSION

Computer assisted hip arthroplasty for restoring function and improving implant longevity for patients with high activity and/or modified anatomy is certainly a step forward toward the future of hip arthroplasty. After 10 years of clinical use, both the biomechanical evaluation and results from clinical experience with this intra- and extramedullary custom concept have shown great promise. However, longer term clinical results in young patients are needed, as is further research in the biomechanical field, including the expected bone remodeling around the stems by finite element analysis, and the evaluation of the patient hip function after total hip arthroplasty using gait analysis or accelerometry during everyday activities.

Reference List

1. Chandler HP, Reineck FT, Wixson RL, Mc Carthy JC (1981) Total hip replacement in patients younger than thirty years old: a five years follow-up study. *J. Bone Joint Surg. (Am.)* 63-A:1426-34.

2. Collis DK (1984) Cemented total hip replacements in patients who are less than fifty years old. *J. Bone Joint Surg. (Am.)* 66-A:353-9.

3. Dorr LD, Luckett M, Conaty JP (1990) Total hip arthroplasties in patients younger than 45 years. *Clin. Orthop.* 260:215-9.

4. Dorr LD, Takei GK, Conaty JP (1983) Total hip arthroplasty in patients less than forty five years old. *J. Bone Joint Surg. (Am.)* 65-A:474-9.

5. Halley DK, Wroblewski BM (1986) Long term results of low-friction arthroplasty in patients 30 years of age or younger. *Clin. Orthop.* 211:43-50.

6. Sharp DJ, Porter KM (1985) The Charnley total hip arthroplasty in patients under age 40. *Clin. Orthop.* 201:51-6.

7. Stauffer RN (1982) Ten-year follow-up study of total hip replacement with particular reference to roentgenographic loosening of the components. *J. Bone Joint Surg. (Am.)* 64-A:983-90.

8. White SH (1988) The fate of cemented total hip arthroplasty in young patients. *Clin. Orthop.* 231:29-34.

9. Malchau H, Herberts P (1998) Prognosis of total hip replacement in Sweden. Proceedings of the 65th annual meeting of the American Academy of Orthopaedic Surgeons.

10. Boeree NR (1993) Baniister. Cemented total hip arthroplasty in patients younger than 50 years of age. *Clin. Orthop.* 287:153-9.

11. Collis DK (1991) Long-term (twelve to eighteen-year) follow-up of cemented total hip replacements in patients who were less than fifty years old. A follow-up note. *J. Bone Joint Surg. (Am.)* 73-A:593-7.

12. Judet R, Siguier M, Brumpt B, Judet T (1978) A non cemented total hip prosthesis. *Clin. Orthop.* 137:76-84.

13. Robertson DD, Walker PS, Hirano SK (1988) Improving the fit of press-fit stems. *Clin. Orthop.* 228: 134-40.

14. Mont MA, Maar DC, Krackow KA, Jacobs MA, Jones LC, Hungerford DS (1993) Total hip replacement without cement for non-inflammatory osteoarthritis in patients who are less than forty-five years old. *J. Bone Joint Surg. (Am.)* 75-A:740-51.

15. Glassman AH (1990) Porous coated total hip replacement in young patients. Read at the annual meeting of the American Academy of Orthopaedic Surgeons, New Orleans, Louisiana, Feb. 8.

16. Rubin PJ, Leyvraz PF, Aubaniac JM, Argenson JN, Esteve P, Deroguin B (1992) The morphology of the proximal femur: a three dimensional radiographic analysis. *J. Bone Joint Surg. (Br.)* 74-B:28-32.

17. Noble PC, Alexander JW, Lindahl LJ (1988) The anatomic basis of femoral component design. *Clin. Orthop.* 235:148-65.

18. Ramaniraka N, Rakotomanana L, Rubin PJ, Leyvraz PF (1998) Influence of the extramedullary parameters on the stem stability and the stress transfer. Proceedings of the 11th annual symposium of the International Society for Technology in Arthroplasty.

19. Argenson JN, Pizzetta M, Essinger JR, Aubaniac JM (1992) Symbios custom hip prosthesis: Concept, realization and early results. *J. Bone Joint Surg. (Br.)* 74-B (Supp. 2):167.

20. Argenson JN, Simonet JY, Aubaniac JM (1993) The indications for cementless custom prostheses in congenital hip dislocation. *J. Bone Joint Surg. (Br.)* 75-B (Supp. 1):113.

21. Argenson JN, Aubaniac JM (1994) Preoperative planning of total hip reconstruction for congenital dislocation of the hip using custom cementless implants. Journal of the Southern Orthopaedic Association, 3:11-18.

22. Husmann D, Rubin PJ, Leyvraz PF, DeRoguin B, Argenson JN (1997) Three-dimensional morphology of the proximal femur. *J. Arthroplasty*, vol 12, n°4:444-50.

23. Argenson JN, Hostalrich FX, Essinger JR, Aubaniac JM (1992) Preoperative planning in designing custom made hip prosthesis. *J. Bone Joint Surg. (Br.)* 74-B (Supp. 2):180.

24. Aubaniac JM, Argenson JN, Pizzetta M (1990) Addressing the anteversion problem in severe CDH and primary or secondary dismorphic, with Egoform and Symbios custom made prosthesis. 3rd Annual International Symposium of Custom Made Prosthesis, 3-5 October.

25. Argenson JN, Ettore PP, Aubaniac JM (1997) Revêtement des tiges fémorales non cimentées. Etude comparative clinique et radiographique. Revue de Chirurgie Orthopédique, vol. 83 (Supp. 2):44-5.

26. Kerjosse R, Tamby I. La situation démographique en 1999. Mouvement de la population. Démographie société in INSEE. Résultats 1999.

27. Amstutz HC, Markolf KL, McNeice GM, Gruen TA (1976) Loosening of total hip components: cause and prevention. The hip: proceedings of the fourth open scientific meeting of the hip society. Mosby, ST Louis, pp. 102-16.

28. Ballard WT, Callaghan JJ, Sullivan PM, Johnston RC (1994) The results of improved cementing techniques for total hip arthroplasties in patients less than fifty years old. *J. Bone Joint Surg. (Am.)* 76-A:956-964.

29. Harris WH, McCarthy JC, O'Neill DA (1982) Femoral component loosening using contemporary techniques of femoral cement fixation. *J. Bone Joint Surg. (Am.)* 64-A.

30. Joshi AB, Porter ML, Trail IA, Hunt LP, Murphy JC, Hardinge K (1993) Long term results of Charnley low-friction arthroplasty in young patients. *J. Bone Joint Surg. (Br.)*, 75-B:616-23.

31. Mulroy RD, Harris WH (1990) The effect of improved cementing techniques on component loosening in total hip replacement. An 11-year radiographic review. *J. Bone Joint Surg. (Br.)* 72-B:757-60.

32. Indong OH, Carlson CE, Tomford WW, Harris WH (1978) Improved fixation of the femoral component after total hip replacement using a methacrylate intramedullary plug. *J. Bone Joint Surg. (Am.)* 60-A:608-13.

33. Solomon MI, Dall DM, Learmonth ID, Davenport MD (1992) Survivorship of cemented total hip arthroplasty in patients 50 years of age or younger. J Arthroplasty, 7 (Suppl).

34. Huten D (1996) Luxation et subluxation des prothèses totales de hanche. In Cahiers d'Enseignement de la SOFCOT:19-46. Expansion Scientifique Française, Paris.

9   Clinical Results with the Omniflex HA Femoral Stem

Joaquín Sánchez-Sotelo, MD, PhD and Miguel E. Cabanela, MD

INTRODUCTION

Periprosthetic osteolysis caused by the effects of wear particles on bone is noted to be one of the most common failure modes of hip arthroplasty (1, 2). It is theorized that wear-related bone loss might be prevented by decreasing the amount of debris produced by hip arthroplasty components, or by limiting the access of particles to the bone-implant interface.

The effectiveness of the seal at the implant-bone interface varies with the strategy chosen for component fixation. Incomplete sealing may allow the formation of access pathways along which debris may migrate, potentially resulting in more extensive osteolysis (3, 4, 5). Hydroxyapatite (HA) coatings are commonly used for the fixation of uncemented femoral components. Several studies have shown satisfactory results with this type of surface treatment (6-12). However, it has been suggested that osteolysis can occur when HA particles detach from the stem surface. The osteolysis may be caused by bone loss stimulated through the same mechanisms activated by other particulate debris, or by third body wear produced by debris migrating to the joint space.

To the authors' knowledge, no study has focused solely on the role of HA coating in generating femoral osteolysis. In order to perform a rigorous assessment of the prevalence of femoral osteolysis associated with femoral components that have a HA coating, it is imperative that the many variables known to influence the development of osteolysis be well controlled. Therefore, we conducted a retrospective study of patients who underwent primary hip replacement with insertion of an Omniflex HA-coated femoral component (Osteonics Corporation, Allendale, NJ).

MATERIAL AND METHODS

Patients

Between January 1991 and August 1993, 68 primary total hip arthroplasties were performed at our institution in 61 patients using Omniflex HA-coated femoral components (Osteonics Corporation, Allendale, NJ) and Osteonics acetabular components were implanted.

Forty implants were implanted in men. The average average age at the time of surgery was 54 years (range, 23 to 66 years), and the mean average weight of the patients in the HA group was 82 kg (range, 47 to 131 kg). The most frequent diagnosis was osteoarthritis, but no patients had inflammatory arthritis. The anterolateral surgical approach was used in 31 hips and the posterior approach in 34. Three hips were approached through a trochanteric osteotomy. Demographics and diagnoses can be found in Table 1.

Implants

The HA stem is straight and wedge-shaped in both the anteroposterior and mediolateral planes and incorporates a circumferential HA coating on the proximal third. A distal polished cobalt-chrome tip was used to centralize the stem and provide additional distal mediolateral stability. The acetabular components used were the Dual Geometry (Osteonics Corporation, Allendale, NJ) in 47 hips and the PSL (Osteonics Corporation, Allendale, NJ) in 21 hips. Screws were used to augment the fixation of the acetabular component in 22 cases. The mean median diameter of the acetabular components was 54mm (range, 44 to 62mm). The

Hips	68
Hips in male patients	40 (59%)
Age (years) [†]	54 (23-66)
Weight (kg) [†]	82 (47-131)
Height (cm) [†]	172 (149-190)
BMI (kg²/cm) [†]	27.9 (17.9-37.9)
Underlying diagnosis	
OA	49 (72%)
AVN	7 (11%)
CDH	9 (13%)
LCPD	3 (4%)
SCFE	–
Femoral head diameter	
22mm	9 (13%)
28mm	59 (87%)

BMI: Body Mass Index. OA: Osteoarthritis. AVN: Avascular necrosis. CDH: Congenital hip dysplasia. LCPD: Legg-Calve-Perthes disease. SCFE: Slipped capital femoral epiphysis. UHMWPE: Ultra-high molecular weight polyethylene.
[†] Median (minimum-maximum).

Table 1 – Demographics of the Study Group.

diameter of the prosthetic femoral head was 28 in 59 cases and twenty-two in 9 cases.

Evaluation

Data regarding the outcome of all procedures was collected prospectively at three months, one, two and five years postoperatively and every five years there after and was collated retrospectively at the time of the study. Modified Harris hip scores were derived from the clinical data (13).

Immediate postoperative and all subsequent radiographs were reviewed. Any geographic area of decreased bone density that caused scalloping of the endosteal cortex and was not observed in the initial postoperative radiograph was interpreted as osteolysis. The area of osteolysis was measured and recorded by size and location according to the three acetabular zones described by DeLee and Charnley (14) and the seven femoral zones described by Gruen (15). If a single osteolytic lesion spanned two zones or more, each zone was recorded as being involved in the lytic process. Femoral osteolysis was graded according to Goetz et al. (5) as mild if it occupied one or two femoral zones or had an area of less than 2.5 square centimeters, moderate if it occupied three, four or five zones or had an area of 2.5 to ten square centimeters, and severe of it occupied at least six zones or had an area of more than

ten square centimeters. Acetabular osteolysis was classified as mild if it occupied one zone or measured less than one square centimeter, moderate if it occupied two zones or had an area of one to three square centimeters, and severe if it occupied three zones or measured more than three centimeters.

Radiolucent lines were also measured in each of the acetabular and femoral zones. Femoral component fixation was categorized using the criteria described by Engh et al. (16) as osseointegration, stable fibrous fixation, or loosening. Radiographic loosening of the acetabular component was defined as a continuous radiolucent line at the bone-implant interface or any change in the position of the component over time. The angle of abduction of the acetabular component was measured as the angle between a line drawn along the face of the cup and a line drawn connecting the inferior margins of the ischial tuberosities. Linear polyethylene wear was determined according to the method of Livermore et al. (17) comparing the measurement on the initial postoperative radiograph with that on the most recent follow-up radiograph. The known diameter of the femoral head was used to correct for magnification. Heterotopic ossification was graded according to the criteria of Brooker et al. (18)

Statistical Analysis

Univariate, revision-free survival rates and 95 per cent confidence intervals were estimated using the Kaplan-Meier survival method (19) for four different end-points: revision for aseptic loosening, mechanical failure (which included both revision for aseptic loosening and radiographic loosening), distal osteolysis and mechanical failure or femoral osteolysis. The calculation of survival with no aseptic loosening was performed as follows: if only the acetabular component was revised, the femoral component was considered stable and was followed until the latest follow-up evaluation or until it was known to have been revised. A significance level of ≤ 0.05 was considered to be statistically significant.

RESULTS

Reoperations and Complications

Ten reoperations were performed in 10 patients 2 to 9 years after the index total hip arthroplasty.

One femoral component was revised for aseptic loosening 2 years postoperatively, and another was revised for osteolysis 6.5 years after the initial arthroplasty. At the time of the revision surgery, the polyethylene liner was changed in the first case. In the second case, the acetabular component was revised for pelvic osteolysis. The remaining reoperations included revision of the acetabular component (4 cases), exchange of the polyethylene liner (1 case), removal of a trochanteric claw (1 case) and internal fixation of a B1 femoral periprosthetic fracture (1 case). One additional periprosthetic fracture was treated elsewhere. Bone grafting for osteolysis was required in 2 cases on the acetabular side and 3 cases on both the acetabular and the femoral side.

Intraoperative fractures of the calcar occurred in 6 cases. These fractures were recognized intraoperatively, were stabilized with circumferential wiring, and healed uneventfully. Three hips had a single episode of postoperative dislocation that was successfully treated with no additional surgery. One additional hip dislocated after revision surgery for bone grafting and liner exchange, but did not require further surgery.

Follow-up

Of the original cohort of 68 hips included in the study, at most recent follow-up, a total of 2 femoral components were revised or removed for the reasons detailed above. Four additional patients (4 hips) died with their implants in place. Thus, at most recent follow-up, there were 62 hips with a surviving femoral component in living patients that were followed for two to nine years.

The median follow-up time was 6.7 years (range, 2.4 to 9.1 years) for surviving femoral components in living patients who had least two years clinical follow-up at most recent evaluation. The most recent follow-up was composed of an exam for 45 hips, a written questionnaire for 18 hips in the HA group, and a phone questionnaire for 5 hips.

Clinical Results

The median preoperative Harris hip score, in the 47 hips in which it was possible to calculate, was 55 points (range 29 to 77). The median change in Harris hip score was an improvement of 36 points (range -8 to 66), $p < 0.01$. Preoperatively, the charts

of 60 of the 68 hips (88%) with pain indicate the pain was described as moderate or severe. At most recent evaluation, none of the hips with a surviving femoral component that were still being followed were classified as moderately or severely painful. Clinical results are shown in Table 2.

	HA-Coated*
Clinical follow-up (years)	6.7 (2.4-9.1)
Harris hip score	
Preoperatively	55 (29-77)
Most recent	98 (69-100)
Radiographic follow-up (years) ‡	6.2 (2-9)
Polyethylene wear rate (mm/year)	0.17 (–0.1-0.6)
Femoral osteolysis	
Zones 2,3,4,5 or 6	0
Any zone	11
Mild	7
Moderate	4
Severe	–

* Median (minimum-maximum). ‡ For living patients with surviving femoral components, seven hips had less than two years of radiographic follow-up.

Table 2 – Clinical and Radiographic Results.

Radiographic Results

The latest radiographs were revised reviewed for all patients, both living and deceased. Only seven of the surviving HA coated stems in living, unrevised patients had less than two years of radiographic follow-up. For surviving femoral components in living patients at most recent follow-up at a minimum of two years, the mean median radiographic follow-up was 6.2 years (range, 2 to 9 years). This difference was statistically significant (p=0.001).

At the latest radiographic examination, femoral osteolysis had developed in 11 cases. Osteolysis was always limited to zones 1 and 7. Osteolysis was categorized as mild in 7 and moderate in 4 cases. One HA-coated femoral component was revised for aseptic loosening.

The median rate of polyethylene wear in this series was 0.17 millimeters per year (range, – 0.1 to 0.6 millimeters). Two acetabular components were revised for loosening, 3 were revised for wear, and 1 liner was exchanged for wear; all cases had associated acetabular osteolysis. One additional component was radiographically loose.

Acetabular osteolysis was present in seven hips. It was mild in 2 cases, moderate in 3 cases and severe in 2 cases. There was no heterotopic ossification in 61 hips. Four hips had grade I heterotopic ossification, and 3 hips and had grade III.

Survivorship Analysis

The survival rate of the femoral component with no revisions for aseptic loosening at ten seven years was 98.5% (95% confidence interval, 93.5 to 100%). The survival rate for mechanical failure (revision for aseptic loosening or radiographic aseptic loosening) of the femoral component at ten seven years was 79.398.5% (95% confidence interval, 93.5 to 100%). The seven-year survival rate for distal osteolysis (in zones 2, 3, 4, 5 or 6) was 100%, and the survival rate for mechanical failure of the femoral component or for distal osteolysis was 95.8% (95%confidence interval, 88.5 to 100%). Table 3 shows the survival rates for the femoral component.

End point	
Revision for aseptic loosening	98.5 (93.5-100)
Mechanical failure †	98.5 (93.5-100)
Osteolysis	
Zones 1 or 7	75.7 (60.6-93.2)
Zones 2, 3, 4, 5 or 6	100
Mechanical failure † or osteolysis in zones 2, 3, 4, 5 or 6	95.8 (88.5-100)

The 95% confidence intervals are given in parentheses.
† Radiographic loosening or revision for aseptic loosening.

Table 3 – Survival Rates for the Femoral Component.

DISCUSSION

Presently, part or all of the surfaces of many uncemented femoral components are covered with a HA coating. The relationship between HA coating and femoral osteolysis has not been fully determined. HA coating has been shown in a experimental model to seal the periprosthetic interface preventing the access of wear debris particles. (20) Avoidance of periprosthetic particle migration is in turn expected to decrease osteolysis. (4) However, some authors have reported substantial osteolysis around HA coated components (21, 22).

These osteolytic lesions have been attributed to detachment of HA particles from the surface, which result in either third body wear or direct macrophage stimulation through mechanisms similar to those described for other particulate material. (21, 23)

Although particle access to the periprosthetic interface is believed to be critical in the development of osteolysis (4), the process of osteolytic bone resorption is also determined by the level of an individual's reaction to wear particles, as well as by the particle load generated in each arthroplasty. The amount of wear debris production is related to the characteristics of the bearing surfaces and several other factors, such as patient age, weight, height, activity, underlying diagnosis, design features, and surgical technique.

The results of our study suggest that a proximally located circumferential HA coating on the femoral component increases the survivorship of the implant, potentially reduces the incidence of osteolysis, and appears to eliminate distal osteolysis. None of the sixty-eight hips in this study developed osteolysis in Gruen zones two to six. Polyethylene wear rates were determined by the method of Livermore *et al.* (17). Although HA particulate material found at the periprosthetic tissue of retrieved implants has been implicated in third body wear (21, 22, 24), we did not find any increase in polyethylene wear. This is in accordance with the findings of Bauer *et al.* (25), who reported less femoral head surface damage in the presence of HA, which suggested no evidence of third body wear with HA-coated stems.

Figure 1 shows a preoperative radiograph of a 54 year-old man with severe osteoarthritis in his right hip. Figure 2 shows the same patient immediately after surgery, and Figure 3 show the same patient 11 years after surgery. Proximal remodeling around the femoral stem and some stress shielding can be observed. There may be some osteolysis in the proximal femur; however, the patient is completely asymptomatic.

Our results show that a proximally located, circumferential HA coating results in excellent implant survival free of mechanical failure and osteolysis. The information available at present does not indicate that the use of HA-coated femoral components increases polyethylene wear. It does indicate that HA coating is effective for both implant fixation and prevention of distal osteolysis.

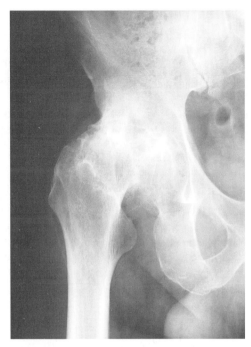

Figure 1 – Preoperative A/P radiograph of the right hip of a 54 year-old man with severe osteoarthritis.

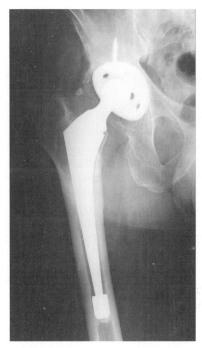

Figure 3 – A/P radiograph of the same patient 11 years after the procedure. Note the proximal femoral remodeling around the stem, some stress shielding, and possibly some osteolysis in the proximal femur. The patient is completely asymptomatic.

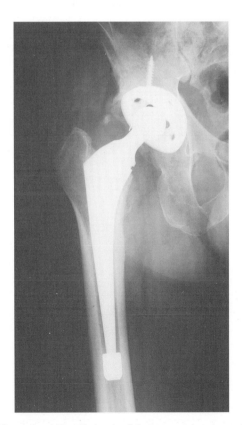

Figure 2 – A/P radiograph of the same patient immediately after uncemented total hip arthroplasty with an Omniflex HA stem.

Reference List

1. Howell GE, Bourne RB (2000) Osteolysis: etiology, prosthetic factors, and pathogenesis. *Instr. Course Lect.* 49:71-82.

2. Harris W (1995) The problem is osteolysis. *Clin. Orthop.* 311:46-53.

3. Bobyn JD, Jacobs JJ, Tanzer M *et al.* (1995) The susceptibility of smooth implant surfaces to peri-implant fibrosis and migration of polyethylene wear debris. *Clin. Orthop.* 311:21-39.

4. Schmalzried T, Kwong L, Jasty M (1992) Periprosthetic bone loss in total hip arthroplasty: The role of polyethylene wear debris and the concept of the effective joint space. *J. Bone Joint Surg. Am.* 74(6):849-63.

5. Goetz DD, Smith EJ, Harris WH (1994) The prevalence of femoral osteolysis associated with components inserted with or without cement in total hip replacement. A retrospective matched-pair series. *J. Bone Joint Surg. Am.* 76(8):1121-9.

6. Capello WN, D'Antonio JA, Feinberg JR, Manley MT (1997) Hydroxyapatite-coated total hip femoral components in patients less than fifty years old. Clinical and radiographic results after five to eight years of follow-up. *J. Bone Joint Surg. Am.* 79(7):1023-9.

7. D'Antonio JA, Capello WN, Manley MT Feinberg JR (1997) Hydroxyapatite coated implants. Total hip arthroplasty in the young patient and patients with avascular necrosis. *Clin. Orthop.* 344:124-38.

8. D'Lima DD, Walker RH Colwell Jr. CW (1999) Omnifit-HA stem in total hip arthroplasty. A 2 to 5 year followup. *Clin. Orthop.* 363:163-9.

9. Geesink R, Hoefnagels N (1995) Six-year results of hydroxyapatite-coated total hip replacement. *J. Bone Joint Surg. Br.* 77 (4):534-47.

10. McNally SA, Shepperd JA, Mann CV, Walczak JP (2000) The results at nine to twelve years of the use of a hydroxyapatite-coated femoral stem. *J. Bone Joint Surg. Br.* 82 (3):378-82.

11. Tonino AJ, Rahmy AI (2000) The hydroxyapatite-ABG hip system: 5 to 7 year results from an international multicentre study. The International ABG Study Group. *J. Arthroplasty.* 15 (3):274-82.

12. Vedantam R, Ruddlesdin C (1996) The fully hydroxyapatite-coated total hip implant. *J. Arthroplasty.* 11(5):534-42.

13. Harris WH (1969) Traumatic arthritis of the hip after dislocation and acetabular fracture: Treatment by mold arthroplasty. An end-result study using a new method of result evaluation. *J. Bone Joint Surg. Am.* 51:737-55.

14. DeLee JG, Charnley J (1976) Radiological demarcation of cemented sockets in total hip replacement. *Clin. Orthop.* 121:20-32.

15. Gruen TA, McNeice GM, Amstutz HC (1979) Modes of failure of cemented stem-type femoral components: A radiographic analysis of loosening. *Clin. Orthop.* 141:17-27.

16. Engh CA, Massin P, Suthers KE (1990) Roentgenographic assessment of the biologic fixation of porous-surfaced femoral components. *Clin. Orthop.* 257:107-28.

17. Livermore J, Ilstrup D, Morrey B (1990) Effect of femoral head size on wear of the polyethylene acetabular component. *J. Bone Joint Surg. Am.* 72 (4):518-28.

18. Brooker AF, Bowerman JW, Robinson RA, Riley Jr. LH (1973) Ectopic ossification following total hip replacement: Incidence and a method of classifcation. *J. Bone Joint Surg. Am.* 55:1629-32.

19. Kaplan EL, Meier P (1958) Nonparametric estimation from incomplete observations. J Am Statist Assn. 53:457-81.

20. Rahbek O, Overgaard S, Lind M, *et al.* (2001) Sealing effect of hydroxyapatite coating on peri-implant migration of particles. An experimental study in dogs. *J. Bone Joint Surg. Br.* 83 (3):441-7.

21. Bloebaum RD, Beeks D, Dorr LD, *et al.* (1994) Complications with hydroxyapatite particulate separation in total hip arthroplasty. *Clin. Orthop.* 298:19-26.

22. Bloebaum RD, Dupont JA (1993) Osteolysis from a press-fit hydroxyapatite-coated implant. A case study. *J Arthroplasty* 8 (2):195-202.

23. Capello WN, D'Antonio JA, Manley MT, Feinberg JR (1998) Hydroxyapatite in total hip arthroplasty. Clinical results and critical issues. *Clin. Orthop.* (355):200-11.

24. Bloebaum RD, Bachus KN, Rubman MH, Dorr LD (1993) Postmortem comparative analysis of titanium and hydroxyapatite porous-coated femoral implants retrieved from the same patient. A case study. *J. Arthroplasty* 8(2):203-211.

25. Bauer TW (1998) Severe osteolysis after third-body wear due to hydroxyapatite particles from acetabular cup coating (letter; comment). *J. Bone Joint Surg. Br.* 80 (4):745.

10 Radiographic Analysis of HA-coated Hip Femoral Components at 10-15 Years of Follow-up

Jean-Alain Epinette, MD, Michael T. Manley, PhD and Philippe Massin, MD

"X-rays never make mistakes ; we makes mistakes, or we expect more than X-rays can provide".

INTRODUCTION

Whether or not an implant is being successfully integrated into the host bone can only be judged from X-ray films. Radiographic evidence can often be obtained well before there are clinical manifestations and is of paramount importance for predicting the eventual outcome of the arthroplasty. However, the appropriate analysis of radiographic changes has become more complicated as far as cementless implants are concerned. Bone is a living structure, and because these implants are no longer shrouded in PMMA, there is close and intimate contact between the implant and the host bone, and a need for the elastic bone tissue to learn to live with the rigid implant. Hence, when analyzing X-ray films, it is imperative to recognize the different patterns and to differentiate between the straightforward osseous reactions that occur as part of the bone's biomechanical adaptation to the implant and lead to lasting fixation and the radiographic signs that herald the forthcoming failure of an implant.

The availability of a simple, reliable, and rapidly applicable radiographic assessment that would be applicable for cementless implants was needed in order to carry out any follow-up of total hip replacements (THR). Charles Engh and Philippe Massin (1) were the first to distinguish between the radiographic patterns produced by the "cementless" type of hip arthroplasty and those seen with the PMMA-cemented ones. The authors were mainly concerned with demonstrating bone ingrowth, and their work essentially consisted of a systematic comparison of the histological findings in retrieved implants with the associated radiographic features. For the femoral components, criteria were derived that reflect direct or indirect changes in the bone-implant system, and this assessment is known as the "Engh and Massin score" (E&M). Later on, a proposal for a new radiographic scoring system (so-called the ARA score) had been published in 1995 by some of us (2). The ARA score is based upon a systematic comparison between the clinical results and the radiographic changes upon more than 3,000 cementless stems followed during a period of 12 years. In addition, the retrieved specimens produced valuable histopathological information indicating why the implants failed. The work also allowed for the features or combinations of features observed via the ARA score to be used as prognostic indicators of implant failure.

In this chapter, we will report on radiographic results of a prospective continuous series of HA-coated Omnifit and Omniflex stems with a minimum of 10 years follow-up. The aim of the study was first to describe the rates of the various changes in these two different types of stems. Then these figures allowed us to compute and compare the two current radiographic scores for the same clinical cases to obtain a better understanding and a more accurate definition of the radiographic features suggested by Charles Engh. Finally, a systematic comparison of the radiographic changes over time with the related clinical outcomes of the implants led us to anticipate a novel approach in radiographic assessment of cementless implants.

MATERIAL AND METHODS

The HA-Coated Stems

The two stems used in the present study were the HA-Omnifit and the HA Omniflex (Stryker-Osteonics, Allendale, USA).

The Omnifit femoral prosthesis utilized had a dense, 50-micron surface treatment with pure highly crystalline hydroxyapatite applied circumferentially to the proximal one-third of the stem. The implant was a collarless, straight titanium alloy femoral stem with normalization steps on the anterior and posterior surfaces. It has a grit-blasted and roughened surface. The proximal 40% is coated with HA applied by a plasma-spray technique. The HA coating was a 50-micron thick (range 45-65 microns), full density coating (porosity < 20%). The content of HA after spraying was $\geq$ 95%, the crystalline phase of HA after spraying was $\geq$ 70%, the tensile bond strength $\geq$ 65 MPA, and fatigue life > 10 raised to 7 cycles at 8.3 MPa. This stem can be defined as a large, long, and rigid stem, with an expected proximal fixation due to the proximal coating.

The HA Omniflex stem has the same proximal HA coating as the Omnifit stem with similar characteristics. However, it the distal geometry is different from that of Omnifit stem. Distally, the stem has a tip ranging between 10 and 22mm that can be trimmed to the exact shape of the bone shaft so as to fill it perfectly without, however, producing a stable bond with the host bone at this level. At the time of the surgery, these two stems required a systematic previous progressive reaming, providing a "line to line" exact fit for both the proximal and the distal part of the implant. (fig. 1a, b)

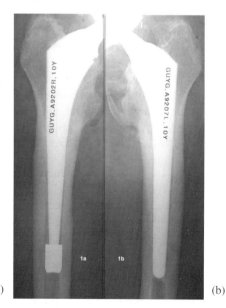

(a)   (b)

Figure 1 – HA Omniflex a) *versus* HA Omnifit; b) stems in the same 58 year old patient who underwent a bilateral replacement in 1992. The unique difference between these two proximally HA-coated stems involves the "distal tip" of the Omniflex.

The Series

From June 1987 until June 1992, 737 primary hip replacements in 649 patients were performed as a consecutive series by one of us (JAE) at the Bruay Clinic (France), including 623 HA Omnifit stems (84.5%) and 114 HA Omniflex stems (15.5%). A third type of Omnifit stem, the shorter Omnifit FC stem, began to be used later in 1992 and, hence, could not be enrolled in the study. All these stems were matched with either the titanium plasma-sprayed Arc 2f cup (1987-1989), or the HA-coated Arc 2f cup from 1990 in almost all cases (98.1%). The exceptions included 14 cups from various designs: 3 bipolar implants, 5 porous press fit cups, 4 HA threaded cups, and 2 cemented ones. Bearings were PE in all cases. A bearing head diameter of 32mm was used in the very first cases in 67 hips (9.2%); all other hips received a 28mm head. Indications for the use of HA-coated implants were broad, with no limitations due to age, aetiology, or shape of the medullary canal. Only poor bone quality with unacceptable primary fixation at the time of the trial led to us of a cemented femoral component; this occurred in less than 5% of cases.

Methods

The clinical course of each patient was evaluated preoperatively, early postoperatively (five to ten weeks), at six months, one year, and yearly thereafter. The entire study was carried out at the CRDA (Center of Research and Documentation in Arthroplasty) located in Bruay, France. At the various post-implantation follow-up periods, those patients able to travel to the clinic received clinical and radiographic review. Those unable to attend because of advanced age or a disability unrelated to the operated hip were evaluated by telephone interview for pain, function and the retention of their implants. All clinical data and radiological images were stored for both retrieval and analysis in a computerized hip database, (OrthoWave, ARIA, Bruay, France) (3). Any visible change of the component was measured on sequential radiographs (fig. 2). The description of the various radiographic assessment parameters follows the subdivision of the femur devised by Gruen (4), with a total of 14 zones, 7 of which apply to the A/P film, and 7 of which apply to the lateral view. Zones 1, 8, and 14 were divided by three and named "a", "b", and "c" in order to permit a more

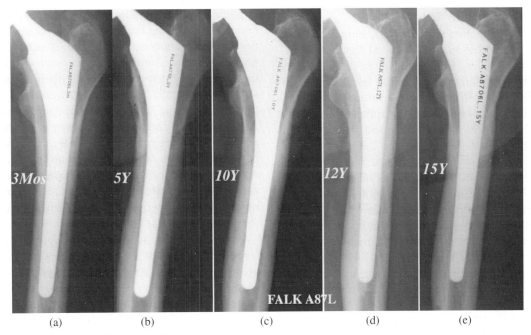

(a)   (b)   (c)   (d)   (e)

Figure 2 – Typical serial films in a 52 year old male at 3 months, then 5, 10, 12, and 15 years postoperatively. Clinical scores are 100 points (HHS) and 18 points (MDA). At 3 months (a), intimate bone contact, endosteal ossification at the tip (which may be due to the healing of the reaming). At 5 years (b), cortical thickening in zone 5, which will not change afterwards. At 10 years, an osteolytic cyst was observed at the proximal portion of the femur, involving both medial and lateral areas, with no increase at 12 and 15 years. At the latest follow-up of 15 years (e), excellent clinical results were obtained (HHS =100 points), while radiographically the stem remains stable and well fixed.

precise description of patterns. The 7th zone was divided by two (7a and 7b). These four upper zones stop at the demarcation between the HA-coated and the uncoated part of the stem, while zone 1a is located under the greater trochanter and zone 7b corresponds to the calcar zone.

The StatWave statistical module of OrthoWave allows a direct assessment of percentages regarding any type of radiographic pattern, as well as any comparison with clinical data including the related statistical tests (Chi square, analysis of variance, non parametric tests, t-tests). The program also automatically computes the two radiographic scores (E&M and ARA) and allows comparison with the two clinical current scores, both the Harris Hip score (HHS) (5) and the Merle d'Aubigné score (MDA) (6).

At the time of the review of all hips remaining "on file", some patients were unwilling or unable to come to the clinic and thus underwent a phone interview. Via telephone, we could make sure the prosthesis remained in place with no particular clinical impairment; we have no recent x-rays for these cases. For a second group of patients who did visit the clinic, the films were of poor quality, or some films were missing. However, even in cases where the films were of poorer quality, we were able to confirm that there was no evidence of radiological loosening, although these films did not allow us to perform a precise and valid assessment of radiographic patterns. In a third group, clinical and radiological assessments could be performed appropriately. In order to make this radiological analysis consistent, only the cases from this third group were enrolled in the present study.

Assessment Of Radiographic Changes

It is critical to assess the various radiographic patterns with a definition that would be as precise as possible. Often this can be extremely challenging. The selected patterns recorded in the current study are based upon the definition by Engh and Massin (1) with the addition of slight modifications and some new patterns as described in the first proposal of the ARA score (2). Their definition and assessment are detailed and discussed by the authors in another chapter of this book.

The following is a listing and summary of the various changes, and the means we used to assess them.

Reactive and Lucent Lines

A strict distinction must be made between "lucent lines" and what Engh first called "reactive lines". *Lucent lines* are radiolucent lines (dark lines on the negative films) of greater or lesser width, paralleled by a thin dense line, surrounding the prosthetic stem or the cement mantle. These lucent lines represent what is referred to as a "radiographic void". The gap along the metal-cement, cement-bone, or even metal-bone interface may be more than 3mm wide. *Reactive lines* consist of a thin, dense line approximately 1mm away from the implant metal, with identical bone density on both sides of the line. There is no radiographic void, hence, no fibrous tissue along the metal-bone interface, as seen in the case of lucent lines. Naturally, any existing line on HA-coated areas denotes a particular predictive prognosis that differs from the lines that can be seen on uncoated areas; this difference was taken into account in the study.

Cancellous Condensation

Engh uses the terms "bony bridges" and "spot welds" to describe streaks or spots of bone that bridge the space between the implant and the endosteal surface of the femoral cortex. Endosteal remodeling can be "none", "moderate" or "marked" according to Engh's definition.

Pedestal Formation

In Engh's description, a pedestal is a shelf of new endosteal bone next to the stem tip. The radiographic density of the newly formed bone equals that of the cortex, with a clear demarcation resembling an upside-down egg cup. The pedestal is said to be stable if the shelf is in direct contact with the metal of the stem tip, and to be unstable if there is a lucent line between the shelf and the stem. The main problem resides in the distinction between a pedestal (which, in proximally fixed devices, is fundamentally a bad sign) and cancellous endosteal condensation at the stem tip. A true pedestal should have well-defined borders. Radiographic changes at the tip of the stem would be defined as "none", "endosteal ossification", "stable pedestal" or "unstable pedestal".

Cortical Hypertrophy

The phenomenon consists in an external thickening of the cortex, without any periostitis or reaction of the adjacent soft tissues being involved. It can be difficult to demonstrate because of the different rotation, on different radiographic films, of an oval femur with irregular cortices. Careful patient positioning and comparative screening of radiographs are essential. In routine practice, true "cortical thickening" is very obvious, since it produces a smoothly bordered "bump" that disrupts the contour of the femur. The location in one or several zones of these cortical thickenings is of major interest in analyzing the reaction of the surrounding bony structures to the new conditions of load, and was recorded as isolated in zone 5, or isolated in zone 3, or again circumferential, i.e., described as involving at least two Gruen zones, generally at the mid shaft.

Calcar Remodeling

Two processes should be distinguished. The first is atrophy, which denotes the occurrence of a bone defect. The second is cancellization, which means a change in the bone pattern. Cancellization cannot be readily quantified using conventional radiographic techniques. Any objective determination of the amount of cancellization would require densitometry. Atrophy, on the other hand, can be readily measured. Its significance is a function of the degree of bone change observed. Conversely, "droplet" osteolysis or "calcar cavitation" (the phenomenon described as "scalloping" by North American authors) should be considered in the context of lytic and cavitating processes. In the present study, we recorded these calcar changes as "none", "moderate", i.e., leading to a bone loss that should be assessed between 20% and 60%, and "marked" over 60% of bone loss.

Subsidence, Stem Migration and Varus Tilt

Migration is measured in terms of the level of the proximal lateral corner of the stem in relation to the superior tip of the greater trochanter. The term "moderate" migration is used to denote subsidence by between 2 and 5mm; anything over 5mm would be qualified as "severe" migration. Tilting into varus is calculated in terms of the angle between the femoral canal axis and the axis of the neck of the implant. A varus tilt of between 2° and 5° would be described as moderate; a tilt by > 5° would be termed severe.

Osteolysis, Cavitation, and Foreign Body Granulomas

We speak about "cavitation" or "scalloping" of the calcar in case of little droplets located either inside the calcar area or at the lateral part of the neck of the stem, immediately below the greater trochanter. Osteolysis would be noticed as "moderate" if a unique cyst reaches the upper part of the coated body of the stem, and involves less than 50% of the coated area. If this osteolysis involves more than one cyst and/or is in contact with more than 50% of the coated area, or again if a cyst, even isolated is located distally, we have to term it as "severe" osteolysis.

Ectopic ossifications at the periphery of the joint were recorded as usually by using the five Brooker grading system (7), i.e., none, slight, moderate, marked or bony bridge.

RESULTS

Demographics

At the time of the study, of a total of 737 hips that were implanted before June 1992, 498 hips (67.6%) in 444 patients remained "on file", while 14 hips (1.9%) in 13 patients were lost to follow-up; 204 hips (27.7%) belonged to 177 patients who died for non hip-related reasons either before or after the tenth year. In the latter case, these hips could be enrolled. Regarding revisions and failures, 2 retrievals in 2 patients for infection (0.27%) and 6 retrievals in 6 patients (0.81%) for secondary accidental fractures were considered to be due to non hip-related reasons. Implant failure with retrieval of the two components occurred in 2 cases (in 2 patients; 0.27%), while in 4 cases (in 4 patients; 0.54%) femoral failure was isolated with retrieval of the stem. Conversely, in 7 cases (in 7 patients; 0.95%) retrieval involved only the acetabular cup or bipolar with retention of the stem.

With respect to the radiographic analysis, of the 737 implanted hips, 620 femoral components could be radiographically reviewed with a minimum follow-up of ten years. One hundred and six stems could not be properly assessed by valid films. Hence, the remaining 514 hips in 445 patients could be enrolled in the present study, with complete and understandable radiological follow-up, including 447 Omnifit, 57 Omniflex and 10 short stems (Omnifit FC). The number of this FC stem was considered as non significant for statistical tests and, thus, was excluded from the study.

Therefore, all results hereafter will concern only these 504 HA-coated Omnifit and Omniflex stems.

The average age at the time of surgery was 62.1 years (range, 18-86 years). Four cohorts were defined according to age: less than 40 years in 16 hips (3.1%), between 40 and 59 years in 167 hips (32.5%), between 60 and 79 years in 319 hips (62.1%), and over 80 years in 12 hips (2.3%). There were 183 males receiving 213 hips (41.4%), and 262 females receiving 301 hips (58.6%). The average BMI was 26.7 (SD: 4.62). Only 39% of cases were considered normal weight; mild obesity was recorded in 41% of cases, medium obesity in 19%, and severe obesity in the remaining 1%. Aetiology was mainly osteoarthritis in 85.8% of hips, followed by avascular necrosis of the femoral head in 10.1%, and rheumatoid arthritis in less than 2%. CDH was 2.1%, while no fresh fracture or revision cases were enrolled in the study.

Radiographic Changes

Lines

The meaning of lines surrounding the implant as previously noticed, is different according the coated or the non coated areas. On the proximally coated zones, "no line" could be recorded in 44.8% of cases, while in 54.6% of cases, a reactive line was noticeable in zone 1a, under the greater trochanter. This line under the greater trochanter was found to be extended upon zone 1b in 3 cases (0.6%). No reactive line extended over 50% of the coated area was ever noticed.

Around the smooth medial-distal areas, 60% of cases demonstrated a reactive line, under fifty per cent of the global surface in 32% *versus* 28% over fifty per cent of the surface. No lucent line was ever noticed either around coated or smooth areas of the stems. Interestingly, with the Omniflex, a significant difference at p = 0.05 was computed regarding the lines around coated zones according to the type of stem with a higher rate of lines under the greater trochanter. Conversely, the line around smooth areas had a higher rate of "no line" in Omniflex (61.4%) as compared to Omnifit (37.3%) (p = 0.01).

A breakdown according to Gruen zones provides percentages of reactive lines for the whole series. The percentages in parentheses are the percentages for Omnifit *versus* Omniflex stems. The percentages are: 30% (28% *versus* 40%) in Z1a; 1% (1% *versus* 2%) in Z1b; 0% in Z1c; 9% (9%

versus 9%)) in Z2 ; 37%(38% *versus* 28%) in Z3 ; 51%(56% *versus* 21%) in Z4 ; 35%(36% *versus* 30%) in Z5 ; 9% (9% *versus* 11%) in Z6 and 0% in Z7ab.

Endosteal Remodeling

This radiographic pattern is highly dependent on various parameters, mainly the shape of the medullary canal and the location of the stem, and whether or not it contacts the cortices. This remodeling was recorded as none in 2.6% of cases, "moderate" in 29.1%, and "marked" in the remaining 68.3% (fig. 3).

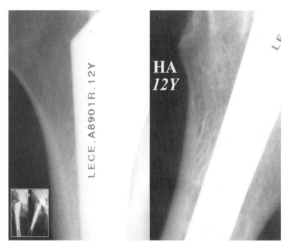

Figure 3 – Close view at 12 years on AP and lateral films of the upper HA-coated portion of a Omnifit stem implanted in 1989. The long lasting effect of the bioactive coating is demonstrated by the intimate bone-metal contact.

A breakdown according to Gruen zones provides percentages of bone condensation for the whole series as follows ; percentages in parentheses are the percentages for Omnifit *versus* Omniflex stems. The percentages are: 0% in Z1a and Z1b ; 8% (8% *versus* 11%) in Z1c ; 54% (54% *versus* 58%) in Z2 ; 23% (24% *versus* 17%) in Z3 ; 19% (19% *versus* 19%) in Z4 ; 26% (28% *versus* 17%) in Z5 ; 64% (63% *versus* 72%) in Z6 ; 10% (9% *versus* 19%) in Z7a ; and 2% (2% *versus* 2%) in Z7b.

Changes At The Tip Of The Stem

No change was recorded at the tip of the stem in the majority of cases (76.4%), while in 21.9% of cases, some endosteal ossification was noticed as a part of the global endosteal remodeling. Conversely, a so-

called "unstable pedestal" was demonstrated in 8 cases (1.6%) all belonging to the Omnifit group. However, no significant difference was demonstrated between the two types of stems at p = 0.05.

Interestingly, none of these eight pedestals (eight patients) ever jeopardized the clinical results, as all of them demonstrated excellent clinical scores at 18 points (MDA) and 100 points (HHS). These pedestals were mainly found in young and active patients with an average age of 54.4 years (7 patients under 60 years) *versus* 62.1 years in the population as a whole. Six were female (75%) and two were male, the gender in favor of female patients compared to the whole population was significant at p = 0.01.

The evolution of these pedestals was critical, since in all cases, the bone formation arose after the fifth year (average: 8.9 years) and followed a dense and active formation of endosteal bone formation around the medial and distal parts of the stem, with primarily endosteal ossification at the tip, subsequently demonstrating progressive change to a typical pattern of stable pedestal (fig. 4). The

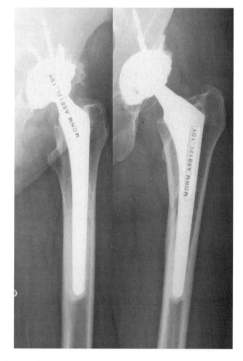

Figure 4 – Typical patterns of bone remodeling at 10 years post operatively in a HA proximally coated Omnifit stem, with endosteal ossification increasing over time down the distal portion of the stem, finally embedding the metallic smooth surface of a very well fixed implant. Changes at tip do not correspond to formation of a pedestal, but to endosteal ossification, with no disparaging prognosis.

frontier between endosteal ossification and stable pedestal, even double checked for each case, was always been difficult to assess, especially with respect to the newly generated digital films.

Cortical Thickening

No cortical thickening was noticed in 67.9% of cases, while an isolated thickening upon zone 5 was present in 16.1% of the cases, and a global circumferential thickening in more than one zone was found in 14.8% of the cases. Isolated thickening upon zone 3 existed in 6 cases (4 patients), i.e., in 1.2% (5 Omnifit and 1 Omniflex) (fig. 5).

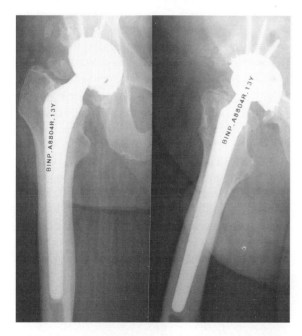

Figure 5 – Excellent long lasting clinical result (HHS: 100, MDA: 18) in a 65 year old male with a HA Omnifit stem. AP and lateral films at 13 years postoperatively confirm intimate bone apposition all around the stem, no migration, and no osteolysis, despite severe wear of the PE acetabular insert, and no calcar change. The pedestal at the tip does not mean there is any instability; conversely, it participates in the global endosteal ossification. The isolated cortical thickening in zone 5 is frequent and denotes the adaptation of the femoral shaft under load.

We paid special attention to these isolated zone 3 thickenings that occurred for all 6 cases after 5 years, with no change hereafter. There was no correlation with age, sex or obesity. The fixation of the stem was assessed in all cases as achieved, with no pending migration or tilting. Clinically, pain was "none" in all cases. Again the characteristics of this pattern were difficult to address, since the case

with the Omniflex stem the pattern seemed to be more a progressive deformation in a Pagetoid-like femoral bone than a typical pattern of external thickening. On the other hand, the five remaining thickenings produced a dense intra and extra medullary bone condensation.

The comparison between the two stems for each pattern seemed of interest, since the Omniflex is supposed to be more flexible. In fact, the percentages of cortical thickening for the Omnifit and the Omniflex stems, respectively, were none in 66.6% and 73.7%, isolated in zone 5 in 18.1% and 1.8%, circumferential in 14.1% and 22.8% and, finally, isolated in zone 3 in 1.2% and 1.7%. The chi square tests applied for each pattern from the two stems were highly significant in the case of "isolated thickening in zone 5 at p = 0.01, and were non significant in all the other cases

A breakdown according to Gruen zones provides percentages of bone condensation that were respectively for the whole series as follows. Percentages in parentheses are the percentages for Omnifit *versus* Omniflex stems. Percentages were 0% in Z1a, Z1b and Z1c; 11% (10% *versus* 19%) in Z2; 6% (6% *versus* 9%) in Z3; 1% (1% *versus* 0%) in Z4; 22% (25% *versus* 8%) in Z5; 15% (14% *versus* 19%) in Z6; 0% in Z7a and b.

Calcar Changes

The meaning of the calcar changes is hard to define as again this pattern depends on various parameters, including the neck-diaphyseal angle, the shape of the proximal part of the metaphysis, the weight of the patient, and the type of the stem. We could through the current study compare two collarless stems that differ only by one parameter, i.e., the supposed higher elasticity of the Omniflex.

On the whole, no change was recorded in 44.3% of cases, while 35.6% demonstrated a "moderate" atrophy and 20.1% a "marked" atrophy. No hypertrophy was recorded in the whole population. The chi-square tests demonstrated more calcar changes in the more elastic stem, i.e., the Omniflex, with a significant difference at p = 0.01 between the two stems. Thus, the percentages for the Omnifit and the Omniflex the percentages respectively were 41.2% (Fit) *versus* 22.8% (Flex) with "no change", 34.0% *versus* 47.4% with "moderate" atrophy and 18.8% *versus* 29.8% with "severe" atrophy. Conversely, no significant difference according to the analysis of variance or non parametric tests could be found with respect to age or body mass index (BMI).

Migration, Subsidence

Some of our patients experienced non hip related traumatic fractures leading to subsidence of the stem and revision and thus were not included in the series. A unique case of unexpected atraumatic subsidence at 3 years postoperatively was recorded in a 58 year old male who received an Omnifit stem in 1989. This led to reoperation and exchange of the stem; excellent results were obtained with the new HA Omnifit at 11 years of follow-up. In all cases of the present series, no pending femoral subsidence or migration has been demonstrated.

Cavitation and Osteolysis

We must stress that the main result observed through the current study is the total lack of distal osteolysis. However, some cases demonstrated either a cavitation (scalloping) of the calcar (27.6%, associated or not with a cyst adjacent to the neck of the stem located under the greater trochanter), or a proximal and limited osteolysis (12.9%). Finally, at ten years of minimum follow-up, 59.5% had no pattern of bone reaction to debris or foreign particulates. Additionally, none of our cases could radiographically be suspected of proximal bone loss resulting from any kind of stress shielding.

As expected, no significant difference at p = 0.05 was computed between the two types of stem, as the proximal geometry is similar. In addition, some cross correlations between the absence of any kind of cavitation or osteolysis and various parameters were carried out. The difference between the group without any modification (Group A) and the group with cavitation or lysis (Group B) was statistically significant according to patient age, gender, and wear of the PE liner. Patients belonging to group A were older at 63.6 years of average age *versus* 60.1 years (t-test: .001; Mann-Whitney: .0001). Cavitation and osteolysis were more frequent in males at p = 0.05 (Chi-square). There was wear of the PE liner (Chi square at .001), with likely more osteolytic reactions in cases that pointed out more visible patterns of wear. Conversely, no significant difference between the groups A and B was demonstrated at p = 0.05 according to aetiology (osteoarthritis *versus* necrosis), head diameter (28mm *versus* 32mm), or final global clinical score.

We paid specific attention to the 69 hips in 61 patients that demonstrated proximal osteolysis. The first change that occurred was a reactive line starting at the shoulder of the stem, below the greater trochanter; this occurred before the first year. Subsequently, either a little cyst appeared between the metal and the line, or the line travels distally, generally at the fifth year going down the angle at the lateral aspect of the stem at the demarcation between the non-coated and the coated area, reaching the "body" of the stem (fig. 6). At the

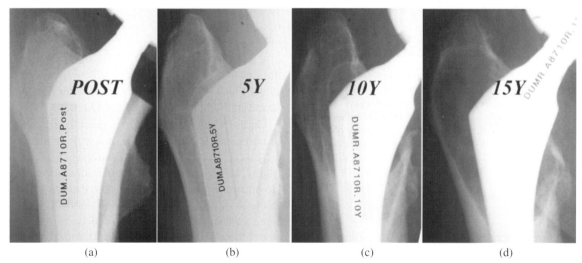

(a)   (b)   (c)   (d)

Figure 6 – Typical evolution of "creeping osteolysis" over time due to PE debris at the upper portion of a HA Omnifit stem implanted in 1987 in a 56 year old female. Close bone contact between metal and bone postoperatively (a); at 5 years (b) a small droplet of osteolysis at the calcar zone, and an extensive line at the shoulder of the stem; at 10 years (c), a typical lytic area reaching the HA-coated zones medially and laterally. Note the dense bone sealing the shaft and preventing distal migration of particles. At 10 years (d), an enormous cyst of osteolysis involving the entire area under the greater trochanter, and the upper medial portion of the femur. This case is pending reoperation for grafting, despite an excellent lasting clinical result (HHS:100 points, MDA:18 points)

same time, the cyst grows and tends to develop under the greater trochanter. The limits of the cyst are well defined by a sclerotic line, which is very different from the patterns of the bone loss due to stress shielding. In all cases, the surrounding bone at the lower part of the lytic lesion is very dense and is a real barrier. In less than 5% of cases, these lytic lesions extend more than 1cm down the lateral, anterior, and posterior parts of the body of the stem. In all other cases, at the current follow-up of the study, this lytic lesion remains limited at the very proximal area. In no case to date have these proximal cysts ever jeopardized the fixation of the stem. In our whole experience, we simply reoperated on three of them to exchanging the bearings, while leaving the components in place, performing a synoviectomy and grafting the cavities with satisfactory results in all cases. In two cases, the acetabular component was a bipolar, and in one case a Ti-coated Arc 2f cup.

Ectopic Ossifications

According to the well defined Brooker classification (7), ectopic ossifications were none in 56.0% of cases, while 19.4% were "slight", 14.9% were "moderate", 8.0% were "marked" and 1.7% of cases demonstrated a real "bony bridge". On the whole, three quarters of the hips did not experience any significant ectopic bone formation.

Finally, these ectopic ossifications were very important (marked or bony bridges) in 51 hips (in 48 patients). In this particular group, we paid attention to the relationship with age, gender, aetiology, or clinical results obtained. Age and aetiology were non significant. Conversely, these patients were largely males (76.5%; significant at p = 0.001). Interestingly, no relationship between these ectopic ossifications and pain or range of motion could be significantly assessed. Moreover, the hip flexion averaged 125 degrees in this group (SD:16.91), while more than ninety per cent flexed over 110 degrees, and zero hips were less than 70 degrees. Only 5 cases (10%) had a flexion between 70 and 90 degrees.

Radiographic Scores

According to the two currently used radiographic scores in cementless stems, we would like to report on the numeric assessment obtained by the entire series of 504 cases at 10-15 years of radiographic follow-up, then perform a breakdown by the type

of stem and, finally, carry out a comparison between the radiographic scores and the clinical assessment for each of the stems.

Engh and Massin Score

This score comprises two numeric values defining the fixation score and the stability score, combined to get the "total" numeric score, leading to the "global" score graded in four levels.

The first level is the fixation score (–7.5 up to 10). This score averaged 8.03 (–2.5 up to 10, SD 2.727) for the whole series, with only one hip under 0 (score:-3). Mean values were respectively 8.0 and 8.1 for the Omnifit and the Omniflex stems, without any significant difference at 0.05 (Error risk, t-test, Mann& Whitney tests). The second level is the stability score (–23.5 up to 17). This score averaged 8.03 (3 up to 17, SD 3.486) for the whole series, with no hip under 0. Mean values were respectively 10.7 and 13.1 for the Omnifit and the Omniflex stems, with a significant difference in favor of the Omniflex (Error risk, Mann& Whitney), while not significantly different at .05 according to the t-test. The Third level is the total score (–31 up to 27): This score averaged 19.04 (5.5 up to 27, SD 4.448) for the whole series, with no hip under 0); Mean values were respectively 18.8 and 21.1 for the Omnifit and the Omniflex stems, with a significant difference in favor of the Omniflex at .001 (Error risk), and at .001 (Mann& Whitney), while not significantly different at .05 according to the t- test. The fourth level is the global score. Ingrowth was confirmed in 98.2% of cases and "suspected" in the remaining 1.8%, since no hip was graded "fibrous encapsulation" or "unstable". The breakdown according to the type of prosthesis did not demonstrate any significant difference at p = 0.05 (chi square test) between the Omnifit and the Omniflex stems.

ARA Femoral Score

This assessment collects various penalties of different weights from the recorded abnormal patterns, which are subtracted from the initial optimal value of 6 points, leading to a numeric score from 0 up to 6 and a grading system from poor (0 to 2), fair (3), good (4) and excellent (5 to 6). The total score averaged 4.2 (0 up to 6, SD 1.439) for the whole series, with only nine hips at 0 . Mean values were respectively 4.2 and 4.0 for the Omnifit and the Omniflex stems, without any significant difference at 0.05 (Error risk, t-test, Mann

& Whitney tests). The global score results were excellent in 49.2% of hips, and good in 25.2%, while fair in 12.2% and poor in the remaining 13.4%. The breakdown according to the type of prosthesis did not demonstrate any significant difference at p = 0.05 (chi square test) between the Omnifit and the Omniflex stems. Thus according to this ARA score, 67 hips were graded "poor" in 59 patients, mainly due to a high rate of osteolysis (67.4% of proximal lysis) and modifications at the tip of the stem (34.8% of cases) in this group.

Relationship With Clinical Results

Comparisons between the E&M score and the Harris Hip Score (HHS) did not demonstrate any significant correlation at .05 according to the Student-Fisher (t) test. Similarly, we could not state any conclusion while comparing the average HHS obtained by the two groups of "ingrowth confirmed" *versus* "suspected", mainly due to the low rate of the latter group. Similarly, no significant correlation could be found when comparing the ARA score to the HHS score. In addition, average values of HHS in each of the four groups "excellent" down to "poor" gave, respectively, values of 97.3, 98.8, 98.4 and 98.8 points, and could not be assessed as significant.

We paid specific attention to the group of hips graded "poor" through the ARA score. In fact, none of the 59 related patients experienced any pain, or any specific functional impairment. To date, none of the films belonging to this group led us to think about any pending failure of the arthroplasty.

DISCUSSION

For the past twenty years, since we began implanting cementless prostheses in 1982, we have tried to understand how the bony structures surrounding a metallic implant could react, and how, through a careful and detailed analysis of radiographic films, a reliable information on the fate of the implants could be derived. After the first period of porous coated stems, we entered fifteen years ago a new era of the "bioactive" implant by using hydroxyapatite-coated stems. The aim of this study was to report at a minimum follow-up of 10 years on a significant prospective radiographic study of more than 500 hundred of fully documented cases,

with respect to two different proximally HA-coated stems, i.e., the Omnifit and the Omniflex femoral implants. Such a detailed study should been carried out using the OrthoWave database, which is able to simultaneously provide any kind of clinical or radiological data, an automatic computation of any scoring assessment, as well as a direct connection to the statistical module and the catalogue of related images.

An encouraging "balance sheet" at the 15-year experience with bioactive coatings

The first lesson we learned from the study was an excellent and promising overview of radiological results with 100% of "bony ingrowth confirmed or suspected", and a very stable relationship between the implant and the host bone over time. Despite the normal degradation of hydroxyapatite over a certain number of years, the fixation afforded by the HA coating has withstood the test of time, and the bony attachment to the microstructured (grit blasted) metallic substrate of these two stems appeared to be of valuable reliability (fig. 7). The excellent results afforded by the two stems participating in the study correspond with other radiographic studies presented in other chapters of this book as well as in the literature (8-18).

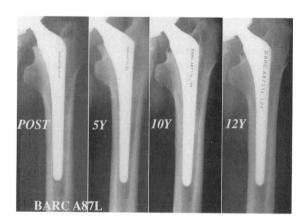

Figure 7 – Serial films postoperatively, then at 5, 10 and 12 years, of a HA Omnifit stem implanted in 1987 in a 66 year old male (osteoarthritis). At the latest follow-up, an excellent clinical result can be observed. The radiographs denote excellent bony apposition onto the HA-coated zones, no migration or varus tilt. Apart from a limited area of osteolytic cysts due to PE debris at the calcar zone and at the shoulder of the stem, this is a typical picture of "mute x-rays" at 12 years.

Radiographic Changes Remain Difficult To Assess In Cementless Femoral Components

The second lesson we learned was an update of our knowledge of radiographic changes and their possible meanings.

The "Lines" surrounding any implant

Whatever any controversial argument regarding the "lines" surrounding any implant, the presence of a reactive line against a surface that provides for bone ingrowth is always a bad sign, since it shows that, upon the involved area, there is neither a bond between the implant and the host bone nor an appropriate stress transfer pattern. It is, however, normal to find reactive lines against the "smooth" (uncoated) parts of the prosthesis. Whether reactive lines are seen along implant surfaces that do not provide for bone ingrowth depends essentially on the shape of the medullary cavity and the fit of the stem, as well as on the elasticity gradient of the host bone, which shows individual differences related to patient age and build. The reactive line seen at the most proximal part of the posterior surface of the stem (at the proximal end of Zone 1-Zone 1A) constitutes a special pattern that is not clearly explained. We still consider this line a response to the elasticity gradient produced by the difference between the rest of the femur and the greater trochanter, which is "pulled about" by the gluteal muscles. The pattern is frequently seen, and is not, to our way of thinking, predictive of failure. However, it may be the manifestation of incipient osteolysis, and, as such, should be monitored very carefully.

The endosteal remodeling

Regarding the endosteal remodeling (or cancellous condensation), there is no consensus on what this condensation signifies ; however, it may be assumed that the phenomenon reflects an attempt, by the local host bone, to adapt to and improve the stability of the implant, by replacing the elastic cancellous bone by rigid endosteal bony tissue. We have routinely observed cancellous condensation at a site immediately distal to the HA covered portion of the implant. The process is seen where the uncoated portion of the implant starts and tends to progress distally, causing densification of the bone segment involved. Sometimes the phenomenon is observed in the most distal part of the HA-covered

portion ; it is uncommon at the proximal coated part of the stem, where most of the load transfer takes place. This suggests that cancellous condensation is not an automatic manifestation of stress transfer, but evidence of a difference in elasticity between the implant and the host bone, which the bone tries to compensate for by becoming stiffer. Cancellous condensation has sometimes been seen at the tip of the stem; at that site, it reflects the same bone response as at the more customary proximal locations. It may be difficult to distinguish from pedestal formation.

The changes at the tip of the stem

Regarding the changes at the tip of the stem, as demonstrated in one quarter of cases, the main problem resides in the distinction between a pedestal (which, in proximally fixed devices, is fundamentally a bad sign) and cancellous condensation at the stem tip, or simply the "healing" of a distal cortical defect left behind after reaming. Regularly, these pedestals, as often demonstrated in our cementless, non HA-coated stems, where known as the best indicator of failure of proximal fixation. In these cases, the pedestal was, as a rule, associated with an extensive sclerotic line surrounding the proximal stem portion and, often, the entire stem. The triad of radiographic signs was basically completed by calcar hypertrophy, which also represents an attempt by the bone to compensate for the poor stress transfer pattern resulting from the absence of a sound bond between the implant and the host bone. However, the few cases of pedestals shown in our series were never associated with any lack of proximal fixation or clinical impairment or pain, and would be seen simply as a part of a general bone remodeling at the tip of the stem over years. Thus the meaning of these patterns would not be as pejorative as assessed by Engh.

The cortical thickenings

With respect to cortical thickenings, a number of different hypotheses have been put forward to account for the diaphyseal remodeling of the implant-bearing bone segment over time. For a long time, this external remodeling was considered undesirable. It was thought that it reflected an irritation of the bone by contact with the metal stem tip, which could give rise to the well-known complaint of thigh pain. Over the years, we have arrived at a fundamentally different interpretation of the phenomenon – we believe this reaction is not one of irritation of the host bone by the implant stem. After all, this thickening is generally seen in the absence of bone-metal contact. Indeed, it is extremely rare to see cortical hypertrophy at a site where there is contact between the metal tip and the host bone. In the clinical examination of our patients, we have never observed thigh pain or tenderness over the site of cortical hypertrophy. To our way of thinking, this remodeling is yet another sign of the adaptation of the host bone to the changed biomechanical conditions obtained after the insertion of a prosthesis.

In light of our radiographic assessment, it would seem reasonable to consider isolated hypertrophy in Zone 5 as a "neutral" sign of straightforward adaptation of the medial cortex to the compressive stress pattern to which the bone is exposed. Overall or circumferential thickening, on the other hand, reflects a major adaptive response by the bone. In our experience with porous or HA-coated implants, isolated cortical hypertrophy in Zone 3 was always a bad sign that might reflect a varus displacement of the prosthesis and might herald thigh pain. This pejorative assessment was not confirmed in the 6 cases of isolated Zone 3 hypertrophy belonging to the current study, since no pending migration or varus tilt was demonstrated in very well fixed stems, with no pain or functional impairment. Finally, these thickenings participated in a dense, intra and extra medullary bone condensation. Again, the meaning of this specific pattern would not be as pejorative as previously assessed.

The calcar structure

It would be challenging to address the fate of the calcar structure over time, with or without a collar. Moreover, there is no consensus regarding the use of an implant collar resting on the calcar. However, both advocates and opponents would admit that partial (moderate) atrophy is evidence of a change in the stress line pattern, with medial stress-shielding produced by the lines running from the metaphyseal portion of the prosthetic stem to the pelvis, *via* the neck of the implant. Although, in biomechanical terms, there is stress- shielding, the process is nowhere near as detrimental as it is at the greater trochanter. In spite of the fact Engh considered a moderate degree of calcar atrophy to be a favorable sign indicating proximal fixation of the implant stem, in the light of the present study, it seems hard to conclude that this "moderate"

atrophy can or cannot mean any successful proximal fixation, as our 44% of "no change at calcar" cases demonstrated excellent proximal fixation . Marked atrophy, on the other hand, was considered as a sign that the implant has tilted into a greater or lesser degree of varus. In these cases, atrophy was supposed to result from any genuine osteolysis as a result of excessive stress. Again, none of the 20% of our "marked" atrophy cases demonstrated any sign of pending varus tilt or implant migration, and the predictive meaning of this marked atrophy seems to remain unanswered. Elasticity of the stem, level of the cut and anatomy of the upper part of the femur, in varus or valgus, should be the most important parameters to consider, with no real impact on the upcoming behavior of the stem fixation.

Subsidence

Absence of any subsidence in the long run as demonstrated in our study, answers some questions about the ultimate fate of the femoral fixation. Secondary migration also generally involves different scenarios, which may be associated. The first, loss of "adhesion", means a breakdown of the metal-bone interface. This argument is frequently advanced by the opponents of HA coating, who maintain that the HA layer may eventually dissolve completely. With hydroxyapatite, the gradual loss of coating over the years may, of course, be a major problem. However, we feel that if the implant has been inserted with adequate stability, the initial coating may be gradually replaced by newly formed bone, which would then be in contact with the microtextured metal on the implant surface, thus ensuring lasting fixation in the host bone. This is why the metal substrate that is to receive the HA coating must be properly prepared by grit blasting. This is why so-called "augmentation" features such as grooves or steps should be provided, to optimize the implant's hold in the bone and to counteract any tendency to subside.

Secondly, subsidence may also be induced by a change in the shape of the bone surrounding the implant. Apart from periprosthetic accidental fractures, subsidence may be caused by lytic lesions resulting from foreign body granulomas. The pattern observed is one of "blown-out" bone, with thin cortices. We have never encountered this problem with our HA-coated stems, since a few cases presenting a progressive proximal osteolysis could be successfully treated by simple grafting and exchange of the bearings. Conversely, with cemented stems, this osteolysis forms part of the general problem of implant loosening.

Thirdly, a potential risk of migration would arise with the problems posed by cylindrical femora in the elderly, with a gradual transformation of the femoral canal over the years. We can only express the hope that bone remodeling in contact with the HA coating, and the biomechanical interchange between the implant and the host bone, will lead to a mutually stable system. However, to date we have routinely used HA-coated stems in very elderly patients (over 80 years of age) and have achieved encouraging results, with excellent osteointegration, and no subsidence of any kind in this particular patient population.

Osteolysis, cavitation, and foreign body granulomas remain at the front of the stage, as a critical concern regarding the outcome of our implants. Nonetheless, osteolysis needs to be considered apart from the bone remodeling facing the implanted stem, since it does not constitute a reaction of the host bone surrounding the metallic implant, as a mutual adaptation content-container. Conversely, this phenomenon is a reaction of the bone to a foreign aggression by some particulate or debris, or an unexplained chemical process that would secondarily jeopardize the fixation of the stem. Thus, when assessing the results of a given femoral component with respect to this osteolytic concern, we can only comment on the shape of the stem that may or may not provide access to particulates, and on the ability of getting an efficient bone-metal bonding that will act as a real barrier to prevent pathways for these particulates.

The scalloping of the calcar would not be termed as real osteolysis, since this limited reaction should be considered as belonging to the periphery of the regular joint space ; it is more a bearing surfaces problem than a stem concern. Hopefully, this issue might be largely resolved by using new hard-on-hard bearings.

Osteolysis was defined for us as lytic granulomas reaching the surface of the body of the stem on the HA-coated areas. The high rate of proximal osteolysis at 12.9% demonstrated by the two stems analyzed in the present study is critical. The shape of the upper part of the stem, which incorporates an oblique and straight contour of the lateral part of the neck instead of a "shoulder", creates a space under the greater trochanter that one might describe

as a "funnel for particles". Systematic comparison of this specific pattern in other types of prostheses would be of major interest and some studies about this issue are currently underway.

In addition, the total absence of distal osteolysis is extremely encouraging and confirms the efficiency of the seal provided by the HA coating and leading to bone condensation at the frontier between the cyst and the host bone. We know that particulates likely use pathways either through the gap between implant and bone, or directly through the structures of cancellous bone. The HA-coated implants discourage particle migration because they do not provide a gap for the particles to migrate into. The absence of any gap combined with bone condensation helps prevent the growth of osteolysis. Hence, we spoke about "creeping" osteolysis, which at this point is more a problem involving bearings and particulates than a stem concern. We believe there is no need to exchange the stem if the fixation remains secure. In our experience with these cases of proximal osteolysis, grafting has been sufficient.

Do the radiographic changes confirm the expected improvements afforded by new designs ?

Engineers often think about improvements regarding the shape and design of their implants. However, it is often difficult to confirm clinically the merits of new features worked out in their laboratories. Fortunately, the published clinical results on almost all HA femoral components are excellent. Thus, it is difficult to clearly comment on the effects of these new designs. The current study gave us the opportunity to compare two stems for which the overall geometry is identical, with the exception of the distal tip. The Omnifit stem is long and rigid, and the Omniflex is long and flexible, due to a thinner medial distal tip. This unique difference allows statistical comparisons in a consistent way. Additionally, the distal tip is supposed to obtain close contact distally between the metal and the surrounding bone.

As expected, the number of reactive lines observed around the medial distal part of the stem was significantly lower in the more flexible stem, confirming the hypothesis according to a bone-metal gradient of elasticity that causes these reactive lines. Additionally, the higher rate of lines below the greater trochanter seen with the Omniflex stem leads us to expect that this more important elasticity of the stem would be at variance with the elasticity of the gluteal muscles. With the Omniflex stem, the consequence of a higher elasticity of the stem in the metaphysis was also demonstrated by a higher rate of calcar atrophy, perhaps due to a better transfer of loads from the stem directly toward the pelvis, causing stress shielding in the calcar zone.

The bone-metal contact provided by the distal tip of the Omniflex stem never generated any specific kind of modification at the tip of the stem. This confirms that the hypothesis that a metal-bone contact would provide "bony irritation", which could give rise to the well-known complaint of thigh pain cannot be supported by any genuine proof; this hypothesis should most likely be abandoned.

On the whole, radiographic patterns appear to confirm through the current study that radiographic analysis might validate some biomechanical theory applied to specific designs. A better knowledge of radiographic patterns and systematic comparisons between different types of the currently implanted femoral components would certainly help to participate in the evolution of designs and hence handle in a better way the outcome of any given implants.

Radiographic assessment:
Do we need any scoring system?

Charles Engh and Philippe Massin (1) were well-advised to distinguish the radiographic patterns produced by the "cementless" type of hip arthroplasty from those seen with the PMMA-cemented ones. The authors were mainly concerned with demonstrating bone ingrowth, and their work consists essentially of a systematic comparison of the histological findings in retrieved implants with the associated radiographic features. For the femoral components, criteria were derived that reflect direct or indirect changes in the bone-implant system. These fundamental studies produced a new insight into the radiographic features of implants designed to be in direct contact with the host bone, and allowed a better understanding of cementless joint replacement techniques. However, some aspects of the dual score require comment, and this numerical score seemed difficult to use in a practical way, mainly because, in all series, 100% of the cases demonstrated bony ingrowth either "confirmed" or

"suspected". In addition, the allocation of positive or negative points by a purely binary "yes-no" decision can lead to the loss of important nuances. Some of the signs observed (e.g., metal particle shedding) apply to one type of implant only. Other signs require further differentiation (to reflect the different prognostic significance of a reactive line *versus* a lucent line) or a different meaning according to the related locations. Some signs, such as cortical hypertrophy, and particularly osteolysis, are not taken into account at all. The total range of the score is from –31 to +27, and the actual figure produced may be difficult to understand. In fact, this score was intended to provide a guide to histopathological diagnosis from the X-ray films, which was fundamental during the first era of cementless implants.

This exercise had to be taken one step further with the ARA score by trying to establish a system based on the analysis of serial radiographs of any type of cementless prosthesis (with or without HA) that would permit the assessment of the success or failure of the host bone's adaptation to the implant. The score provided by such an assessment would make it possible to judge whether this adaptation was ideal (with every prospect of implant longevity), whether it was suboptimal, or whether it was so poor as to suggest that clinical failure was only a matter of time. The system would, in fact, be a radiographic application of the ACT (Alternating Compression Tension) theory initially proposed by Schneider (19). Practically, the aim was to find a system similar to the MDA score devised by Merle d'Aubigné and Postel that awards between 0 and 6 points for each parameter rated with regard to assessment of radiographic data.

In the analysis of hip arthroplasty radiographs, the questions to be answered were, 1) Have there been any changes as compared with the postoperative films?, and 2) If so, are the changes normal, or are they warning signs of threatening failure/evidence of established implant failure? Where there is no change in the surrounding bone, under conditions of normal physical activity, the implant/host bone system may be considered to be well adjusted, with adequate fixation and a good stress transfer pattern. Any signs that may subsequently appear could be either "neutral", reflecting nothing more than an adaptive process, or "adverse".

The comparative analysis of these two scoring systems carried out in the present study demonstrated that if the E&M score is not very selective and consistently provides excellent results, the ARA score is more "sensitive", and would therefore provide lower results given the same data. Two main reasons explain why this score can be biased with respect to the behavior of the stem itself is that some patterns were considered to be "warning signs", such as the modifications at the tip of the stem or the cortical thickening in zone 3, and thus considerably lowered the global score despite no real pejorative clinical. Secondly, cavitation of the calcar or any type of osteolysis, however important because they can lead to failure, are not to be considered as any bone reaction to the stem itself, and normally are not to be taken into account while assessing the result of the femoral component itself.

Are scoring assessments valuable for radiological data?

Certainly the answer would be positive, since the outcome studies in hip arthroplasty need X-rays to be taken into account, and a numerical scoring system is the only way to evaluate one's own data, compare it with other series, and finally assess it with regard to the behavior of different designs. However, the goal of this assessment must be defined. Does one want to anticipate the behavior of the femoral component itself, or the global outcome of the arthroplasty? The behavior of the stem depends only on the bony reactions, while the fate of the prosthesis must take into account some foreign adverse effects such as osteolysis or any unexpected problems, e.g., fracture of a ceramic head.

CONCLUSION

Maurice Muller is accustomed to saying that X-rays are of fundamental interest as far as evaluation of arthroplasty is concerned. A prospective systematic assessment of thousands of films can nowadays be carried out due to great improvements in computerized databases and imaging systems. However, the collection of data needs to be precisely defined, and as quoted by Michael Freeman some time ago (20), the exact definition of radiographic patterns remains terribly difficult. Therefore, the value of each pattern, according to its type, location, or combination, must be assessed well in order to provide valuable information. This

information is critical for comparing the results of different implants, for confirming or refuting any mechanical theory leading to expected improvements, and for assessing objective results of our prostheses in the long run.

The current study of more than 500 HA-coated femoral implants with a 10 to 15 years of radiological follow-up gave us the opportunity to confirm the excellent long lasting fixation afforded by two types of HA-coated stems, the Omnifit HA and the Omniflex HA, as well as the lack of any adverse effects due to the presence of hydroxyapatite coating. These radiographic results go together with the very encouraging survival rates and the excellent clinical results obtained from these two femoral components, as well as the results published in other chapters of this book or in the literature regarding HA-coated arthroplasty.

Reference List

1. Engh CA, Massin P, Suthers KE (1990) Roentgenographic assessment of the biologic fixation of poroussurfaced femoral components. *Clinical Orthopaedic* 257:107-27.

2. Epinette JA, Geesink RGT (1995) Radiographic assessment of cementless hip prostheses: ARA, a proposed new scoring scoring system – in Cahiers d'Enseignement de la SOFCOT: "Hydroxyapatite Coated Hip and Knee Arthroplasty", *L'Expansion scientifique*, Ed. Paris, France, 51:114-26.

3. http://www.orthowave.net

4. Gruen TA, McNeice GM, Amstutz HC (1979) "Modes of failure" of Cemented Stem type femoral components. A Radiographic Analysis of Loosening. *Clinical Orthopaedics* 141:17-27.

5. Harris WH (1969) Traumatic arthritis of the hip after dislocation and acetabular fractures: treatment by mold arthroplasty. An end – result study using a new method of result evaluation. *J. Bone Joint Surgery* 51A, 4:737-55.

6. Merle d'Aubigne R, Postel R (1954) Functional results of hip arthroplasty with acrylic prosthesis. *J. Bone Joint Surg. Am.* 36:452-75.

7. Brooker AF, Bowerman JW, Robinson RA, Riley RH (1973) Ectopic ossification following total hip replacement: incidence and a method of classification. *J. Bone Joint Surgery* 55-A:1629-31.

8. Geesink RG (2002) Osteoconductive coatings for total joint arthroplasty. *Clin. Orthop.* (395):53-65.

9. Palm L, Jacobsson SA, Ivarsson I (2002) Hydroxyapatite coating improves 8- to 10-year performance of the link RS cementless femoral stem. *J. Arthroplasty* 17(2):172-5.

10. D'Antonio JA, Capello WN, Manley MT, Geesink R (2001) Hydroxyapatite femoral stems for total hip arthroplasty: 10- to 13-year follow-up. *Clin. Orthop.* (393):101-11.

11. D'Antonio JA, Thomas SJ, Bischak TL (2001) Hydroxyapatite: a noncemented fiction. *Orthopedics* 24(9):857-8.

12. Oosterbos CJ, Rahmy AI, Tonino AJ (2001) Hydroxyapatite coated hip prosthesis followed up for 5 years. *Int. Orthop.* 25(1):17-21.

13- McNally SA, Shepperd JA, Mann CV, Walczak JP (2000) The results at nine to twelve years of the use of a hydroxyapatite-coated femoral stem. *J. Bone Joint Surg. Br.* 82(3):378-82.

14. Tonino AJ, Rahmy AI (2000) The hydroxyapatite-ABG hip system: 5- to 7-year results from an international multicentre study. The International ABG Study Group. *J. Arthroplasty* 15(3):274-82.

15. Bauer TW, Schils J (1999) The pathology of total joint arthroplasty. I. Mechanisms of implant fixation. *Skeletal Radiol.* 28(8):423-32.

16. D'Lima DD, Walker RH, Colwell CW Jr (1999) Omni-fit-HA stem in total hip arthroplasty. A 2- to 5-year follow-up. *Clin. Orthop.* (363):163-9.

17. Nilsson KG, Karrholm J, Carlsson L, Dalen T (1999) Hydroxyapatite coating *versus* cemented fixation of the tibial component in total knee arthroplasty: prospective randomized comparison of hydroxyapatite-coated and cemented tibial components with 5-year follow-up using radiostereometry. *J. Arthroplasty* 14(1):9-20.

18. Capello WN, D'Antonio JA, Manley MT, Feinberg JR (1998) Hydroxyapatite in total hip arthroplasty. Clinical results and critical issues. *Clin. Orthop.* (355):200-11.

19 Schneider R (1985) La biomécanique de la prothèse totale de hanche. *Acta Orthop. Belg.* 51:196-209.

20. Freeman MAR (1999) Radiolucent Lines: A Question of Nomenclature. *J. Arthroplasty* 14:1-2.

11   Ten-Year Results of the PRA Stem

Roland Petit, MD

INTRODUCTION

The earliest studies of hydroxyapatite (HA) coatings had shown that implants obtain stable fixation as a result of a dynamic response by the host bone (1). The osteoconduction brought about by HA manifests itself in early bone formation, with rapid contact being achieved between the host bone and the implant; the intimate bond thus formed will firmly anchor the implant in the bone (2, 3, 4).

Under physiological conditions, bone is constantly being remodeled, which allows it to adapt itself to the stresses to which it is exposed. Removing the femoral head and neck, and replacing these anatomical structures with a femoral and an acetabular component, will considerably alter the physiological stress transfer pattern. The introduction of the metallic implant will result in a dynamic mechanical adaptation of the bone structure in the hip bone and in the femur. On the evidence of the studies cited above, it may be assumed that sound biological fixation of the implant in the host bone may have a beneficial influence on the process of adaptation to the new stress pattern.

The design, in 1987, of a new femoral component was intended to reflect the lessons learnt from the frequent failures of cementless implants (5, 6, 7) as well as the hopes raised by the introduction of HA coatings. The device thus produced was the PRA stem, which has been in clinical use since 20 January, 1988.

The early results were very encouraging, and were published in the literature (8,9). Readers were, however, warned that longer follow-up would be required before a final verdict could be given. By now, more than 13 years have passed since the first implantations of this device, and the

time has come to take stock and see what the follow-up, at more than ten years, of the patients managed with a PRA stem has shown.

MATERIAL AND METHODS

The PRA Stem

The PRA stem (fig. 1) is characterized by its pronounced proximal flare and distal taper. In the coronal plane, the stem is straight. The neck-shaft angle is 130°. The anterior and posterior aspects of the stem have grooves bordered crests with a quarter-circle section, to provide excellent contact with the cancellous host bed over a large developed surface. This produces less stress per unit of sur-

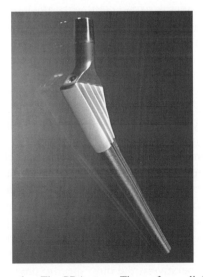

Figure 1 – The PRA stem. The surface relief allows good penetration into the cancellous bone, and provides an increased developed contact surface between the implant and the host bone.

face area at the implant-bone interface than is the case with stems that do not feature a macrointer-lock. The PRA stem is collarless. The HA coating involves only the proximal one-third of the stem, while the rest of the stem has a mat surface. The device (Fournitures Hospitalières Industrie, Quimper, France) is made of grit-blasted anodized titanium alloy.

The implant design features were based upon the following considerations:

1) Stress should be transferred in the metaphysis. The metaphyseal flare given to the stem ensures optimal metaphyseal fill, and leaves a layer of cancellous bone standing around the implant. This design feature derives from studies (10, 11, 12) of the stress transfer patterns in implanted femurs.

2) The distal part of the stem should be excluded as much as possible from the transfer of stresses, so as to prevent the thigh pain reported (13) with some cementless implants fitting to tightly in the reamed canal.

3) The stresses per unit surface area should be reduced. This was why the stem was designed with grooves, which increase the contact surface area and thereby decrease stress (12). However, it was essential to ensure that the depth and the shape of the grooves were such as to allow complete contact with the host bone.

4) Initial fixation of the implant should be in the metaphysis. For this reason, the HA coating was confined to the proximal one-third of the stem, so as to obtain osseointegration in the metaphysis before any fixation might occur in the more distal part of the stem. With this pattern, the host bone's adaptation to the new stress transfer pattern starts in the metaphysis.

Prior to the insertion of PRA stem, the bone bed must be carefully prepared with broaches, to prevent any tendency of the implant to go into varus as a result of the pronounced superolateral contour of the intraosseous portion of the device. The stem is then press-fitted into the femur. With this technique, excellent rotational stability has always been obtained, and the shape of the stem rules out distal migration of the implant. The excellent primary stability thus produced means that sound secondary osseointegration should consistently be obtained.

Postoperatively, the only specific precaution to be observed is the avoidance of full weight-bearing (walking without a walking aid). The osseointegration of the implant is preceded by the fracture of bony trabeculae. This means that the very firm seating obtained at surgery is followed by an initial phase of slightly reduced stability, which accounts for the slight distal migration of the implant during the first three postoperative months described by Scott & Freeman (14) and by Søballe *et al.* (15). Because of this phenomenon, patients are required to use two aids for the first five weeks, so as to partially unload the operated hip. As shown by histological studies of retrieved specimens (16), this period corresponds to the time during which bone will be laid down on the implant surface. After five weeks, full weight-bearing may be resumed. This policy has never resulted in any problems. The maximum distal migration seen on the customary radiographs has been 1mm.

The PRA stem has very many indications. However, it is very rarely used in cylindrical femurs with thinned-out and poorly vascularized cancellous bone, whose potential for restoration is uncertain.

Implants Used

On the acetabular side, a variety of implants were used. HA-coated cups did not become available until 21 October 1988, which is why, in the first half of 1988, non-HA-coated cups were used. Of the 32 cementless non-HA-coated cups implanted, 12 were threaded patterns, eleven were press-fit, and nine were expansion cups. The 53 HA-coated cups used were all of the threaded type. Two PRA stems were used at revision arthroplasties in which the cup was left *in situ*.

PRA stems

The stem was available in six sizes (numbered 3 to 8). Size 3 was used only once, in a dysplastic femur. Size 8 was used only once as a primary device. In the other two instances, it was used at revision THR; in one case, it was not large enough to guarantee stable fixation. The other sizes (nine times Size 4, 17 times Size 5, 30 times Size 6, 27 times Size 7) reflect the usual spread of dimensional patterns encountered in the femur.

Femoral heads and necks

All the femoral heads used in this series were made of alumina ceramic. Initially, 32-mm diameter heads were used. This policy was subsequently changed in favour of 28-mm heads, which have since been the only size used. The neck lengths were: 28 short, 39 medium, and 20 long.

Patients

The series comprised 87 hips in 83 consecutive patients operated on between 20 January 1988 and 21 June 1991. There were 51 women (61.5%), three of whom had bilateral hip replacements; and 32 men (38.5%), of whom one had a bilateral arthroplasty. The mean patient age in the series was 57.6 years (range: 28 to 71 years). This reflects our policy to use this type of implant in patients who have a reasonable long life expectancy.

Preoperative co-morbidity

As regards general problems, four of the patients (5 hips) were obese. One patient had chronic renal failure and was on dialysis. Eight of the patients had difficulty walking because of problems related to the contralateral hip; three patients had knee problems. Twenty-eight hips (32.2%) had local problems: seven had sequelae of developmental dysplasia of the hip (DDH), while 24 (27.6%) had undergone prior surgery.

Indications

Osteoarthritis (OA) was the most frequent condition necessitating THR. Seventy-four hips were affected, mainly by the primary simple form of the disease. Avascular necrosis of the femoral head accounted for seven arthroplasties. Five hips suffered from rheumatoid arthritis (RA). One patient had sequelae of tuberculosis of the hip, which was a rare indication.

Primary	52
Dysplastic	7
Post-traumatic	2
Sequelae of DDH	9
Protrusio acetabuli	2
Sequelae of hip disease in childhood	2

Table 1 – Forms of OA in the patient material.

Twenty-four of these hips had undergone prior surgery. One had had internal fixation for a fracture of the femoral neck, and two had undergone a shelf procedure for dysplasia. These operations had not significantly changed the conditions under which arthroplasty had to be performed. Some of the prior operations, however, did make THR more complicated. These involved 9 proximal femoral

osteotomies (3 McMurray procedures, 5 varus osteotomies, and, above all, one Sujioka osteotomy); 2 Chiari osteotomies; 5 cemented double cup arthroplasties; and 4 total hip replacements (1 cemented, and 3 cementless).

Ten-year review of the patients

In 68 patients (72 hips), a review could be performed at ten years from arthroplasty; in 20 of these patients (23 hips), this review was by telephone interview. Nine patients (9 hips) had died, three of them before the fifth year post-arthroplasty. Apart from the one fatality in the immediate postoperative period, there were no deaths related to the hip replacement. Three patients (3 hips) were lost to follow-up. Three PRA stems had to be revised. Thirty-one patients were seen at ten years from arthroplasty, 19 at eleven years, 14 at twelve years, and eight at 14 years.

Died	9	10.3%
Lost to follow-up	3	3.5%
Failure	3	3.5%
Telephone interview	23	26.4%
Reviewed at centre	49	56.3%
Total	87	100%

Table 2 – Ten-year review.

RESULTS

Complications

Local Complications

Complications at surgery (Table 3) comprised four calcar fissures, of which three were managed with screw fixation, and one greater trochanter fracture, which was treated with cerclage.

The postoperative complications were more serious. One failure occurred when the patient was first allowed out of bed. This was a revision case, in which the Size 8 stem chosen proved insufficient to stably fill the void left by the removal of a cemented implant. The failure was attributable to operative error. There were two postoperative dislocations, which were readily managed with closed reduction. Two haematomas were experienced, of which one was resorbed and the other evacuated surgically, without any further complications in either case. There were seven instances of periprosthetic ossification. Of these seven, five were

	N	%	Remarks
Complications at surgery			
Vascular injury	0	–	
Nerve injury	0	–	
Calcar fissure	4	4.6%	3 × managed with screw fixation
Femoral shaft fracture	0	–	
Fracture of greater trochanter	1	1.1%	1 Cerclage
Early postoperative complications			
Postoperative dislocation	2	2.3%	Closed reduction
Stem loosening	1	1.1%	Revised
Isolated DVT	4	4.6%	Medical treatment
Pulmonary embolism	2	2.3%	1 Caval filter
Thrombosis of aortic bifurcation	1	1.1%	Extraction of white thrombus
Haematoma	2	2.3%	1 Evacuated
Wound dehiscence	0	–	
Superficial infection	0	–	
Deep infection	0	–	
Periprosthetic ossification	7	8%	
Late complications			
Dislocation	1	1.1%	
Non–traumatic migration	0	–	
Secondary fracture	0	–	
Daily pain	3	3.5%	See text
Stem loosening	1	1.1%	Revised
Cup loosening	9	10.3%	Revised
Haematogenous infection	1	1.1%	Implants removed

Table 3 – Summary of complications (n = 87)

Brooker (17) Class II, and two were Brooker Class III.

The late complications encountered necessitated 13 reoperations (14.9%). One stem and cup revision for loosening in a case of osteolysis took place five years after the index arthroplasty. A polyethylene (PE) debris granuloma had been noted more than one year earlier. One implant was removed for haematogenous infection in a case of septicaemia with endocarditis. The implant had been *in situ* for five years, without giving any trouble. In the other cases, only the cup was revised. Of the 32 non-HA-coated cups, 21.8% were revised (five threaded and two press-fitted patterns). Of the 53 threaded HA-coated devices, 5.6% (3 cases) required revision. Three patients had daily residual pain, without any evidence of loss of fixation or stability of the femoral stem. One of these patients had undergone multiple prior surgeries for the sequelae of DDH, and one female patient, who died eleven years after arthroplasty, was on chronic dialysis and had severe osteoporosis. The third patient had a history of head injuries and had undergone two cup revisions without success ; the cause of the pain could not be established. There was one late dislocation, which did not recur.

In all, there were three PRA stem failures. One occurred immediately after surgery, and was due to an error on the part of the surgeon, who failed to obtain sufficient stability of the stem inserted. The second failure was due to late haematogenous infection. These two failures were not attributable to the implant as such. Only one case of loosening of an initially stable PRS stem was a genuine implant-related failure ; in this case, loosening was the result of a spread of the osteolytic lesions caused by PE debris.

It should be noted that revision for instability of the acetabular component was performed in 21.8% of the non-HA-coated cups, whereas only 5.6% of the HA-coated sockets required revision for instability.

Systemic Complications

Apart from one case of postoperative delirium tremens, the complications encountered were mainly of a thromboembolic nature. There was one massive, fatal pulmonary embolism in the immediate postoperative period, and another pulmonary embolism, which responded to treatment, but was complicated by femoral nerve palsy on the uninvolved side, caused by a haematoma in the femoral triangle. The functional outcome was excellent. There were four deep vein thromboses, which cleared up and left no sequelae. One obliteration of the aortoiliac bifurcation by white thrombus occurred as a manifestation of the patient's previously unknown intolerance to low molecular weight heparin. The thrombus was immediately extracted, and there were no sequelae.

Clinical Results

Using the Charnley system of walking categories, 45 hips were rated as being Category A, 32 as Category B, and 10 as Category C. For the clinical assessment, the scoring system devised by R. Merle d'Aubigne and M. Postel (MDA) (18) was used in all cases. This system rates the intensity of pain, range of movement (mobility), and walking ability (function), with a range, in each category, from six points (best) to one point (poorest). The Harris Hip Score was established retrospectively, from the patients" charts, for the preoperative situation, and at clinical examination for the final review.

Pain

Pain was the chief complaint for which THR had been sought. Fifty-four hips (62%) were very painful (MDA score: 0 to 1). Another 25 hips (28.7%) were painful enough to prevent walking (MDA score: 2). At the latest examination, 60 patients (83.3%) had no pain; nine patients (12.5%) scored 5. In three of these cases, the pain was in the buttock; in three, at the level of the greater trochanter; while in the remaining three it was impossible to determine whether the pain was in the hip region or whether, in actual fact, the patients concerned had low-back pain. Three times, there was radiographic evidence of an unstable cup. The three patients (4.2%) who scored 3 or 4 had a long history of co-morbidity. None of the patients in the study had thigh pain.

Mobility

Pre-arthroplasty, only 17 hips (19.5%) had a full ROM. In 53.6% of the cases. Dressing was difficult; half of these patients had a fixed deformity. At ten years, mobility was found to be better than 90° of flexion and 40° of abduction in 64 (88.8%) of the 72 patients reviewed. In seven cases, the score was 5; and in one case, it was 4. All of these were patients who had suffered from DDH.

Function

The Function score rates both the patient's walking ability and the stability of the hip.

Prior to arthroplasty, 90.8% of the patients were severely limited in the distance they could walk, even with a walking aid. At the latest review, 57 hips (79.1%) had unlimited walking ability without the patients needing walking aids, while eleven patients (15.7%) required an aid for walking long distances. Five patients, who were in Charnley categories B or C, did not have satisfactory hip stability.

Rating with the Harris Hip Score (HSS) gave a mean preoperative score of 42.3, while the mean score at the latest review was 94.3. Excellent results (scores of between 98 and 100) were seen in 40 cases (55.5%). Twenty-four patients (33.3%) had Good results (scoring between 80 and 97); while seven (9.7%) scored between 60 and 79, and were consequently rated Fair. There was only one Poor result, in a patient with major co-morbidity. Table 4 gives a summary of the scores as a function of the Charnley categories. Co-morbidity is clearly seen to be a factor affecting the results of arthroplasty.

	A	B	C
HHS (pre-arthroplasty)	42.9	43	35.2
HHS (at latest review)	96.0	93.6	87.0

Table 4 – Harris Hip Score *versus* Charnley Categories.

Assessment using the MDA score showed a different distribution: 84.1% of the results were rated Excellent or Very Good; 12.5% were rated Good; while 3.4% were rated Fair. Regardless of the scoring system used, the patients" lives were significantly improved, from the sixth month post-arthroplasty onwards; this improvement was durable, and still seen at the latest review.

Radiological Results

The radiological results following the implantation of a PRA stem were assessed in 53 patients, who had been followed up since their hip replacement. The outstanding feature was the stability over time of the implants. Radiologically evident osseointegration of the HA-coated implants was obtained not later than the sixth month post-arthroplasty;

any voids initially seen between the implant and the host bone had been filled in by that time.

"Radiological silence" (fig. 2)

In 41.8% of the patients reviewed, the radiographic pattern of the hip had remained unchanged out to the latest follow-up at ten or twelve years. This is what we call "radiological silence". In these patients, the implant-bone interface did not show any defects, and neither the cortex nor the cancellous bone was altered (fig. 3).

The only change indicative of an adaptation of the bone structure to the new stress pattern was the appearance of trabecular reinforcements in the form of bridges running obliquely downwards from the host bone to the implant, especially in Gruen (6) Zones 2, 3, 5, and 6. This trabeculation was sometimes seen in the distal zone, and was interpreted in the same way.

Changes Observed In The Other Patients

Most of the changes observed provided evidence of host bone biological activity.

Distal lucent lines

These were thin lucent lines rarely more than 1.2mm in width, most frequently found in Zone 4, but running into Zones 3 and 5 in 40% of the cases. In some instances they were bordered by a sclerotic

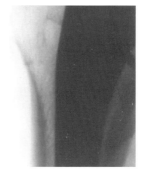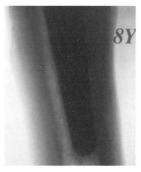

Figure 3 – The bony trabeculae reproduce the force line pattern. Any such trabeculae in the metaphyseal zone are not seen before six months post-arthroplasty. In Zone 4, they tend to appear at a late stage.

line running around the stem tip. These lucent lines were carefully followed over time. Their time course never gave cause for concern. Of the 15 lucent lines that had appeared in Zone 4 or in Zones 3, 4, and 5, during Year-1 radiographic follow-up, eleven were monitored for ten years. In five patients, these lucent lines were replaced by a normal bone pattern; in four patients, by linear cancellous densification in intimate contact with the implant; in two patients, they remained unchanged and without any further progression. Three distal lucent lines appeared in the fifth year

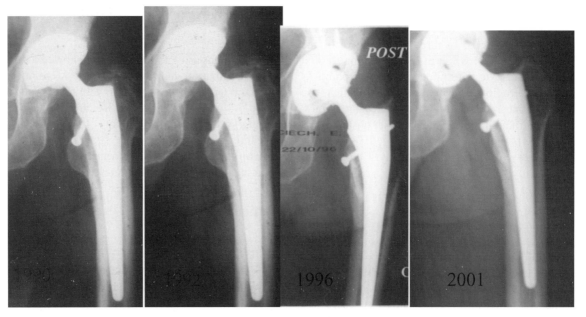

Figure 2 – Radiological silence. No change, at 13 years, from the 2-year pattern. The screw was inserted for the management of a femoral neck fissure at implantation, and shows the absence of distal stem migration.

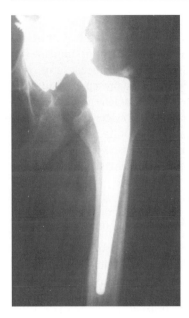
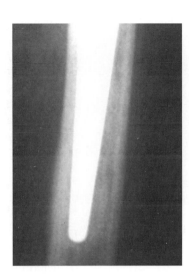
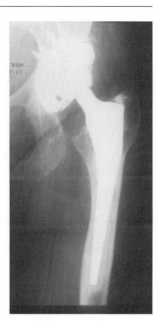

Figure 4 – Distal lucent lines were not associated with changes in proximal osseointegration. The lucent line shown here was eventually replaced by cancellous densification, at three years.

from arthroplasty; of these, one remained, while the other two filled in (fig. 4).

These lucent lines probably bear witness to the elastic adaptation of the host bone to the tip of the rigid implant. In none of the cases was there any change in the bone-implant interface anywhere else along the stem, and the patients concerned did not have any clinical symptoms.

Proximal lucent lines

One lucent line in Zone 1 had appeared during the first year post-arthroplasty, and was no longer seen at further follow-up. The other lucent line was seen at the five-year review. It involved Zones 1 and 7, and showed up, at the latest follow-up, as a PE debris granuloma.

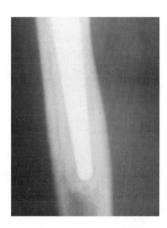

Figure 5 – Cancellous densification with segmental ballooning of the shaft. The patient was asymptomatic.

Distal cancellous densification was not seen at the one-year review. Two patterns of this kind were seen at five years. By the ten-year review, one had remained unchanged, while the other had disappeared. Cancellous reinforcement, with bridging between the cortex and the implant, as described above, was a common finding (fig. 5).

Pedestals always were of the stable type. The only pattern seen was a half-pedestal against the lateral cortex; most of these formations were not very dense, and many were temporary features: four had disappeared by the latest follow-up. At ten

years, there were three stable pedestals and there lateral shelves that were not very dense. There was no evidence of medullary canal occlusion (fig. 6).

Cortical thickening in Zone 6 was seen in one patient, as early as Year 1; it did not progress thereafter.

Thinning of bone was an extremely rare finding. Three cases had radiological evidence of discreet osteoporosis at the latest follow-up; one of these patients had generalized osteoporosis.

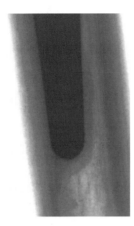

Figure 6 – The most pronounced pedestal seen in the series. There were no clinical symptoms.

Osteolysis was seen in seven cases (13.2%), as defects in the calcar (typical scalloping), and defects in the trochanteric region, three times with posterolateral spread. In all of these cases, there was evidence of insert wear; in three cases, revision had to be performed for cup loosening. At surgery, a foreign body granuloma containing large numbers of PE wear particles was found at the level of the acetabulum, as well as a granuloma along the posterior aspect of the stem extending over a distance of 3 to 5 cm.

Implant migration was not observed in any of the cases.

Engh score. This score was obtained at the latest radiological examination. It showed all the implants to have been osseointegrated. Four cases scored between 16 and 20, 16 between 21 and 24, and 33 between 20 and 27.

ARA score (20). Rating with this score also gave good results, since 31 cases scored 6; 13 scored 5; and 6 scored 4.

In all, the radiological follow-up of these patients did not show anything that could have given cause for concern, other than the seven cases of osteolysis in the form of granulomas where there had been wear of the PE insert. In all the other cases, there was evidence of osteoconductivity around the implant. None of the radiographs showed instability of the PRA stem.

The radiological results of the cups in the 53 patients for whom follow-up radiographs were available at the ten-year review were equally good as far as the HA-coated cups were concerned. Of the 28

HA-coated threaded cups, only one had a Zone 3 lucent line. Osteolysis was seen in three cases, but was not considered to be endangering implant stability. Two implants were revised because of osteolysis, and do not figure in the present study. Of the six threaded cups originally implanted in the patients reviewed at ten years, only two were still *in situ*; one of the two had a Zone 3 lucent line. The six expansion cups were remarkably stable. Of the eight press-fit cups, four had lucent lines, though never in Zone 2.

Implant Survival

For the 87 cases in the study, cumulative survival (calculated using the Kaplan-Meier method) could be determined out to eleven years, since 42 hips were still "alive" at the end of the eleventh year. Following the policy of the Scandinavian registries, it was decided to apply the term 'revision" only to reoperations involving the exchange of at least one of the two major components in direct contact with the host bone (*ie* the cup and/or the stem), while the exchange of an acetabular insert or a femoral head would not be considered to be a "revision".

Using this definition, there were two stem failures, one in the first and one in the fifth year post-arthroplasty, that may be attributed to the implant itself; in addition, there was one revision required for intercurrent causes (haematogenous infection), in the fifth year. As regards the purely implant-related failures, they accounted for two cases (2.3%) out of a total of 87 hips, and comprised one operative error (inappropriate choice of stem size) and one failure of implant fixation. This means that the failure rate at ten years of the HA fixation of the PRA stem was 1 case in 87 (1.15%).

When these data were used to plot the survival curves, the cumulative survival rates at eleven years, using different endpoints, were observed to be 95.25% ± 0.0414 for hip replacement failure (all causes); PRA stem failure, 96.45 ± 0.0333; and HA fixation failure (aseptic loosening), 98.75 ± 0.0243.

DISCUSSION

Following up these arthroplasty patients for more than ten years has been instructive in several respects.

Observation of Osseointegration

The initial design concept was based upon the results of experimental studies (1), and upon the clinical results obtained in the short term (2, 3, 4, 21). There is evidence that HA-coated implants are rapidly, reliably, and lastingly osseointegrated, providing that sound primary stability has been achieved (22). This was borne out by all the PRA stems and all the HA-coated acetabular components in the present study. Only one PRA stem and three cups had to be revised. All of these components showed clinical and radiological evidence of osseointegration; their late loosening had been the result of the extension of PE debris granulomas.

Adaptation of the Host Bone

Continuous bone remodeling, and the adaptation of the host bone to the changed stress transfer pattern following the insertion of an implant, often manifest themselves in the formation of downward-sloping trabecular bridges. These bridges link the host cortex to the implant and visualize the force lines at these sites. The findings around the stem were paralleled by the patterns observed around the cup. In a smaller number of cases, there was cortical thickening, cancellous densification, or lateral pedestal-like half-shelf formation. These patterns were not permanent; they would come and go, without the stability of the implants being affected in any way.

No Thigh Pain

Thigh pain is a notorious problem in cementless stems without an HA coating (5, 6), which has given cementless hip arthroplasty a bad name. The pain is due to the frequently observed instability of the stem, as evidenced by extended lucent lines, and to mid-shaft stress risers resulting from exclusively diaphyseal stabilization and proximal stress shielding (13). In our series, thigh pain was not observed, even though some of the stems were in slight varus. It is difficult to decide how much of this was due to the reduced dimensions of the distal part of the stem, and how much was attributable to the quality of the metaphyseal fixation obtained thanks to the HA coating. Most of the PRA stems showed evidence of osseointegration; a small number had a distal lucent line. There was no difference with regard to thigh pain between these two groups. Absence of thigh pain has been reported in the literature to be a feature of the majority of HA-coated stems (23, 24, 25).

Resorption of the HA Coating

Where implants have been retrieved for breakage, it has been seen that this resorption is never complete. No conclusions with regard to this phenomenon can be drawn from our study; however, the time *in situ* (13 years in the case of the patients with the longest follow-up) should have been long enough for resorption to occur. It was encouraging to see that the radiographic patterns had not changed in any way.

Reasons for Revision

Apart from one late haematogenous infection, the only reason for the revision of the HA-coated implants was foreign body granuloma formation as a result of PE wear debris. These granulomas produce extensive periprosthetic osteolysis in the effective joint space (26). In all the cases of granuloma formation in the present study, there was radiographic evidence of PE insert wear. However, PE insert wear was not consistently associated with granuloma formation. Often, evidence of wear is seen several years before granulomas are observed on the radiographs. Only continued monitoring will tell.

Sealing Function of HA Coating

The view that the intimate contact between the host bone and the implant may act as a barrier to the spread of PE debris was borne out in the present study. In the cases of revision for cup loosening as a result of granuloma formation, periprosthetic femoral osteolysis was found to be confined to the most proximal portion of the stem. It never exceeded 1cm in length, except on the posterior aspect of the stem, where it was sometimes found to extend to a length of 3-4 cm. Meticulous curetting and grafting of the osteolytic lesions appeared to result in excellent stability, although follow-up to date has been short.

HA and Infection

Since there were no early infections in the present study, no conclusions can be drawn. The only infection observed was spread by the bloodstream, in a patient with septicaemia complicated by the presence of several septic foci. When the implants were removed, they were found to be perfectly stable. The condition of the hip was one of suppurating arthritis, without any evidence of bone infection, especially at the implant-bone interface. This suggests that the intimate contact between the biologically active host bone and the HA-coated device protects against the spread of the septic process at this site.

CONCLUSION

This consecutive series of the first 87 PRA stems at a follow-up of between ten and 13 years showed the device to give excellent and very durable results. The consistency with which osseointegration was achieved marks an important improvement on the results obtained with non-HA-coated cementless devices. The outcomes were markedly better than those obtained by the author using cemented implants or non-HA-coated cementless stems (27). This suggests that the PRA stem should be liberally used in the management of femurs that still have their basic trabecular pattern. However, these stems may cost slightly more than cemented devices, which means that they would not be used in patients with limited life expectancy in whom there are no contraindications to the use of cement.

Notwithstanding its many obvious qualities, the PRA stem has the disadvantage of being very bulky in the metaphysis, which may make its correct insertion difficult in some cases. Work is in progress to reduce the proximal bulk of the device in order to facilitate surgery without, however, compromising the long-term results.

Osteolysis in the wake of PE particle granuloma formation was the worst complication in the series. In order to bring this problem under control, the entire bearing combination will need to be addressed. The new PE materials have not been around for long enough to allow their utility to be assessed. Metal-metal bearing combinations hold promise, although their surface hardness is such as to make them prone to scoring. Alumina-alumina combinations have been in use for a considerable time, and have been found to produce markedly less wear debris; such debris as is produced has never been known to affect implant longevity (28).

There is reason to believe that the clinical and radiological results obtained will remain stable in the very long term. However, all the patients managed with the PRA stem will need to be meticulously followed up to detect any problems that may arise; and implant designers will need to consider any new findings concerning the biological processes that govern the way in which the host bone manages to live with the implant.

Reference List

1. Geesink RGT, De Groot K, Klein CPAT (1988) Bonding of bone to hydroxyapatite implants. *J. Bone Joint Surg.* 70-B, 1, 17-22.

2. Furlong RJ, Osborn JF (1991) Fixation of hip femoral prostheses by hydroxyapatite ceramic coating. *J. Bone Joint Surg.* 73-B, 741-5.

3. Hardy DCR, Frayssinet P, Guilhelm A, Lafontaine MA, Delince PE (1991) Bonding of Hydroxyapatite-coated Femoral Prostheses. *J. Bone Joint Surg.* 73-B, 732-40.

4. Cartillier JC, Balay B, Charlet C, Machenaud A, Semay JM, Setiey L, Vidalain JP (1989) Intérêt de l'hydroxyapatite de calcium dans la fixation précoce d'un implant sans ciment, premiers résultats cliniques. *Rev. Chir. Orthop.* 75, Suppl. n° 1, 138-9.

5. Barrack RL, Jasty M, Bragdon C, Haire T, Harris WH (1992) Thigh pain despite bone ingrowth into uncemented femoral stems. *J. Bone Surg. Br.* 74-B, 507-10.

6. Campbell ACL, Rorabeck CH, Bourne RB, Chess D, Nott L (1992) Thigh pain after cementless hip arthroplasty. *J. Bone Joint Surg. Br.* 74-B, 63-6.

7. Wykman A, Olsson E, Axdorf G, Goldie I (1991) Total Hip Arthroplasty. A comparison between cemented and press-fit noncemented fixation. *J. Arthroplasty* 6, 19-29.

8. Petit R (1992) La prothèse de hanche PRA. *Orthop. Traumatol.* 2, 239-46.

9. Petit R (1995) The PRA prosthesis. Biomechanical principles and clinical experience. In Cahiers d'enseignement de la SOFCOT n°51, Hydroxyapatite coated hip and knee arthroplasty, 239-44, Epinette JA, Geesink RGT, Expansion Scientifique Française, Paris,

10. Oh I, Harris WH (1978) Proximal strain distribution in the loaded femur: an *in vitro* comparison of the disribution in the intact femur and after insertion of different hip-replacement femoral components. *J. Bone Joint Surg.* 60-A, 75-85.

11. Dambreville A (1991) Prothèses de hanche sans ciment. La fixation élective métaphysaire. Principe. Avantages et inconvénients. *Rev. Chir. Orthop.* 77, suppl. n°1: 147

12. Spotorno L, Romagnoli S (1987) Teoria e risultati radiografici e clinici dello stelo CLS. *Min. Ort. Traum.* 39, 321-5.

13. Engh CA, Bobyn JD, Glassman AH (1987) Porous coated hip replacement: the factors governing bone ingrowth, stress shielding, and clinical results. *J. Bone Joint Surg.* 69-B, 45-55.

14. Scott G, Freeman MAR (1995) Migration studies on cemented, press-fit and hydroxyapatite coated femoral stems. In Cahiers d'enseignement de la SOFCOT, n°51, Hydroxyapatite coated hip and knee arthroplasty, 110-3, Epinette JA, Geesink RGT, Expansion Scientifique Française, Paris.

15. Søballe K, Toksvig-Larsen J, Gelinek J, Fruensgaard S, Hansen ES, Ryd L, Lucht U, Bünger C (1995) RSA studies on HA coated and porous coated implants. In Cahiers d'Enseignement de la SOFCOT, n°51, Hydroxyapatite coated hip and knee arthroplasty, Pages 105-9, Epinette JA, Geesink RGT, Expansion Scientifique Française, Paris.

16. Frayssinet P, Hardy DCR, Tourenne F, Rouquet N, Delince P, Bonel G (1995) Osseointegration of plasma sprayed coated hip implants in humans. In Cahiers d'Enseignement de la SOFCOT, n°51, Hydroxyapatite coated hip and knee arthroplasty, Pages 149-57, Epinette JA, Geesink RGT, Expansion Scientifique Française, Paris.

17. Merle d'Aubigné R (1990) Cotation chiffrée de la fonction de la hanche. *Rev. Chir. Orthop.* 76, 371-4.

18. Brooker AF, Bowerman JW, Robinson RA, Riley RH (1973) Ectopic ossification following total hip replacement: incidence and a method of classification. *J. Bone Joint Surg.* 55-A, 1629-31.

19. Gruen TA, McNeige GM, Amstutz HC (1979) Modes of failure of cemented stem type femoral components. A radiographic analysis of loosening. *Clin. Orthop.* 141, 17-27.

20. Epinette JA, Geesink R and the AGORA Group (1979) Radiographic assessment of cementless hip prostheses: ARA, a proposed new scoring system. In Cahiers d'Enseignement de la SOFCOT, n°51, Hydroxyapatite coated hip and knee arthroplasty, Pages 114-26, Epinette JA, Geesink RGT, Expansion Scientifique Française, Paris.

21. Epinette JA, Duthoit E, Carlier Y, Poison R. (1987-1992) Prothèse totale de hanche. Le cotyle ARC2F; à propos de 2850 cas avec un recul maximum de cinq ans. 67ème Réunion annuelle de la SOFCOT, Paris, 10-13 novembre 1992.

22. Petit R (1999) The use of hydroxyapatite in orthopaedic surgery: a ten-year review. *Eur. J. Orthop. surg. Traumatol.* 9, 71-4.

23. Vidalain JP and the ARTRO group (1995) The Corail system in primary hip arthroplasty. Seven-year experience of the ARTRO Group. In Cahiers d'Enseignement de la SOFCOT, n°51, Hydroxyapatite coated hip and knee arthroplasty Pages 193 à 203, Epinette JA, Geesink RGT, Expansion Scientifique Française, Paris.

24. Epinette J-A (1995) HA coated Omnifit stems in primary hip replacement surgery: seven-year experience. In Cahiers d'Enseignement de la SOFCOT, n°51, Hydroxyapatite coated hip and knee arthroplasty, 215-26, Epinette JA, Geesink RGT, Expansion Scientifique Française, Paris.

25. Nourissat Ch, Adrey J, Berteaux D, Gueret A, Goalard Ch, Hamon G (1995) The ABG standard hip prosthesis: Five-year results. In Cahiers d'Enseignement de la SOFCOT, n°51, Hydroxyapatite coated hip and knee arthroplasty, 227-38, Epinette JA, Geesink RGT, Expansion Scientifique Française, Paris.

26. Schmalzried TP, Jasty M., Harris WH (1992) Periprosthetic bone loss in total hip arthroplasty. *J. Bone Joint Surg.* 74-A, 849-63.

27. Petit R (1996) Cinq années d'expérience des prothèses totale de hanche revêtues d'hydroxyapatite. in "Actualités en Biomatériaux", Volume III, Mainard D, Merle M, Delagoutte JP, Romillat (Ed), 187-96.

28. Bizot P, Nizard R, Charon Ph, Sedel L, Witvoet J (1997) Prothèse totale de hanche pour nécrose atraumatique de la tête fémorale. Résultats d'une série de 70 PTH alumine-alumine à 9 ans de recul moyen. *Rev. Chir. Orthop.* 83, suppl II, 48.

12   Long-Term Results with the HA-coated Arc2f in Primary Hip Surgery

Jean-Alain Epinette, MD, Michael T. Manley, PhD and Etienne Duthoit, MD

INTRODUCTION

Acetabular replacement is a challenging procedure in Hip Arthroplasty. The implanted cup and its fixation interfaces must cope with the stresses imposed by patient activity as well as stresses imposed by neck impingement at the extremes of motion. For many years, a stable fixation alone was considered as the ultimate goal in acetabular arthroplasty. Nowadays, complex problems as wear, migration of particles, and osteolytic lesions tend to be the major concern. A number of "hot" issues remain unanswered, and must be handled through long term follow up of the various solutions proposed by designers, afforded by the industry, and validated by surgeons. We would like to contribute to the debate by reporting a continuous series of 602 HA-coated screw Arc2f cups implanted by two of us (JAE-ED) at two institutions from 1989 to 1991 in primary hip surgery with a minimum follow-up of 10 years and a maximum of 13 years. The overall implant design remained unchanged throughout. We attempt to answer some important questions, such as the potential for threaded components to obtain a long lasting reliable fixation, the use of additional screws, the real rate of osteolysis and its relationship with wear, and finally compare the results with this threaded cup to results of press fit cups reported in the literature.

The design of our implant began after disappointing results were reported with the first generation of threaded cups (1, 2, 3, 4). These lacked provisions for bone attachment and thus had limited prospects for long-term "biological" fixation. In 1987, we hypothesized that a combination of the principle of screw-type fixation with an ingrowth surface on a hemispherical cup might prove an ideal solution and provide substantially better clinical results than were observed with earlier threaded components. These design considerations were realized in the Arc2f cup, where the "2f" designation is understood to stand for the ability to provide two fixation interfaces, primary fixation in the form of the equatorial threads, and secondary fixation in the form of a well characterized ingrowth surface.

Initially, the cups were covered with plasma-sprayed commercially pure titanium (CpTi). Various authors have studied retrieved specimens with this type of coating and found the amount of bone ingrowth into the porous surface to be rather disappointing: Even the most encouraging reports showed only 20-30% of the available surface to be covered by attached bone (5, 6, 7). We believed the use of a hydroxyapatite (HA) coating would be the most reliable means of achieving secondary –and lasting – "bioactive" fixation (8, 9, 10). We also believed sufficient data existed to suggest that HA could enhance the rate at which apposition occurs. This enhanced apposition rate appeared to be related to the gradual transformation of the HA crystals into newly formed bone, which in turn remained in apposition to the microporosities of the underlying metal. The use of the roughened titanium surface was abandoned near the end of 1988 in favor of an HA coating. In all other aspects, the first and second generations of the Arc2f were identical.

In general, the Arc2f cup appears to comply with Schneider's ACT (Alternating Compression Tension) theory (11) by providing, enhanced bone-implant bonding to a bioconductive ongrowth surface, reduced micromotion between cup and bone due to the preferential stabilization of the cup at the periphery by threads and enhanced rigidity of the hip bone through the use of cranial screws. This system protects against the detrimental effects of stress transfer by ensuring that the stability of the bone-implant system can withstand the tensile/compressive forces produced by patient activity (12).

MATERIAL AND METHODS

The Arc2f component (Stryker Howmedica Osteonics Corp., Allendale, NJ) has a thin cutting, double-start thread incorporated into the periphery of the shell. The threaded peripheral section of the Arc2f component consists of a true multiple-start thread (as opposed to the buttress-like threads of most previous designs). The implant is fabricated from titanium alloy (Ti-6Al-4V), and is coated with a 50 micrometer thick layer of hydroxyapatite (> 90% hydroxyapatite minimum) plasma-sprayed onto a roughened substrate (fig. 1). The polyethylene liners (Vecteur Orthopedic, Paris, France) matched with the Arc2f cup during the study consisted initially of compression molded ultrahigh molecular weight polyethylene (UHMWPE), followed later by regular machined UHMWPE. Both liners now are replaced with highly crosslinked "Crossfire" liners (Stryker Howmedica Osteonics Corp., Allendale, NJ) as part of contemporary orthopaedic practice. During insertion, the component is screwed into the reamed acetabulum with a small ratcheting wrench. Supplementary fixation was achieved in all surgeries by the placement of three or four bone screws through holes in the shell into the ilium.

Early on we recognized that even the most carefully prepared acetabulum will have some local gaps and imperfections that prohibit full contact being made across the entire area of the replacement cup. Therefore, we advocated the packing of the reamed acetabulum with the small particles of bone obtained during reaming in order to provide a moldable interposition layer of autologous bone graft. This approach was used in all the surgeries. The Arc2f cup was used in a wide variety of indications, since it gave good primary fixation even in poor bone stock and in revision cases. We used the cup in all cases where primary reconstructive stability was not a problem (i.e., in all primary replacements) as well as in almost all revisions (9, 13, 14).

Between January 1989 and December 1991, 602 HA-coated Arc2f threaded cups were implanted as

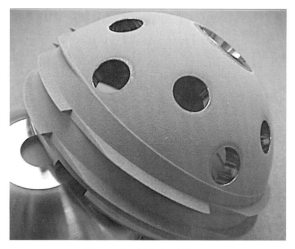

Figure 1 – HA Arc 2f cup:
HA-coated hemispherical cup with thin peripheral thread.

a consecutive multicenter series in 593 patients either at the Bruay Clinic or at the Henin-Beaumont Clinic (France) by two of us (JAE & ED). The cups had been mainly matched with a HA-coated femoral component (487 hips with a Omnifit-HA stem, Stryker Howmedica Osteonics Corp., Allendale, NJ, USA *versus* 108 hips with a Corail stem, De Puy, Warsaw, In, USA) while only 7 HA cups were implanted against a cemented stem. Bearing surfaces in 503 cases consisted of a metallic head (CrCo) and in 99 cases an alumina ceramic head against a hooded (10°) polyethylene liner sterilized using gamma irradiation in air. The head diameter was 28 mm in all cases. The most common cup size was 52 mm (29%) followed by 50 mm (28%), 48 mm (18%) and 54 mm (13%), while 12% were 56 mm and over in diameter. Additional fixation was afforded by complementary screws (generally three upward screws) in all cases.

The clinical course of each patient was evaluated pre-operatively, then early (five to ten weeks), at six months, at one year and yearly thereafter. All clinical and radiological data, as well as radiographs, were stored and computed in a custom computerized hip arthroplasty database known as OrthoWave, developed under the aegis of the CRDA (Imaging Center and Clinical Research in Arthroplasty, Bruay, France). For all pre- and post-operative evaluations, clinical assessment was performed using both the Harris scoring system (HSS) (26) and the Merle d'Aubigné-Postel assessment (PMA) (29, 30, 31). In the report on our results, we assumed that each hip "lives its own life", and thus gave counts of "hips" rather than "patients". A patient who underwent a bilateral replacement for instance can experience pain in a given hip and be painfree on the other side, or can be consider as a success on one hip and a failure on the opposite side. The "unit of follow-up" was thus each operated hip, independent of the patient undergoing uni or bilateral hip replacement.

With respect to the radiographic assessment, anteroposterior and lateral radiographs of the 375 hips with updated films at 10 years minimum follow-up were evaluated for both bone changes and for cup migration. In the remaining 29 cases, films were missing or were not useable for precise evaluation due to poor technical quality. This study focuses on the 375 complete radiographic dossiers. At the pre-surgical and at all follow-up patient evaluations, anterior-posterior and lateral radiographs of each involved hip were taken. All radiographs were converted to digital files for storage and later analysis using a film digitizer (VXR-12, Vidar Systems Corp., Herndon, VA.). All clinical data and radiological images were stored for both retrieval and analysis in a computerized hip database, (OrthoWave, ARIA, Bruay, France). Any visible migration of the acetabular component was measured on sequential radiographs using the teardrop line as a vertical datum and a vertical line drawn through the base of that teardrop closest to the cup as a horizontal datum.

Three acetabular zones, based on the DeLee-Charnley model (57), were delineated so that apparent radiographic changes from visit to visit for each patient could be documented. Each acetabular implant was evaluated for radiolucencies, regions of increased bone density, component migration, and osteolytic lesions. Osteolysis was assessed as "severe" if it exhibited progressive evolution, extended to more than 50% of the surface of the shell, or was not immediately adjacent to the surface of the shell but had distinct boundaries. Osteolysis was assessed as "moderate" if none of the previously mentioned "severe" characteristics was observed. A third category of lytic lesions was added, described as "mild" to characterize some minor lytic cysts located at the periphery of the cup, especially onto zone 1 of Charnley and De Lee, described as "droplets" in reaction to polyethylene debris, and similar to the "scalloping" of the calcar at the proximal aspect of the femoral metaphysis.

Acetabular interface stability was determined using a modification of Engh's criteria (16, 58). The designation "stable bone ingrown" was used for components that did not migrate and did not show radiolucencies in fifty percent or more of any fixation zone. The designation "stable fibrous ingrown" was used for components that did not migrate but showed radiolucencies in all three zones, and the designation "unstable" was used for cups that migrated three millimeters or more and showed radiolucencies in all three zones.

For the span of the minimum ten year study, we calculated survivorship based on implants revised for aseptic loosening. In addition, we calculated the overall mechanical and combined failure rates using the criteria of Capello *et al.* (27).

RESULTS

Clinical Results

Demographic analysis of the population at the beginning of the study showed that sixty-one per cent of the patients were female. The mean patient age at the time of surgery was 65.8 years with a range of twenty-one to eighty-eight years. Computation of the Body Mass Index (BMI: Average 26.5; 14.3-47.6) revealed an optimum weight in only 38% of patients. Mild obesity was exhibited by 43% of patients, and medium or severe obesity was exhibited by 19% of patients. The etiology of hip disease was mainly osteoarthritis (87.5%) and avascular necrosis (9.3%). Only 37% (224 hips) of the study population had no other significant disabling problem (Class A) according to Charnley classification (24).

At the time of this report, of a total number of 602 implanted cups, data from a total of 408 hips were available for follow-up analysis, including 4 isolated femoral failures while the non failed cup had been left in place. From the original patient cohort there were 173 non-hip related deaths. Twelve cups underwent revision, 2 for deep infection, 6 for accidental traumatic fracture, and 4 for aseptic loosening, including two isolated cup failures and two retrievals of both femoral and acetabular components. Only 8 patients (1.33%) from the total cohort were lost to follow-up (Table 1). Clinical and radiological results reported in the present paper cover only patients reviewed both clinically and radiologically at 10 year minimum follow-up. Of the 404 cups remaining "on file", 383 satisfied this criterion. We were unable to review the remaining 21 hips for a variety of non-arthroplasty related co-morbidities. However, these patients were contacted by telephone to ascertain the status of their hip arthroplasty. None indicated that their hip had been revised elsewhere. Therefore, we report detailed clinical and radiographic follow-up of these primary 383 hips with complete clinical review at a minimum ten years, but we encompass the whole population of 602 cases when discussing survivorship.

Archiving	Number	%
On file	404	67.11
Lost to follow-up	8	1.33
Dead	174	28.9
Retrieved due to infection	2	0.33
Retrieved due to fracture	6	1
Global failure	2	0.33
Acetabular isolated failure	2	0.33
Femoral isolated failure	4	0.66
Total	602	100

Table 1 – Breakdown of the 602 HA Arc2f series according to archiving status at the time of the study.

At 10 year of minimum follow-up, pain was noted as "none" in 377 cases (93.3%) and "slight" in the remaining 7 cases. No "moderate" or "severe" pain was recorded. Walking distance was unlimited in 81.4% of cases, and a single patient was limited to indoor activities. This latter patient is a 93 year old female with excellent function in the operated hip, but who suffers from mobility impairment due to a severe and disabling osteoarthritis in the contralateral hip. The use of stairs was considered as "normal" in 70.3% of cases, and in 29.7% as "able" when using a banister or by any other method. The mean Harris pain score was 5.1 out of a maximum of 44 preoperatively and up to 43.9 points (40-44; SD: 0.257)postoperatively. Mean range of motion

(ROM) score was 8.3 preoperatively up to 9 points postoperatively. Mean function score out of a maximum of 47 points was 21.4 preoperatively, with up to 44.6 measured postoperatively (range 32 to 47; SD: 4.085). We noted that the function score mean was highly dependent on the patient's pre-operative hip classification as mean function score was 46.4 points in the Charnley A patient cohort as opposed to 42.4 in the Charnley B or C cohorts (p = 0.001 using both t-test and Mann Whitney test).

The mean Harris hip score (HHS) value was 35 (range 7 to 91) out of a maximum of 100 preoperatively rising to a mean value of 97.56 points (range 85 to 100, SD 4.096) at 10 years. Before the operation, 92.5% of hips were considered as "poor", 6.3% as "fair" and 1.2% as "good" according to this Harris score, while at 10 years 62.8 % were assessed as "excellent" (i.e. $\geq$ 98 points), and 37.2 % were "good" (i.e., total score between 80 and 98 points). No hip in the 10 year follow-up group was assessed as "poor" or "fair". Results computed according to Merle d'Aubigné (PMA) assessment demonstrated similar gains as follows: scores (out of 6) were preoperatively 1.6 for Pain, 4.9 for Range of Motion, and 1.7 for Function. At ten years mean scores were 6 (Pain), 6 (ROM) and 5.4 (Function). Mean combined PMA score was 8.27 out of a maximum of 18 points preoperatively (0.6% "Good", 4.8% "Fair" and 94.6 % "Poor"). At ten years, the mean combined PMA score was 17.38 points (ranged 13 to 18; SD 1.08) and could be characterized as 73.55% "Excellent" (18 points), 25.62% "Good" (15-17 points) and two cases graded "Fair" (0.8 %). Considering only those patients with a pre-operative Charnley classification of "A" (a way of gauging the results of the hip intervention alone), we calculated a mean of 99.38 /100 (HHS) and 17.85/100 (PMA). More than 85% of Charnley A patients had an assessment of "Excellent" at the ten year interval (Tables 2 and 3).

Assessment	Pain		Motion		Function		Total	
	Pre	10 year	Pre	10 year	Pre	10 year	Pre	10 year
HHS	5.1	43.9	8.3	9	21.4	44.6	35	97.56
Max value (HHS)	*/44*	*/44*	*/9*	*/9*	*/47*	*/47*	*/100*	*/100*
MDA	1.6	6	4.9	6	1.7	5.4	8.27	17.38
Max value (MDA)	*/6*	*/6*	*/6*	*/6*	*/6*	*/6*	*/18*	*/18*

Table 2 – Mean values of clinical results of the HA Arc2f series updated with 10 year minimum follow-up (N:383).

Assessment	HHS		MDA	
(in %)	*Pre*	*10 year*	*Pre*	*10 year*
Excellent	0	62.8	0	73.55
Good	1.2	37.2	0.6	25.62
Fair	6.3	0	4.8	0.8
Poor	92.5	0	94.6	0

Table 3 – Global results of the HA Arc2f series clinically reviewed at 10 year minimum follow-up (N:383).

Radiological Findings

As a general observation, comparison of films at sequential follow-up intervals showed, in a few cases, an increase in bone density adjacent to the implant, most frequently around the threads in Zone 3 of DeLee and Charnley (25). However, no adverse bone remodeling was found around an Arc2f component in any zone, which led us to characterize the vast majority of radiographs as "mute" (fig. 2a,b,c).

(b)

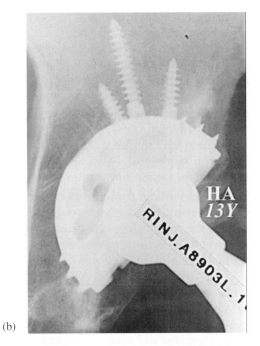

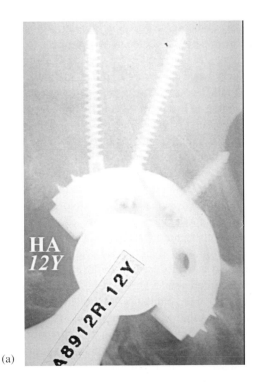

(a)

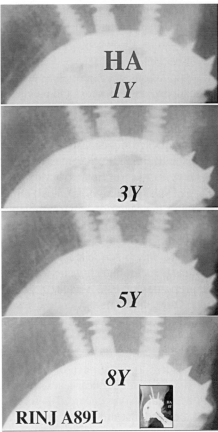

(c)

Figure 2 – Typical films demonstrating excellent long lasting fixation obtained with the HA-coated cup respectively at 12 years (a) and at 13 years (b) postoperatively in the same patient. Serial close views of this patient's left hip at 1, 3, 5, and 8 years (c) reveal intimate contact between the metallic surface of the cup and the surrounding bone with no change over time.

With respect to the orientation of the acetabular component, the abduction of the cup was between 40 and 45 degrees in 47% of cases, while less than 40 degrees in 39% and greater than 45 degrees in the remaining 14 %. This degree of abduction was never in our experience correlated with a higher risk of radiological failure. It is always challenging to state the precise anteversion based upon 2D films. Normally the cup anteversion at the time of the surgery, was chosen in a range of 10 up to 25°, so as to match as best as possible any femoral antetorsion.

We paid a particular attention to the radiographic changes at the interface as well as density changes in the surrounding bony structures. No reduction in bone density was noted visually in any zone. Examination for radiolucent lines showed "no line" in 99% of cups and a line extending more than fifty percent of a single zone in the other 5 cups. No lucent lines were found adjacent to the cancellous bone screws. Comparison of postoperative and ten-year plus radiographs showed no cups had tilted or migrated. No broken screws were observed except a single screw that failed at the time of surgery with no additional change further on.

Osteolytic lesions were defined as any enclosed area of reduced bone density in the pelvis with distinct boundaries.

At ten years follow-up, 373 hips (97.6%) showed no evidence of osteolysis. Four hips (1.0%) showed a small "droplet" of decreased radiographic density in zone 1, described as "mild" osteolysis, this "droplet" was similar to the "scalloping" osteolysis seen in the calcar of femurs implanted with HA-coated stems as reported by Capello *et al.* (27). These authors proposed that these benign local osteolyses are due to entrapped polyethylene particles concentrated in one area due to the excellent sealing properties of HA. Finally 5 hips (1.3%) showed pelvic "moderate" osteolytic lesions. No cases of severe osteolysis were observed, nor were osteolytic lesions observed around any of the screws. All five "moderate" osteolytic lesions were directly adjacent to the surface of the implant. In three of the five "moderate" cases, radiographic patterns of lytic lesions occurred before the first year of follow-up, but did not experience any visible progression after the first year. In these five hips, the osteolysis did not extend along the bone screws. Harris Hip scores regarding these five moderate "osteolytic cases" were comprised between 96 and 100 points (fig. 3). The overall osteolysis

rate with the Arc2f component at 10 years, including the aforementioned cases with moderate osteolysis, remained below 2%.

With respect to the wear rate of the Arc2f cup liners, it is extremely difficult to define the real periphery of the metallic implant from a single X-ray view . However, as a simple check, we found 33% of cases without any visible wear based upon a Charnley equatorial linear wear based method, and 45% of "mild" wear, (1mm of linear wear), 21% of "moderate" wear (2-3mm) and 1% of "severe" wear (over 3mm of linear wear). No correlation between these crude wear measures and patient factors could be demonstrated. All of the surviving HA-coated Arc2f acetabular components were found to be stable at 10 year minimum follow-up. According to Engh's criteria, 98.67% were classified as "stable bone ingrowth". There were no "fibrous stable" or "unstable" implants.

Complications and Cumulative Survival Rates

No serious intraoperative complications were experienced in the series, and in particular there were no cases of sciatic nerve palsy or vascular injury stemming from screw placement. With respect to Arc2f failure rate, twelve cups were revised. Six revisions were performed following traumatic pelvic fracture after a fall. Two revisions were due to a deep infection leading to an exchange of the implants upon a two stage surgery. The four remaining cases were mechanical failures. The first involved a 52 year-old, active patient who experienced sudden pain and functional limitation at ten years; limited osteolysis and a loose cup were revealed at revision. The second involved a heavy, 61 year-old female who experienced moderate pain at 8-years leading to revision in another clinic. The third failed cup belonged to a young 43-old male whose primary lesion was osteonecrosis, and in whom the results were excellent during ten years. This patient then experienced unexpected pain, limitation of functional abilities, global lucent line with limited osteolysis, leading to a revision with simple exchange of the cup at 10-year, and a satisfactory result so far at 13-years from the first surgery. The fourth patient was a 77-year old female who underwent a revision at the eleventh year for excessive wear against an alumina head matched with a Corail stem, while clinical results had been quoted as excellent until the tenth year follow-up.

(a)

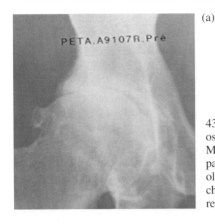

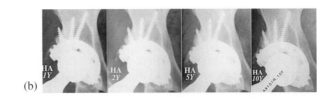

(b)

Figure 3a, b – One of the radiographic changes recorded as "osteolysis" in a 43 years old female patient who received a HA-coated Arc 2f in 1991 further to osteoarthritis (a) with excellent clinical result at 10 years of follow-up (HHS:100; MDA:18). Serial radiographs at 1,2,5,10 years postoperatively (b) show a typical pattern of bone loss over the top of the cup that obviously might be noticed as osteolysis. However, this radiographic pattern seen at the first year experienced no change over years, and is absolutely identical 10 years later on. Some questions regarding osteolysis remain unanswered as in this specific case.

Thus, the aseptic loosening rate in this series (3 cups in three patients) was 0.5%. No implants were found to be unstable radiographically, and the mechanical failure rate was 0.5% as well. Similarly, with no revision for osteolysis, and one for excessive wear, the combined failure rate at ten years was 0.66%.

With respect to the cumulative survivorship analysis, our series may thus be taken to have twelve retrievals, of which four cases at 6, 8, 10 and 11 years, may be considered as "implant-related mechanical failures". Three of these failures were resulting from loose fixation and lack of bone bonding provided by the HA interface, and the fourth was a revision due to excessive wear provoked by an inappropriate head. There were no instances of cup migration and no clinical failures for pain or osteolysis. Considering the 602 cases global series with 93 hips remaining at risk at 11 years, we calculated a cumulative probability of survival of 96.85% ± 0.026 while considering all retrievals (excluding isolated femoral revisions with cup left in place) due to any cause. The cumulative probability of survival rises to 99.16% ± 0.0225 if one uses only aseptic loosening as the endpoint (Table 4).

DISCUSSION

Hydroxyapatite-coated joint replacements have come a long way since they were generally lumped together with all other cementless techniques. Threaded ring types of acetabular components fell into disrepute following the unacceptable failure rates demonstrated by the smooth components that belonged to the first generation of threaded cup designs. Therefore, our contemporary report on a series of HA-coated threaded acetabular compo-

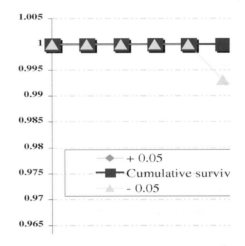

Table 4 – Survivorship analysis in 602 HA Arc2f cups in primary hips, with 93 patients remaining at risk at 11 year of FU, and considering all types of retrieval as endpoint. Graphical analysis is provided with confidence interval additional curves at plus and minus 0.05. Survival rate at 0.9685 rises 0.9916 when considering only mechanical failures. The "worst case scenario" rate at minus 5% (for mechanical failures as endpoint) should be 0.9691 at 11- year.

nents followed for a minimum of ten years is somewhat unique. In the present study, we provide clinical and radiological data obtained on a series of 383 cases clinically reviewed at 10-year minimum follow-up and exhibiting excellent overall results. To summarize, this series has an average Harris Hip Score of 97.6 points, a mechanical failure rate at less than 1%, a migration rate of zero, and an osteolysis rate less than 2% at 10 years. Our cumulative survival rate was 99.16% at the eleventh year using revision for aseptic loosening as the endpoint. In the vast majority of cases, serial radiographs demonstrated an absence of bony changes, which led us to use the term "mute" radiograph (Table 5). These results compare favorably with best published failure rates (3, 5, 15).

N clinically assessed at 10 year minimum FU	383
N radiographically reviewed at 10 year minimum FU	375
Global Harris Hip Score at 10 year	97.56 points /100
Harris Hip Score in "Charnley A" cohort	99.38 points /100
Global Merle d'Aubigné-Postel Score	17.85 points /18
Migration rate	0%
Osteolysis rate	1.33 %
N of retrievals (any cause)	12 (1.99%)
Mechanical failure rate (Combined)	4 (0.66 %)
Hydroxyapatite failure rate (Primaries)	3 (0.50 %)
Cumulative survivorship analysis rate at 1 year (MF)	99.16% ± 0.0225

Table 5 – Specific figures of the HA Arc2f series at 10 year minimum follow-up.

Success or failure of an acetabular component seems to be very sensitive to design. Our design philosophy uses peripheral threads to minimize shear stresses at the bone-implant interface, particularly in Zone 3 (25). The thread of the Arc2f is very thin and is a true cutting thread that cuts its way into the bone bed. This is in contrast to other "threaded" designs, especially of the previous generation, which essentially have thread-like buttresses into which bone may or may not grow, depending on each patient's biomechanics and biology. Because the threads of the Arc2f cut into the host bone in an efficient manner, we have been able to use the device in all manner of indications, including patients with brittle bone, dysplasia, protrusio, as well as in revision applications (8, 13, 14).

The use of secondary screw fixation is perhaps more controversial in view of claims that such screws are only of short-term benefit and could serve as conduits for debris, thereby leading to local osteolysis. We believe that screws contribute to initial stabilization by prohibiting cup rotation and increasing cup pull-out strength, although admittedly, neither of these eventualities is common. However, screws have an additional benefit, as espoused by Schneider, where he argues that inserting screws along the lines of the forces acting on the joint enhances the rigidity of the cancellous bone around the acetabulum (11). We also believe that a principal function of the secondary fixation screws is to prevent cup migration over the long term. Divergent lines of force obtained by the screws insure that the cup is held firmly in place and cannot migrate along any line, because the extended center-lines of the screws intersect. Our observed migration rate of zero after following more than 2,600 Arc2f cup implantations over

fourteen years encourages us to continue with the philosophy of peripheral threads combined with secondary screw fixation.

The quality of mechanical interlock remains critical to the outcome of shell fixation. Using a similar shell with a plasma sprayed CPTi porous coating, we obtained roughly similar clinical and radiographic results (13). The biologic fixation of these components was excellent. We have previously reported that the overall performance of these titanium coated components was indistinguishable from the current series of HA-coated components insofar as Harris Hip score values and mechanical failure rates are concerned (13). Nonetheless, the overall radiographic appearance of the HA-coated components is somewhat more satisfying in the sense that no lines were seen in Zone 3, and that the HA coating appeared to be more conducive to an eventual filling-in of initial bone-implant gaps.

Lastly, as others have noted, HA-coated devices appear to be more likely to maintain a direct bone-implant interface without the interposition of any degree of fibrous tissue (fig. 4a,b). A recent radiostereometric study (RSA) dedicated to "migration and wear of HA-coated press-fit cups in revision hip arthroplasty" (33), by Nivbrant *et al.*,

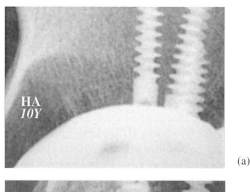

(a)

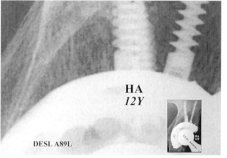

(b)

Figure 4 – Two typical samples of "biological" fixation provided by hydroxyapatite, even in the long run at 10 and 12 years postoperatively, with intimate contact between metal and bone well demonstrated in these two close views of HA-coated Arc 2f cups.

indicates that despite extensive use of morsellized grafts, HA cups displayed the smallest degree of migration reported so far in revision acetabular surgery. Additionally, they maintained stability up to 2 years after surgery. Previous RSA studies in porous coated press fit cups displayed increased proximal migration in association with the development of radiolucent zones and accelerated wear in some designs, which may dramatically jeopardize the long term results of these implants (34-36). Conversely, in experimental models HA when compared to titanium has repeatedly shown superior osteoconductive properties, even in compromising circumstances (37-40).

In the above mentioned study (27), RSA was carried out in 29 consecutive acetabular revisions operated on because of aseptic loosening using HA-coated ABG cups (SHO, Rutherford, NJ, USA), and morselized bone graft. After 2 years, 89% of the interface seemed to be in direct contact with living bone, which is superior to the mean 59% bone-cup contact found earlier in press-fit cups with a porous titanium coating (35). Additionally, the authors noted that despite forceful impaction, if the press fit cup did not contact the bottom of the acetabulum, a very tight peripheral rim fit could be expected, which seemed to stabilize the implant more reproducibly during the postoperative period. Interestingly, this specific concept is the one employed by a HA-coated threaded cup that gets sound primary stability from a "very tight peripheral rim fit" (fig. 5).

As an additional contribution to this study regarding the rate of wear experienced by this Arc2f cup, we would like to report on a specific retrospective wear study that was performed by Martell *et al.* (32) assessing the comparative performance of compression molded *versus* machined UHMWPE in otherwise identical metal backed HA-coated Arc2f cup on 112 THRs implanted between January '89 and December '90 The study attempted to determine the effect of machining *versus* molding of acetabular inserts on wear using a previously validated computerized measure of in vivo wear. There was no significant difference in the age, sex, height, weight, diagnosis or Charnley classification between the two groups, a 28mm CoCr bearing was used in all cases. In 50 hips, the liner was made by direct compression molding of GUR 1120, while in the remaining 62 hips the liner was machined from a large slab of GUR 1120. Linear and volumetric wear rates were calculated for both groups from scanned sequential radiographs using a two dimensional edge detection based algorithm. A comparison for significant difference in wear rate per year between the molded and machined hips was calculated using the Student's non-paired t-test.

The acetabular inclination angle was not significantly different between the two groups (molded = 43.2° and machined = 44.4°) The machined polyethylene linear wear rate was 0.137 mm/yr ± 0.178, while the volumetric wear rate was 84 cubic mm/yr

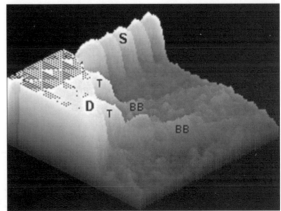

(b)

Figure 5 – Close view of the peripheral threads of an Arc2f cup at 10 years confirming an efficient mechanical interlock afforded by threads (a), which may be a fundamental asset toward a long lasting bone bonding, as demonstrated by bony bridges that bond peaks of threads to the surrounding bone. This radiographic pattern can be pointed out through a 3D-like picture provided by Imagika Software (b) showing the metallic dome (D), the screw (S), the threads (T) and the bony bridges (BB).

(a)

± 82. The linear wear rate for direct compression molded polyethylene was 0.136 mm/yr ± 0.217, with volumetric wear of 98 cubic mm/yr ± 96. These differences were not significant at the 95% level (linear wear rate p = 0.97, volumetric wear rate p = 0.42). In addition, this study addresses concerns regarding the potential for third body wear in HA coated implants. All acetabular components and all but two stems were HA coated but the wear rates reported in this study were consistent with those published for metal on polyethylene hip articulations, which suggests that HA coating plays no role in accelerating or retarding wear rates.

Osteolysis remains a major concern in acetabular replacement, and especially for uncemented cups. The rate of osteolysis exhibited in this series is relatively low, especially compared to rates exhibited by other series (16). There are several possible advantages this device possesses that may limit the formation and progression of osteolytic lesions. The intimate and robust initial fixation of the implant in the host bone combined with a HA coating appears to substantially limit the formation of fibrous tissue, which may be a conduit for particulate debris. The simple yet robust design of the locking mechanism used in this implant may reduce backside wear and reduce the likelihood of contact stress "hot-spots" developing due to deformation of the liner. Lastly, the essentially waterproof nature of the locking mechanism at the equator may prevent issue of joint fluid between the backside of the liner and the inner surface of the shell, thus preventing osteolytic cyst development near screw holes resulting from the "pumping effect" (17, 18, 19). Note that in this series, neither the screw holes nor the screws themselves were associated with osteolysis formation or progression (fig. 6a, b, c). More recently, we have begun to use a ceramic-ceramic bearing in the Arc2f component (Trident Arc2f, Stryker Howmedica Osteonics, Allendale, NJ) which may lead to a further reduction in the already low osteolysis rate using this cup design.

Finally, the success achieved with this Arc2f implant suggests that early threaded designs that performed poorly did so because no provision for long-term stability in the form of secondary fixation was provided. We have provided for such fixation *via* the use of screws and HA coating. Furthermore, it should also be noted that the means of achieving primary fixation for the present design is *via* a true cutting threaded, which was not always the case in most of the first generation threaded components (5, 13, 20, 22). Our experience with this cup would suggest that HA-coated threaded cups are appropriate in all cases (either regular or difficult hips) and also in revision cases. Moreover, the use of threads and additional screws did not lead to any kind of problem or complication. We naturally cannot state on the absolute need of addi-

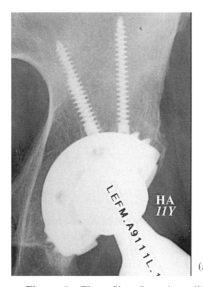 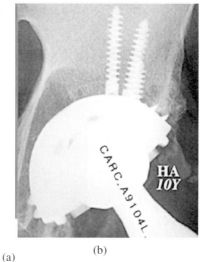 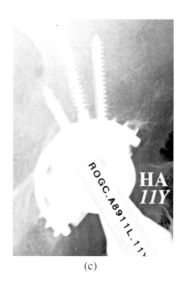

(a)   (b)   (c)

Figure 6 – Three films from three different patients at 11(a), 10(b) and 11(c) years postoperatively. In each case the polyethylene liner is severely worn, yet there is no pattern of osteolysis over the metallic dome or around the screws. The excellent "water tight" locking mechanism of the liner into the Arc2f metallic shell, as well as the intimate bone bonding provided by the HA coating, might explain the lack of osteolysis in this Arc2f series, despite the presence of screws and screw holes.

tional screws with the Arc2f as data without screws is not available. However, our 10 year + experience with the actual combination threads and screw provided results as good as any in the literature (fig. 7a, b) (34).

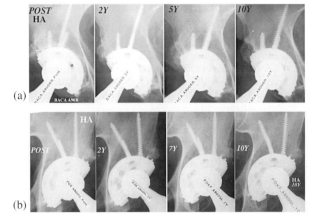

Figure 7a, b – Serial films from the first year until the 10-year radiographic control in two cases, which denote the usual follow-up of this HA-coated screw cup, with excellent stable mechanical and biological fixation, as well as no radiographic change over time, leading us to speak about "mute X-rays".

Reference list

1. Perez RE, Rodriguez JA, Deshmukh RG, Ranawat CS (1998) Polyethylene wear and periprosthetic osteolysis in metal-backed acetabular components with cylindrical liners. *J. Arthroplasty* 13(1):1-7.

2. Bruijn JD, Seelen JL, Veldhuizen RW, Feenstra RM, Bernoski FP, Klopper PJ (1996) High failure rate of cementless threaded acetabular cups: a radiographic and histologic study in the goat. *Acta Orthop. Scand.* 67(2):133-7.

3. Yahiro MA, Gantenberg JB, Nelson R, Lu HT, Mishra NK (1995) Comparison of the results of cemented, porous-ingrowth, and threaded acetabular cup fixation. A meta analysis of the orthopaedic literature. *J. Arthroplasty* 10(3):339-50.

4. Fox GM, McBeath AA, Heiner JP (1994) Hip replacement with a threaded acetabular cup. A follow-up study. *J. Bone Joint Surg. Am.* 76(2):195-201.

5. Manley MT, Capello WN, D'Antonio JA, Edidin AA, Geesink RG (1998) Fixation of acetabular cups without cement in total hip arthroplasty. A comparison of three different implant surfaces at a minimum duration of follow-up of five years. *J. Bone Joint Surg. Am.* 80(8):1175-85.

6. Bauer TW, Stulberg BN, Ming J, Geesink RG (1993) Uncemented acetabular components. Histologic analysis of retrieved hydroxyapatite-coated and porous implants. *J. Arthroplasty* 8(2):167-77.

7. Galante JO, Jacobs J (1992) Clinical performance of ingrowth surfaces. *Clinical Orthopaedics* 276:41-9.

8. Geesink RG, Hoefnagels NH (1995) Six-year results of hydroxyapatite-coated total hip replacement. *J. Bone Joint Surg. Br.* 77(4):534-47.

9. Epinette J.A (1993) Hydroxylapatite-Coated Implants for Hip Replacement : Clinical Experience in France – In: Geesink RGT, Manley MT (eds) Hydroxylapatite Coatings in Orthopaedic Surgery, Raven Press, pp. 227-48.

10. Geesink RGT, de Groot K, Klein CPAT (1988) Bonding of bone to apatite-coated implants. *J. Bone Joint Surg. Br.* 70B, 1:17-21.

11. Schneider R (1985) Biomechanics of Hip Prostheses. *Acta Orthop. Belg.* 51:196-209.

12. Huiskes R (1987) Finite element analysis of acetabular reconstruction. Noncemented threaded cups. *Acta Orthop. Scand.* 58(6):620-25.

13. Duthoit E, Epinette JA, Carlier Y (1995) The Arc2f Cup: Biomechanics and Interface; Systematic study of HA-coated Vs. Porous Textured Components. In: Cahiers d'Enseignement de la SO.F.C.O.T: "Hydroxyapatite Coated Hip and Knee Arthroplasty", L'Expansion scientifique Ed. Paris, France, n° 51, pp. 176-82.

14. Poison R, Epinette JA, Carlier Y, Duthoit E, Tillie B (1995) Seven years experience with the Arc2f Cup in Acetabular Revision Surgery, Operative Strategy and Results. In: Cahiers d'Enseignement de la SO.F.C.O.T: "Hydroxyapatite Coated Hip and Knee Arthroplasty", L'Expansion scientifique Ed. Paris, France, n° 51, pp. 291-301.

15. Havelin LI, Vollset SE, Engesaeter LB (1995) Revision for aseptic loosening of uncemented cups in 4,352 primary total hip prostheses. A report from the Norwegian Arthroplasty Register. *Acta Orthop. Scand.* 66(6):494-500.

16. Zicat B, Engh CA, Gokcen E (1995) Patterns of Osteolysis around total hip components inserted with and without cement. *J. Bone Joint. Surg.* 77A:432-9.

17. Schmalzried TP, Jasty M, Harris WH (1992): Periprosthetic bone loss in total hip arthroplasty. Polyethylene wear debris and the concept of the effective joint space. *J. Bone Joint Surg. Am.* 74(6):849-6.

18. Schmalzried TP, Akizuki KH, Fedenko AN, Mirra J (1997): The role of access of joint fluid to bone in periarticular osteolysis. A report of four cases. *J. Bone Joint Surg. Am.* 79(3):447-52.

19. Whiteside LA (1995) Effect of porous-coating configuration on tibial osteolysis after total knee Arthroplasty. *Clin. Orthop.* (321):92-7.

20. Delaunay CP, Kapandji AI (1996) Primary total hip arthroplasty with the Karl Zweymuller first-generation cementless prosthesis. A 5- to 9-year retrospective study. *J. Arthroplasty* 11(6):643-52.

21. Cartillier JC and the Artro Group (1995) The contribution of Hydroxyapatite; Study of implants of identical geometry with and without hydroxyapatite coating; In: Cahiers d'Enseignement de la SOFCOT "Hydroxyapatite Coated Hip and Knee Arthroplasty", L'Expansion scientifique Ed. Paris, France, n° 51, pp. 165-8.

22. Pupparo F, Engh CA (1991) Comparison of porous-threaded and smooth-threaeded acetabular components of identical design. Two-to-four-year results. *Clin. Orthop.* 271:201-6.

23. D'Antonio JA, Capello, WN (1995) HA-Coated Hip Implants: U.S. Experience; A Multicenter Study with three-Five year follow-up. In: Cahiers d'Enseignement de la SOFCOT "Hydroxyapatite Coated Hip and Knee Arthroplasty", L'Expansion scientifique Ed. Paris, France, n° 51, pp. 249-56.

24. Charnley J (1972) The long-term results of low-friction arthroplasty of the hip performed performed as a primary intervention. *J. Bone Joint Surg.* 54-B(1):61-76.

25. DeLee JG, Charnley J (1976) Radiological demarcation of cemented sockets in total hip replacement. *Clin. Orthop.* 121:20-32.

26. Harris WH (1969) Traumatic arthritis of the hip after dislocation and acetabular fractures: treatment by mold arthroplasty. An end-result study using a new method of result evaluation. *J. Bone Joint Surg.* 51A:737-55.

27. Capello WN, D'Antonio JA, Feinberg JR, Manley MT (1997) Hydroxyapatite-coated total hip femoral components in patients less than fifty years old. Clinical and radiographic results after five to eight years of follow-up. *J. Bone Joint Surg.* 79-A:1023-9.

28. Livermore J, Ilstrup D, Morrey B (1990) Effect of femoral head size on wear of the polyethylene acetabular component. *J. Bone Joint Surg.* 1190, 72A, 4, 518-28.

29. Merle d'Aubigne R (1970) Cotation chiffree de la hanche. *Rev. Chir. Orthop.* 56:481-6.

30. Merle d'Aubigne R (1990) Cotation chiffree de la fonction de la hanche. *Rev Chir Orthop* 76:371-4.

31. Postel M, Kerboul M, Evrard J, Courpied JP (1985) Arthroplastie totale de hanche. Paris, Springer-Verlag.

32. Martell JM, Epinette J-A, Leopold S, Edidin AA (1999): In Vivo Performance of Compression Molded versus Machined UHMWPE in Otherwise Identical Metal Backed HA Coated Acetabular Components, *Trans. Orthop. Res. Soc.,* 24.

33. Nivbrant B., Kärrholm J. (1997) Migration and wear of Hydroxyapatite-coated pressfit cups in revision hip arthroplasty: A radiostereometric study. *J. Arthroplasty,* 12:904-12.

34. Epinette J-A, Manley MT, D'Antonio JA, Edidin AA, Capello WN (2003) A Ten Year Minimum Follow-up of a Consecutive Series of 418 Hydroxyapatite-coated Threaded Cups: Clinical, Radiographic, and Survivorship Analyses with Comparison to the Literature. *J. Arthroplasty,* 18(2):140-8.

13 Minimum Ten-Year Follow-up of the Hydroxyapatite-Coated Atlas Cup

Alain Dambreville, MD

INTRODUCTION

The Atlas cup (1) is a press-fit acetabular component (fig. 1). It consists of a hemispherical shell made of a titanium alloy (TiAl6V4) with a split in the lower part to provide elasticity. The titanium shell is very thin (2.5mm), so as to allow a maximal thickness of polyethylene (PE) to be inserted. The first cups of this pattern, used between July 1987 and December 1989, were of grit-blasted titanium alloy and did not have a hydroxyapatite (HA) coating. Since then, an HA-coated pattern has been used.

In 1995, we performed a comparative study (2) of the porous titanium versus the HA-coated pattern and found the HA-coated cup to be superior. The present study reflects the follow-up period of more than ten years that has elapsed by now. The investigation described herein was a prospective study of a consecutive series of the first 151 HA-coated Atlas cups used, at primary arthroplasty, between 8 January 1990, and 27 September 1991.

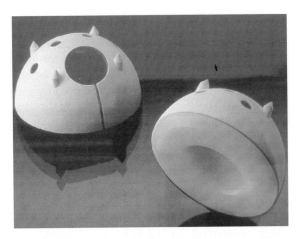

Figure 1 – The Atlas Acetabular component.

MATERIALS AND METHODS

All the acetabular components used in the study were HA-coated Atlas cups. The Atlas cup is made of titanium alloy (TiAl6V4). It is hemisperical and has a split that provides elasticity. The cup size chosen is 2mm greater than the diameter of the final reamer. As the cup is impacted into place, the split closes; when the insert is placed in the cup, the split opens up again and produces a strong press-fit effect (3).

The stability of the insert is ensured by the circumferential clamping action of the cup around the peripheral cylindrical portion of the insert. This design counteracts any tendency of the insert to tilt (3) (fig. 2).

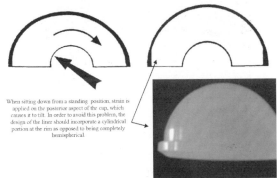

When sitting down from a standing position, strain is applied on the posterior aspect of the cup, which causes it to tilt. In order to avoid this problem, the design of the liner should incorporate a cylindrical portion at the rim as opposed to being completely hemispherical.

Figure 2 – Stability of the liner. When sitting down from a standing position, strain is applied on the posterior aspect of the cup, which causes it to tilt. In order to avoid this problem, the design of the liner should incorporate a cylindrical portion at the rim as opposed to being completely hemispherical.

The thickness of the cup shell is limited to 2.5mm, so as to allow a maximal thickness of PE to be inserted.

The femoral heads used were 22-mm diameter in 145 cases, and 26-mm diameter in six cases. Like the thin shell, these small heads allowed a greater thickness of PE to be used. The PE insert was always at least 10mm thick.

On the femoral side, a PSM stem (HA-coated in the metaphyseal portion) was used in 147 cases; the remaining four cases were managed with a variety of cementless implants.

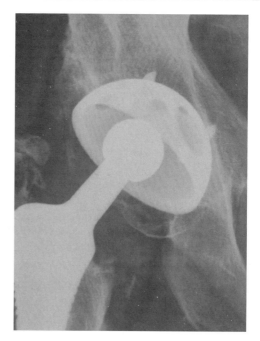

Figure 5 – Polyethylene wear of 1.5mm in an Atlas cup at 11-years follow-up; there is no osteolysis.

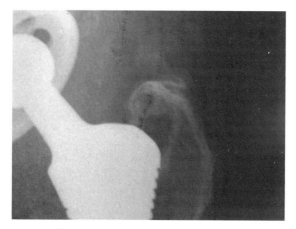

Figure 3 – Osteolytic femoral cysts were in all cases limited to a small area under the greater trochanter

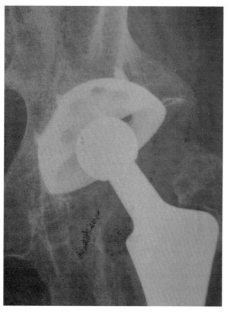

Figure 4 – An Atlas cup radiographic control at 11 years postoperatively: no wear. The importance of the polyethylene thickness should be noted.

The study described herein was a prospective study of a consecutive series of 151 primary hip replacements performed at our center between 8 January 1990 and 27 September 1991. The mean patient age was 62 years (range, 25 to 82 years). Of the patients, 78 were women, and 73 men. There were 72 right and 79 left hips. In 129 cases, the indication for arthroplasty was primary osteoarthritis (OA) of the hip; eleven patients had developmental dysplasia of the hip (DDH); two had rheumatoid arthritis (RA); and two had osteonecrosis.

Twelve patients died, and 16 were lost to follow-up. Fourteen patients were reoperated on: one for infection, three for dislocation, four for failure of the stem to obtain primary stability, four for metallosis caused by the deterioration of the titanium femoral head, and two for cup loosening. This left 109 patients for review in the present study, at a follow-up of eleven years post-arthroplasty in 61 cases, and of ten years in 48 cases. For the clinical assessment, the MDA scoring system was used. The radiographic assessment was concerned with the detection of lucent lines, cysts, and evidence of loosening, on the A/P and the lateral films. Wear was measured on the A/P hip films using the Charnley method, (4) taking magnification into account. Cumulative survival out to eleven years could be calculated, with the Kaplan-Meier method, for the 151 hips that had undergone replacement.

RESULTS

The one revision for deep infection occurred in the first year. The two instances of cup loosening were at six years and nine years, respectively. The first of these two cases was that of a female patient who had had several falls. At revision surgery, a deep notch was seen in the posterior part of the acetabular rim, which was interpreted as evidence of impingement. The other case had to be revised because the patient had fallen and sustained a fracture of the acetabular fossa, with loosening of the implant. This was, therefore, a case of intercurrent trauma necessitating revision.

In the 109 cases that were followed up, the MDA pain score was 6 in 95 cases, 5 in 10 cases, and 4 in 5 cases. The MDA mobility score was 6 in 98 cases, 5 in seven cases (who had slight stiffness), and 4 in 4 cases (whose hips were stiff). The MDA function score was 6 in 93 cases (patients walking normally), 5 in 7 cases (slight limp), and 4 in 9 cases (limp). Seven of the last-mentioned nine patients were DDH cases.

Radiography showed a total absence of any periacetabular cysts. In the femur, there were 15 cysts, all of which were confined to the greater trochanter (fig. 3); there were no extensive cysts and no extensive lucent lines.

At the level of the cup, non-progressive lucent lines of less than 3mm width were seen in Zone III in seven cases (6.2%). There were no extensive lucent lines.

Wear (Figures 4 and 5) was 0mm in eleven cases, 0.5mm in 31 cases, 1mm in 42 cases, 1.5mm in 16 cases, 2mm in seven cases, and 2.5mm in one case. Mean wear was 0.90mm. The mean annual wear rate in this series was 0.82mm/year.

Mean cumulative survival was calculated, with the Kaplan-Meier method, for the 151 hips in the series. It was calculated out to eleven years, since 78 of the hips were still "alive" by the end of that time. The seven stem failures were not included in the analysis, since the study was concerned with cup survival. Also, following the policy of the Scandinavian registries, it was decided to apply the term "revision" only to reoperations involving the

exchange of at least one of the two major components in direct contact with the host bone (i.e., the cup and/or the stem), while the exchange of an acetabular insert or a femoral head would not be considered to be a "revision".

There were three failures involving the Atlas cup, one each in the first, the fifth, and the ninth year post-operatively. Two were revisions for 'intercurrent' reasons (one deep infection in the first year, the other as a result of an accidental fracture at nine years). Only in the case of the cup that needed revising at five years was failure of the implant fixation to blame. Thus, when analyzing cup failure as such, the rate was 1.98% (3/151 cups). This figure comprises the two failures not attributable to the implant as such, and one failure of implant fixation. The failure rate of the HA fixation of the Atlas cup at ten years was thus 0.66% (1/151 cups).

When these data were used to plot the survival curves, the cumulative survival rates at eleven years, using the different endpoints, were seen to be 96.95% ± 0.0269 for cup replacement (all causes), and 99.18% ± 0.0159 for cup mechanical failure.

DISCUSSION

There were two instances of cup loosening. The ten-year survival, taking cup failure as the endpoint, was 99.18%. Four cases of metallosis were associated with the use of titanium femoral heads (5). This type of deterioration remained rare (3.4%) over the period for which the patients were followed up. It is not impossible that further cases of metallosis may be encountered at a later stage of the in-service life of the implants.

The absence of macrophage-filled cysts around the cup provided evidence of the firm seating of the PE insert in the cup shell. The insert fixation system by circumferential clamping in the cup proved efficient in the clinical study, as it had done previously in a retrieval study (6). In that study, no macroscopic or microscopic evidence of backside deterioration of the inserts was found after more than ten years post-operatively. These results were certainly due, in some measure, to the absence of microfretting between the insert and the shell thanks to the stable seating of the insert, and to the great thickness of the polyethylene. Another factor was the size of the femoral heads used. Most of the heads were 22-mm diameter ones, and this size is known to produce little wear debris and, consequently, little macrophage reaction. The findings in this study thus bear out Charnley's low-friction theory.

Lucent lines around the cup were rare (6.2%) and confined to Zone III. It is interesting to recall that, in a comparative study in 1995, (1) we found the non-HA-coated Atlas cups to be associated with a 40% rate of Zone III lucent lines.

Many authors (7, 8, 9, 10, 11) have described the barrier to the migration of PE wear particles provided by the intimate contact, without any interposed fibrous tissue, between the host bone and a circumferential HA coating on the implant. It would appear that, in the case of the implants used in the present study, this barrier effect resulted in any femoral cysts being confined to the greater trochanter.

Linear polyethylene wear was slight (0.8mm/year). While Bloebaum *et al.* (12) have voiced concern over possible third-body wear by dislodged HA particles becoming embedded in the PE bearing surface, this study showed that a good quality HA coating does not constitute such a hazard.

While Nashed *et al.* (13) Bankson *et al.* (14) and Hernandez *et al.* (15) reported major wear in metal-backed cups, this contradicts the work of Markel *et al.* (16) and Callaghan *et al.* (17), who found low wear rates. Wear is a multifactorial phenomenon, with PE quality, PE thickness, femoral head quality, patient's level of physical activity, component positioning, and other factors each playing a role. Under the conditions of use described in this study, there appears to be no cause for concern about accelerated PE wear.

CONCLUSION

This study, with more than ten years follow-up, suggests that HA-coated metal-backed cups are reliable, provided that the PE insert has been firmly seated in the shell and is of sufficient thickness. The HA coating was found to be effective in terms of providing secondary stabilization of the implant and in terms of limiting the migration of PE wear particles.

Reference List

1. Dambreville A (1992) Le cotyle ATLAS. *Eur. J. Orthop. Surg. Traumatol.* 2:111-4.

2. Dambreville A, Lautridou P (1995) Comparison of two series of THR: hydroxyapatite versus porous coated. Cahiers d'Enseignement de la SOFCOT, 51:159-65.

3. Dambreville A, Lautridou P (1996) Les cotyles impactés. *Eur. J. Orthop Surg. Traumatol.* 6:217-22.

4. Charnley J, Halley DK (1975) Rate of wear in total hip replacement. *Clin. Orthop.* 112:170-9.

5. Dambreville A, Rolland Jacob G (2001) Têtes en titane implanté et métallose. *Rev. Chir. Orthop.* 87, Suppl. 6, 2S87.

6. Dambreville A (2001) Assessing the stability of metal back acetabular inserts. A microscopic study of explants. *Eur. J. Orthop. Surg. Traumatol.* 11:213-8.

7. Bauer TW (1995) Hydroxyapatite coatings The histology of bone apposition and the mechanisms and consequences of coating metabolism. *Cahiers d'Enseignement de la SOFCOT*, 51:136-41.

8. D'Antonio JA, Capello WN (1995) HA-coated hip implants: US experience. A multicenter study with three-five year follow-up of the Omnifit stem. *Cahiers d'Enseignement de la SOFCOT*, 51:249-56.

9. Epinette JA (1995) HA-coated Omnifit stems in primary hip replacement surgery: seven years experience. *Cahiers d'Enseignement de la SOFCOT*, 51:215-26.

10. Frayssinet P, Hardy D, Tourenne F, Rouquet N, Delince P, Bonel G (1995) Osteointegration of plasma sprayed HA coated hip implants in humans *Cahiers d'Enseignement de la SOFCOT*, 51:142-8.

11. Søballe K, Toksvig-Larsen S, Gelineck S, Fruensgaard S, Hansen ES, *et al.* (1995) RSA studies on HA coated and porous coated implants. *Cahiers d'Enseignement de la SOFCOT*, 51:105-9.

12. Bloebaum RD, Beeks D, Dorr LD, Savory CG, Du Pont JA, Hofmann AA (1994) Complications with hydroxyapatite particulate separation in total hip arthroplasty. *Clin. Orthop.* 298, 19-26.

13. Nashed RS, Becker DA, Gustilo RB (1995) Are cementless acetabular components the cause of excess wear and osteolysis in total hip arthroplasty. *Clin. Orthop.* 317,19-28.

14. Bankston AB, Cates H, Ritter MA, Keating E, Faris PM (1995) Polyethylene wear in total hip arthroplasty. *Clin. Orthop.* 317, 7-13.

15. Hernandez JR, Keating EM, Faris PM, Meding JB, Ritter MA *et al.* (1994) Polyethylene wear in uncemented acetabular components. *J. Bone Joint Surg.* 76B, 263-6.

16. Markel DC, Huo MH, Katkin PD, Salvati EA (1995) Use of cemented all-polyethylene and metal-backed acetabular components in total hip arthroplasty. A comparative study. *J. Arthroplasty*, Suppl 10, S1-S7.

17. Callaghan JJ, Pedersen DR, Olejniczak JP, Goetz DD, Johnston RC (1995) Radiographic measurement of wear in 5 cohorts of patients observed for 5 to 22 years. *Clin. Orthop.* 317:14-8.

HA IN HIP REVISION
SURGERY

1 Experimental Data Regarding Macroporous Biphasic-Calcium Phosphate Ceramics: Can they replace bone grafting?

Norbert Passuti, MD, Joël Delécrin, PhD and Gérard Daculsi, PhD

INTRODUCTION

Bone grafts are frequently used in orthopaedic surgery. On the one hand, the risks and difficulties of autograft harvest and of the other the potential risks of allografts (viral hepatitis, acquired immune deficiency syndrome) led us to consider using bone substitutes. If orthopaedic surgeons had a reliable and effective implantable material available, the need to use autogenous or bank bone would be diminished and even abolished. The calcium phosphates and their composites (autogenous bone, collagen, fibrin glue) with a calcium phosphate ceramic base, show considerable potential and have obvious value for bone reconstruction (13).

Biological apatite crystals are the principal constituents of bones and teeth. These apatites belong to the large chemical family of calcium phosphates A large part of these calcium phosphates are of interest biologically because they make up the mineralized fraction of calcified tissues and may also be the precursors of mature crystals during the process of mineralization (5). The problems raised by different grafts in bone led orthopaedic surgeons to look for a biocompatible material, capable of being rapidly replaced by bone or of being incorporated in new bone (osteocoalescence). In 1892 Dressmann used Plaster of Paris (calcium sulfate) as a substitute in bone cavities. This was studied further by Martin in 1894 and Kofmann in 1925, and more recently by Bahn in 1966 and Peltier and Jones in 1978 (14). However, it seems that while the *in vivo* biotolerance of calcium sulfate is satisfactory, on the other hand its resorption is too fast to get a simultaneous replacement by bone. The synthetic calcium phosphates might satisfy the needs of numerous areas of bone surgery (peridontology, maxillo-facial surgery, orthopedics,

otorhinolaryngology) (17). These well defined chemical materials are formed by ceramic methods, using the process of frittage and prepared in this way constitute immediately usable biomaterials.

The principal property of calcium phosphate ceramics, hydroxyapatite (HA), beta tricalcium phosphate (beta TCP), a mixture of HA and beta TCP called bicalcium phosphate (BCP), is comparable to the mineral phase of bone (14). Their *in vitro* and *in vivo* biocompatibility have been proven (26), but in comparison with the other biocompatible biomaterials, the calcium phosphates are bioactive ceramics (5). They take part in exchanges between the cells and neighboring tissues in contrast to the bioinert ceramics, such as alumina. The bioactivity has been recently defined as the property of inducing specific biological reactions.

Calcium Phosphate Ceramics

Due to their chemical and crystal similarity to the biological apatite crystals, the principal constituents of calcified tissues, the synthetic calcium phosphates have been extensively studied and in the last 20 years have started to be used in clinical application.

Manufacture

They are prepared using classical ceramic techniques. The basic constituents are prepared by chemical synthesis and presented as a powder. Forming them for clinical utilization requires different procedures. After calcination (heating to the region of 900°C) the powder is compacted and then heated to between 1100°C and 1300°C. This last thermal treatment, called frittage, has the double aim of consolidating and increasing the density of the piece being compacted. In the case of the calcium phosphate ceramics, maintenance of some porosity is necessary to conserve the properties of bioactivity and osteoconduction of the implant. There are two type of porosity, microporosity and macroporosity. Microporosity (pore diameter less than 10 microns) is due to spaces persisting between crystals of the biomaterial after frittage. Macroporosity (pore diameter being 100 and 500 microns) is created deliberately in order to encourage penetration of cells and living tissue. It is obtained by adding hydrogen peroxide, naphthalene microspheres or a wax skeleton, which disappears during calcination, leaving pores of the desired volume in the material. It is also possible to obtain a porous calcium phosphate ceramic by changing other biological substances.

Chemical Properties

The calcium phosphate ceramics are part of a large class of apatites characterized by the formula $M_{10}(XO_4)_6Z_2$. The apatites form a large range of compounds. Numerous substitutions of the calcium, phosphate or hydroxyl are possible. These different substitutions modify the properties of the calcium phosphates, in particular their solubility (14). Flouro-apatite, obtained by substituting the HO^- by the F^-, has much less solubility than hydroxyapatite, while the presence of CO_3^{2-} and Mg^{2-} increases the solubility of hydroxyapatite. With tricalcium phosphate, substituting the Ca^{2+} by Mg^{2+} diminishes the solubility.

Hydroxyapatite (HA): $Ca_{10}(PO_1)_6(OH)_2$

This phosphate of calcium is the nearest relation to the biological apatite crystals. However, the atomic ratio (1.6) is longer than that in powdered bone, dentine or dental enamel. Of all the calcium phosphate biomaterials, pure hydroxyapatite is the least soluble.

Beta tricalcium phosphate (bTCP): $Ca_3(PO_4)_2$

This is characterized by a calcium phosphate atomic ratio of 1.5. bTCP is more soluble than pure HA.

The biphasics (BCP)

Biphasic products are mixtures of HA and betaTCP. Their chemical properties depend on the proportions of these two constituents in the mixture, which allows control of the speed of resorption and bone substitutions of the ceramic. The higher the HA/TCP ratio, the less the solubility of the biphasic.

Physico-Chemical Properties

Density

The density depends on the conditions of pressure and temperature of the frittage. The higher the pressure and temperature the greater the density.

Porosity

Two types of porosity can be distinguished: microporosity, corresponding to the spaces between the crystals which allows the circulation and ex changes with biological fluid, and macroporosity, created by the addition of porogenic agents which encourage bone in-growth.

Dissolution properties (10)

The properties of dissolution depend on the characteristics of the ceramic, such as (a) the physical form (block/granule/powder), (b) porosity, (c) the composition (Ca/P), (d) crystallized structure, (e) the crystalinity (size and perfection of the crystals) and the specific surface. Other factors including pH and the composition of the solution in which the calcium phosphate is immersed also influence the solubility of the ceramic. The relative order of solubility of some calcium phosphate compounds is as follows (14): ACP»DCP>TTCP>aTCP >cTCP»HA. This order may, however, be modified by ionic substitutions.

Biological Properties

Numerous studies have shown the biocompatibility of the calcium phosphates with a lack of local or systemic toxicity, inflammation, or foreign body reaction (12). Another property of calcium phosphate ceramics is their bioactivity, which is their capacity to bond with the bone tissue without fibrous interposition (17). Following physico-chemical exchanges, an extremely strong bond is formed between the implant and the host bone. This bond is shown by the impossibility of removing the implant without breaking either the ceramic or the bone with the fracture rarely occurring at the interface (27). This very strong bond is also produced with materials having a bioactive surface, such as bioglasses and vitroceramics, but the interface composition varies depending on the nature of the implant (16). It is now recognized that all the calcium phosphates, even hydroxyapatite, are absorbable, but in varying degrees according to the chemical and physico-chemical characteristics just described. The discrepancy between some studies can be explained by the differences in materials studied or techniques utilized (25). In contact with biological fluid, all calcium phosphates undergo biodegradation/bioresorption, resulting in changes in the physico-chemical properties of the material (disintegration, changes in porosity, dissolution, formation of new phases, phase transformation). Two types of factors influence this biodegradation (6), physico-chemical characteristics of the material, such as composition, microporosity, mode of fabrication, and biological factors, such as the degree of bony contact, type of bone, species of animal, age, sex.

The mechanisms leading to this biodegradation bioresorption are the combination of three processes: physical (abrasion, fracture, disintegration), chemical (dissolution, local increase in the concentration of calcium and phosphate ions, leading to the formation of new phases (ACP, DCPD, OCP, impure HA)), and biological (reduction in pH due to cellular activity, which increases the biodegradation of calcium phosphates).

The degradation may be of two types: infra or extracellular (9). Intracellular degradation corresponds to particle phagocytosis (1), while extracellular degradation is a process of dissolution which can occur with or without the presence of cells (physico-chemical equilibrium). The cell types involved in the extracellular degradation have now been established. They are multinucleated giant cells resistant to tartaric acid phosphatase (1). However, since their brush border is slightly different from that osteoclasts, many authors have preferred since the start of the 1990'S to call them osteoclast-like cells. It seems now that there is a consensus that these resorption cells should be considered as true osteoclasts (1). The process of calcium phosphate degradation starts by extracellular dissolution on the surface of the material liberating ceramic aggregates. These aggregates are then incorporated in the cytoplasm of the phagocystic cells and dissolved by acid attack or enzymatic processes (5).

The result of the biodegradation of the ceramic is an increase in the local concentration of calcium and phosphate ions. Following this rise, precipitation of the biological apatite microcrystals incor-

porating the ions present in the fluids (Ca^{2+}, MG^{2+}, Na^+, CO_3^{2-}, HPO_4^{2-}, *etc*) take place on the surface and between the grains of the ceramic. It takes place in a milieu that is rich in proteins and ends in the formation of needle-shaped biological apatite crystals resembling those of bone. This precipitation is a purely physico-chemical phenomenon of the equilibrium with the biological fluids (5). Only thereafter, when the material is in contact with bone tissue, does true osteogenesis occur around and within the macropores of the implant. True bone, characterized by osteocysts and a mineralized matrix, appears in the biomaterial. Haversian remodeling can take place and turn over with resorption/apposition as in classical bone may be produced.

The calcium phosphate ceramics are osteoconductive. That is to say, they serve as a framework within which the bone can grow. They allow the growth of vessels and osteoprogenitor cells arising from the host bone. However, the calcium phosphates are not osteoinductive since they do not stimulate the non-differentiated cells to convert phenotypically into chondroprogenitor or osteoprogenitor cells. Most studies of calcium phosphate ceramic implantations in extraosseous sites have shown that these materials do not induce bone formation (26). However, some authors have seen the presence of bone tissue when the implants have been placed intramuscularly or subcutaneously (18) (fig. 1).

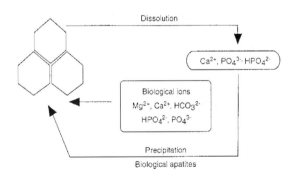

Figure 1 – Schematic representation of the portial disolution of the ceramic crystals and te formation of the biological apatite microcrystals.

Commercial Products

The characteristics given here are taken from the literature, except for Triosite™, which has been analyzed during this study.

Hydroxyapatite

The first hydroxyapatite was developed by Jarcho. This was durapatite, a dense ceramic with a compression resistance in the order of 935 MPa (13). It is now sold as Periograf™, Alveograf™ and Calcitite™. Other synthetic hydroxyapatites have also been marketed: Calcid™, Cerapatite™, Ceros™ and Synatite™. The products are presented as blocks or cylinders with an overall porosity varying between 30 and 60% for the first three (the porosity of Calcid™ has not been detailed in the data sheet). Their resistance to compression is in the region of 15 MPa with a porosity of 45%.

Tricalcium Phosphates

Biosorb™ and Calciresorb™ have been used in humans since 1992 and 1990 respectively, either as granules or blocks. The porosity is between 30 and 45% for Biosorb™ and 45% for Calciresorb™. The compression resistance is 10 to 15 MPa for implants with a porosity of 45% and > 30 MPa for implants with a porosity of 30%.

Biphasics

The first biphasic product developed was Triosite™ (8). Composed of 60% hydroxyapatite and 40% beta tricalcium phosphate, it has an overall porosity of 70% and compression resistance of 2.6 MPa (23). In clinical application it has been shown to be effective in posterior spinal fusion for internally fixed neurological scoliosis, and to fill cavities left by curettage of benign bone tumours (24). The second biphasic product developed was Biocer™ (blocks) -Biocel™ (granules), which is made up of 75% hydroxyapatite and 25% beta tricalcium phosphate. The standard products have a porosity of 70% and a compression resistance of 1-2 MPa.

Cellular Mechanisms

Implantations of macroporous cylinders in cancellous bone in the rabbit show very rapid (few hours) invasion of the intra-trabecular spaces of the biomaterial by conjunctive tissue without signs of inflammation. The new bone appears very quickly with signs of cellular resorption. Woven bone is formed before lamellar bone by osteoblasts. Osteoblastic activity, in particular cellular migration, is influenced by the presence of absorbed proteins on the surface of the material. However, the biomaterial itself can guide the migration of cells from the adjacent bone. Calcium phosphate ceramics implanted in bone may also serve as a support for the local differentiation of osteoblasts from the precursor cells in the bone marrow. Furthermore, it has been shown that subcutaneous implantation of calcium phosphate ceramics, associated with marrow cells, will give differentiation into mature bone. Transmission electron microscopy of the bone/implant interface shows collagen microfibrils intimately related to the hydroxyapatite crystals and these fibrils invade the inter-granular spaces of the ceramic (microporosity). The biomaterial is thus acting as a support for the deposition of new bone. The resorption of the ceramic appears early by dissolution of the apatite crystals and cellular degradation.

Experimental results suggest that two types of multinucleated cells are involved in the resorption. The first are large cells resembling giant cells and containing more than 20 nuclei. They never have any TRAP activity nor brush borders and phagocytose the hydroxyapatite particles. The second are multi-nucleated cells with 10 nuclei and TRAP activity and a brush border and behave like osteoclasts. Overall after implantation of a macroporous ceramic, the sequences are similar to the early stages of embryonic bone formation or fracture healing. Formation of lamellar bone implies osteoblastic differentiation and resorption is due to osteoclast type multinucleated cells.

Whichever calcium phosphate is considered, the sequences of biointegration of a calcium phosphate implant are identical. Biological degradation due to the cellular components at the implantation site occurs rapidly in the first few days. Some ceramic crystals, surface irregularities and dead cells are phagocytosed by macrophages, proceeding the stage of healing. This phase of active recognition of the implant and intracellular dissolution is also accompanied by extra cellular dissolution. These processes depend on the chemical structure (HA, betaTCP or BCP), on the physical structure (microporosity and size of the phagocytosed particles, macroporosity) and the type of tissue at the implantation site (I). The resorption of the implants should not be too fast so as to allow colonization of the macropores by more or less differentiated mesenchymal cells, which in bone will acquire the specialized features of the osteoblast and allow direct apposition of new bone onto the calcium phosphate surfaces (osteoconduction).

During these steps of colonization and cellular activity, two complementary and simultaneous mechanisms are acting:

In the micropores

Biological fluids (containing calcium, phosphate and carbonate ions) in the intercrystalline spaces of the ceramic are enriched in calcium and phosphate ions liberated by the intra and extracellular dissolution. Crystalline precipitation occurs on an extracellular matrix, creating a new saturation equilibrium. This precipitation leads to the neo-formation of biological apatite crystals, similar to those of the neighboring bone. This process leads to early calcification between the crystals of the ceramic, limiting the ex change processes of diffusion and thus dissolution.

In the macropores

When calcium phosphate ceramics are macroporous, the pre-osseous and osseous cells in the implantation site invade the macropores thanks to the osteoconductor properties of calcium phosphate ceramics. True bone, characterised by a mineralized extracellular collagen matrix, osteoblasts, osteocytes, and neo-vascularisation is seen. The interactions between ceramics and living tissue (degradation, dissolution) are very clearly slowed down. The bone directly apposed on the ceramic surfaces is generally lamellar. Several months after implantation (from the 2nd month) Harvesian bony remodelling takes place, similar to the remodelling of normal bone. It is during this process that implant degradation can take place due to osteoclast like multinucleated cells. This phase of bony remodelling is dependent on the macroporosity and the interconnection between the pores leading to bony colonisation. On the contrary, the promotion of new bone in non-bone sites, or if there is no previous direct contact with bone at the implantation site, can only take place under the influence of induction factors specific to bone tissue (22). The physical phenomena and mechanisms are essential for each of these steps of biological interaction to occur. Our different experimental studies have shown the need for early intimate contact between the implant and bone tissue and satisfactory immobilisation of the construct to prevent micromovements of the interface, which would end up with fibrous encapsulation (7). This fibrous encapsulation limits the development of true bone ingrowth. The calcium phosphate ceramics (commercial and non-commercial) currently made which are macroporous and chemically well defined, have inadequate mechanical qualities to be used in diaphyseal bone or to be used with traction or shearing stresses. On the other hand, ceramics are useful for filling bone cavities or to establish an arthrodesis bridge in the spine. Clearly the kinetics and quality of the bone ingrowth depend in variable degree on the age, sex, type of bone, presence or not of local injection calcium/phosphate metabolism and hormonal factors, as well as the species.

Development of the Mechanical Properties of Biphasic Macroporous Ceramics

The macroporous biphasic composites allow centripetal bony ingrowth by differentiated cells which secure the resorption/ingrowth processes. The favorable pore size for bone formation should be greater than 100 to 200 microns, but the resulting mechanical properties are insufficient. In fact, the resistance to axial compression gives a value in the region of 2.5 to 3 MPa. An animal model has allowed definition of the improvement in the mechanical properties associated with ingrowth by differentiated bone (23). Cylinders of 6 x 6 mm of a biphasic macroporous ceramic were implanted in the distal femur or rabbit and Beagle. After one week in the rabbit and 3 weeks in the dog, the mechanical properties of the ingrown ceramic were multiplied by 2 to 2.5 with compression resistance increased to 5.9 to 6.8 MPa. The improvement in the mechanical dissolution properties with reprecipitation of the apatite crystals and differentiation of bone tissue, was guided by osteoclastic resorption. Furthermore, infrared spectometry showed the appearance of organic composites (collagen, carbonate ions and water), which were not present in the ceramic before implantation. These events are essential because they show the adaptation of the material to bone and this progressive bioactivity goes on a par with an increase in the mechanical qualities which with time approaches that of trabecular bone.

Animal models allow us to define conditions of use in clinical practice. Postero-lateral lumbar vertebral arthrodesis allowed a comparison of the quality of autologous graft arthrodesis with fusion by macroporous biphasic ceramic blocks. Internal fixation by pedicular screws and titanium rods at the L2/L3/L4 level and a follow-up of 9 months allowed a study of the rigidity of these two types are arthrodesis by mechanical tests of the vertebral block on an MTS machine.

The average values of stiffness were higher for the ceramic group ($3.8 \pm 0.7 Nm^2$) than the autologous group ($3.3 \pm 1 \ Nm^2$), but without significant difference. We do not find any significant difference between the average maximum value obtained during rupture in forwards flexion, which were for the autologous us group and the ceramic group respectively, 19.1 ± 4.8 Nm and 17.6 ± 3.7 Nm. This functional evaluation of the use of ceramics for postero-Iateral spinal fusion supported the histological results, having shown the quality of the osteointegration/osteosubstitution kinetic of the biphasic ceramics and showed experimentally the possible value of substituting bone grafts by macroporous biphasic ceramics.

Models of diaphyseal resection in the adult Beagle femur (11) were very demanding for bony ingrowth. Two centimeters diaphyseal femoral resections were replaced by a ceramic cylinder stabilized by a locked intramedullary nail and reviewed histologicaIly at 8 months. With this follow-up the cylindrical blocks of BCP had consolidated over more than 80% of the cortices associated with endosteal and periosteal callous. Bony apposition was similar on the endosteal and periosteal surfaces. The quantitative assessment of bony ingrowth by histomorphometry showed 20-24% of the surface occupied by bone, without statistically significant difference between the blocks and the junctional areas.

CONCLUSION

The calcium phosphate ceramics are bioactive products and the closest relatives to the mineral phases of calcified tissues. For surgical applications it is necessary to assess all the factors that allow one to obtain the best osteointegration for the type of operation planned (filling bone with or without stresses, bone reconstruction). These factors are: chemical factors (HA, beta TCP, HA/BTCP ratio in biphasic BCPS, impurities, ionic substitutions), physico-chemical factors (temperature of preparation, micro and macroporosity, size of crystals), and biological factors (implantation zone, condition of the neighboring tissue, age of patient, importance of calcium/phosphorous metabolism, presence of extracellular proteins).

Current developments call for perfection of hybrid materials linking a macroporous calcium phosphate ceramic with bone marrow cells. These methods have a double interest, on the one hand basic research for long term tissue culture of hematopoietic activity and to better understand the stem cells and osteogenic progenitors, but on the other hand to prepare a hybrid material from the patient's own cells for bone graft.

Reference List

1. Jarcho M (1981) Calcium Phosphate ceramics as hard tissue prosthetics. *Clin. Orthop.* 157:259-78.

2. Daculsi G, Legeros RL, Heughebaert M, Barbieux I (1990) Formation of carbonate apatite crystals after implantation of calcium phosphate ceramics. *Calcif. Tissue Int.* 46:20-7.

3. Klein CPAT, Driessen AA, De Groot K, Van Den Hoof A (1983) Biodegradation behavior of various calcium phosphate materials in bone tissue. *J. Biomed. Mater. Res.* 17:769-84.

4. Nery EB, Legeros RZ, Lynch KL, Lee K (1992) Tissue response to biphasic calcium phosphate ceramic with different ratios of HA/BTCP in periodontal osseous defects. *J. Periodontol.* 63:729-35.

5. Winter M, Griss P, De Groot K, Taga H, Heimke G, Von Digh HJA, Sawai K (1981) Comparative histocompatibility testing of seven calcium phosphate ceramics. *Biomaterials* 2:159-61.

6. Frayssinet P, Trouillet JL, Rouquet N, Autefage A, Delga C, Conte P (1993) Calcium phosphate porous ceramics osseointegration : the importance of a good definition of material specifications. 1er Congress European d'Orthopedie, Paris, 21-23 Avril. *Rev. Chir. Orthop.* 79, Abstract n° 402.

7. Hoofendoorn HA, Renooij W, Addermans LMA, Visser W, Wittibol P (1984) Long-term study of large ceramic implants (Porous hydroxyapatite) in dog femora. *Clin. Orthop.* 187:281-8.

8. Zheng QX, Zhu TB, DuJY, Hong GX, Li SP, Yan YH, Zhang ED (1992) Artificial bone of porous tricalcium phosphate ceramics and its preliminary clinical application. *J. Tongji. Med. Univ.* 12:173-9.

9. Legeros RZ (1988) Calcium phosphate materials in restorative dentistry. A review. *Adv. Dent. Res.* 2:164-80.

10. Van Blitterswijk CA, Grote JJ, Kuijpers W, Daems WTh, De Groot K (1986) Macropore tissue ingrowth: a quantitative and qualitative study on hydroxyapatite ceranlics. *Biomaterials* 7:137-43.

11. Daculsi G, Passuti N (1990) Effect of the macroporosity for osseous substitution of calcium phosphate ceramics. *Biomaterials* Il: 86-8.

12. Basie MF, Chappard D, Grizon F, Filmon R, Delécrin J, Rebel A (1993) Osteoclastic resorption of Ca-P biomaterials implanted in rabbit bone. *Calcif. Tissue Int.* 53: 348-56.

13. Ohgushi H, Goldberg VM, Caplan Al (1989) Heterotopic osteogenesis in porous ceramics induced by marrow cells. *J. Ortop. Res.* 7:568-78.

14. Daculsi G, Corlieu P, Bagot D'arc Maurice, Gersdorff M (1992) Macroporous biphasic calcium phosphate efficiency in mastoid cavity obliteration: experimental and clinical findings. *Ann. Oto Rhin. Laryng.* 101:669-74.

15. Trecant M, Delécrin J, Rorer J, Daculsi G (1994) Mechanical changes in macroporous calcium phosphate ceramics after implantation in bone. *Clin. Mater.* 15:233-40.

16. Uchida A, Araki N, Shinto Y, Yoshikawa H, Kurisaki E, Ono K (1990) The use of calcium hydroxyapatite ceranlic in bone tumor surgery. *J. Bone Joint Surg. Br.* 72:298-302.

17. Takagi K, Urist MR (1982) The role of bone maroon in bone morphogenetic protein-induced repair of femoral massive diaphyseal defects. *Clin. Othop.* 17:226-31.

18. Daculsi G Passuti N, Martin S, Deudon C, Legeros RZ, Raher S (1990) Macroporous calcium phosphate ceramic for long bone surgery in humans and dogs. Clinical and histological study. *J. Biomed. Mater. Res.* 24:379-96.

19. Gründel RE, Chapman MW, Yee T, Moore DC (1991) Autogeneic bone marrow and porous biphasic calcium phosphate ceramic for segmental bone defect in the canine ulna. *Clin. Orthop.* 266:244-58.

20. Burwell RG (1985) The function of bone marrow in the incorporation of a bone graft. *Clin. Orthop.* 200:125-41.

21. Cockin J (1971) Autologous bone grafting-complications at donor site. *J. Bone Joint Surg. Br.* 53-B:153.

22. Daculsi G, Passuti N, Martin S, Le Nihouanen JC, Brulliard V, Delécrin J (1989) A comparative study of bioactive calcium phosphate ceramics after implantation in cancellous bone in the dog. *Rev. Chir. Orthop.* 75:65-71.

23. Flatter TJ, Lynch KL, Benson M (1983) Tissues responses to implants of calcium phosphate ceramic in the rabbit spine. *Clin. Orthop.* 179-246.

24. Laurie SWS, Kaban LB, Mulliken JB, Murray JE (1984) Donor-site morbidity after harvesting rib and iliac bone. *Piast. Reconstr. Surg.* 73:933-8.

25. Paller D, Young MC, Wiler AM, Fomasier, VL, Jackson RW (1986) Percutaneous bone marrow grafting of fractures and bony defects. *Clin. Orthop.* 208:300-12.

26. Passuti N Daculsi G, Rogez JM, Martin S, Bainvel JV (1989) Macroporous calcium phosphate ceramic performance in human spine fusion. *Clin. Orthop.* 248:169-76.

27. Summers BN, Eisenstein SM (1989) Donor site pain from the ilium. A complication of lumbar spine fusion. *J. Bone Joint Surg. Br.* 71-B:677-9.

2 Hydroxyapatite Granules in Acetabular Reconstruction

Hironobu Oonishi, MD, PhD and Hiroshi Fujita, MD, PhD

INTRODUCTION

Freeze-preserved allografts have been used in cases of massive bone deficiencies during revision total hip arthroplasty. Excellent results have been reported in Europe and in the USA (1-4). Cases using allografts have also been reported in Japan (5), although in Japan materials other than femoral heads, partial femoral condyles and partial tibial plateaus from patients undergoing arthroplasty are still very difficult to obtain. However, increasing interest in bioactive ceramics, particularly in hydroxyapatite (HA) over the past 15 years, has resulted in a significant increase in its clinical application during this period (6-14). Under these circumstances, we began to use sintered HA granules clinically. As a material, sintered HA is not resorbable, binds to the bone physicochemically, and is strong enough as a bone defect filler. We obtained good results in three revision cases by placing fine HA granules (300-500µm) between the bone cement and the bone graft on the deficiencies of the femur in 1984 (Oonishi et al., 1991). In addition, since 1985 massive bone deficiencies have been filled with HA granules (9, 10, 11, 12).

In the first generation (1986-1992), the entire surface of the exposed HA granules at the peripheral deficiencies after filling HA granules in the cavitary deficiency was covered with bone cement to reconstruct stabilized complex. However, spaces were observed between HA granules and nearly bone and the prostheses migrated in the case of enormous wall deficiency to allow stable filling of only HA granules (8-14, 17, 18). Consequently, in the second generation (since 1993), the peripheral segmental deficiency was covered with bulk allografts to gain stable filling of HA granules (14, 17, 18). Since 1995, the Kerboull cross plate was used in some cases to intend to obtain more stable fixation (18, 19).

THE FIRST GENERATION (1986-1992) MATERIALS AND METHODS

Reconstruction Procedures Using HA for Massive Bone Deficiencies in the Acetabulum

The soft tissue and necrotic tissue adhering to the acetabulum are completely removed. At the bone defect site, only the necrotic tissue and inflamed tissues are removed, then HA granules are prepared to fill the defect. HA granules were manufactured by sintering at 1 200°C with a porosity of 35 to 48% (average 42%), then sieved to obtain granules of several sizes (Bioceram P®. Sumitomo-Osaka Cement Co. Ltd. Tokyo, Japan). Granules of 300-600µm (G-2), 0.9-1.2mm (G-4) and 3.0-5.0mm (G-6) are mixed at a ration of 10:45:45. Physiological saline is added to the mixture to increase the mixing density and, due to the porous characteristic of the powder, facilitates the adhesion of granules with one another. This results in firmer adhesion and more stable shape formation. The acetabulum is filled with the mixture. If the same size of HA granules are used, the mixing density decreases, a firmer and more stable filling can't be obtained, and the shape easily breaks.

At this time, a previously determined space for the socket installation is left open. A hemispherical compressor 2mm larger than the outer diameter of the socket is then inserted successively into this space and firmly struck into the acetabulum using a plastic hammer while continuously making adjustments to determine the best socket location (fig. 1a-d). In cases with small and moderate medial wall deficiencies, excluding cases with large deficiencies, HA granules could be filled sufficiently. In other words, even though a large amount of filled HA granules escaped from the defect in the medial wall, the area was sufficiently filled with HA granules without any use of bone plate or other biomaterial to cover the deficiency. Escaped HA granules were protected by the soft tissues and never leaked out from within.

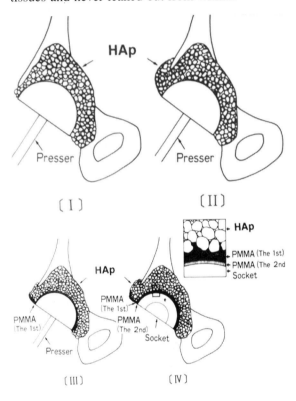

Figures 1a-d – Reconstruction procedures using HA granules for massive bone deficiency in the acetabulum.

When cementing the socket, a 2-3mm thickness of cement in paste-like condition is placed on the entire surface of the acetabulum, immediately after aspirating liquid completely from the HA granules impacted in the acetabulum using an aspirator. The cement is then compressed with a compressor 2mm larger than the outer socket diameter until the cement hardened.

The paste-like cement makes handling easier. During the period between 1986 to 1993, if the margin of the acetabulum had not been sufficiently filled with HA granules, the margin was filled with additional HA granules. When a bone defect

extended over a large area on the superior periphery of the acetabulum and it was not possible to sufficiently fill it with HA granules, additional HA granules were placed in this region and fixed using a 1-2mm thickness of cement.

In 35 cases, the superior peripheral deficiency was covered with bone cement after filling with HA granules. In one case, autograft bone from the iliac bone was used to cover a peripheral deficiency. In addition, all exposed surfaces of HA granules filled around the socket were covered with bone cement.

Before the socket is cemented, the hardened cement surface is dried and the socket is fixed with viscous cement containing a lot of monomer. This procedure facilitates binding the viscous cement to the hardened cement. By using these procedures, the adequate cement thickness around the socket can be kept.

Clinical Cases

Between 1986 and 1992, 9 to 15 years after surgery, we carried out this procedure on 40 hips. The bone loss was assessed according to the AAOS classification of acetabular deficiencies (20). Whole peripheral segmental and cavitary deficiencies with medial walls intact were found in 13 joints (33%), and peripheral cavitary deficiencies over the whole area with the medial wall absent were found in 18 joints (45%). They were very unstable cases after revision surgery. There were 2 men and 38 women, and their ages at operation ranged from 35 to 81 years. The follow-up period was from 8 to 14 years. Our original revision THR was performed because of osteoarthritis in 33 patients, rheumatoid arthritis in five, avascular necrosis of the head of the femur in one, and systemic lupus erythematosus in one. In 36 joints, this was the first revision, in three it was the second, and in one it was the third. Histological studies were performed in the retrieved case.

As for radiographic evaluation, the interface between bone and HA, the interface between bone cement and HA, changes in volume and shape of HA granules, absorption of HA, and movement of the component were carefully observed.

Postoperative Procedures

Partial weight bearing was allowed 4 to 6 weeks after surgery for the stable cases, and for unstable cases, full weight bearing was allowed after 8 to 12 weeks. Very careful and supervised partial weight bearing was allowed 2 to 4 weeks after surgery for the patient with Parkinson's disease.

RESULTS

X-ray Evaluation

When HA granules are firmly packed, a stable filling is attained, similar to a stone wall. Although spaces were observed in areas at the interface between HA granules and bone immediately after surgery, these spaces gradually disappeared within 3 months following surgery. This was probably due to new bone formation into the space between the HA granules, and the subsequent binding with HA granules. Sclerotic bone surrounding loose components changed to cancellous bone over a period of one to three years following revision surgery.

Our radiographic evaluation showed neither morphological changes nor decreases in volume (figs 2, 3, 4, 5) except for some cases with very specific complications. In a case with a considerable cavitary and peripheral deficiency and a medial wall defect, even HA granules were over filled in the medial area of the acetabulum, and the

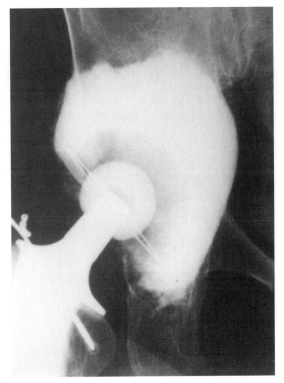

Figure 3 – Patient with systemic lupus erythomatosus at 15 years after revision THR (50 year old female).

socket settled laterally. Not only there were there no detrimental effects radiographically or clinically, but the filled HA granules were also very

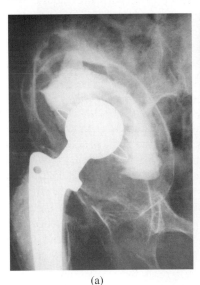 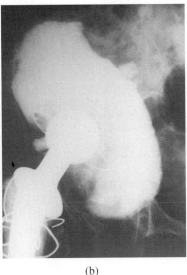 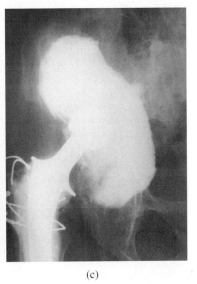

(a) (b) (c)

Figure 2 – Osteoarthritis due to dysplastic acetabulum; the first case in which HA granules were filled in the acetabular massive bone defect.
a – Before revision THR (65 year old female).
b – Immediately after revision THR.
c – 15 years after revision THR (at age 80).

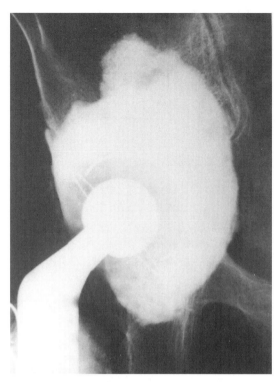

Figure 4 – Fifteen years after revision THR for avascular necrosis of the femoral head (55 year old female).

stable following surgery (figs 6, 7, 8). However, when HA granules were filled into the acetabulum with a huge cavitary deficiency and complete anterior and posterior peripheral deficiencies, and further with medial wall defects, the filled HA granule shape was broken and the socket moved as a result.

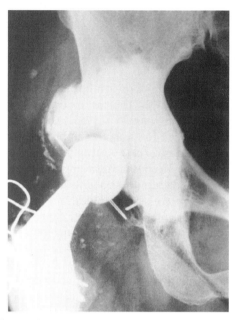

Figure 6 – Fourteen years after revision THR for osteoarthritis due to dysplastic acetabulum (51 year old female).

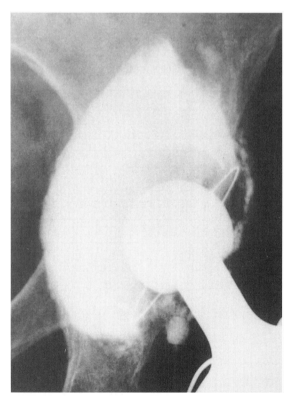

Figure 5 – Fourteen years after revision THR for osteoarthritis due to dysplastic acetabulum (58 year old female).

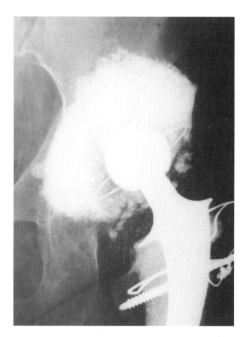

Figure 7 – Fourteen years after revision THR for osteoarthritis due to dysplastic acetabulum (69 year old female).

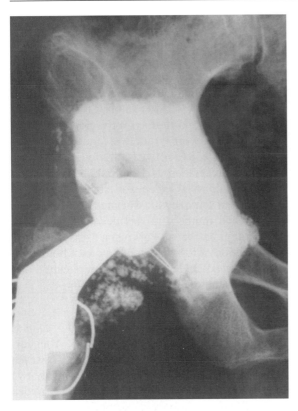

Figure 8 – Fourteen years after revision THR for congenital dislocation of the hip (62 year old male).

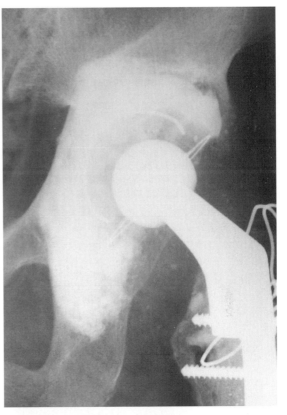

Figure 9 – Five years after revision THR for osteoarthritis due to dysplastic acetabulum. Spaces were observed between HA granules nearly the bone at the latero-superior lesion.

Complications

In two cases, spaces were observed between HA granules near the bone at the latero-superior lesion (fig. 9). The width of the space increased very slowly, but stopped after 5 to 6 years; clinically, there were no problems. We theorized that rather wide spaces were left between the bony base and packed HA granules at surgery, and in the vicinity of these gaps, the bond between bone and HA granules was unstable after surgery. Continuous micromotion most likely occurred right under the bone at these gaps before sufficient bone ingrowth into the spaces was obtained between HA granules or sufficient bonding was obtained between bone and HA. In these cases, if the superior peripheral deficiencies had been covered with an allograft plate, such as a tibial plateau, HA granules could have been filled sufficiently in the superior peripheral region and, as a result, the appearance of the spaces could be avoided.

In two patients after the second revision and in one patient after third revision in the other, the central part of the medial wall was absent and the overall deficiency was too great to allow stable filling of the granules. The packed HA granules broke and the prostheses migrated. In the third revision case, bone formation was very poor because it was the patient's third revision THR. In one of the second revision cases, the patient was obligated, soon after surgery, to continue care of a bedridden relative. Since this occurred within the first two months following surgery, the HA mass could not endure the over 60 kg load. These prostheses began to move at around six months after surgery and continued migrating. In two of them, the prostheses migrated as close as the ilio-sacral joint and stopped there (fig. 10). Osteolysis occurred widely around the mass of HA granules due to the fine HA powder that was produced while the prostheses were migrating. After the prostheses attained and contacted the bone directly near the ilio-sacral joint, migration stopped. At latest review, the two patients could walk with occasional slight or moderate pain, but were obliged to use crutches. The one patient continued to work on a farm. They refused another revision surgery.

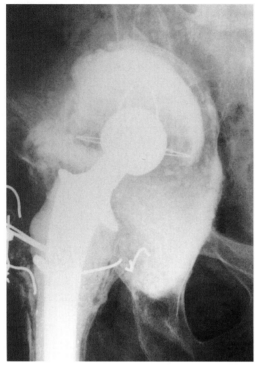

Figure 10 – Two and one half years after third revision THR for osteoarthritis due to dysplastic acetabulum. The socket migrated as close as the ilio-sacral joint.

Clinical Results

As for clinical results, evaluation criteria by Merle d'Aubigné before and after surgery were compared. The categories are as follows.

Pain

Before surgery, one patient was graded 0, two patients were graded 1, seven patients were graded 2, four patients were graded 3, eleven patients were graded 4, eight patients were graded 5, and seven patients were graded 6. After surgery, all patients were graded 6 except two patients who were graded 5, and one patient who was graded 4. Excluding patients developing complications, pain relief was particularly remarkable, and pain was in fact, completely alleviated from all patients. One patient had a fracture at the femur at the time of initial THR and pain continued in a thigh and greater trochanter areas still after revision surgery.

Walking ability

Before surgery, one patient was graded 0, two patients were graded 1, four patients were graded 2, ten patients were graded 3, 12 patients were graded 4, ten patients were graded 5, and only one patient was graded 6. After surgery, twenty patients were graded 6, and thirteen were graded 5, while three patients were graded 4, one patient was graded 3, one patient was graded 2, and two patients were graded 1. The walking ability was markedly improved except for patients with complications of tetraplegia associated with moderate sensory and motor paralysis due to myelopathy, with complication of Parkinson's disease, with complication of RA with contracture of both bilateral knees and ankles, and with complication of a socket loosening after the third revision.

Range of motion (ROM)

Before surgery, all patients were graded 4, 5, or 6, except two patients who were graded 3. After surgery, twenty-eight patients were graded 6, seven were graded 5, and three were graded 4. Only two cases were under 4, one graded 3 and one graded 1. The ROM also improved except for patients with complications of a socket loosening after the third revision and RA with contractures of both bilateral knees and ankles.

Complete evaluation

Before surgery, seventeen patients were graded 11 or less, thirteen patients were graded 12, 13, or 14, nine patients were graded 15, 16, or 17; only one patient was graded 18. After surgery, nineteen were graded 18, fourteen were graded 15, 16, or 17, five were graded 12, 13, or 14, and only two patients were graded 10 and 11. The pain, the walking ability, and the ROM were markedly improved, except for the cases mentioned above. Pain relief was particularly remarkable, and pain was, in fact, completely alleviated from all but one patient.

THE SECOND GENERATION (1992-1997) MATERIALS AND METHODS

In the second generation, since 1992, peripheral segmental deficiencies were covered with allograft from the femoral heads of patients undergoing arthroplasty to allow for stable filling of HA granules. In some cases with a large cavitary deficiency combined with a large peripheral segmental deficiency, a large block of the femoral head was used. Since 1995, latero-superior large peripheral deficiencies were covered with an allograft from the tibial plateau (figs 11a-d).

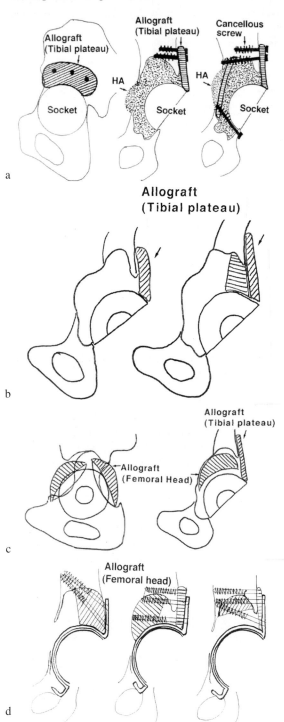

Figure 11a-d – The second generation. Latero-superior large peripheral deficiency was covered with an allograft of tibial plateau.

As a filler in the cavitary deficiency, mixtures of G-4 and G-6 HA granules were filled as in the first generation, and in some cases mixtures of HA granules of 0.9-1.2mm (G-4) and small bone chips at a ratio of 30 to 70 or 50 to 50 were filled. Since 1995, the Kerboull cross plate was used to obtain more secure fixation. The Kerboull cross plate is very useful for supporting weight bearing on the whole area of the filled HA by interposing bone cement in order to prevent the volume change (fig. 11d).

Since 1997, the superior peripheral segmental and cavitary deficiency was filled by bone block to support the Kerboull cross plate and the socket firmly, because in some cases with the superior peripheral segmental and cavitary deficiency, the hook of the Kerboull cross plate had broken.

Clinical Cases

Between 1992 and 1997, 48 hips have been operated on using the procedure. The follow-up period was 3 to 8 years. Of the 48 hips, it was the first revision for 43, in 4 hips it was the second revision, and in 1 hip it was the third revision. They were very unstable cases, with great peripheral segmental and cavitary deficiencies, as in the first generation.

Results and Complications

In general, when the whole peripheral segmental deficiency was covered with allografts, filled HA granules were very stable. In one case filled with mixture of HA granules and bone chips, a slight volume change was observed. However, there were no clinical symptoms, and the change did not increase. There was no difference radiographically between HA alone and mixture of HA and bone chips as fillers when the peripheral segmental deficiency was covered with allografts (fig. 12a-d).

Between 1995 and 1997, Kerboull cross plates were used in 24 patients. In two patients, the hook of Kerboull cross plate broke (10%). In both patients, a considerably great deficiency at the superior periphery involving great cavitary deficiency was covered only with allograft from the tibial plateau, and the patients were obliged to begin a heavy labor 3 to 5 months after surgery. Consequently, when the Kerboull cross plate is used, the superior peripheral deficiency must be filled by bone block to support the body weight.

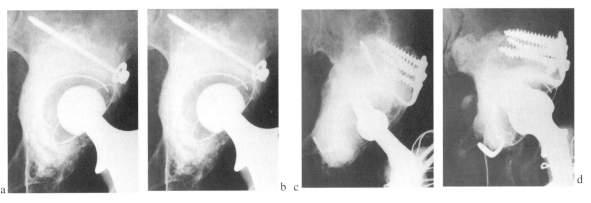

Figures 12a-d – The whole peripheral segmental deficiency was covered with allograft. The cavitary deficiency was filled with mixture of HA granules and bone chips.
Case 1 at one month postoperatively (a) and at 8 years (b).
Case 2 (c) and Case 3 (d), both shown at 6 years postoperatively.

Fate Of HA Granules Filled Into The Cavitary Bone Defect

At the second revision surgery after breakage of a Kerboull cross plate, we found that HA granules had formed a homogeneous mass into the whole depth of about 2cm, and it was difficult to drill a hole through this homogeneous mass, or to cut it with a chisel, because the mass adhered to the bone very firmly. In histological studies, dense bone ingrowth was obtained in the spaces between HA granules to the entire depth of 2cm two years after surgery (fig. 13).

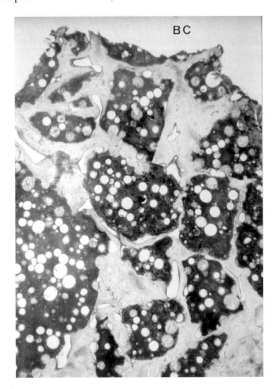
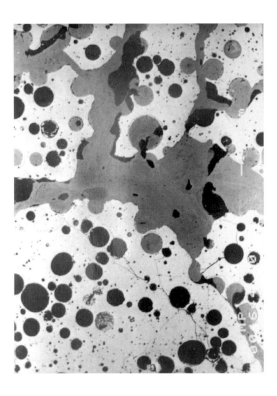

Figure 13 – Non decalcified hard tissue specimen stained by Methylene blue was observed by optical microscopy (a) and the specimen was observed by back-scattered electron image (b).
In a retrieved case (two years after surgery), dense bone ingrowth was obtained in the spaces between HA granules the entire depth of 2cm. The top was fixed with bone cement (BC) around the socket.

As a control in an animal experiment, mixtures of G-4 and G-6 HA granules as in clinical cases were filled into the cavity of 2cm in diameter and 4 cm in length made at the proximal end of the tibia of a goat. Eighteen months after implantation, non-decalcified hard sections were made. A small amount of the new bone had entered from the periphery to the center. Where the surrounding bone was cortical bone, cortical bone entered. When the surrounding bone was cancellous bone, cancellous bone entered. As the quantity of bone ingrowth lessened, some HA granules that filled into the cavity dropped out while making non-decalcified hard tissue specimens, and some HA granules dislodged from the specimens.

In a clinical case, HA granules were filled in the weight bearing area. However, in experimental studies HA granules were filled in the non weight bearing area. From these results, it can be assumed that, in the weight bearing area, a great amount of new bone entered into the spaces of the HA granules, and in the non-weight bearing area, only small amount of new bone entered into the spaces.

DISCUSSION

In Japan, use of HA granules for treatment of massive bone defects is indispensable, as it is still very difficult to obtain allograft. For what is probably the first time ever, we used HA for revision THR that involved massive bone deficiencies. The advantages of HA are 1) immunoreactions can be completely ignored, 2) postoperative morphological changes and volume decreases do not occur if a mixture of adequate granule sizes are packed densely and firmly during surgery, 3) postoperative HA absorption, if any, is small in amount and extremely slow, and moreover, it is bound to bone physicochemically, and 4) there would be less osteolysis by polyethylene wear particles at the interface of the bone. We suppose the reasons for the marked pain relieving effect is that there were neither changes in the shape of packed HA granules, nor movement of the component, as HA granules were packed firmly and stably, bound to the bone physicochemically, and fixed with bone cement mechanically.

The spaces observed in part at the interface between HA granules and bone immediately after surgery gradually disappeared within 3 months.

These phenomena would result from new bone tissues entering into the space between the HA granules encircling the surface of the bony cavity.

After filling HA granules into the cavitary deficiency, the sclerotic bone around the loosened socket changed to cancellous bone over a period of one to three years after revision surgery. This could be because the bone ingrowth into the spaces of HA granules from the surrounding sclerotic bone was obtained, and the HA granules may have physicochemically bound to the entire surface of the sclerotic bone wall. This phenomenon was very similar to bone union after non-union of fracture.

On the retrieved studies, HA granules had formed a homogeneous mass, which was difficult to make a drill hole in or to cut with a chisel, and it adhered to the bone very firmly. Histologically, bone ingrowth was obtained two years after surgery in the majority of the spaces between HA granules to the entire depth of about 2cm. Consequently, if HA granules were filled very firmly and stably, a very strong new acetabulum could be reconstructed.

In the retrieved case, HA granules were filled in the weight bearing area. However, in an animal experiment using a tibia of a goat, HA granules were filled in the non weight bearing area, and much less bone ingrowth into the spaces of HA granules was obtained. Consequently, excellent results can be expected when a mixture of several grain sizes of HA are packed densely and firmly during surgery into the massive defect of the bone in weight bearing area (9).

As occurrence of spaces between HA granules and neighboring bone at the latero-superior lesion (Zone I) was one of the complications, we thought that the filling of HA granules may not have been dense near the bone base at the latero-superior lesion (Zone I), because, the superior peripheral deficiency was covered with bone cement after filling with HA granules. As a result, continuous micromotion probably caused occurrences of the gaps before sufficient bone growth could provide bonding. If the superior peripheral deficiency had been covered by an allograft plate, such as tibial plateau, or allograft block, such as femoral head, the HA granules would probably have filled the spaces more satisfactorily.

In the case of the socket migration, as the central part of the medial wall was absent and the overall deficiency was too great to allow stable filling of the granules, the form packed with granules broke. Moreover, osteolysis occurred widely around the mass of HA granules due to fine HA powders, which were produced while the prostheses were migrating. In order to prevent these complications, in the second generation (after 1992), the peripheral segmental deficiencies were covered by allografts in whole area.

A superior peripheral segmental deficiency was covered by the tibial plateau. The majority of anterior and posterior peripheral deficiencies could be covered when major superior peripheral segmental defects were covered by the tibial plateau. In some cases, both the peripheral and cavitary deficiencies were filled and stabilized by thick allografts to support the load and to shield the HA granules. In some cases, Kerboull cross plates were used.

Bone blocks of allografts have to be fixed stably to the pelvis by screws, and the spaces between bone block and pelvis have to be filled by bone chips to prevent migration of HA granules. If HA granules migrate into the space, physiological bone fusion will be disturbed.

In the 2nd generation, complications due to spaces between granules and the neighboring bony base at the latero-superior lesion of the acetabulum has not been observed, nor has socket migration, although breakage of the hook of Kerboull cross plate was observed in 2 cases.

Reference list

1. Borja FJ, Mmaymneh W (1985) Bone allografts in salvage of difficult hip arthroplasties. *Clin. Orthop.* 197:123-30.

2. Denissen HW, de Groot K, Makkes P.Ch, Van den Hooff A, Klopper PJ (1980) Tissue response to dense apatite implants in rats. *J. Biomed. Mater. Res.* 14:713-21.

3. Gross AE, Lavoie MV, McDermott P., Marks P (1985) The use of allograft bone in revision of total hip arthroplasty. *Clin. Orthop.* 197:115-22.

4. Hoogendoorn HA, Renooij W, Akkermans LMA, Visser W, Wittebol P (1984) Long-term study of large ceramic implants (porous hydroxyapatite) in dog femora. *Clin. Orthop. Rel. Res.* 187:281-8.

5. Itoman M, Sunabe S (1988) Revision total hip replacement supplemented with allogenic bone grafting. *J. of Joint Surgery (Japan)* 7,3:83-93.

6. Jarcho M, Kay JR, Gumaer KI, Doremus RH, Drobeck HP (1977) Tissue, cellular and subcellular events at a bone-ceramic hydroxyapatite interface. *J. of Bioengineering* 1:79-92.

7. McGann W (1986) Massive allografting for sever failed total hip replacement. *J. Bone Joint Surg.* 68A:4-12.

8. Oonishi H (1988) Revision of THR for massive bone defects. *J. of Joint Surg. (Japan)* 7,3:49-60.

9. Oonishi H, Kushitani S, Aono M, Ukon Y, Yamamoto M, Isimaru H, Tsuji E (1989) The effect of HA coating on bone growth into porous titanium alloy implants. *The Journal of Bone and Joint Surgery* 71-B,2:213-6.

10. Oonishi H (1991) Orthopaedic applications of hydroxyapatite. *Biomaterials* Vol.12;171-178, Butterworth-Heinemann Ltd.

11. Oonishi H, Iwaki Y, Kin Y (1997) Hydroxyapatite in revision of total hip replacements with massive acetabular defects. *J. Bone Joint Surg. Br.* 79:87-92.

12. Oonishi H, Fujita H, Itoh S, Kin T, Oomamiuda K (2002) Histological studies on retrieved Ha granules filled in acetabular massive bone defect in revision total hip arthroplasty. *Bioceramics* 14:423-6.

13. Oonishi H, Kushitani S, Murata N, Saito M, Maruoka A, Yasukawa E, Tsuji E, Sugihara F (1991) Long term bone growth behavior into the spaces of HAp granules packed into massive bone defect cavity, Bioceramics, Vol. 6, Butterworth-Heinemann Ltd., 157-61.

14. Oonishi H (1995) Long term clinical results after revision total hip arthroplasty by using HA, J. of Joint Surgery (Japan) 14,II;51-64.

15. Oonishi H, Kushitani S, Yasukawa E, Iwaki H, Hench LL, Wilson J, Tsuji E (1997) Particulate bioglass compared with hydroxyapatite as a bone graft substitute. *Clinical Orthopaedics and Related Research* No 334, 316-25.

16. Oonishi H, Hench LL, Wilson J, Tsuji E, Kin S, Yamamoto T, Mizokawa S (2000) Quantitative comparison of bone growth behaviour in granules of Bioglass®, A-W Glass-Ceramics, and Hydroxyapatite, *J. Biomed. Mater. Res.* 51:37-46.

17. Oonishi H, Iwaki Y, Kin N (1997) Hydroxyapatite in revision of total hip replacements with massive acetabular defects. *J. Bone Joint Surg. [Br]* 79-B:87-92.

18. Oonishi H (2000) Reconstruction of the hip-revision surgery of acetabulum with massive bone defects; material. *OS Now Orthopaedic Surgery (Japan)* 5:144-52.

19. Kerboull M (1985) La reconstruction du cotyle, Arthroplastie total de hanche, edited by Postel M. *et al.* Springer-Verlag. Berlin Heidelberg 89-96.

20. D'Antonio JA, Capello WN, Borden LS (1989) Classification and management of acetabular abnormalities in total hip arthroplasty. *Clin. Orthop.* 243:126-37.

3   The Use of the OP-1 Implant in Reconstructive Surgery of the Hip and Knee

Stephen D. Cook, PhD and Robert L. Barrack, MD

INTRODUCTION

The number and complexity in total hip and knee arthroplasty cases continues to increase. Implant loosening and osteolysis related to wear debris generation is the leading cause of total joint component failure and can be associated with massive bone loss. In addition, the incidence of periprosthetic fractures is steadily increasing probably related to progressive osteoporosis adjacent to implants. The use of graft material to restore bone stock and promote bone healing and implant stabilization is a crucial part of total joint arthroplasty, especially in the revision situation. The added surgical time, limited supply and morbidity associated with the autogenous bone graft harvest has resulted in the use of various types of allograft bone in the vast majority of cases. Contained defects are effectively managed with morselized cancellous allograft. While allograft bone can heal defects, ingrowth does not occur from the defect to a porous ingrowth surface (fig. 1). This can compromise component stability if extensive defects are present. In addition, when there is a need for immediate structural support, cortical allografts are often used, which have a much slower rate of incorporation.

Allograft bone is an attractive alternative to autograft bone because it supports bone formation, supply is less limited, and large structural restorations are possible. However, allograft bone has only a fraction of the osteoinductive capacity of autograft bone (4) and a lowered capacity to incorporate with host bone (5-7). Cortical allografts have the added disadvantage of slower incorporation and a higher rate of nonunion compared to cancellous allograft (8, 9). Nonetheless cortical strut grafts are widely utilized in conjunction with hip arthroplasty when biomechanical support is required. Allograft also carries a small risk of disease transmission and requires extensive testing of donors. Some methods of sterilization such as high dose radiation and freeze-drying compromises the mechanical properties of allograft bone.

Recent research has centered on the use of osteoinductive materials such as osteogenic protein (OPs) or bone morphogenetic proteins (BMPs) to aid in the healing of bone. These proteins either alone or in combination with other regulatory molecules, induce new bone formation (10-16) Osteogenic proteins are members of the transforming growth factor-β (TGF-β) super family of proteins involved in the cascade of cellular events of tissue formation and regeneration including stem cell commitment, differentiation, and proliferation (12). Osteogenic proteins have been produced in highly purified form from the bones of a variety of species and have been found to induce bone formation at ectopic and orthotopic sites in small and large mammals (12, 17-19). The most recent advance in the development of OPs is the cloning

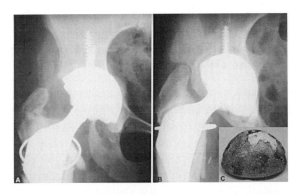

Figure 1 – Revision cementless acetabular component placed against morselized allograft (a). Two years later the patient underwent re-revision for aseptic loosening (b). Minimal bone was adherent to the component at the dome (c).

and expression of recombinant human bone proteins. Recombinant human osteogenic protein-1 also referred to as bone morphogenetic protein-7 (rhOP-1, rhBMP-7) and bone morphogenetic protein-2 (rhBMP-2) have been proven safe and efficacious in improving and accelerating bone healing in orthotopic animal models (20-25). Osteogenic protein-1 has also been shown in a randomized, prospective study to heal tibia fracture nonunions clinically and radiographically equivalent to autogenous iliac crest bone graft (26).

An osteogenic protein-1 device (OP-1 Implant, Stryker Biotech, Hopkinton, Massachusetts) consists of 3.5 milligrams of rhOP-1 combined with one gram of highly purified bovine bone derived Type I collagen. The carrier does not have cartilage or bone inductive properties (27). The final preparation is freeze dried and sterilized by gamma irradiation. The device is reconstituted with sterile saline at the time of surgery producing approximately 4 cc of a granular graft material that offers no structural capacity.

The use of an OP-1 Implant alone or in conjunction with autograft or allograft bone offers many potential advantages. Containment of the OP-1 Implant at the site may be enhanced by combination with the bone graft material, resulting in greater and better localized new bone formation. When a structural graft is required or if a bone defect volume is large, the use of the OP-1 Implant alone may not be satisfactory since it has no structural integrity. Under such circumstances there would be a substantial advantage to enhancing the healing potential of the autograft or allograft material so that extensive bone formation and mechanical strength could be achieved more rapidly and reliably. In addition to better defect healing bone ingrowth to a porous surface may be enhanced with the use of the OP-1 Implant. This should speed the rehabilitation process and shorten the time of protected weightbearing and attendant functional disability for the patient.

PRECLINICAL EVALUATION OF THE OP-1 IMPLANT

Morselized Autograft and Allograft Bone with an OP-1 Implant

Bilateral, critical size, osteoperiosteal segmental defects were surgically created in mid-ulna of 24 adult male dogs (28). Either autograft bone, allograft bone or OP-1 Implant alone or various combinations of the OP-1 Implant mixed with allograft or autograft bone were implanted in the segmental bone defects. Combinations used included 67% bone graft/ 33% OP-1 Implant, and 33% bone graft/67% OP-1 Implant. Healing of the defects was assessed radiographically, and in biomechanical and histologic studies at twelve weeks postoperative.

The use of the OP-1 Implant alone or any combination of autograft or allograft bone and the OP-1 Implant improved radiographic, mechanical and histologic healing of the critical sized defects compared to autograft or allograft bone alone (table 1). Earlier and greater volume of new bone formation was observed with the presence of the OP-1 Implant. The amount of new bone, degree of remodeling and graft incorporation was proportional to the amount of rhOP-1 implanted. Histologically only 22% of defects treated with allograft bone alone completely healed while 67% of defects treated with autograft bone alone were completely healed at twelve weeks. Defects treated with the OP-1 Implant alone or any combination of bone graft and the OP-1 Implant healed 93% of cases at twelve weeks. These differences were significant at $p < 0.05$. The highest radiographic grade, histologic grade and mechanical strength was achieved with the use of 33 percent allograft/67 percent OP-1 Implant, although no significant differences in healing were observed among the groups containing the OP-1 Implant. Defects treated with any amount of the OP-1 Implant obtained two times the mechanical strength obtained by autograft bone alone at twelve weeks postoperative.

Cortical Allograft with the OP-1 Implant

Fourteen adult male dogs underwent bilateral onlay allograft strut procedures to the mid-femur utilizing stainless steel cables. (29) In each animal one femur received the OP-1 Implant interposed between the graft and host bone while the contralateral femur strut graft served as an untreated control. The animals were studied with biweekly radiographs and histologic and microradiographic evaluation at sacrifice periods of at four, eight and twelve weeks postoperative. The radiographic results showed that the healing of cortical strut

Treatment Group	3	1 Radiographic	2 Histologic	Mechanical
Allograft	At least one cortex bridged	3/9	2/9	0.15 ∀ 0.30 (9)
	All cortices bridged	0/9		3%
67% Allograft/33% OP-1 Implant	At least one cortex bridged	6/6	5/6	1.60 ∀ 1.43 (6)
	All cortices bridged	5/6		38%
33% Allograft/67% OP-1 Implant	At least one cortex bridged	6/6	6/6	3.18 ∀ 1.68 (6)
	All cortices bridged	6/6		74%
Autograft	At least one cortex bridged	5/9	6/9	1.33 ∀ 1.42 (9)
	All cortices bridged	4/9		31%
67% Allograft/33% OP-1 Implant	At least one cortex bridged	5/6	5/6	2.76 ∀ 1.69 (6)
	All cortices bridged	5/6		64%
33% Allograft/67% OP-1 Implant	At least one cortex bridged	5/6	6/6	2.85 ∀ 1.40 (6)
	All cortices bridged	5/6		66%
OP-1 Implant	At least one cortex bridged	5/6	5/6	2.74 ∀ 1.60 (6)
	All cortices bridged	5/6		64%

1. Number of defects/sample size.
2. Number of defects healed histologically/sample size.
3. Maximum torque to failure (Nm) (mean ∀ SD, (sample size)) and % intact ulna strength.

Table 1 – Radiographic, Histologic and Mechanical Testing Evaluation of Defect Healing with the OP-1 Implant and Bone Graft at 12 weeks.

grafts to the femur was improved and accelerated by the addition of the OP-1 Implant (Table 2). The OP-1 Implant treated sites also had significantly greater histologic and microradiographic grading scores at all time periods. Rapid formation of new bone and graft incorporation was observed in sites treated with the OP-1 Implant.

While cortical strut allografts were shaped intraoperatively to fit the femur, immediate post-operative radiographs often revealed that areas of nonconformity existed. Histologic sections demonstrated that extensive new bone completely filled gap regions between the host and the strut graft as early as four weeks postoperative in sites treated with the OP-1 Implant. In control struts the gaps were slower to fill and were not completely filled with new bone at eight weeks postoperative. Strut healing with the OP-1 Implant at four weeks postoperative was radiographically and histologically superior to control sites at eight weeks.

Acetabular Defects with the OP-1 Implant

Acetabular defect healing and bone ingrowth from an acetabular defect into a porous coating was evaluated. Six canines underwent bilateral total hip arthroplasty with a cementless press-fit porous coated acetabular component. A defect 8mm in diameter and 5mm in depth was created in the superior weight-bearing area of each acetabulum. The right defects of each animal were filled with the OP-1 Implant. Each contralateral defect was filled with either allograft bone, left empty (defect healing control), or no defect was created (porous ingrowth control). The degree of defect healing and bone growth into the porous acetabular component surface was quantified histologically and radiographically at six weeks postoperative.

The osteogenic bone protein device was successful in achieving complete healing of the

Postoperative Weeks	Control Mean ± SD (Sample Size)	OP-1 Mean ± SD (Sample Size)	p value
2	0.04 ± 0.13 (14)	0.86 ± 0.07 (14)	0.0005
4	0.82 ± 0.54 (14)	2.50 ± 0.59 (14)	0.0001
6	0.80 ± 0.82 (10)	3.30 ± 0.89 (10)	0.0002
8	1.88 ± 0.63 (4)	4.13 ± 0.06 (4)	0.0194
All times	0.65 ± 0.75 (42)	2.30 ± 1.33 (42)	0.0001

Grade:
0 = No visible new bone formation.
1 = Minimal new disorganized bone.
2 = Disorganized new bone bridging graft to host.
3 = Organized new bone of cortical density bridging both ends.
4 = Loss of graft-host distinction.
5 = Significant new bone formation and remodeling.

Table 2 – Radiographic Grading of Cortical Strut Graft Healing with the OP-1 Implant.

acetabular defects such that the percent cancellous bone volume was not significantly different from the control hips in which no defect was present. In addition, bone growth into the porous acetabular cup surface was comparable to that which occurred without a defect present. The OP-1 Implant treated defects healed more completely (37% bone density) than allograft bone (23%) or empty defect (14%) ($p < 0.05$) and achieved a bone density equivalent to the no defect controls (34%). Bone ingrowth also occurred to a significantly higher degree in the OP-1 Implant (37% bone ingrowth) compared to the allograft (18%) or empty defects (16%) ($p < 0.05$) achieving a degree of ingrowth equivalent to the no defect controls (30%)

DISCUSSION

Preclinical studies have demonstrated that the osteoinductive capacity of autograft and allograft bone can be improved with the addition of the OP-1 Implant. Although the OP-1 Implant is effective alone, its use with bone graft materials in hip and knee reconstructive surgery appears to be an ideal combination. The combination of autograft or allograft bone with the OP-1 Implant consistently improved the amount and rate of new bone formation compared to bone graft alone. Earlier graft incorporation and consolidation of the new bone and graft was also observed. In addition to the healing of large defects, the OP-1 Implant can be expected to improve component fixation by enhancing the amount of bone ingrowth.

The use of morselized autogenous and allogenic bone graft in combination with the OP-1 Implant performed similarly in preclinical studies. However, the complications associated with the donor site can be eliminated by using allograft without reducing the efficacy of the bone graft in the clinical situation. Aside from the risks of bleeding and infection, patients frequently complain of more postoperative pain from the autograft donor site than the primary operative site following a major reconstructive procedure (30, 31). The clinical cases to date suggest efficacy of allograft bone with the OP-1 Implant in promoting new bone formation and graft incorporation (fig. 2). The clinical use of the OP-1 Implant at the interface of a porous coated acetabular device exhibited extensive new bone formation in histologic evaluation of tissue retrieved at revision surgery (fig. 3). These results are also consistent with preclinical studies that indicate the OP-1 Implant may be efficacious in promoting earlier and greater bone ingrowth or implant apposition (23).

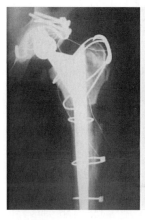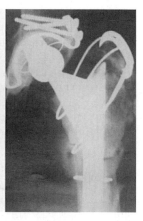

Figure 2 – The OP-1 Implant with morselized allograft bone was placed at the host bone interface of a proximal femoral allograft in a re-revision of a Charnley hip replacement (left). The initial revision had also utilized a proximal femoral allograft due to severe bone loss but failed due to periprosthetic fracture. The radiographic appearance at six months (right) postoperative displayed significant new bone formation in the area where the OP-1 Implant was placed.

Both the quantity and the quality of the graft incorporation was improved based on objective grading of plain x-rays, microradiographs and histology. The overall scores were significantly higher in the rhOP-1 treated group and the subscores for new bone formation and graft incorporation were significantly higher as well. Most importantly, the time course of healing was significantly accelerated. Clinical application of the OP-1 Implant with a cortical allograft strut demonstrated new bone formation at twelve weeks postoperative (fig. 4). Consolidation of the new bone and graft was observed at later time periods. Enhancement in strut healing was observed clinically in spite of the more challenging biologic environment compared to the preclinical studies. Improving and speeding the course of cortical strut graft healing would be of substantial clinical benefit in providing earlier biologic and mechanical stability to the construct. These benefits should lower the risk of graft nonunion and shorten the time of protected weight-bearing and attendant functional disability for the patient.

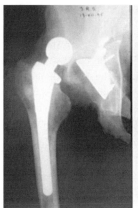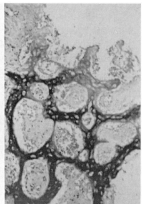

Figure 3 – A noncemented total hip replacement was performed for osteoarthritis due to a previous hip fracture. At surgery an OP-1 Implant was placed at the interface of the porous coated acetabular cup and host bone. At four weeks postoperative the patient dislocated and was unstable after closed reduction (left). At revision surgery bone from the acetabular bone-prosthesis interface was obtained and examined histologically. Histologic evaluation revealed extensive new bone formation (right). A transition from mesenchymal tissue to mature mineralized bone through an osteoid zone with prolific osteoblasts was observed.

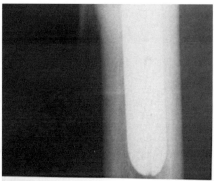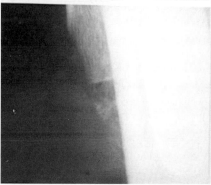

Figure 4 – Immediate postoperative radiographic appearance at the distal end of a cortical strut allograft in which the OP-1 Implant was placed in a revision total hip arthroplasty (top) and three month radiographic appearance (bottom) showing new bone formation in the area where the OP-1 Implant was placed.

Preclinical study also demonstrated healing of structural cortical strut allografts to the femur was enhanced by the addition of the OP-1 Implant.

The OP-1 Implant, either alone or in combination with bone graft, appears to be an attractive alternative to autograft bone. The use of rhOP-1 in combination with morselized or structural allograft appears to be an ideal combination. Further work has shown the OP-1 Implant to be equally as effective when used with bone graft substitute materials such as calcium phosphate and calcium sulfate materials. Compared to autograft bone alone, new bone formation and graft incorporation is improved with the use of the OP-1 Implant. However, in any clinical application, an osteogenic protein cannot overcome a poor biological or biomechanical environment. Implant stability must be present as well as absence of infection. Osteogenic proteins require a viable cell source and vascularity, as well as mechanical stability, to induce bone formation and remodeling. Failure to provide the prerequisite biologic and mechanical conditions will likely result in failure of the graft material to promote healing or bone ingrowth. In addition, maintenance of the osteogenic protein at the implantation site and delivery by an appropriate carrier material are essential for successful osteoinduction.

Reference List

1. Brady OH, Garbuz DS, Masri BA, Duncan CP (1999) The treatment of periprosthetic fractures of the femur using cortical onlay allograft struts. *Orthop. Clin. North Am.* 30:249-57.

2. Emerson RH Jr, Malinin TI, Cuellar AD, Head WC, Peters PC (1992) Cortical strut allografts in the reconstruction of the femur in revision total hip arthroplasty. A basic science and clinical study. *Clin. Orthop.* 285:35-44.

3. Head WC, Malinin TI, Mallory TH, Emerson RH Jr (1998) Onlay cortical allografting for the femur. *Orthop. Clin. North Am.* 29:307-12.

4. Gazdag AR, Lane JM, Glaser D, Forster RA (1995) Alternatives to autogenous bone graft: efficacy and indications. *J. Amer. Acad. Orthop. Surgeons* 3:1-8. Heiple KG, Chase S, Herndon C (1963) A comparative study of the healing process following different types of bone transplantation. *J. Bone Joint Surg.* 45-A: 1593-616.

5. Hooten JP, Engh CA, Heekin RD, Vinh TN (1996) Structural bulk allografts in acetabular reconstruction: analysis of two grafts retrieved at post-mortem. *J. Bone Joint Surg.* 78-B:270-5.

6. Pelker R, Friedlaender GE, Markham TC (1983) Biomechanical properties of bone allografts. *Clin. Orthop.* 174:54-7.

7. Schwarz N, Schlag G, Thurnher M, Eshberger J, Dinges H, Redl H (1991) Fresh autogenic, frozen allogenic, and decalcified allogenic bone grafts in dogs. *J. Bone Joint Surg.* 73-B:787-90.

8. Burchardt H (1983) The biology of bone graft repair. *Clin. Orthop.* 174:28-42.

9. Enneking WF, Burchardt H, Puhl JJ, Piotrowski G (1975) Physical and biological aspects of repair in dog cortical-bone transplants. *J. Bone Joint Surg.* 57A:237-52.

10. Celeste AJ, Lannazzi JA, Taylor RC, Hewick, RM Rosen V, Wang EA, Wozney JM (1990) Identification of transforming growth factor-beta superfamily members present in bone inductive protein purified from bovine bone. *Proc. Natl. Acad. Sci. USA* 87:9843-7.

11. Ozkaynak E, Rueger DC, Drier EA, Corbett C, Ridge RJ, Sampath TK, Oppermann H (1990) OP-1 cDNA encodes an osteogenic protein in TGF-beta family. *EMBO J.* 9:2085-93.

12. Sampath TK, Coughlin JE, Whetstone RM, Banach D, Corbett C, Ridge RJ, Ozkaynak E, Oppermann H, Rueger DC (1990) Bovine osteogenic protein is composed of dimers of OP-1 and BMP-2A, two members of the transforming growth factor-beta superfamily. *J. Biol. Chem.* 265:13198-205.

13. Stevenson S, Cunningham N, Toth J, Davy D, Reddi AH (1994) The effect of osteogenin (a bone morphogenetic protein) on the formation of bone in orthotopic segmental defects in rats. *J. Bone Joint Surg.* 76-A: 1676-87.

14. Urist MR (1965) Bone formation by autoinduction. *Science* 150:893-9.

15. Urist MR, Mikulski A, Lietze A (1979) A solubilized and insolubilized bone morphogenetic protein. *Proc. Natl. Acad. Sci. USA* 76:1828-32.

16. Wang EA, Rosen V, Cordes P (1988) Purification and characterization of other distinct bone inducing proteins. *Proc. Natl. Acad. Sci. USA* 87:9484-8.

17. Sampath TK, Maliakal JC, Hauschka PV, Jones WK, Sasak H, Tucker RF, White KH, Coughin JE, Tucker MM, Pang RH (1992) Recombinant human osteogenic protein-1 (hOP-1) induces new bone formation in vivo with a specific activity comparable with natural bovine osteogenic protein and stimulates osteoblast proliferation and differentiation *in vitro. J. Biol. Chem.* 267:20352-362.

18. Urist MR, Delange RJ, Finerman GA (1983) Bone cell differentiation and growth factors. Science 220:680-6.

19. Wozney JM, Rosen V, Celeste AJ, Mitsock LM, Whitters MJ, Kriz RW, Hewick RM, Wang EA(1988) Novel regulators of bone formation: Molecular clones and activities. Science 242:1528-34.

20. Cook SD, Baffes GC, Wolfe MW, Sampath TK, Rueger DC (1994) Recombinant human bone morphogenetic protein-7 induces healing in canine long-bone segmental defect model. *Clin. Orthop.* 301:302-12.

21. Cook SD, Baffes GC, Wolfe MW, Sampath TK, Rueger DC (1994) The effect of recombinant human

osteogenic protein-1 (rhOP-1) on healing of large segmental bone defects. *J. Bone Joint Surg.* 76A:827-38.

22. Cook SD, Dalton JE, Tan EH, Whitecloud TS, Rueger DC (1994) *In vivo* evaluation of recombinant human osteogenic protein (rhOP-1) implants as a bone graft substitute for spinal fusions. *Spine* 19:1655-63.

23. Cook SD, Rueger DC (1996) Osteogenic protein-1. Biology and applications. *Clin. Orthop.* 324:29-38.

24. Cook SD, Wolfe MW, Salkeld SL, Rueger DC (1995) Effect of recombinant human osteogenic protein-1 on healing of segmental defects in non-human primates. *J. Bone Joint Surg.* 77A:734-50.

25. Gerhart T, Kirker-Head C, Kriz MJ, Schellin S, Wang E (1991) Healing segmental defects in sheep using recombinant human bone morphogenetic protein (BMP-2). *Trans. Orthop. Res. Soc.* 16:172.

26. Friedlander GE, Perry CR, Cole JD, Cook SD, Cierny G, Muschler GE, Zych GA, Calhoun JH, LaFore AJ, Yin S (2001) Osteogenic Protein-1 (Bone Morphogenetic Protein-7) in the treatment of Tibial Nonunions. *J. Bone Joint Surg.* 83A (Suppl. 1):151-8.

27. Sampath TK, Reddi AH (1981) Dissociative extraction and reconstitution of extracellular matrix components involved in local bone differentiation. *Proc. Natl. Acad. Sci. USA* 78:7599-603.

28. Salkeld SL, Patron LP, Barrack RL, Cook SD (2001) The Effect of Osteogenic Protein-1 on the Healing of Segmental Bone Defects Treated with Autograft and Allograft Bone. *J. Bone Joint Surg.* 83A:803-16.

29. Cook SD, Barrack RL, Santman M, Patron LP, Salkeld SL, Whitcloud TS (2000) Strut healing to the femur with recombinant human osteogenic protein-1. *Clin. Orth.* 350: 50-60.

30. Cockin J (1973) Autologous bone grafting-complications at the donor site. *J. Bone Joint Surg.* 53-B:153.

31. Younger EM, Chapman MW (1989) Morbidity at bone graft donor sites. *J. Orthop. Trauma.* 3:192-5.

4   Management of Severe Acetabular Defects Using a Hydroxyapatite-Coated Reconstruction Ring

Bruno Balay, MD and the ARTRO Group

INTRODUCTION

When there has been acetabular component loosening with severe segmental or cavitary bone defects, a threaded or screw-fixed cup cannot be adequately stabilized. There is agreement in the literature that such cases should be managed with reconstruction associating grafting (to restore the deficient bone stock) and a reinforcement ring (to enhance the strength of the construct and improve graft compression). We report herein the experience of the ARTRO Group with the Octopus cementless ring (fig. 1), in the management of some cases of cup loosening with extensive loss of bone stock.

MATERIALS AND METHODS

Description of the Implant

The Octopus is a modular device that is assembled from three parts (fig.2). The base constitutes the actual ring. It is made from commercially pure titanium and can be molded to the anatomical configuration required. It provides anatomical fit and

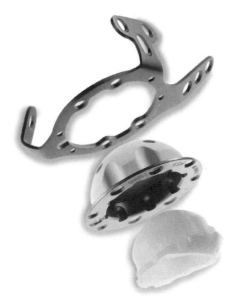

Figure 2 – Octopus: base, HA-coated cup and PE insert.

mechanical support. The base has a hook to engage the superior margin of the obturator foramen, and two iliac lugs to allow its fixation in healthy bone stock. This design ensures that the construct can be given the appropriate acetabular inclination and anteversion. The cup is attached to the base with

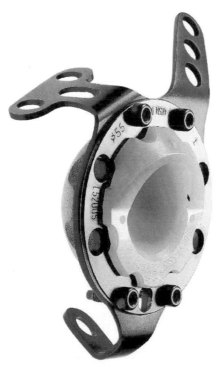

Figure 1 – Octopus: 50-mm and 55-mm diameter.

four screws. In order to enhance the stability of the construct, cancellous screws may be introduced through a number of equatorial and radial holes. The cup fits into the center of the base and compresses the bone grafts placed in the reconstructed acetabulum. It is coated with hydroxyapatite (HA), a material well known for its biocompatibility and osteoconductive properties. The insert is made of polyethylene (PE), and comes in two versions (anti-dislocation or reorientation). It accepts femoral heads of 22mm, 28mm, or 32mm diameter.

Surgical Technique

The Octopus ring may be introduced through any of the customary surgical approaches. The incision must be wide enough to provide exposure of both columns and the acetabular roof.

The failed cup is removed, as is all the cement used with the previous implant and any interposed fibrous tissue. Next, the extent of the bone defects is assessed, and the need for a reconstruction ring is confirmed.

In order to obtain correct implant positioning, acetabular roof defects must be repaired. This is done using a screw-fixed corticocancellous graft onto which the superior lug will be applied. An inclination of between 40 and 45 degrees with respect to the inter-ischial-tuberosity line will provide a good stress pattern in the graft and will reduce the pull-out forces acting on the obturator foramen hook. A malleable trial base is provided for use as a pattern, to establish the amount of iliac lug molding required to suit individual patient.

The pattern is then transferred, on an anvil, to the definitive base. The definitive base is inserted, with the superior and posterior lugs fixed in healthy bone. The stability of the construct is tested. Corticocancellous bone grafts are inserted between the ring and the defective columns, and any cavitary defects are filled with morselized bone. The cup is fixed to the base with screws. Additional screws are inserted through the holes provided, in order to enhance stability.

The chosen PE insert (with an anti-dislocation shoulder, or a reorientation pattern) is placed in the cup, and orientated in such a way as to provide optimal stability (fig. 3).

The Series

The series comprised 75 revisions performed between 1989 and 30 June 2000. This may appear

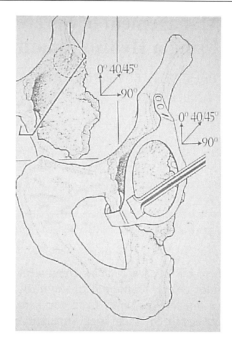

Figure 3 – Reconstruction of superior defect using a corticocancellous graft. Ring inclination 40° to 45°.

to be a very small number of revisions over a ten-year period; however, as will be explained below, our indications for cementless reconstruction are still very restrictive. The patients in the study had Paprosky (1) Type 3A and 3B bone defects. In 81% of the cases, the underlying disease was osteoarthritis (OA) (Table 1).

Aetiology	N
OA	61
Rheumatoid	3
Infection	2
Dysplasia	2
Fracture	7
Total	75

Table 1 – Breakdown of patient population by aetiology (N = 75; 1989-2000).

The mean patient age was 71.9 years, and mean follow-up was 6.4 years. Regarding the Charnley classification (2), 45% of hips were graded A, 21% were graded B, and 34% were graded C. Twelve patients had been revised once in the past, and another twelve had been revised twice in the past. In 60% of the cases, only the cup was loose. In 30%, both components were affected. In 52 cases, both components were exchanged; in 22, this was done routinely. Thirty-eight hips were revised to a cementless HA-coated stem (KAR, the long-stemmed version of the Corail; TDK; or Reef, a prosthesis with a screw-locked stem).

All the patients were followed up with clinical and radiological examination. Clinically, the Postel-Merle d'Aubigné (MDA) scoring system (3) was used, notwithstanding its known drawbacks, in particular the way in which comorbid conditions (Charnley categories B and C) will affect the rating of a perfect hip. Radiologically, cup migration was calculated using Ranawat's triangle plotted on the postoperative film and on subsequent follow-up radiographs. (fig. 4).

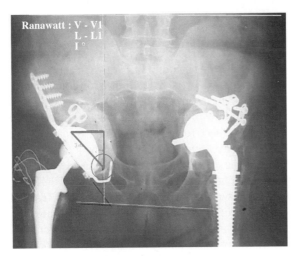

Figure 4 – Construction of Ranawat's triangle (to assess migration).

The condition and osseointegration of the bone graft, the presence of lucent lines, PE wear, and the presence of periprosthetic ossifications (with Brooker grading (4) of any ossifications found) were also studied.

RESULTS

Complications

One strikingly severe complication was peroneal nerve palsy, which occurred in five cases (8%) and never completely remitted, with three patients suffering definitive and total deficit. The rates of haematoma and DVT were respectively 4% and 2.7%. Dislocation occurred in 10% of the cases before the third month, and 2.7% after the third month.; one patient, whose cup was excessively vertical, had to be re-revised to a standard cup18 months after the index revision. There were four

cases (5.3%) of early infection, and 2 cases (2.7%) of late infection. One of these patients was reoperated on without exchange of the implant; one underwent successful two-component revision; one had a Girdlestone; and one could not be reoperated on because of his poor general condition. There were eleven cases (14.7%) of loosening, of which eight were mechanical in origin. They were managed with revision to a cemented ring in three cases (one Kerboull ring, two cemented Octopus devices); in two cases, it was possible to implant a standard cup at revision for loosening. Three patients were in such poor general health that they could not be revised. Breakage of the acetabular device occurred in 2 cases (2.7%). One fracture of the greater trochanter was recorded at the time of surgery.

Clinical Outcome

Of the 75 hips managed with the cementless Octopus reinforcement ring, 15 were in patients who died, and seven in patients who were lost to follow-up. This left 53 cases available for analysis. Improvement was observed, especially with respect to pain, where the MDA score went from 1.5 to 5.3. In terms of activity, the results went from 1.6 up to 3.4: However, this improvement was particularly noticeable in Charnley Category A patients, whose freedom from involvement of other joints meant that they were able to gain three points (improving from 1.6 to 4.3). Mobility went from 4.4 up to 5.4. The mean global MDA score went from 7.6 to 14.1, which marked an over-90% improvement compared with the pre-revision baseline.

Of the patients in the study, preoperatively, 53% were poor, 41% were fair, and 6% were grade good. Conversely, 66% had an excellent (36%) or a good (30%) clinical outcome, against 28% of fair and 6% of results graded poor.

Radiological Outcome

Plotting Ranawat's triangle (5) on the serial radiographs gave a picture of ring migration, with an error margin of 3mm to take account of differences in pelvic positioning for successive radiographs. In 62% of the cases, the ring was found to be exactly where it had been on the immediate postoperative radiograph. There were nine (17%) instances of greater than 3mm (4 to 16mm) of migration. All of these were seen in the first 16 months and were associated with collapse of the graft. These patients had evidence of secondary stabilization and of radiographic osseointegration at the ring/graft and the graft/host bone interface, as well as healing within the graft. In seven (13%) patients, breakage of one of the lugs (usually the superior one), or screw breakage, was seen during this initial migration. These fixation device failures did not affect secondary integration. Where such failures occurred, they were seen on average within the first 12 months. Initial mechanical stability must be obtained with the ring and the screws used for its fixation. The titanium hardware is subjected to major forces, which may cause hardware fractures in cases of non-osseointegration and would also account for the lug breakages observed in cases of graft collapse. In order not to unduly weaken the lugs, it is recommended that all the molding required be performed in one attempt (fig. 5).

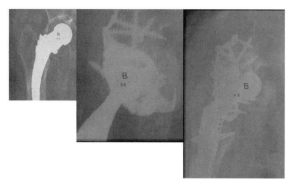

Figure 6 – Acetabular destruction in a hip with a bipolar PE cup. Reconstruction with an Octopus. Poor primary stability ; implant disassembly at three months.

Three (5.7%) Zone III lucent lines less than 2mm and six over 2mm (11.3%) were seen in hips that otherwise had satisfactory "radiological integration". These lines were evidence of the natural pull-out forces acting on the device. In order to counteract these forces, the obturator foramen hook must be correctly positioned, and the inclination of the cup must be close to 40°. In the series overall, mean cup inclination was 47°.

There was only one (2%) Brooker Class III periprosthetic ossification ; in 90% of the cases, no ossifications were seen. PE wear was calculated using Charnley's method. Mean wear was found to be 1.6mm, maximum wear was 3mm.

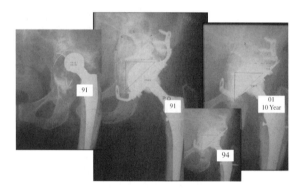

Figure 5 – Type 3 acetabular destruction. Postoperative radiograph. Ring migration during the first year with proximal displacement by 12 mm and fracture of the superior lug (four-year radiograph shown here). Secondary stabilization with no further migration of the ring ; good radiological integration at ten-years follow-up.

Survivorship analysis

The cumulative survival rate could be plotted until the sixth year with an initial number of 75 cases, and 35 hips remaining "at risk" at this period of time, this rate was 91% ± 0.069 with retrieval for any cause as endpoint.

DISCUSSION

In any cementless acetabular reconstruction following cup loosening with Paprosky Type 3A or 3B segmental and cavitary bone defects, the surgeon will be faced with three types of challenges – anatomical, mechanical, and biological (fig.7).

In eleven cases (21%), there was breakage and migration of the hardware. Among the causes of integration failure were infection, which accounted for three cases, and excessively vertical positioning of the ring, which led to three failures. In the remaining cases, no actual cause could be established. One case had had insufficient primary stability ; one patient had poor-quality bone stock ; and one device was excessively vertical. All of these factors would be likely to adversely affect the integration of the graft (fig. 6).

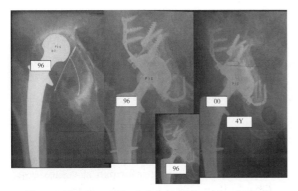

Figure 7 – Type 3B defects with proximal displacement. Postoperative radiograph. Four-year radiograph: no loosening, good osseointegration.

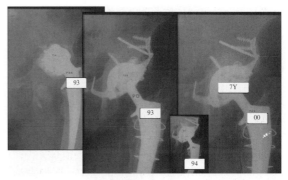

Figure 8 – Type 3B defects following loosening of a McKee cup. Postoperative and one-year radiographs show 40° inclination of the ring. Seven-year radiograph: no loosening, sound appearance of the graft.

The Anatomical Challenge

If a lasting result is to be obtained, the reconstruction must restore the physiological center of rotation of the hip. A slight cephalad displacement of the center of rotation is acceptable and will not adversely impact on the survival of the component, provided that undue lateralization is avoided (6, 7). However, this pattern is never encountered in hips with severe bone defects following cup loosening, which means that a reconstruction ring will need to be used. Lowering the center of rotation in an attempt to restore a physiological pattern may be to blame for the increased rate of peroneal nerve palsies (4% of lasting deficit in our study) in patients who may have undergone multiple prior revisions. (In our study, 16% had been revised more than three times previously).

The loss of bone stock is made up with grafting. In view of the severity of the defects encountered, allografts will need to be used. We tended to use frozen bank bone early in our series; later on, a change was made to irradiated bank bone from the blood transfusion center.

There are many papers on the use of cemented reinforcement rings. The reported success rates of excellent and good results are in the vicinity of 70%. Our findings reported herein were of the same order of magnitude (fig. 8).

We also found that in re-revisions (seven patients in our study), a standard cup could be used in 43% of the cases (with macroscopically viable allografts). This finding is particularly important, since it suggests that, at least in some patients, "implant de-escalation" may be possible. This possibility, which does not exist with cemented rings, prompted us to go on using cementless reinforce-

ment rings in appropriately selected patients (fig. 9).

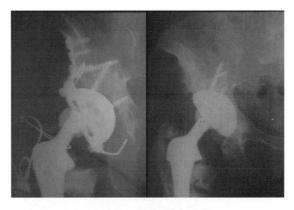

Figure 9 – Reconstruction following Type 3A defects: ring excessively vertical. Implant disassembly at 14 months with hook torn off. Revised to press-fit cementless cup.

The Mechanical Challenge

Excellent primary stability must be obtained, since otherwise secondary osseointegration will not occur. If fixation is inadequate, or where the quality of the bone stock is poor (severe osteoporosis), other ways of managing the patient's hip will need to be sought. We agree with Wasielewski (8) that at least part of the posterior column should still be intact, to give stability. We look upon this structure as a safety barrier. Ring positioning, at between 40° and 45° of inclination, is also very important. Another essential condition is the reconstruction of the acetabular roof using corticocancellous bulk grafts (fig.10).

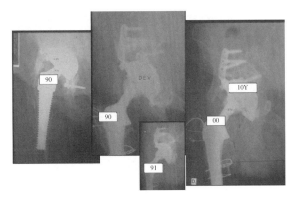

Figure 10 – Type 3B defects following loosening of a cementless cup. Major reconstruction using bone graft. Graft collapse during the first year. Follow-up radiograph at ten years: no evidence of secondary loosening.

The Biological Challenge

This is still the most difficult of the three. However, grafting is vital if the defective bone stock is to be restored. Autograft material is frequently not available in sufficient quantities. Also, experimental studies (Kienapfel *et al.* (9), Heiple *et al.* (10)) have shown that, while autografts tend to heal more rapidly into the host bone, the long-term pattern is not very different from that obtained with frozen allografts (Heiple *et al.* (10), Delloye *et al.* (11)).

The incorporation of structural allografts is inconsistent. Judet *et al.* (12) reported a 40% rate of radiological incorporation; Lazennec *et al.* (13) found a rate of 84%; while Pascarel *et al.* (14) found 82% of the grafts to have been incorporated. Allografts may resorb: Lazennec *et al.* (13) found resorption in 18% of the cases, and Lachiewicz and Hussamy found 36% of grafts to have resorbed.

Morselized bone grafts appear to consolidate more predictably and to be less prone to resorption. Thus, Schimmel and Slooff (15) found an osseointegration rate of 93%; Lachiewicz and Hussamy (16), of 100%; while Massin *et al.* (17) reported a 12% rate of osseointegration failure following graft site resorption, in the case of a cemented reinforcement ring.

In the recent literature on reconstructions using a ring, bone grafts, and a cemented cup, the reported rate of actual or potential failures is around 19% (18, 19). However, there are no figures to document the fate of acetabular reconstructions using a cementless ring. In our series, the rate of non-osseointegration was 17%. The question is

what happens histologically at the interface between the HA-coated cup and the allograft on the one hand, and the interface between the allograft and the host bone on the other hand. Hardy and Frayssinet (20) and Silverton *et al.* (21) feel that there may be osseointegration between the graft and the host bone; however, this may be only partial. As regards the cup-graft interface, the only histological studies that we have performed to date were in specimens retrieved for failure, and are therefore of very limited information value.

Given all these uncertainties, we must restrict our indications. It is our policy to use the device only in patients who still have at least 50% of bone stock onto which the ring may be fixed (fig. 11).

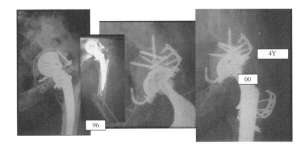

Figure 11 – Type 3B defects with proximal displacement and protrusion. Postoperative and four-year radiographs. Partial graft Resorption graft and ring radiologically well osseointegrated.

CONCLUSION

It is our current policy to use the Octopus reinforcement ring only in patients have at least 50% of their bone stock preserved, including at least part of the posterior column. We feel that under these conditions, and providing that sound primary stability can be obtained, everything that can be done will have been done to give secondary osseointegration a chance. If primary stability cannot be obtained, a cementless reconstruction is absolutely contraindicated.

Acetabular reconstructions may deteriorate in the long term. However, as shown in our series, re-revisions is possible after the failure of a cementless revision, and may, at least in some cases, allow implant de-escalation.

Reference List

1. Paprosky WG, Perona PG, Lawrence JM (1994) Acetabular defect classification and surgical reconstruction in revision arthroplasty. A 6 year follow-up examination. *J. Arthroplasty*, 9:33-44.

2. Charnley J (1979) Numerical grading of clinical results. In: Low Friction Arthroplasty of the Hip, edited by Charnley J, Berlin, Heidelberg, New-York: Springer-Verlag. 20-4.

3. Merle d'Aubigne R (1970) Cotation chiffrée de la fonction de la hanche. *Rev. Chir. Orthop.* 56:481-6.

4. Brooker AF, Bowerman JW, Robinson RA, Riley Jr LH (1973) Ectopic ossification following total hip replacement: Incidence and a method of classification. *J. Bone Joint Surg. Am.* 55:1629-32.

5. Ranawat CS, Dorr LD, Inglis AE (1980) Total hip arthroplasty in protrusio acetabuli of rheumatoid arthritis. *J. Bone Joint Surg. Am.* 62:1059-65.

6. Russotti GM, Harris WH (1991) Proximal placement of the acetabular component in total hip arthroplasty. A long-term follow-up study. *J. Bone Joint Surg. Am.* 73:587-92.

7. Weber KL, Callaghan JJ, Goetz DD, Johnston RC (1996) Revision of a failed cemented total hip prosthesis with insertion of an acetabular component without cement and a femoral component with cement. *J. Bone Joint Surg. Am.* 78:982-94.

8. Berzins A, Sumner DR, Wasielewski RC *et al.* (1996) Impacted particulate allograft for femoral revision total hip arthroplasty. *In vitro* mechanical stability and effects of cement pressurization. *J. Arthroplasty* 11(5):500-6.

9. Kienapfel H, Sumner DR, Turner TM, Urban RM, Galante JO (1992) Efficacy of autograft and freeze-dried allograft to enhance fixation of porous coated implants in the presence of interface gaps. *J. Orthop. Res.* 10:423-33.

10. Heiple KG, Chase SW, Herndon CH (1963) A comparative study of the healing process following different types of bone transplantation. *J. Bone Joint Surg. Am.* 45:1593-1610.

11. Delloye C, Verhelpen M, D'Hemricourt J, Govaerts B, Bourgois R (1993) Morphometric and physical investigations of segmental cortical bone autografts and allografts in canine ulnar defects. *Clin. Orthop.* 282:273-92.

12. Judet T, De Thomasson E, Paukovic J, Arnault O (1994) Reconstruction of acetabular insufficiency in initial total hip endoprosthesis surgery using a massive autograft. *Acta Chir. Orthop. Traumatol. Cech.* 61(1):29-33.

13. Lazennec JY, Laudet CG, Roger B, Feron JM, Guerin-Surville H (1990) Cartilaginous and bony anatomy of the human cotyloid cavity: preliminary study for the analysis of the specific dynamics of cotyloid cornua. *Bull. Assoc. Anat. (France)* 74(226):21-27.

14. Pascarel X, Liquois F, Chauveaux D, Le Rebeller A, Honton JL (1993) utilization des anneaux endocotyloïdiens de Müller dans la chirurgie de révision des prothèses totales de hanche. A propos de 141 cas avec un recul minimal de 5 ans. *Rev. Chir. Orthop.* 7:357-64.

15. Slooff TJ, Buma P, Schreurs BW, Schimmel JW, Huiskes R, Gardeniers J (1996) Acetabular and femoral reconstruction with impacted graft and cement. *Clin. Orthop.* 324:108-15.

16. Lachiewicz PF, Hussamy OD (1994) Revision of the acetabulum without cement with use of the Harris-Galante porous-coated implant. Two to eight year results. *J. Bone Joint Surg. Am.* 76:1834-9.

17. Massin P, Bocquet L, Huten D, Badelon O, Duparc J (1995) Observations radiographiques et histologiques d'allogreffes autoclavées et non autoclavées dans la métaphyse fémorale inférieure de chien. *Rev. Chir. Orthop.* 81:189-97.

18. Gill TJ, Sledge JB (2000) The management of severe acetabular bone loss using structural allograft and acetabular reinforcement devices. *J. Arthroplasty* 15:1-7.

19. Massin P, Duparc J (1995) Total hip replacement in irradiated hips. A retrospective study of 71 cases. *J. Bone Joint Surg. Br.* 77, 847-52.

20. Hardy D, Frayssinet P (1991) Bonding of HAC coated femoral prothesis. *J. Bone Joint Surg Br.* 73:732-9.

21. Silverton CD, Rosenberg AG, Sheinkop MB, Kull LR, Galante JO (1995) Revision total hip arthroplasty using a cementless acetabular component. *Clin. Orthop.* 319:201-8.

5 The Use of the Hydroxyapatite-Coated Arc2f Cup in Acetabular Revision Surgery

Jean-Alain Epinette, MD, Michael T. Manley, PhD and Bruno Tillie, MD

INTRODUCTION

For years, the use of acrylic cement has been a conventional fixation method for orthopaedic implants. For revision surgery in the acetabulum, cement has used been used as the method of fixation for revision implants and has been used in innovative techniques such as fixation of cups into reinforcement rings and as the stabilization medium for impacted bone graft. As an alternative to cement, porous and hydroxyapatite-coated implants are showing positive results in achieving direct bone-implant bonding and preservation of bone stock in the revision acetabulum.

Any revision surgery of a failed acetabular component is always a major challenge, as bone reconstruction must be taken into consideration in addition to hip balance. Although the similar principles for choosing an implant configuration apply to revision surgery as much as to primary arthroplasty (i.e., good primary mechanical fixation combined with an interface that produces secondary stability via osseointegration), the host bone in revision cases is almost always of poorer quality. This makes the correct choice of implant and operative strategy extremely important.

As an update to a previously published study about the use of Arc2f in revision surgery (1, 2), we report our experience up to 13-year follow-up with a hydroxyapatite-coated threaded hemispherical acetabular component used routinely in the revision setting. One hundred sixty cases had more than 5 years of minimum follow-up and were enrolled in this cohort. The goal of the study was to sum up the results and complications experienced with the Arc2f cup used in revisions, and to compare this particular cementless option to other procedures, such as cemented cups with impacted grafting and acetabular reinforcement rings and cages reported in the literature. In addition, we tried to point out the potential benefits afforded by hydroxyapatite as a bioactive coating with regard to bone loss and grafting procedures.

MATERIAL AND METHODS

The Arc2f component (Stryker Howmedica Osteonics Corp., Allendale, NJ) has a thin cutting, double-start thread incorporated into the periphery of the shell, is fabricated from titanium alloy (Ti-6Al-4V), and is coated with a 50 micrometer thick layer of hydroxyapatite (> 90% hydroxyapatite minimum) plasma-sprayed onto a roughened substrate. The polyethylene liners (Vecteur Orthopedic, Paris, France) matched with the Arc2f used during this study consisted first of compression molded ultrahigh molecular weight polyethylene (UHMWPE), followed by regular machined UHMWPE. Both liner types are now replaced with highly cross linked Crossfire™ polyethylene-(Stryker Howmedica Osteonics Corp., Allendale, NJ). During insertion, the component was screwed into the reamed acetabulum with a small ratchet wrench. Supplementary fixation was achieved in all surgeries by the placement of three or four bone screws through holes in the shell into the ilium.

The study described included 160 cases operated on between january 1989 and December 1996, as a consecutive series performed by two of us (JAE-BT) either at the Bruay-Clinic or the Bon Secours-Clinic (Bruay-Labuissière-Arras, France). Outcome analysis was determined using the OrthoWave Hip Data System, under the aegis of the Imaging Center and Orthopaedic Research in Arthroplasty (CRDA-Bruay-France). At surgery, the condition of the acetabulum was defined using the Paprosky Grading system (3). While reporting on our results, we considered that each hip "lives its own life", and thus we prefer give counts of "hips" rather than "patients". For example, a patient who underwent bilateral revision replacement can experience pain in a given hip and be pain-free on the other side, or can be considered as a success on one hip and a failure on the opposite side. In the series, the "unit of follow-up" was the operated hip, whether the patient underwent single side or bilateral revision hip replacement.

With respect to the series, the type of surgery was a revision of both the femoral and acetabular implant in 99 hips, and isolated acetabular revision in 59 hips. A HA-coated Arc2f cup was implanted in all hips with the overall average size of 56mm. The most common cup size was 58mm (in 22% of hips), followed by 56mm size (in 18%), and both 52mm and 62mm in 14%. The maximal size 66mm had been fitted only in 5 hips, i.e., 7% of revisions.

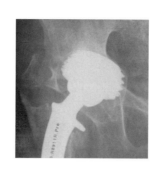
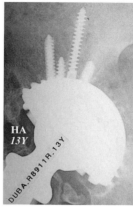

Figure 1 – "Regular" case of revision subsequent to loosening and migration of a smooth threaded ring in a 66 year old female (a). Excellent clinical and radiological results at 13 years postoperatively with bony ingrowth, no reactive or lucent line over the dome or the screws, no migration, no osteolysis (b).

RESULTS

Demographic analysis of the patient population showed a female predominance with 103 hips (64.4%) and a mean patient age of 68.34 years (range 25-93 years). The indication for revision was failure of a cemented cup in 64 (40%) cases, migration of a threaded (smooth) cup in 53 (33.1%) cases (fig. 1), and failure of a uni or bipolar hip replacement in 21 (13.1%)cases. Three (1.9%) hips were failed porous press fit cups, and 4 (2.5%) were loose Arc2f cups. In 5 hips (3.1%), arthroplasty was performed in order to convert a Girdlestone pelvic osteotomy (fig. 2). The reason for revision was recurrent dislocation in 10 cases (6.3%).

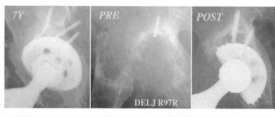
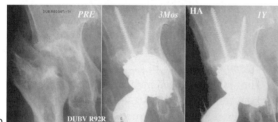
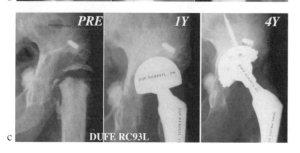

Figure 2 – Three cases of severe bone loss due to revisions following removal of the implants due to previous septic loosening. The mechanical fixation afforded by the threads of the Arc 2f cup with additional upwards screws allow these "extreme" cases to be dealt with through a procedure that remains simple and preserves the surrounding structures. a – Serial X-rays showing the initial failed cementless cup in an obese 66 year old male, then Girdlestone procedure and finally post op film; b – Preop status after prior removal of an infected cemented cup, radiological result postoperatively and one year later; c – Tremendous bone loss in a young male following deep infection and retrieval of the implants as well as the upper portion of the femur, temporary acetabular reconstruction with bipolar cup, followed by insertion of the Arc 2f cup with excellent fixation at 4 years postoperatively.

Using the Paprosky grading system, we recorded 28.6% of cases to have Type I deficiencies, with minimal deformity, no migration, and bone loss localized in minimal areas; 13.4% had Type IIa, 9.8% had Type IIb, and 13.7% had Type IIc. Finally, 16.8% exhibited Type IIIa, and 17.6% Type IIIb, with major destruction of the acetabular rim and supporting structures.

At the time of the current study, 116 hips (72.5%) remained "on file", while 28 patients (30 hips; 18.8%) were deceased and one patient (1 hip; 0.6%) lost to follow-up (table 1). Five (3.1%) isolated femoral recurrent failures involved isolated stem failures with no cup-related clinical or radiological issues and are to be added to the "on file" hips since the non-failed cup was retained in place. Eight cups failed and led to recurrent revision, including three for deep infection (1.9%), three for (1.9%) isolated mechanical failures, one combined femoral and acetabular failure (0.6%) and one (0.6%) clinical failure. The clinical failure did not undergo re-operation due to the poor general health status of the patient.

Clinical and radiological analysis addressed only those patients specifically reviewed clinically and radiologically for this study. Of the original 160 cases, data from 121 hips were available for follow-up analysis at the time of this report. The

Status	N	%
On file	116	72.5
Lost to Follow-Up	1	0.6
Deceased	30	18.8
Revision due to infection	3	1.9
Combined femoral and acetabular failure	2	1.2
Isolated acetabular failure	3	1.9
Isolated femoral failure	5	3.1
Total	160	100

Table 1 – Archiving status at the time of the study for the 160 cases series at 5-13-year follow-up.

average follow-up was 8.12 years. The clinical results thus report the 121 "on file" hips reviewed at 5 to 13 year follow-up, while survivorship analysis and rate of complications take into account the whole series of 160 cases. Radiographic analysis of the results was performed using standard anterior posterior and lateral views and comparing the serial radiographs with the immediate postoperative films. The quality of fixation of the cup was judged in terms of the presence or absence of a progressive lucent line, of graft osteolysis, screw breakage, or a change in the orientation of the implant (figs 3 and 4).

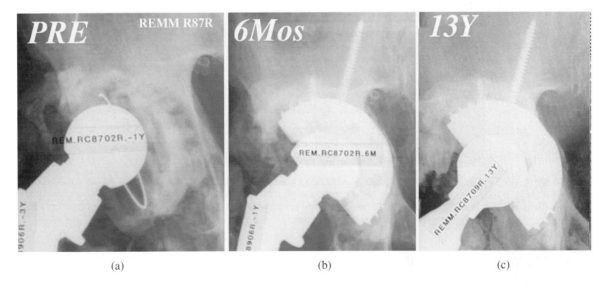

(a)   (b)   (c)

Figure 3a, b, c – Excellent Arc 2f results at 13 years in a 69-year old male who had a failed cemented cup in 1980 that led to severe bone defects graded Paprosky 3a (a), a revision in 1987 with an Arc2f cup and additional grafting (b). 13 years later, although the stem had to be exchanged in the meantime, X-rays of the acetabular side demonstrate no radiographic changes, no migration, no reactive or lucent line around the dome or the screws (c), while the clinical result is good with total lack of pain.

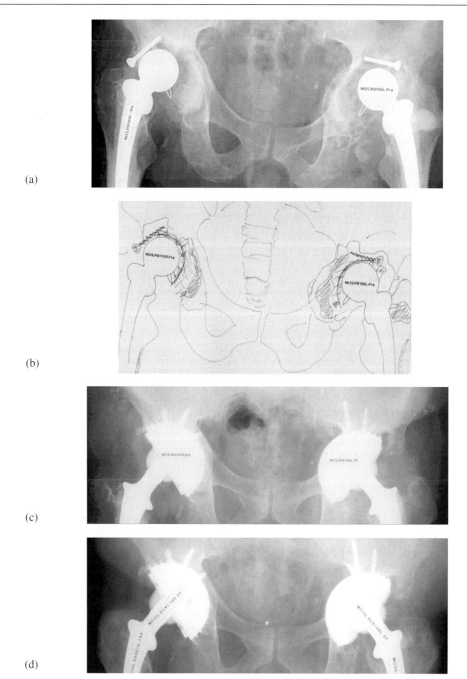

(a)

(b)

(c)

(d)

Figure 4 – The use of a "Jumbo" Arc2f cup is sometimes necessary due to the poor general health of the patient. This case involves a "light" procedure, as in this 79-year old male experiencing a bilateral cemented loose cup with severe bone loss graded 3b (a, b). A bilateral jumbo cup was fitted to achieve secure primary stability, with no graft added (c). Excellent pain-free results at the 5-year follow-up (d) with no radiological change and no migration or tilting, as compared to the postop films.

Complications

Re-operations were associated with 22 cups (13.75%) in 22 patients. Re-revisions required removal of the metal shell (Table 2). This classification, discriminating between "reoperations" and "re-revision" follows the recommendations of the Swedish Register (4).

Preoperatively, neither vascular nor nerve injury was recorded within the whole 160 surgeries, and the use of bone screws as routine procedure had not led to any apparent problems. Postoperatively, haematomae were associated with 4.1% hips. A dislocation occurred in 6 hips (3.75%), including 4 recurrent dislocations leading to re-operation. Re-operation in three of these hips consisted of a simple exchange of a neutral cup liner for a hooded one with the cup itself left *in situ*. One dislocation required re-revision due to a mal-oriented acetabular component. Deep infection occurred in 7 patients (4.38%). Of these, 4 hips resolved after a single debridement-lavage, while three hips required removal of the implant. Of these, two were converted to Girdlestone osteotomy. There were 5 isolated femoral revision after femoral loosening while cups were retained.

Complications	N	%
• Reoperations without cup revision	9	5.6 %
• Isolated femoral revision	5	3.1%
• Cup Revisions, of which:	8	5 %
- Revised for Deep infection	3	1.9 %
- Revised for recurrent dislocation	2	1.3 %
- Revised for Mechanical Failure	3	1.9 %

Table 2 – Breakdown of complications leading to reoperations, with or without retrieval of the cup.

There were eight cup re-revisions (5%). These included the 3 deep infections (1.9%) leading to retrieval of implants and Girdlestone procedure in two cases, and one two-stage revision for the third patient, 2 recurrent dislocations (1.3%) in which a modular stem was fitted at the same time as a tripolar cup, and 3 cup loosenings (1.9%) due to a mechanical failure of the cup. These latter three hips with mechanical failure were analyzed separately. The first case was a 65-year old female, who underwent a revision in 1990 for a failed primary cemented stem with severe osteolysis matched with a failed Morcher polyethylene cup graded Paprosky IIc. A HA regular Omnifit stem was implanted with a HA-Arc2f cup. The reason for re-revision at 6-year was mainly due to loosening and subsidence of the stem. This patient underwent a re-revision surgery and received a Wagner uncemented stem. There were few bony lesions associated with the Arc2f cup. It was exchanged simply with a HA coated Atlas expansion cup with no additional reinforcement structure.

The second case was a 69-year old female with a loose cemented cup graded Paprosky IIIa, who received an Arc2f together with grafting the acetabular roof with a block of allograft bone secured by screws. This graft resorbed and the cup tilted and migrated. It was re-revised after 28 moths postoperatively with a Muller reinforcement ring and cemented cup. The third re-revision case involved a heavy 93 kg 51-year female (BMI:38.7), who had a primary cemented cup and stem for inflammatory lesions in 1988. These were revised in 1990 due to a loosening and cavitation graded Paprosky IIb. A HA-Arc2f was fitted with bony reconstruction with morselized allografts. Clinical results were satisfying until sudden pain and functional impairment in the fifth post-operative year. Radiographs showed cup migration and loosening at the dome of the reconstructed acetabulum. The cup was revised.

RESULTS

Clinical Results

It was difficult to assess clinical results in the traditional sense with these revision cups, as this particular cohort of patients had various preoperative problems and functional impairment, some of which related to the stem and some to multiple lesions of soft tissues. We report on 133 cases, clinically and radiologically followed-up at five year minimum after the operation. Some patients, deceased after the fifth year, were included in the series at their final follow-up visit.

According to Harris Hip Score (HHS) (5) and Merle d'Aubigné and Postel (MDA) (6, 7) score, pain was "none" in 115 hips (86.5 %°, "slight" in 13 hips (9.8%), "moderate" in 4 hips and severe in the remaining unique case (0.8%). The hip graded as "severe" pain is pending femoral re-revision but has a well fixed and radiographically stable cup. Additionally, the 4 "moderate" painful hips involve 4 patients with major extra-articular lesions, mainly low back pain. All of these moderate pain patients are classified as Charnley C group.

For the entire group, walking distance was unlimited in 64.8% of hips, with only 4 patients limited to "indoor activities". This functional impairment had been checked as resulting from cardiac or poor general health in 2 cases, a recent femoral fracture in one, and finally a severe neurological lesion due to spinal disease in the latter.

For overall performance, preoperatively, the mean Harris pain score was 4.6 out of a maximum of 44 points, and postoperatively it was up to 42.7 points (20-44). Mean range of motion scores were 7.9 (out of a possible 9 points) preoperatively up to 8.9 points (6-9) postoperatively. Mean Function scores out of a maximum of 47 points were 19.5 preoperatively, up to 42.1 postoperatively (range 22 to 47). Mean HHS values were respectively 32.33 (range 5-96) out of a maximum of 100 preoperatively, up to 93.7 points (range 51 to 100, SD 9.39). Before the operation, 91% of hips were considered "poor" and 8% "fair" and 1% "good", according to the Harris score, while at 5-13 years, 45 % were assessed as "excellent" (i.e. ≥ 98 points), 47 % were "good" (i.e. total score between 80 and 98 points), 5% were "fair" (i.e. between 60 and 79 points), and 3 % were "poor". Results computed according MDA assessment demonstrated similar gains as follows: scores (out of 6) were preoperatively at 1.5 for Pain, 4.7 for Range of Motion, and 1.3 for Function, up to 5.78, 5.84 and 4.68, respectively. Mean MDA values recorded at 7.5 out of a maximum of 18 preoperatively reached at 5-13 year evaluation 16.3 points (ranged 10 to 18; SD 1.919) postoperatively.

Survivorship analysis relates to the 160 patients from the 5- to the 13-year follow-up and can be drawn until the seventh-year, since at this period of time 39 hips remained "on file", which allows statistically valuable report. Using Kaplan-Meier survivorship analysis, the acetabular cumulative survival rate, taking into account retrieval for any cause as endpoint was 92.15% ± 0.0487. Cumulative survivorship, taking into account aseptic loosening as endpoint was 95.02 ± 0.0508 (fig. 5).

Radiographic Results

The position of the cup was analyzed with reference to a tangent to the teardrop. An abduction angle of 40° to 50° was obtained in 82% of the cups. The cups inserted in this revision group tended to be placed slightly more vertical than those implanted at primary arthroplasty. In this series, 16% were over 45°inclination while 2% were under 40° inclination. No cups had an inclination angle greater than 55°. Of the cups that survived, only one experienced migration and tilting. This implant remains pain free.

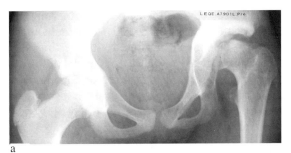

a

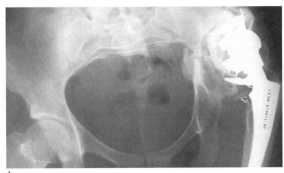

b

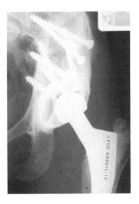

c

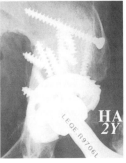

d

Figure 5 – Multi-revision in an 86-year old female, first operated on in 1973 with implantation of a cemented cup that failed (a). She was revised in '76, re-revised in '82 (b), re-re-revised in '88 with a huge Schneider reinforcement ring and Judet stem (c), which failed again and finally re-re-re-revised in 1993 with a HA-coated Arc 2f cup. Post op films demonstrated the ability to treat such hugely damaged hips with a regular cup in order to prevent "implant escalation". Good radiological and clinical results at 2-years (MDA 5/6/3, HHS: 86) with slight pain and full ROM (d).

There were few lucencies or reactive lines between the implant and the native or grafted bone bed in the series. Interestingly, 85% of cases did not experience any line around the dome of the cup, while 6% showed lines in limited areas. Nine percent showed lines all around the surface (fig. 6). Conversely, 100% of screws were "line free" and no screws broke. This finding is in line with all the observations indicating the absence, very possibly due to the use of HA, of any fibrous tissue reaction between the bone and the implant.

A common finding following revision for major bone defects in the present study was a progressive lack of density of the graft in response to mechan-

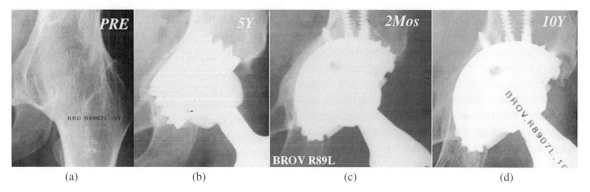

(a)   (b)   (c)   (d)

Figure 6 – Serial films of a revision case successfully treated with a HA-coated Arc2f cup at 10-year follow-up in a 45-year old female who had a fusion for Pott disease in her youth (a). First implantation of a smooth threaded ring in 1994, which failed 5 years later (b), leading to a re-revision with a HA-coated Arc2f cup in 1989 (c). At the 10-year clinical follow-up, the MDA score was 6/6/6 and the HHS was 100 points. Radiologically, there was no migration and no reactive or lucent line around the dome or the screws. There was excellent osseointegration of the grafts with optimal transmission of loads, as demonstrated by the lack of any modification of bone density all around the cup, including zone 3 (d).

ical loading. This phenomenon was not progressive and did not affect function. The pattern seen may give cause for concern and be thought to herald cup loosening. However, the non-progressive nature of the phenomenon suggests that it was caused by a lack of mechanical strength on the part of the graft, which settled when weight-bearing was resumed. The finding underscores the importance of achieving direct contact between the cup and the host bone, and of avoiding implant interfaces supported only by bone grafts.

DISCUSSION

Surgical Technique

In the operative strategy for the revision acetabulum, it is difficult to draw up hard and fast rules, since bone defects vary widely, both in size and in distribution. A careful study of the pre-operative films should enable the surgeon to foresee difficulties and identify potential pitfalls. Great attention should be paid to correcting limb length discrepancy, to establishing whether the center of

rotation of the hip can be restored, and to the support and fixation of the cup and the position of screws used for graft fixation. The risk of cup protrusion or extrusion (e.g., by a superior osteophyte) should not be underestimated. Pre-operative radiographs may also be used to judge the amount of grafting that will be required. Approach is very much a matter of the individual surgeon's preference and does not affect the reconstruction of the acetabulum or the implantation of the cup.

Unlike some reinforcement rings, the Arc2f cup does not necessitate wide exposure of the peri-acetabular bone and trochanteric osteotomy is not routinely required. We have always used a posterior lateral approach and tried to preserve any remnants of the posterior capsule. Extraction of the original acetabular component may be difficult; great care should be taken not to damage the bony rim, especially when trying to obtain a purchase to lever out the cup. If there are problems, it is certainly preferable to drill a row of holes into the cup liner in order to permit its removal piecemeal. Following acetabular debridement and exposure of the rim, the bone, which is invariably corticalized, should be carefully reamed to produce a bleeding bone bed.

In this series, the attempt was made to insert these cups at an abduction angle of 40 to 50° and an anteversion angle between 10 and 15°. The cup was screwed in by means of its peripheral thread until contact with the acetabulum or the bone graft and a peripheral border flush with the acetabular rim. Lasting implant stability is predicated upon sound primary fixation. We routinely use supplemental screws to augment fixation. While screws may be used as a matter of principle for minor defects, they are mandatory in severe osteoporosis or in cases of major bone defects. The screws may be directed towards the acetabular roof, the upper part of the two columns, and the base of the sacro-iliac joint. The medial wall and the anterior column should be avoided. Our aim is to achieve cortical fixation, and to use as many screws as possible. As a rule, between 3 and 5 screws were inserted. Whenever possible, we attempted to reinsert the remnants of the posterior capsule. Postoperative limitations were limited weight-bearing for the first six weeks, and the use of walking aids for the first three months after surgery.

The Need For Primary Mechanical Fixation

The requirement for a minimum three-point support to allow the Arc2f thread to grip bone was met in virtually all cases. In all patients, the stability obtained appeared to be vastly superior to that achieved with an impacted press-fit cup. We determined that supplemental screw fixation, which is routinely used in primary surgery, is mandatory in revisions, since in revision arthroplasties these supplemental screws can make a major contribution to primary implant fixation. The 6.5mm diameter screws have a better hold in the bone, but may be difficult to angle because of the tight fit through the screw holes in the cup. Primary fixation is vital; where it was found to be inadequate, especially when the posterior column and the weight-bearing dome were compromised, the technique must be reviewed. The situation may be addressed by using a "jumbo" cup or a different type of reconstruction with a reinforcement ring. In this series, we did not encounter any intra-operative adverse events and there were no complications produced by the use of the supplemental screws. Our data suggests that the use of this Arc2f cup can be recommended in all cases belonging to I up to IIIa Paprosky type defects (fig. 7). Some type IIIb cases can be handled if threads allow a sufficient primary stability to be attained. In a few cases we could not obtain this stability and fitted a reinforcement ring with cemented cup. However, at present the Arc2f cup covers more than 98% of our revision surgeries.

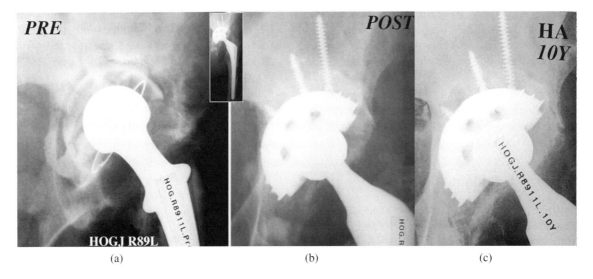

(a)   (b)   (c)

Fig. 7 – HA revision case with the Arc2f cup at 10-year follow-up in a 52-year old male first operated on in 1976 with a cemented hip leading 13 years later to a tremendous bone loss and severe migration (fig. 7a); The comparison between the post op film in 1989 (fig. 7b) and the 10-year control (fig. 7c) demonstrates no migration, no reactive or lucent line, and excellent remodeling of the allografts around the dome.

Restoration Of Hip Center And Use Of Jumbo Cups

Restoration of the center of rotation is one of the main goals of any hip arthroplasty. However, in reconstruction cases we have always given priority to the achievement of primary implant stability, even if this meant accepting a less than optimal center of rotation (fig. 4). We prefer to have maximum direct contact between the cup and the native host bone in order to limit the load-bearing role of any bone grafts used. As a result, the average size of the cup chosen for insertion was larger than the size required in primaries, i.e. mean of 56mm in revision cases *versus* 52mm in primary cases. Of interest, the use of Jumbo cups was infrequent, since only 21% of cases were over 60mm in size.

Grafting Policy

Grafting was widely used at the beginning of our experience with this cup. At the time, it was our policy to graft even minor defects. Since then, concerns with allograft have led to a change in this policy. Minor defects, in which grafts are just a "filler" without any load-bearing function, are now left ungrafted or are filled with bone substitute. This approach is justified by histological studies of osseointegration at HA-coated interfaces which have shown that even substantial gaps (of up to ca. 2mm) between the HA and the host bone can be overcome due to the osteoconductive properties of hydroxyapatite (8). Such osseointegration has never been found to be accelerated or encouraged by the use of bone allografts (9). Thus we attempt to avoid grafts, and try to get at least 50% of direct contact between HA-coating and the host bone. In severe bone losses, we prefer use jumbo cups in contact with the host bone rather than placing a cup of regular size on a bed of allografts.

It was encouraging to see that the results of revision surgery in cases of simple loosening were identical, in terms of pain and mobility, to those of primary arthroplasty. Unlike many other authors, we found a low rate of recurrent loosening of 4.8% in the more complex cases. This very encouraging finding appears to be related to the design of the Arc2f, whose equatorial thread and supplementary screw fixation produce sound primary stability, which is a prerequisite for graft incorporation and for bone bonding to the coating material.

Surgical Options And Results From A Review Of Literature

With regard to the most recently published series about acetabular revision surgery, a complete review (10) of the "use of cancellous allograft in revision total hip arthroplasty", by Leopold *et al.*, summarized the clinical results of numerous techniques. We should roughly provide some comparative figures related to three main techniques: (1) acetabular impaction allografting with cement, (2) cancellous allograft and acetabular reconstruction rings or cages, and finally (3) cementless cups with or without cancellous allograft.

Impaction allografting and cemented cups

Impaction allografting may allow new bone formation and bone stock reconstruction when allograft is impacted into place and stabilized with polymethylmetacrylate cement. According to Leopold (10), the bone graft appeared to unite and remodel, but clinical and radiographic failure rates have varied widely from 11% to 31% (11-13). The follow-up published by Scheurs in 1988 pointed out 5 revisions and 5 additional radiographic failures in a cohort of 60 patients, i.e., a 16.7% failure rate at a mean of 11.8 years. However, these authors recently updated their data (14) in 69 acetabular reconstructions with 94% of overall survival rate at an average of 12.3 years. Shinar and Harris (15) assessed long term results of bulk structural autologous grafts and allografts with cemented cups in complex arthroplasty including various forms of congenital dysplasia and revision of acetabular failed components.

Despite grafting, cemented cups functioned well for the initial five to ten years. In 70 hips with a mean follow-up of 16.5 year, 36% were revised for aseptic loosening and 26% had radiographic evidence of loosening, while only 39% were "rigidly fixed in place". An additional RSA study about migration of the acetabular component two years after revision using impacted morselized allograft and cemented cups published by Ornstein *et al.* (16) confirmed early severe migration (95% in the proximal direction) in a consecutive 21 cases series of revisions due to mechanical loosening, with 30% of components still migrating in at least 1 direction between 1.5 and 2 years postoperatively.

Reconstruction rings or cages

The advent of acetabular reconstruction rings or cages has dramatically improved the chances of success when used with cemented cups in addition to cancellous grafts.

Kerboull *et al.* reported recently (17) a survival rate of 92.1% at 13 years in a 60 consecutive cases series with severe bone loss (grade III and IV according to the AAOS grading system) treated with bulk allograft bone supported by the Kerboull reinforcement acetabular device. Another French study by Massin *et al.* (18) assessed the results using the Muller ring in addition to allografts in 81 cemented acetabular revision arthroplasties at a mean follow-up of 8 years. According to these authors, reconstruction of severely destroyed acetabula using this method gave satisfactory results within the first decade. However, hip function could not be reliably maintained over 10 years with a cumulative survival rate of 72% at 10 years, down to 55% at 11 years. Mechanical failures were related to resorption of weight bearing structural bone grafts. Two studies by Garbuz *et al.* (19, 20) advocated the use of reinforcement rings. At a mean 7 year follow-up, the only factor that was clinically significant for success in Type 2B defects (*ie* non-contained defects) was choice of acetabular component. The re-revision rate in the group treated with structural allografts that supported more than 50% of the cup was 45%, while in hips that received roof rings with cemented cups, the success rate was 100%. The authors recommend the use of allograft bone in revision acetabular surgery; however, when structural grafts are required, every attempt should be made to achieve more than 50% support from host bone. If this is not possible, then a roof reinforcement ring with a cemented cup may be the best solution. Interestingly, Gill et al recently confirmed this assessment (21) with 37 acetabular reconstructions covering more than 50% of the socket with major structural pelvic bone loss at an average follow-up of 7.1 years. In this series, one hip was revised for septic failure, 2.7% were "definitively" loose, 5.4% "probably" loose, and 10.8% "possibly" loose. A novel approach was carried out by the French ARTRO group, who reported (22) on the HA-coated Octopus device that is a metallic reinforcement cage to be used in severe bone losses with morselized bone grafts and a HA-coated socket. Their results are somewhat encouraging; however, the fate of grafts apposed to hydroxyapatite coatings is unpredictable so far as limited histologic data are available from post mortem retrieval

studies to indicate that bone healing and graft incorporation indeed occur (23).

Cementless implants

The results of series using cementless implants have been rather disappointing in the very first period of so-called "smooth first generation cups". However at present, many studies, according to Leopold *et al.* (10) support the cementless hemispherical cup as the gold standard acetabular revision technique, even in patients with combined cavitary and segmental defects (24-31) provided there is an intact posterior column and weight bearing dome. Cementless fixation in these cases appears extremely durable with aseptic loosening occurring in less than 2% of patients in a series from Dorr (24) and Lachievicz (26). Leopold (27) followed 138 consecutive cementless acetabular revisions at a mean follow-up of 10.5 years and found a survival rate of 84% at 11.5 years. Chareancholvanich *et al.* (28) in a 5 to 11-year study in 40 porous cups in revision pointed out 13% failures that led to re-revision, of which 5% were caused by aseptic loosening. Most of the authors of the cementless published series assessed the results of the porous coated Harris-Galante cup and recommended substantially oversized cups (up to 66mm diameter) in order to obtain direct acetabular support. This is similar to Dearborn (29), who reported on 24 hips in a 7-year follow-up study showing no acetabular components revised and none loose radiographically. Also, Jasty (30), with the use of jumbo components with 70 up to 80mm outer diameters, showed at 10-year average follow-up 1 revision for septic reasons, while none of the remaining cups experienced any aseptic loosening.

The use of hydroxyapatite as a coating material may be considered as a major advance, since HA is very biocompatible. Unlike PMMA cement, it does not cause thermal damage or otherwise compromise the patient's bone stock. However, published series regarding revision acetabular arthroplasty using HA-coated cups are few. A recent radiostereometric study (RSA) dedicated to "migration and wear of HA-coated press-fit cups in revision hip arthroplasty" (31), by Nivbrant *et al.*, indicates that despite extensive use of morselized grafts, HA cups displayed the smallest degree of migration reported so far in revision acetabular surgery. Additionally, they maintained stability up to 2 years after surgery. Previous RSA studies in porous coated press fit cups displayed increased proximal migration in association with the development of radiolucent zones and accelerated wear in some designs, which may dramatically jeopardize the long term results of these implants (32-37). Conversely, in experimental models HA when compared to titanium has repeatedly shown superior osteoconductive properties, even in compromising circumstances (38-39). In the above-mentioned study (31), RSA was carried out in 29 consecutive acetabular revisions operated on because of aseptic loosening using HA-coated ABG cups (SHO, Rutherford, NJ, USA), and morselized bone graft. After 2 years, 89% of the interface seemed to be in direct contact with living bone, which is superior to the mean 59% bone-cup contact found earlier in press-fit cups with a porous titanium coating (40). Additionally, the authors noted that despite forceful impaction, if the press fit cup did not contact the bottom of the acetabulum, a very tight peripheral rim fit could be expected, which seemed to stabilize the implant more reproducibly during the postoperative period.

CONCLUSION

An analysis of the different series shows the crucial importance of primary stability, with a direct contact between the cup and the host bone. As previously demonstrated in primaries (41), in revision arthroplasty optimum stability can be achieved with screws inserted in a fan pattern using a peripheral thread on the cup, as afforded by the Arc 2f cup. This has been widely used as a routine procedure in our practice, addressing all types of bone defects, from the Grade I of the Paprosky assessment up to Grade IIIa and almost all Grade IIIb, with the use of larger cups.

Our Arc2f results with 160 cups at a follow-up between 5- and 13-year showed a mechanical failure rate of 1.9%, a mean Harris Hip score of 93.7 points and a cumulative survival rate of 95.02% at the seventh year with aseptic loosening as endpoint. These results compare favorably with the more successful revision hip series in the literature. Cementless Porous hemispherical press fit cups were assessed by Leopold *et al.* (10) as the "gold standard acetabular revision technique", even in patients with combined cavitary and segmental defects. The tight peripheral rim fit identified in the RSA study carried out by Nivbrant (31) as giving

superior results with HA-coated press fit cups can more readily be obtained by threads. This suggests that a potentially better primary fixation can be obtained with the Arc2f cup than with a press-fit design; a suggestion supported by our results in this revision series. We suggest that HA-coated threaded acetabular components constitute a credible alternative to the use of press-fit cups, cemented cups and bone allografts in the revision setting.

Reference list

1. Poison R, Epinette JA, Carlier Y, Duthoit E, Tillie B (1995) Seven years Experience with the Arc 2f Cup in Acetabular Revision Surgery; operative strategy and results; In J.A. Epinette, RGT Geesink, Hydroxyapatite-coated Hip and Knee Arthroplasty, pp291-301; Cahiers d'Enseignement de la SOFCOT (English Version); L'Expansion scientifique Ed. Paris, France (51).

2. Duthoit E, Epinette JA, Carlier Y (1995) The Arc 2f Cup: Biomechanics and Interface; Systematic Study of HA-coated Vs. Porous textured components; In JA Epinette, RGT Geesink, Hydroxyapatite-coated Hip and Knee Arthroplasty, pp 176-182; Cahiers d'Enseignement de la SOFCOT (English Version); L'Expansion scientifique Ed. Paris, France (51).

3. Paprosky WG, Perona PG, Lawrence JM (1994) Acetabular defect classification and surgical reconstruction in revision arthroplasty. A 6-year follow-up evaluation. *J. Arthroplasty* 9(1):33-44.

4. http://www.jru.orthop.gu.se

5. Harris WH (1969) Traumatic arthritis of the hip after dislocation and acetabular fractures : treatment by mold arthroplasty. An end result study using a new method of result evaluation. In *J. Bone Joint Surg.* 51A, 4, 737-55.

6. Merle d'Aubigné R (1990) Cotation chiffrée de la fonction de la hanche. *Rev. Chir. Orthop.* 76, 371-4.

7. Postel M, Kerboul M, Evrard J, Courpied JP (1995) Arthroplastie totale de hanche. In Paris, Springer-Verlag.

8. Epinette JA (1993) Hydroxylapatite-Coated Implants for Hip Replacement : Clinical Experience in France. In RGT Geesink, M. Manley, Hydroylapatite Coatings in Orthopaedic Surgery, pp. 227-248. New York, Raven Press.

9. Søballe K, Hansen ES, B-Rasmussen H, Pedersen CM, Bünger C (1992) Bone graft incorporation around Titanium-alloy and Hydroxyapatite coated implants in dogs. *Clin. Orthop.* 274, 282-93.

10. Leopold SS, Jacobs JJ, Rosenberg AG (2000) Cancellous allograft in revision total hip arthroplasty. A clinical review. *Clin. Orthop.* (371):86-97.

11. Azuma T, Yasuda H, Okagaki K, Sakai K (1994) Compressed allograft chips for acetabular reconstruction in revision hip arthroplasty. *J. Bone Joint Surg.* 76B: 740-4.

12. Schreurs BW, Slooff TJ, Buma P, Gardeniers JW, Huiskes R (1998) Acetabular revision with impacted

morselized cancellous bone graft and cement: A 10-to 15-year follow-up of 60 revision arthroplastie. *J Bone Joint Surg.* 80B: 391-5.

13. Sloof TJ, Buma P, Schreurs BW, Schimmel JW, Huiskes R, Gardeniers J (1996) Acetabular and femoral reconstruction with impacted graft and cement. *Clin. Orthop.* 324:108-15.

14. Welten ML, Schreurs BW, Buma P, Verdonschot N, Slooff TJ (2000) Acetabular reconstruction with impacted morcellized cancellous bone autograft and cemented primary total hip arthroplasty: a 10- to 17-year follow-up study. *J. Arthroplasty* 15(7):819-24.

15. Shinar AA, Harris WH (1977) Bulk structural autogenous grafts and allografts for reconstruction of the acetabulum in total hip arthroplasty. Sixteen-year-average follow-up. *J. Bone Joint Surg. Am.* 79(2):159-68.

16. Ornstein E, Franzen H, Johnsson R, Sandquist P, Stefansdottir A, Sundberg M (1999) Migration of the acetabular component after revision with impacted morselized allografts: a radiostereometric 2-year follow-up analysis of 21 cases. *Acta Orthop. Scand.* 70(4):338-42.

17. Kerboull M, Hamadouche M, Kerboull L (2000) The Kerboull – Acetabular reinforcement device in major acetabular reconstructions; *Clin. Orthop.* (378):155-68.

18. Massin P, Tanaka C, Huten D, Duparc J (1998) Treatment of aseptic acetabular loosening by reconstruction combining bone graft and Muller ring. Actuarial analysis over 11 years. *Rev. Chir. Orthop. Reparatrice Appar Mot* 84(1):51-60.

19. Garbuz D, Morsi E, Gross AE (1996) Revision of the acetabular component of a total hip arthroplasty with a massive structural allograft. Study with a minimum five-year follow-up. *J. Bone Joint Surg. Am.* 78(5):693-7.

20. Garbuz D, Morsi E, Mohamed N, Gross AE (1996) Classification and reconstruction in revision acetabular arthroplasty with bone stock deficiency. *Clin. Orthop.* (324):98-107.

21. Gill TJ, Sledge JB, Muller ME (2000) The management of severe acetabular bone loss using structural allograft and acetabular reinforcement devices. *J. Arthroplasty* 15(1):1-7.

22. Balay B. and the ARTRO Group (1995) Use of the Corail System in Acetabular Component Revision; In J.A. Epinette, R.G.T. Geesink, Hydroxyapatite-coated Hip and Knee Arthroplasty, pp. 283-290; Cahiers d'Enseignement de la SOFCOT (English Version); L'Expansion scientifique Ed. Paris, France (51).

23. Heekin RD, Engh CA, Vinh T (1995) Morselized allograft in acetabular reconstruction. A postmortem retrieval analysis. *Clin. Orthop.* 319:184-90.

24. Dorr LD, Wan Z (1995) Ten years of experience with porous acetabular components for failed cemented total hip arthroplasty. *Clin Orthop.* 319:191-200.

25. Jasty M (1998) Jumbo cups and morselized graft. *Orthop. Clin. North Am.* 29:249-54.

26. Lachiewicz PF, Poon ED (1998) Revision of a total hip arthroplasty with a Harris-Galante porous-coated acetabular component inserted without cement: A follow-up note on the results at five to twelve years. *J. Bone Joint Surg.* 80A:980-4.

27. Leopold SS, Rosenberg AG, Bhatt RD (1999) Cementless acetabular revision: Evaluation at an average of 10.5 years. *Clin. Orthop.* 369:179-87.

28. Chareancholvanich K, Tanchuling A, Seki T, Gustilo RB (1999) Cementless acetabular revision for aseptic failure of cemented hip arthroplasty. *Clin. Orthop.* (361):140-9.

29. Dearborn JT, Harris WH (2000) Acetabular revision arthroplasty using so-called jumbo cementless components: an average 7-year follow-up study. *J. Arthroplasty* 15(1):8-15.

30. Jasty M (1998) Jumbo cups and morselized graft. *Orthop. Clin. North Am.* 29(2):249-54.

31. Nivbrant B, Kärrholm J (1997) Migration and wear of Hydroxyapatite-coated pressfit cups in revision hip arthroplasty: A radiostereometric study. *J. Arthroplasty* 12:904-12.

32. Silverton CD, Rosenberger AG, Sheinkop MB, Kull LR, Galante JO (1996) Revision of the acetabular component without cement after total hip arthroplasty: A follow-up note regarding results at seven to eleven years. *J. Bone Joint Surg.* 78A:1366-70.

33. Sutherland CJ (1996) Treatment of type III acetabular deficiencies in revision total hip arthroplasty without structural bone graft. *J. Arthroplasty* 11:91-8.

34. Woolson ST, Adamson GJ (1996) Acetabular revision using a bone-ingrowth total hip component in patients who have acetabular bone stock deficiency. *J. Arthroplasty* 11:661-7.

35. Silverton CD, Rosenberg AG, Sheinkop MB *et al.* (1995) Revision total hip arthroplasty using a cementless acetabular component. In *Clin. Orthop.* 319:201.

36. Nivbrant B, Kärrholm J, Onsten I (1996) Migration of porous pressfit cups in hip revision arthroplasty. In *J. Arthroplasty* 11:390.

37. Maloney WJ, Peters P., Engh CA, Chandler H (1993) Severe osteolysis of the pelvis in association with acetabular replacement without cement; *J. Bone Joint Surg.* 75A:1627.

38. Søballe K, Hansen ES, Brockstedt-Rasmussen H, Jorgensen PH, Bunger C (1992) (Tissue ingrowth into titanium and Hydroxyapatite-coated implant during stable and unstable mechanical conditions. *J. Orthop. Res.* 10(2):285-99.

39. Søballe K, Hansen ES, Brockstedt-Rasmussen H (1992) Bone graft incorporation around titanium-alloy and Hydroxyapatite-coated implants in dogs. *Clin. Orthop.* 274:82.

40. Tisdel C, Goldberg V, Parr J (1994) The influence of Hydroxyapatite and tricalcium-phosphate coating on bone growth into titanium fiber-metal implants. *J. Bone Joint Surg.* 76A:159.

41. Epinette JA, Manley MT, D'Antonio JA, Edidin AA, Capello WN (2003) A 10-Year Minimum Follow-up of Hydroxyapatite-Coated Threaded Cups: Clinical Radiographic and Survivorship Analyses with Comparison of the Literature. *J. Arthroplasty* 18(2):140-8.

6   Acetabular Revision Using Cementless Hydroxyapatite-Coated Components

Alfons J. Tonino, MD, PhD, Mathijs van der Linde, MD, Will Meijers, MD and Jelle Schaafsma, MD

INTRODUCTION

The problem of aseptic loosening is nearly always accompanied by important loss of bone stock. Apart from the clinical symptoms, such as pain and decreased range of motion, the anatomic centre of rotation has migrated medially and proximally, with subsequent loss of leg length. To restore the loss of bone stock, conventional techniques with plain cementation have yielded poor long term outcomes (Kershaw et al. 1991 (1), Iorio. 1995 (2), Raut et al. 1995 (3), 1996 (4).

Other combinations with cemented cups and bulk grafts, bulk or morselized grafts with bipolar prosthesis or uncemented cups, have all been tried with varying success (Harris and Penenberg 1987 (5), Wilson et al. 1989 (6), Gates et al. 1990 (7), Jasty and Harris 1990 (8), Mulroy and Harris 1990 (9), Hooten et al. 1994 (10), Marti et al. 1994 (11), Papagelopoulos et al. 1995 (12), Garbuz et al. 1996 (13), Shinar and Harris 1997 (14)).

However, the use of morselized bone grafts with and without anti protusio cages has proven to be more reliable for the long term, with survival percentages between 81%-95% at 10 years follow up (Schreurs et al. 1998 (15), Schreurs et al. 2001 (16), Van der Linde and Tonino 2001 (17)). One of the causes for the large difference of reported results is the difference in interpretation of the acetabular defects. As the AAOS classification defines only qualitative aspects and not quantitative, most series are quite different from the beginning. Sutherland (1996 (18)) well understood these problems, and quantified the amount of superior migration of the failed hip center as a measure of the extent of bone loss. In our opinion, there is almost always a combination of a cavitary and a segmental bone defect, which makes a clean classification of these bone defects very arbitrary.

Although the best method for revising the deficient acetabulum is not known, it has become increasingly obvious that to achieve long-term cup fixation in the structurally-deficient revision acetabulum, the primary goal is to achieve a certain but sufficient amount of stability on host bone.

As new bone bonding surfaces like hydroxyapatite (HA) have repeatedly shown to promote bone ongrowth (Geesink et al. 1995 (19), Capello et al. 1998 (20), Tonino et al. 2000 (21), Garcia et al. 1998 (22), Tonino et al. 1999 (23)) and to stabilize the prosthetic components securely and reliable, it was tempting to perform acetabular revision with a HA-coated component under the hypothesis that the HA coating could theoretically compensate for the reduced amount and vitality of the host bone bed. As fixation by bone ongrowth to the new cup must come directly from the host bone, much larger cups than the original size must be implanted. We report here the intermediate results of 81 consecutive hip revisions, in which 59 cups were revised for aseptic loosening with a cementless HA coated acetabular component.

PATIENTS AND METHODS

Between October 1990 and march 1999, 81 consecutive hip revisions were performed. In 66 of them, the acetabular cup was revised with a HA-coated component. Of the other 15 hips, only the stem (14 x) was revised, while in one patient, apart from the stem revision, the acetabular component was revised using the technique with morselized bone grafts and a an anti protusio cage (17).

Of these 66 hips, 7 hips presented with a deep infection and are the subject of a separate study. Therefore, 59 hips were left with aseptic loosening of the acetabular component revised with a HA-coated cup and are the subject of this paper.

The mean age of these patients at their first THA operation was 57.1 years (range 26-80 years). The mean age of the patients at the index cup revision operation was 70.7 years (range 39-90 years). The diagnosis at the first hip arthroplasty was osteoarthrosis (52 cases), rheumatoid arthritis (3 cases),femoral neck facture (3 cases) and one patient with osteonecrosis. Seven hips had a prior acetabular revision.

The mean Harris hip score was pre-operatively 38.7 (range 4-71 points) while the pre-operative Merle d'Aubigné score was 8,2 (range 2-14 points). Of the 59 cups that were revised, 40 were originally cemented, and 19 were uncemented; 15 of the 59 cups had been inserted at another hospital. The mean size of the index cup was 50mm (range 44-58).

Operative technique

All procedures were done by 3 of the authors (AT,WM, and JS) in a normal operation room with vertical flow. No body exhaust suits were worn. Prophylactic anticoagulants were administered, and prophylactic antibiotics were given after a deep culture was obtained. A straight lateral anterior approach was used with the patient supine in 37 cases (AJT) and with the patient in lateral decubitus in the other cases (15 by WM, and 7 by JS).

Trochanteric osteotomy was needed once. When it was necessary to remove a loosened stem (46 cases), this was performed before the loosened acetabular cup was taken out. Much attention was given to remove all debris and granulomatous tissue. The acetabular bone stock was then classified according to the location and severity of bone loss using Paprosky's classification (24-25) as well as the AAOS classification. According to Paprosky's classification, there were no type I defects, 7 type II defects and 52 type III defects. According to the AAOS classification, 12 hips had a peripheral or central segmental defect, 7 had only cavitary defects, and 40 had combined defects.

The acetabulum was then shaped into a hemisphere using hemispherical reamers. All defects, contained and not contained, were subsequently filled with morselized bone grafts from our bone bank. The stability of a trial component was then tested. If stability was good, 2 spikes were used, but no screws. When stability was not good, mostly

because of peripheral segmental bone loss, screws were used (38 cases). In a few cases where the acetabular wall became more or less elastic after reaming, the shell that was inserted was an over-sized component in relation to the diameter of the last reamer used (figs 1 , 2 and 3). The mean cup size was upgraded from 50mm to 62mm (range 50-70mm). All patients were mobilised immediately after the operation with controlled, partial weight bearing. Further weight bearing was mainly determined by the femoral construct.

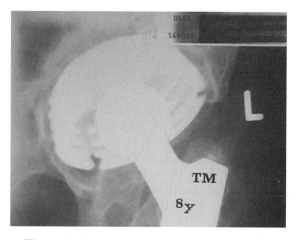

Figure 1 – Case R38: 8 years after uncemented screw cup (size 58) with major bone column loss, Paprosky 3b and AAOS grade III in a rheumatoid patient.

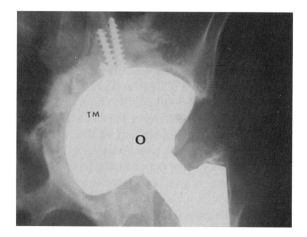

Figure 2 – Case R38: directly postoperative; the position of the cup is at the anatomic centre anchored with 3 screws in host bone; cup size 70. Large amounts of morselized bone is used to fill all defects.

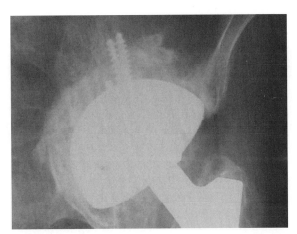

Figure 3 – Case R38: five years after cup revision. No cup migration or screw breakage or radiolucent lines MDA score 664.

Follow up

All 59 patients were included in a prospective follow up study using the Merle d'Aubigné functional scoring system and the Harris functional scoring system. They were reviewed clinically and radiographically at 3, 6, and 12 months after surgery, and yearly thereafter. All radiographic changes were evaluated by one of the authors (M. van de L) who is a skilled orthopaedic surgeon in total knee surgery but who did not perform any of the hip revisions. We used the criteria in the literature for radiographic failure (Azuma *et al.* 1994 (26), Hooten *et al.* 1994 (10), Zehnter and Ganz 1994 (27)), noting radiolucencies, migration and tilting of the cup, and breakage of a screw. Migration of the cup or change in its angle of inclination was determined with the M.E. Müller template, comparing the direct postoperative AP radiograph with the radiographs taken at follow-up (Zehnter and Ganz 1994 (25)). The X-line of the template was oriented to the distal edge of each teardrop and the vertical line bisected the ipsilateral teardrop. The widths of the radiolucencies at the metal backed cup bone interface in each of the three zones of DeLee and Charnley (28) were measured. Radiographic failure was defined either as migration of more than 2mm in any direction, or as progressive radiolucent lines exceeding 2mm in all zones. Breakage of screws was also defined as failure. The acetabular components were considered definitively loose if component migration or change in position occurred or screws were broken.

RESULTS

Complications were seen in 7 cases (9.6.%) and divided between surgeons as follows: two for AT, three for WM and two for JS. There were 5 dislocations, of which 3 were early and 2 late (i.e., after more than 1 year post operatively). All 5 cases also had stem revision at the same time. Only one dislocation (early) could be managed conservatively, while the other four had to be re-operated. In three of those cases, the acetabular component was left in place. One time, a longer neck length was sufficient, once a reorientation of the insert, and once a reorientation of the femoral stem. The fourth case (late dislocation) was revised 7.1 years after the index revision with exchange of the complete acetabular component; however, it had to be cut out by chisel because of the good fixation. There was one peroneal lesion that did not heal, and one late sepsis occurred in a patient who died 3.4 years after the cup revision.

No patient was lost to follow up, which was concluded in August, 2001. Of the seventeen patients who died before this date, two reached the 5 year follow up. They all showed excellent results with a mean Merle d'Áubigné score at one year post operatively of 14.5. Preoperatively, this figure was 8.0. All the seventeen acetabular components showed bone ongrowth, and none showed any migration or any change of position of the hip centre at the last follow up.

The mean duration of follow up of the 42 living patients was 4.6 (range 1.0-10.1 years). The mean Merle d'Aubigné score at follow up was 14.1 (range 9-18), and the mean Harris score was 80.6 (range 14-100). The inclination of the acetabular components as measured on a standing AP radiogram was between 40° and 55° in 88% of the hips, in 4% of the hips the angle was 55° or more, while in 8% of the hips the angle was 40° or less.

All 59 acetabular components showed osseointegration, i.e., bone ongrowth to the titanium substrate, except for one case, where a radiolucent line next to a radiodense line persisted in all 3 DeLee and Charnley zones. This patient, with rheumatoid arthritis, had primary THA elsewhere in 1986 with a cemented Lubinous SP prosthesis and an all polyethylene cemented cup. There was minor bone loss (Paprosky grade 2c and AAOS classification grade II); so the new HA cup could be firmly inserted with spikes, and no screws were needed for fixation (operated by JS). The hip functioned well for one year, after which the patient started complaining about pain in the groin. At two years follow-up, the scintigraphy showed a persistent elevated level of Technetium 99 isotope uptake, which is pathognomic for no bone ingrowth. She was re-operated elsewhere, where it was found that the cup was loose.

One other case (figs. 4A, 4B, 4C) is also of specific interest. A man born in 1940 developed an avascular femoral head necrosis after longstanding alcohol abuse. He was operated in 1977 with core decompression and grafting of the femoral head with a tibial autograft. However, the femoral head necrosis progressed and, in 1980, he received a THA with an uncemented Mittelmeier prosthesis. He did reasonably well for several years, but returned in 1993 with progressive symptoms of pain and diminished walking distance. Both cup and stem showed lack of bone ongrowth, and both components were revised in 1994 using the uncemented HA-coated ABG hip system. He did well for six years, until he was involved a serious, high speed traffic accident in June, 2000, incurring a fracture of the ramus inferior ossis pubis at that side. From that time on, he started to have progressive symptoms from this hip, and also developed radiological signs of loosening. The Technetium 99 isotope uptake became elevated, so the cup was revised 6.9 years after the index revision; at operation it was definitively loose.

From one of the cases (figs 5A, B, C) that died from cardiac failure, the cup with the adjoining pelvis could be harvested post mortem 2 years and seven months after the revision, because written consent was obtained during the patient's life. The cup was macroscopically stable and fixed in the acetabulum, but at histology, all three DeLee and Charnley sections showed no bone contact in the superior-anterior areas, because at the time of surgery, all anterior-superior bone ring support was already deficient. Only in the posterior-inferior part of the sections was there full bone ongrowth to the cup in a percentage that varied from 37% to 43%. The mean percentage of bone-implant contact was 11% for DeLee and Charnley section I, 10% for section II, and 20% for section III (fig. 5C.).

On the whole, the survival rate for this HA-coated cup was 98.8% after a mean follow up of 4.6 years when we take aseptic loosening as end point (95% - 100% confidence interval). The prognostic survival rate for the cup at 10 years is 94.4% (95% confidence interval between 83.8% and 100%).

DISCUSSION

It is interesting to observe that, even in acetabular revision cases where the bone stock may be significantly diminished, or where only a small remainder of the host bone is present, the bone growth onto the HA-coated acetabular component

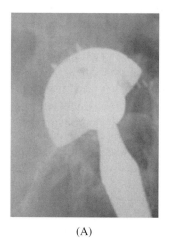
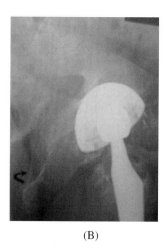
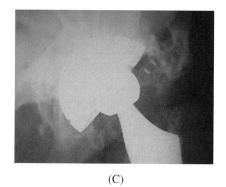

(A)   (B)   (C)

Figures 4A, B and C. – Mittelmeier prosthesis. Both cup and stem show lack of ongrowth (4A). Patient was revised to an uncemented HA-coated ABG hip system. That cup was revised after 6.9 years due to complications from a fracture of the ramus inferior ossis pubis incurred during a high speed traffic accident (4B). During the surgery, the cup was found to be definitively loose (4C).

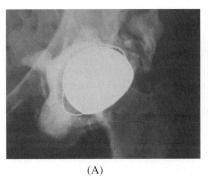

(A)

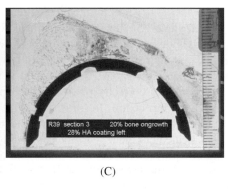

(C)

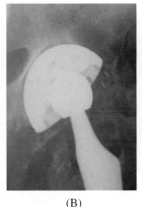

(B)

Figures 5A, B, and C (Case R39) – 18 years after implantation of a Wagner prosthesis for coxarthrosis. The cup is loose (5A). 2 years after revision with the ABG hip system (5B); MDA score 6, 6, 6. Section III deLee and Charnley; there is full bone ongrowth (23%) in the posterior-inferior part of the section, but the mean amount of bone ongrowth for the whole cup is 20% (5C).

can still occur, subsequently resulting in a reliable fixation. From a theoretical viewpoint, it is obvious that a certain amount of immediate mechanical stability of the cup with or without screws must be attained in order to allow the second stage of cup fixation to occur via bone ongrowth. Notwithstanding the fact that compression forces also enhance bone formation from a fibrous interface (Søballe et al, 1993 (29)), the filling of the contained and uncontained bone defects with morselized bone grafts was seen as essential to obtaining primary mechanical stability.

From human autopsy retrieved material, it has been observed that reliable fixation in the elderly occurs when only 20% to 30% of the surface of the acetabular component is covered by bony ongrowth (21). At the same time, this rather low percentage of bone ingrowth may explain the traumatic component loosening after a serious high speed accident as was observed in one of the patients.

As was noted in 15 of the 40 hips classified as AAOS grade III where the newly placed HA-coated component had less than 50% but more than 20% of contact to the host bone (figs 1, 2 and 3), this amount of contact still proved to be sufficient for enduring cup fixation. Also in the presented histology case (fig. 5C) where the surgeon (JS) stated that the anterior-superior wall was totally missing at revision, while there were another three cavitary defects, the amount of host bone contact was less than 50%. This question of what percentage of contact with the host bone is minimally needed for reliable ongrowth can perhaps be

answered, but only on the condition that primary anchorage of the cup is stable.

Nivbrandt and Kärrholm (30) could confirm these excellent results with HA-coated ABG cups for acetabular revision. Although their results are short term (2 years), this implant displayed the smallest migration so far reported in revision hip arthroplasty, even in cases where the cup had less than 50% contact with living bone. To what extent the percentage of bone-implant contact is influenced by the local bone density or osteopenia is still not well known, but a certain relationship seems probable. When there is a positive correlation between the amount of bone ongrowth and the local bone density, medicines like biphosphonates or Fosamax may have a positive influence on the endurance of implant fixation.

In this series the rate of the re-revision for aseptic loosening was low (1/59) and comparable with the best figures for survival after acetabular revision, which are between 81% and 95% after 10 years for cemented revision in combination with morselized bone grafts (15, 16, 17). Also, some other series of cementless acetabular revision show excellent results (Silverton et al 1995 (31), Dorr and Wan 1995 (32)). Therefore, both techniques can give excellent results in experienced hands and could be used alternatively depending on the local situation of available residual bone stock.

But as Dearborn and Harris (33) put it: "If the antero-posterior pelvic dimensions permit a jumbo acetabular component, such a component has the advantages of being an uncemented device with the potential to lower a high hip centre, and thicker polyethylene". So this technique should not be used in pelvic discontinuity, and not in cases with a too high hip centre with fairly small antero posterior acetabular dimensions, because then it is almost impossible to correctly place a large cup and still lower the hip centre. In these cases, the high hip centre must be take precedence, and a smaller uncemented component, or the cemented cup technique with morselized bone grafts and a protusio ring, must used to normalise the hip centre.

CONCLUSION

When we look at the clinical performance of the revised hips, both the Harris Hip Score and the Merle d'Aubigné Score improved significantly, with lasting effects after 5 to 10 years. It is also worthwhile to perform this procedure in the elderly patient who is over eighty years old.

Another point for discussion is the high complication rate reported for extensive cup revisions by various authors (33), (Stiehl *et al.* 2000 (34)). Of course, multiple prior hip surgeries and major column defects are negative factors but most authors are using a posterior approach or routinely perform trochanteric osteotomies. Both are factors leading to a higher dislocation rate.

In our series, where we used the direct lateral anterior approach (Hardinge) and where only once a trochanteric osteotomy was needed, the dislocation rate was rather low (7.5%), and sepsis occurred in only one case.

In summary, it was found that acetabular revision with a large or jumbo HA-coated cup has given very reliable results in cases where host bone support was less than 50%, as is seen in most Paprosky type III and AAOS type III acetabular defects.

Reference list

1. Kershaw CJ, Atkins RM, Dodd CAF, Bulstrode CJK (1991) Revision total hip arthroplasty for aseptic failure. *J. Bone Joint Surg. (Br)* 73:564-8.

2. Iorio R, Eftekhar NS, Kobayashi S, Grelsamer RP (1995) Cemented revision of failed total hip arthroplasty. *Clin. Orthop.* 316:121-30.

3. Raut VV, Siney PD, Wroblewski BM (1995) Cemented revision for aseptic loosening. *J. Bone Joint Surg. Br.* 77:357-61.

4. Raut VV, Siney PD, Wroblewski BM (1996) Revision of the acetabular component of a total hip arthroplasty with cement in young patients without rheumatoid arthritis. *J. Bone Joint Surg. Am.* 78:1853-6.

5. Harris WH, Penenberg BL (1987) Further follow up socket fixation using a metal-backed acetabular component for total hip replacement. *J. Bone Joint Surg. Am.* 69:1140-3.

6. Wilson MG, Hipoor H, Aliaback P, Poss R, Weissman BN (1989) The fate of acetabular allografts after bipolar revision arthroplasty of the hip. J. *Bone Joint Surg. Am.* 71:1469-79.

7. Gates HS, McCollum DE, Poletti SC, Nunley JA (1990) Bone grafting in total hip arthroplasty. *J. Bone Joint Surg. Am.* 72:248-51.

8. Jasty M, Harris WH (1990) Salvage total hip reconstruction in patient with major acetabular bone deficiency using structural femoral head allografts. *J. Bone Joint Surg. Br.* 72:63-7.

9. Mulroy RD, Harris WH (1990) Failure of acetabular autogenous grafts in total hip arthroplasty. *J. Bone Joint Surg. Am.* 72:1536-40.

10. Hooten JP, Engh Jr. CA, Engh CA (1994) Failure of structural acetabular allografts in cementless revision hip arthroplasty. *J. Bone Joint Surg.* 76:419-22.

11. Marti RK, Schüller HM, van Steyn MJA (1994) Superolateral bone grafting for acetabular deficiency in primary total hip replacement and revision. *J. Bone Joint Surg. Br.* 76:728-34.

12. Papagelopoulos PJ, Lewallen DG, Cabanela ME, McFarland EG, Wallricks SL (1995) Acetabular reconstruction using bipolar endoprosthesis and bone grafting in patients with severe bone deficiency. *Clin. Orthop.* 314:170-84.

13. Garbuz D, Morsi E, Gross AE (1996) Revision of the acetabular component of a total hip arthroplasty with a massive structural allograft. *J. Bone Joint Surg. Am.* 78:693-7.

14. Shinar AA, Harris WH (1997) Bulk structural autogenous grafts and allografts for reconstruction of the acetabulum in total hip arthroplasty. *J. Bone Joint Surg. Am.* 79:159-68.

15. Schreurs BW, Slooff TJ, Buma P, Gardeniers J, Huiskes R (1998) Acetabular reconstruction with impacted morsellised bone graft and cement. *J. Bone Joint Surg. Br.* 80:391-5.

16. Schreurs BW, van Tienen TG, Buma P, Verdonschot N, Gardeniers JWM and Slooff TJJH (2001) Favorable results of acetabular reconstruction with impacted morsellised bone grafts in patients younger than 50 years. *Acta Orthop. Scand.* 72(2):120-6.

17. Van der Linde M and Tonino AJ (2001) Acetabular revision with impacted grafting and a reinforcement ring. *Acta Orthop. Scand.* 72(3):221-7.

18. Sutherland CJ (1996) Treatment of type III acetabular deficiences in revision total hip arthroplasty without structural bone graft. *J. Arthroplasty* 11:91-8.

19. Geesink RG, Hoefnagels NH (1995) Six-year results of hydroxyapatite-coated total hip replacement. *J. Bone Joint Surg. Br.* 77:534-47.

20. Capello WN, D'Antonio JA, Manley MT, Feinberg JR (1998) Hydroxyapatite in total hip arthroplasty. Clinical results and clinical issues. *Clin. Orthop.* 355:200-11.

21. Tonino AJ, Rahmy AL (2000) The hydroxyapatite-ABG hip system: 5-7 year results from an international multicentre study. The international AGB Study Group. *J. Arthroplasty* 15:274-82.

22. Garcia Araujo C, Fernandez Gonzalez J, Tonino AJ (1998) Rheumatoid arthritis and hydroxyapatite-coated hip prostheses: five-year results. International ABG Study Group. *J. Arthroplasty* 13:6660-7.

23. Tonino AJ, Thèrin M, Doyle C (1999) Hydroxyapatite-coated femoral stems. Histology and histomorphometry around five components retrieved at *post mortem. J. Bone Joint Surg. Br.* 81:148-54.

24. Paprosky WG and Magnus RE (1994) Principles of bone grafting in revision total hip arthroplasty. Acetabular technique. *Clin. Orthop.* 298:147-55.

25. Paprosky WG, Perona PG, Lawrence JM (1994) Acetabular defect classification and surgical reconstruction in revision arthroplasty. A 6-year follow-up evaluation. *J. Arthroplasty* 9:33-44.

26. Azuma T, Yasuda H, Okagaki K, Sakaik (1994) Compressed allograft chips for acetabular reconstruction in revision hip arthroplasty. *J. Bone Joint Surg Br.* 76:740-4.

27. Zehntner MK, Ganz R (1994) Midterm results (5,5-10 years) of acetabular allograft reconstruction with the acetabular reinforcement ring during total hip revision. *J. Arthroplasty* 5:469-79.

28. DeLee JG and Charnley J (1976) Radiological demarcation of cemented sockets in total hip replacement. *Clin. Orthop.* 1976; 121:20-32.

29. Søballe K, Hansen ES, Brockstedt-Rasmussen H, Bünger C (1993) Hydroxyapatite coating converts fibrous tissue to bone around loaded implants. *J. Bone Joint Surg. Br.* 75-B:270-8.

30. Nivbrant B, Kärrholm J (1997) Migration and wear of hydroxyapatite-coated press-fit cups in revision hip arthroplasty. *J. Arthroplasty* 8:904-12.

31. Silverton CD, Rosenberg AG, Sheinkop MB, Kull LR, Galante JO (1995) Revision total hip arthroplasty using a cementless acetabular component. *Clin. Orthop.* 319:201-8.

32. Dorr LD, Wan Z (1995) Ten Years of experience with porous acetabular components for revision surgery. *Clin. Orthop.* 319:191-200.

33. Dearborn JT, Harris WH (1999) High placement of an acetabular component inserted without cement in a revision total hip arthroplasty. *J. Bone Joint Surg. Am.* 4:469.

34. Stiehl JB, Saluja R, Diener T (2000) Reconstruction of major column defects and pervic discontinuity in revision total hip arthroplasty. *J. Artrhoplasty* 7: 849-57.

7 Femoral Component Revision With Hydroxyapatite-Coated Revision Stems

Jean-Christophe Chatelet, MD and Louis Setiey, MD

INTRODUCTION

Revision following major femoral component loosening can be difficult, both in terms of finding a means of stable fixation of the revision implant and in terms of finding viable bone stock. Adequate primary stability must be obtained, in order to allow the restoration of the badly damaged bone around the new implant, and to ensure the sound and lasting integration of the new device. This means that specially designed implants will be required so as to obtain the necessary primary stability and to find a solution to the individual patient's needs. Stability will be a function of the preoperative condition of the femur (granulomas, osteolysis, fractures, implant breakage) and of what happens at revision surgery (inadvertent perforation, fractures, cortical windows, Wagner osteotomy).

Two Corail HA-coated implants are available. The KAR, a long-stem Corail specially designed for revisions, allows most cases of femoral loosening (Paprosky1 Types 2A, 2B, and 3A) to be managed. Where there are major defects following loosening (Types 2C and 3B), or after transfemoral osteotomy, fixation will have to be sought in the diaphysis, and a modular screw-locked device such as the Reef will need to be used so as to obtain sufficiently distal fixation and to reconstruct the femur (figs 1 and 2).

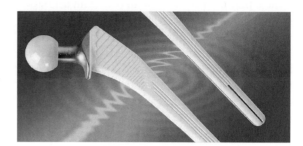

Figure 1 – The KAR prosthesis.

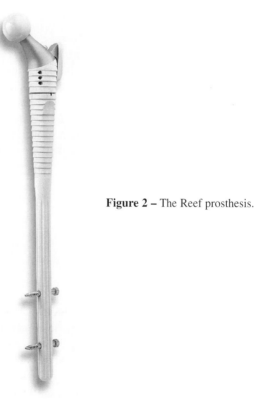

Figure 2 – The Reef prosthesis.

MATERIALS AND METHODS

Implants

KAR prosthesis

The KAR prosthesis a revision device based upon the pattern of the Corail. It has a straight, proximally flared stem of oblong cross-section to provide three-dimensional stability. It always has a collar, which contributes to the proximal stabilization of the implant and serves to compress any bone grafts at the calcar that may have been required to fill medial cortical defects. It differs from the Corail in that it has a 25% longer stem to allow it to bridge bone defects or windows made in the femur to facilitate cement removal. Also, unlike the Corail, the KAR has two distal slots, one in the coronal and one in the sagittal plane. These slots make the device less stiff and prevent stress risers in the cortex at the level of the stem tip; they also prevent distal wedging that can result in stress shielding and thigh pain. After grit blasting, the stem is plasma spray-coated all over with a 150 μm layer of hydroxyapatite (HA).

The horizontal macrotexture applied to the metaphysis counteracts subsidence, while the vertical macrotexturing in the diaphyseal portion guards against implant rotation. These macrotexturing features also increase the contact area with the host bone by 15%. The long KAR stem is made of wrought titanium alloy, and comes in five sizes (12, 14, 16, 18, and 20). Regardless of implant size, the distal diameter is always 11mm.

The Reef Stem

This is a modular locking device with an all-over HA coating. It consists of three parts. The first is a single-piece metaphyseal-diaphyseal part, which has two zones. The metaphyseal zone has the shape of a truncated cone and is flattened in the antero-posterior direction; this zone is 100mm high in all femoral component sizes. It features horizontal macrotexturing, which increases the surface area between the implant and the host bone, and guards against subsidence.

The second part is composed of a cylindrical diaphyseal zone with a slight bow to prevent contact with the anterior cortex of the femur. This zone has vertical macrotexturing, the object being once again to increase the implant-bone interface; the macrotexture also guards against rotation. Depending on the length of the stem, there are between one and three holes for locking with 5mm-diameter screws. The component comes in four lengths, of 225mm, 275mm, 325mm, and 375mm, and in six diameters, of 10mm, 12mm, 14mm, 16mm, 18mm, and 20mm.

The third part is composed of a neck unit, which fits onto the stem with a Morse taper lock and a proximal screw. This system provides for a sound construct, and allows anteversion to be fine-tuned during the trial stage, using marks provided at 10°

intervals. This unit enables the surgeon to perform a perfect reconstruction of the hip in terms of limb length and femoral neck anteversion. The proximal screw is used for the fixation of the construct, and also serves to attach the trochanter wing, which is an optional component. The neck unit comes in two heights, of 25mm and 35mm, either with or without a medial collar. It has horizontal macro-texturing, as well as medial perforations through which cerclage wires or cables may be passed. The unit has a neck, with a 135° neck-shaft angle, and features a Morse taper spigot onto which 28mm-diameter or 22.2mm-diameter ceramic or metallic femoral heads may be fitted.

The lateral wing comes in three sizes, and is also HA-coated. This wing allows the stabilization and fixation of the greater trochanter, and to achieve the necessary offset if tensioning of the gluteals is required.

Surgical Technique

The surgical technique for the insertion of the KAR prosthesis has some specific features that must be borne in mind. As always, preoperative planning is of the utmost importance. In this exercise, templates are used to determine the implant that will give the best fit and fill of the metaphyseal flare of the patient's femur. In the selection of the implant, care must be taken to ensure that the length of the device will be sufficient to bridge any bone defects left behind by loosening or by windows made in the femoral cortex at surgery.

At the preoperative planning stage, the center of rotation and the optimal positioning of the implant will also be determined, so as to enable a normal Shenton line pattern (2) to be restored and to decide on the extent of any calcar grafting that may be required. Cement removal is performed from above, without opening the femur, using a centering device; a mechanical cement extractor may be used to remove the cement plug. This plug may also be removed through an anterior cortical window or a Wagner osteotomy (3), providing that doing so will not jeopardize the primary stability of the KAR prosthesis to be inserted.

Once the loosened implant and all the cement have been removed, the femur is prepared for the implantation of the revision device. In the shaft, this is done with an 11mm diameter rigid reamer. If the trial stem jams prematurely, reaming with a 12mm-dimeter reamer may be required. Proximally, Corail broaches of increasing size are used until sound primary stability can be obtained. The KAR prosthesis requires primary stability both proximally and distally, which means that stability confined to the distal zone will not suffice. It is therefore vital to ensure that the implant also has proximal stability, in the metaphysis, lack of which would adversely affect the implant's in-service life.

Postoperatively, patients are managed along the same lines as those who have undergone primary arthroplasty. If the implant is stable, immediate weight-bearing with two forearm crutches is permitted. If a Wagner osteotomy was used at surgery, weight-bearing will not be allowed for the first 45 days.

The Reef prosthesis requires a detailed preoperative radiographic work-up with a standing A/P film and A/P and lateral views of the entire femur, with a millimeter grid placed over the films. This planning is of the utmost importance, since it allows the extent of bone defects determined, and gives an idea of the possible worsening of the pattern at surgery, as a result of the parlous condition of the bone stock. The required length of the transfemoral osteotomy can be established at this stage, and the length and diameter of the single-piece unit chosen in such a way as to ensure bridging of the osteotomy site and sound locking in healthy bone stock. The first (proximal) screw must be at least 4cm distal to the distal end of the osteotomy.

Within our group, different surgical approaches are in use. In the series reported herein, a Hardinge-Müller approach (4) was used 20 times, while 16 hips were revised through a posterior approach, and 11 via an anterior approach. The implant site is always approached through a wide Wagner (3) transfemoral osteotomy. In cases of comminuted periprosthetic fractures, it may be possible to go through the fracture site. We are against performing a trochanteric osteotomy, since we think that it provides insufficient exposure of the lesions and does not allow the failed implant to be properly retrieved.

At the 1999 symposium of the French Society for Orthopaedic Surgery and Traumatology SOFCOT (5), it was shown that in Stages III and IV (6), trochanterotomy had a 20% non-union rate, and that insufficient exposure was to blame for fractures or inadvertent perforation in 22% of cases. We routinely use a Wagner osteotomy, and have never had problems with non-union. The lid will heal within three to six months. Intravenous

antibiotics are started intraoperatively; before that, swabs are taken for culture, and periprosthetic tissue is removed for intraoperative frozen section. Taking frozen-section specimens was started several years ago, in the light of research by Feldman and Lonner (7), and the results have invariably been confirmed by the further clinical course of our patients.

The presence of fewer than five polymorphonuclear leukocytes per field is considered negative for active infection; if there are more than five PMNs per field, there may well be active infection, and the patient should be put on long-term prophylactic antibiotics. Patients who do not have a history of thromboembolism receive low molecular weight heparins for the first month post-arthroplasty. Anti-inflammatories are used cautiously in our elderly patients, because of the adverse gastrointestinal and renal effects involved.

While, with the KAR prosthesis and with primary hip replacements, immediate resumption of weight-bearing is the rule, we recommend that the patients managed with a Reef device are kept off weight-bearing for between six weeks and two months. The actual time will depend upon the quality of the patient's bone stock, and the quality of the reconstruction. However, some of our very elderly patients have been non-adherent with regard to these instructions, without, however, suffering any ill effects. This suggests that the construct obtained with a screw-locked stem is very sound and sturdy.

Indications

The indications for the KAR prosthesis are revision after femoral component loosening, with or without a cortical window. In terms of the Paprosky classification (1), the types that lend themselves to being managed with this device are 2A, 2B, and 3A. Trochanteric osteotomy or a Wagner osteotomy may be used, providing that they do not jeopardize the primary stability of the revision implant (fig. 3a, b, c). Other possible indications for the use of the KAR prosthesis are pertrochanteric fractures with cerclage of the greater trochanter, periprosthetic fractures, and tumors, osteolysis, and ballooning, providing that stable seating of the implant can be achieved. If the proximal bone defects are too severe, it will be impossible to obtain sufficient stability for a KAR prosthesis. In such cases, fixation will need to be sought more distally, in healthy diaphyseal bone stock.

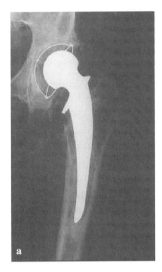
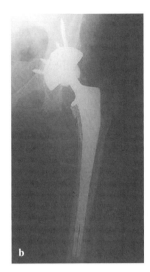
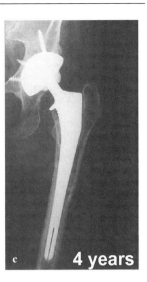

Figure 3a, b, c – Cemented loose stem (a); stability
and osseointegration at four years with a KAR stem (b, c).

When we were designing the Reef prosthesis in the early 1990s, we were convinced of the value of HA in primary arthroplasty because of the osteoconductive properties of the material. We also knew that in revisions for Stages I or II of loosening, HA was beneficial, as proved by the results obtained with the KAR prosthesis. In Stages III and IV, where bone defects are huge, the remaining bone in the metaphysis is often paper-thin and sclerotic. We therefore were not certain that a large reconstruction device would be a solution. Perhaps these sort of femurs were at or beyond the limit of what osteoconduction in response to HA could achieve. We were, however, encouraged to pursue our concept of HA-coated implants, since the 1989 SOFCOT symposium (5) had shown the high failure rate of iterative cemented arthroplasties in the management of Stages III and IV of implant loosening.

The Study

The present study was performed in 242 patients who were followed up with clinical and radiographic investigations. Of these patients, 203 had received a KAR prosthesis, while 49 had been managed with a Reef device.

KAR stem

The first KAR stems were implanted in 1989. Our study includes 203 stem revisions (197 patients) performed between 1990 and 1998, and followed up for a mean of seven years (longest follow-up, 132 months). Of the patients, 54% were men, and 46% women; the mean patient age was 67.9 years. Five patients died of non-hip-related causes; three patients were lost to follow-up. All the remaining patients were followed up clinically and radiographically.

In 78% of the cases, the patients had not previously been revised. In 22%, there had been two or more prior revisions (two revisions in 18%; 3 revisions in 5%). In 53% of the cases, both the cup and the stem were loose. The general condition of the patients was expressed in terms of Charnley categories (8). Fifty-nine percent of the patients were in Category A (120 patients); 18% were in Category B (36 patients), and 23% were in Category C (46 patients). The mean preoperative MDA score (9) of 9.02 showed the severity of the patients' disability. The preoperative radiological bone defect patterns varied widely; most, however, were Paprosky Types 2 and 3. Type 2A was seen in 64 patients, and Type 2B in 58. When we first had the KAR prosthesis, and prior to the advent of the Reef, we used it in all patients with Types 1 (28), 2C (9), 3A (23) and 3B (21).

Reef stem

Forty-nine patients were revised to a Reef stem, between March 1994 and March 2001. Of these 49 patients, 47 were reviewed at the "Fifteen Years of the Corail Prosthesis" symposium. Two patients died in the first year post-arthroplasty, from old age and co-morbid conditions. Mean follow-up was

25 months (longest follow-up, seven years). Of the patients, 60% were women, and 40% men.

The age range was wide (from 17 to 93 years); the mean patient age was 68 years. The majority (27 cases) had SOFCOT (6) Stage III or IV, Paprosky (1) Types 2C or 3, loosening. In terms of Charnley categories, 46% were A, 38% were B, while 16% were Category C. Twenty-seven cases had loose stems. Six of the patients – including the youngest patient in this group (Ewing's sarcoma of the upper end of the femur) – had a primary tumor or secondaries in the femur. Nine patients had peri- or infraprosthetic fractures associated with implant loosening. In this series, there were also two revisions to Reef stems following infection. In one case (see Case 1, below), this was the fourth operation; in the other, revision was required for an MRSA-infected haematoma. There three remaining cases involved malunion and stress shielding. The shortest stem (225mm) was the one used most frequently (22 cases), while the 275mm stem was used in 16 cases, and the longest stem (325mm) was used in the remaining 10 cases. The most frequently used diameter was 12mm (27 cases), followed by the 14mm diameter in 10 cases, and the 10mm in 4 cases. In 35 cases, two screws were used. In 6 cases, one screw was used, and in five cases, 3 screws were used.

In the light of our experience, over the past 15 years, of the use of HA-coated primary implants, we think that for revision, even in Stages III and IV, grafting is not required in the majority of cases. At the start of our learning curve, however, we used allografts in seven cases, autologous bone in one case, and bone graft substitutes in three cases; the substitutes were poorly incorporated. We share the view expressed by most of the other authors who use a Wagner osteotomy that the bone lid is well vascularized since its soft-tissue cover is preserved; this creates optimal conditions for the restoration of the bone stock. Sometimes, when all the bone has gone, the use of bulk allografts may appear to be indispensable; however, we have never resorted to this form of grafting. We prefer to cut the bone lid around the implant into small chips and "petals", with their blood supply left intact, so as to stimulate osteogenesis and healing. Of the 47 cases in this study, 45 required cup revision as well. In 20 of them, a threaded Tropic cup was used, while 13 were managed with a press-fit device. Eight patients had weak gluteals and were at major risk for dislocation; they were, therefore, given a bipolar cup. Four patients received an Octopus reconstruction socket.

RESULTS AND COMPLICATIONS

Clinical Results

The patients' subjective assessment of the outcome following revision to a KAR prosthesis showed the beneficial effects of the procedure: 190/195 were satisfied (144 patients) or very satisfied (46 patients). Five patients were disappointed (dislocation and infection). None of the patients had thigh pain. This was interpreted as a beneficial effect of the distal slots, which prevent stress risers forming at the stem tip. Five patients died of non hip-related causes. One stem subsided and had to be revised. In this particular instance, primary implant stability had been suboptimal, and a femoral fracture had been missed. In all the other cases, results were very encouraging, even though these were revision arthroplasties. The patients were consistently pain-free and had an increased ROM. In this respect, the outcome was comparable to that of a primary arthroplasty.

The global MDA score increased by 6.7, from 9.02 before revision to 15.72 post-arthroplasty (constituent scores: pain 5.45, mobility 4.96, walking 5.37). The MDA score correlated with the Charnley categories. Category A had a mean MDA of 16.46; Category B, of 16.33; and Category C, of 14.6. The complications encountered were typical of revision arthroplasty in general: there were three dislocations; two deep infections, despite routine prophylactic antibiotics for 48 hours; one greater trochanter non-union; as well as seven intraoperative perforations, mainly in cases where the failed implant had been in varus.

Of the 49 patients revised to a Reef stem, two died in the first year from arthroplasty. None of the complications encountered was related to the method of implant fixation. The implant was always screw-locked, and screw breakage was not encountered in any of the cases. Equally, there never was any evidence of cortical reaction around the screws. These observations may be accounted for by the rapid secondary fixation of the implant by new bone formation. Once this fixation has been obtained, the screws cease to have a mechanical function, and there will be "radiological silence" at the screw sites.

The complications encountered were typical of revision surgery; there were three haematomas, and two dislocations. The mean global MDA score went from 7 to 14, the Pain score improved from

1 to 5. Subjectively, the outcome was assessed as follows: 96% of the 47 revision patients were satisfied, while 4% (the two who suffered dislocation) were disappointed.

Radiological Results

KAR Stem

The three features checked on the follow-up radiographs were implant stability, bone defect healing, and osseointegration. The achievement of stability at surgery is of crucial importance. Where primary stability had been obtained, osseointegration was consistently observed, and long-term implant survival was similar to that seen following primary arthroplasty. In the 190 cases followed up, there was no varus tilt, and only three cases of implants had settled at a slightly lower level (<3mm below the original level of implantation). Only one case of subsi-

dence required re-revision. In this case, a femoral crack fracture had been missed at surgery (fig. 4).

Virtually all the bone defects healed. Some of these defects had been there prior to revision, as a result of granulomas, osteolysis, or fractures; others were caused at surgery by inadvertent perforation or when cortical windows or Wagner osteotomies were performed. Cortical windows must be bridged by the implant, with the stem-end slots placed distal to the window level. Transfemoral osteotomies were found to heal within three months, providing the lid was snug against the implant and held in place with wire cerclage. Granulomas were curetted; grafting, however, has been largely abandoned. We believe in the femur's capacity to rebuild around the "stenting" implant, with the stimulus for bone growth coming from the healing of the bone lid. In the case of an isolated granuloma, the lesion may be packed with cancellous bone (fig. 5).

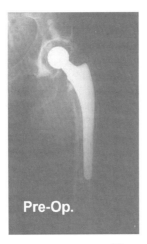 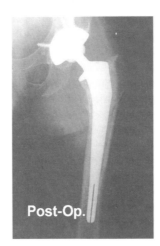 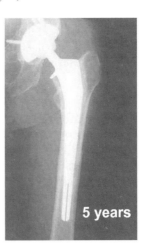

Figure 4 – Osseointegration of a KAR prosthesis at five years.

Figure 5 – Healing of a cortical window around a KAR prosthesis.

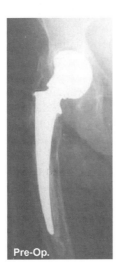 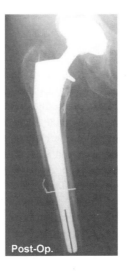 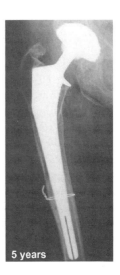

Osseointegration

With stable implants, osseointegration was consistently seen. A change in the bone bed was seen in 65% of the cases, with evidence of periprosthetic ossification in 50% of the cases. In the space between the implant and the femoral cortices, newly formed bony bridges of the kind always seen after primary arthroplasty were noted (21). There was no evidence of stress shielding or lucent-line formation. Osteopenia in the trochanteric region was infrequent (2%); calcar remodeling was more frequently observed (5%), mainly following calcar grafting. Pedestal formation was seen in 4% of the cases, and the same percentage had cortical hypertrophy along the implant stem. Thirty-five % of the cases showed no radiological changes (fig. 6).

Reef Stem

The analysis of the results of the Reef stem required a study of femoral bone lid healing.

Radiologically, signs of bone stock restoration were seen from the second month post-arthroplasty. There were two types of new bone formation – cortical bone formation, and endosteal ossification. The latter consisted of thin trabeculae bridging from the cortex to the implant. Reactive lines or lucent lines were not observed in any of the cases. Cortical bone formation, as shown by thickening of the cortex in the diaphysis and the metaphysis, was seen in 16 cases. Endosteal ossification was observed in 18 cases. Six patients with severe cortical atrophy prior to revision failed to improve their cortical pattern. All the patients concerned were elderly females

with severe osteoporosis. However, even in these patients, the cortical bone lids healed.

The following two case reports give a picture of the problems managed with a Reef prosthesis.

In Case 1, this male patient, born in 1925, had undergone primary hip arthroplasty in 1981. He was revised for loosening in 1994. Postoperatively, he developed an MRSA infection, which failed to clear up with long-term antibiotic therapy. In order to obtain control, we removed the implant and all the wires, and meticulously curetted the soft tissues. Six weeks later, the patient was revised to a Reef prosthesis. He was re-examined at regular intervals, and, following long-term antibiotic therapy, laboratory and scintigraphic investigations showed the infection to have been cured completely. He was entirely pain-free, and radiography showed the reappearance of a healthy bone pattern, especially in Zone 7, where the cortex looked very satisfactory (fig. 7).

In Case 2, this male patient, who was 75 years old in 1997, had been given a cemented self-locking hip replacement 16 years earlier. He had Stage IV loosening associated with a comminuted peri- and infraprosthetic fracture. At revision, a Reef prosthesis was inserted through the fracture site. No supplementary grafts were used. The screw-locked prosthesis acted as a stent around which the metaphysis was reconstructed using titanium bands. The functional outcome was very satisfactory, and the patient finished up pain-free and with a good ROM. The two-year radiographs showed healing of the fracture site, and a very satisfactory restoration of the entire metaphyseal region in Zones 1 and 7 (fig. 8).

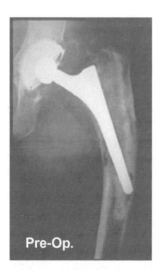
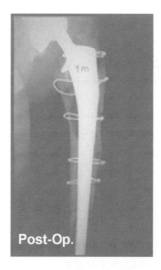
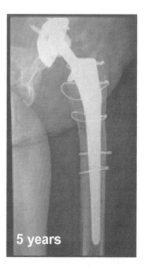

Figure 6 – Reconstruction of a femur around a KAR prosthesis.

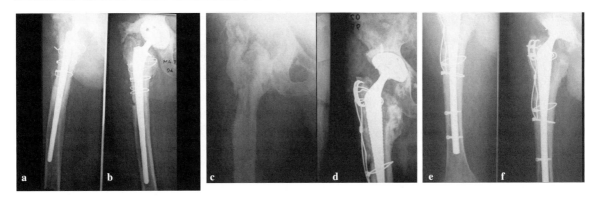

Figure 7a, b, c, d, e, f – Infected THR (7a, b) ; Staged revision (c, d) ;
Patient symptom-free, and radiographs normal, following implantation of a Reef prosthesis (e, f).

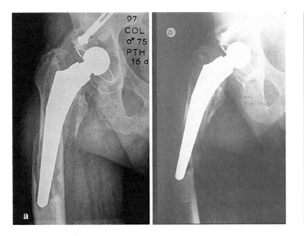

Figure 8a – Loosening and fracture of a cemented THR.

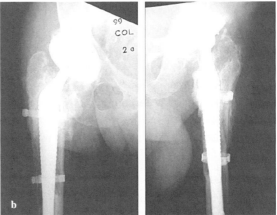

Figure 8b – Revision to a screw locked Reef stem.

DISCUSSION

Literature is plentiful regarding hip revision surgery. However, comparison between published series remains hazardous because of their lack of homogeneity. Whatever the grade of loosening would be, our personal strategy deals in all cases with a "biological" rebuilding of the bone stock. However, other solutions have been put forward such as cemented stem reinsertion, either isolated or combined with bone grafting, or methods stimulating new bone formation around uncemented stems.

Isolated cemented stem reinsertion

Literature reports on various failure rates from 21% at 12 years postoperatively, as published by Harris *et al.* (10), up to 43% with Amstutz (11).

Kerboull (12) reports 82% of excellent and good results. However, at 5-year follow-up, 32% of cases exhibited lucent lines, and 10% of cases were assessed as loose, possibly causing one to assume that the increased likelihood of recurrent loosening increases relative to the extent of the initial bone loss. According to a multicenter study by Huten *et al.* provided at the Sofcot symposium in 1999 (13), survival rates at 8 years according to the Sofcot-Vives (6) classification were 95% in cases with grade I lesions, down to 84% in the grade II and III groups. The latter authors did not recommend isolated cemented stem reinsertion in the most severe cases belonging to grade IV of this classification, as well as in young patients. Despite progress in terms of cementation techniques, for Pierson (14), the loosening rates remain over 20% at 5 years, whatever lesion grade.

Cemented stem reinsertion associated with allografts

These grafts can be either morcellized or massive allografts. Ling *et al.* in Exeter (15, 16) are used to cementing a stem in a compacted bone bed composed of morcellized impacted allografts. However, Gie (17) reports on a subsidence rate of 20% with respect to the cement mantle and the stem itself. Kerboull (18, 19) prefers to cement a stem into a massive allograft embedded in the living host bone, according to a procedure known as intussusception allografts technique; however, this technique depends on the availability of massive allografts, as well as evidence of the harmlessness of these grafts.

The last solution consists in stimulating new bone formation all around an uncemented implant

However, this bony ongrowth needs as a prerequisite a stable implant lying directly on living bone, without any additional allografts. According to a multicenter study reported by Dujardin (20), based upon 803 femoral revisions, the thickness of metaphyseal cortices increases in cases of HA-coated implants when compared to cemented or non hydroxyapatite-coated uncemented stems. In the case of an unstable stem, the bone stock becomes worse. Conversely, in the case of stable stem

secured by distal screws, the new bone formation increases, leading to a paradoxical reaction, since a distal fixation normally generates some radiographic stress-shielding bone loss; in fact, in these cases, the bony formation would be considered as a bone healing process (21). As a matter of fact, we never noticed in our experience any screw-related problems, which tends to confirm a successful metaphyseal bone formation stabilizing the proximal aspect of the stem. Nevertheless, a secure diaphyseal fixation at a healthy portion of the femur would be expected without the use of hydroxyapatite in press-fitted stems, as with the Wagner implant (22, 23), which is supposed to fix distally, it being said that stress shielding and thigh pain may occur in such a distal fixation. In addition, the valgus neck-diaphysis angle of the latter stem at 145 degrees can medialize the shaft and lead to a decreasing lever-arm resulting in a higher risk of dislocation (24).

We firmly believe new bone formation can exist only if primary stability is achieved, and direct contact between a living host bone and a stable implant can be obtained. The primary mechanical stability, if not obtained at the metaphyseal level, involves for us a distal locking of the stem. In addition, an intimate contact between the host bone and the metallic device is favored by a transfemoral approach. This osseous flap must be osteotomized in parts if necessary in order to provide a close contact with the metallic stem. By properly selecting the implant and ensuring an appropriate

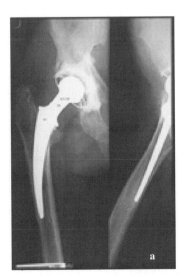
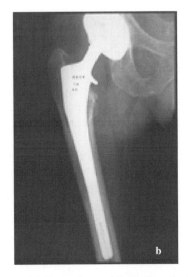
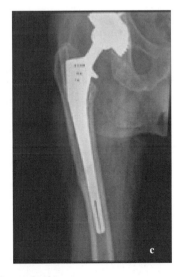

Figure 9a, b, c – Stability and osseointegration of a KAR prosthesis:
previous loose cemented stem (a); excellent result at seven years (b, c).

fit of the implant to the type of the bone defect, a bone reconstruction of the proximal portion of the femur in revision surgery is possible without the need for additional grafting.

The present study has provided encouraging evidence of the reliability of long HA-coated stems in revision arthroplasty. The KAR prosthesis must be stably seated at surgery. If this stability is achieved, osseointegration is consistently seen, and the long-term survival of this revision device is similar to that of primary replacements. The KAR is the key implant in our range of revision prostheses. This long-stem version of the tried and tested Corail is used in the management of the majority of our revision patients. Proper monitoring of arthroplasty patients will allow loosening to be detected at an early stage, and any revisions that may be required become very similar to primary arthroplasties (fig. 9).

Where bone defects are extensive (Paprosky Types 2C and 3B), or if large transfemoral osteotomies are required for the removal of the failed implant, the Reef stem is available, as a modular, screw-locked device that can be anchored very distally to reconstruct the femur. In light of our clinical and radiological results, fully HA-coated screw-locked stems would appear to be a satisfactory option in Stage III and IV loosening. We feel that, in revision implants, all-over HA coating is an essential feature. We have never encountered any screw site problems. Implant integration occurs rapidly, and none of the screw-locked stems has been found to subside. We fully agree with the conclusions of the 1999 SOFCOT symposium on stem revision, according to which "cementless stems must have a macro- or micro-interlock surface design, and should, preferably, be locked with a screw or screws. Interlocking may provide better initial stability, and enhanced long-term fixation (5). At that symposium, the point was made that new bone formation appeared to be maximal in the metaphysis, especially where the implant had sound distal fixation (20).

CONCLUSION

The present study of 252 revisions of failed THRs to HA-coated devices has confirmed the reliability of HA-coated prostheses in revision arthroplasty. No one implant could cater to all the patients. The Corail system, with its long-stem version, the KAR, and the Reef prosthesis, allow the overwhelming majority of problems in stem revision to be appropriately dealt with.

We use the KAR for the bulk of our revisions. Revision surgery is straightforward, without the need for windows or osteotomies. Postoperative management is likewise straightforward. The femur heals around the implant. Cysts require only curetting, without any need for grafting. Load transfer and stability are obtained in healthy bone stock in the metaphysis and diaphysis. If healthy bone stock is encountered only distally, fixation is obtained distally with a screw-locked construct, and the femur is reconstructed proximally. For such cases, the Reef prosthesis is used. The bone will heal around the HA-coated implant, similar to the way in which fracture healing occurs.

The advent of modular cementless prostheses has transformed the outlook for these difficult revisions. We think that all-over HA-coated screw-locked modular stems allow us to cope with extremely difficult patterns. Even in badly damaged femurs, the Reef stem will act as a stent that can be anchored in healthy diaphyseal bone stock, and locked with screws. This provides very sound initial stability, and the stent can be adjusted to obtain the required length and anteversion. Over the weeks, good-quality diaphyseal and metaphyseal bone stock will rebuild around the stent. This new bone formation appears to proceed more rapidly thanks to the presence of HA on the implant; and the healthy look of the bone on the radiographs suggests that the implant will have a long in-service life.

References List

1. Paprosky W, Lawrence J, Cameron H (1990) Femoral defects classification: clinical application. *Orthop. Review*, Suppl 9-16.

2. Lichtblau S (1966) Early recognition of congenital dislocation and congenital subluxation of the hip. An evaluation of Shenton's line. *Clin. Orthop.* 48:181-9.

3. Wagner H (1989) A revision prosthesis for the Hip joint. *Orthopade*, 18:438-53.

4. Pai VS (1997) A comparison of three lateral approaches in primary total hip replacement. *Int. Orthop.* 21(6): 393-8.

5. Migaud H, Courpied JP (2000) Conclusions symposium SOFCOT 1999. RCO, vol. 86, Suppl. I:86-90.

6. Vives P, De Lestang M, Paclot R, Cazeneuve JF (1989) Le descellement aseptique – définitions, classifications.-

Symposium SOFCOT 1988; RCO, Suppl. I, vol. 75, 29-31.

7. Feldman D, Lonner JH, Desal P, Zucherman J (1995) The role of intraoperative frozen sections in revision total joint Arthroplasty. *JBJS A*, vol. 77A, n°12:1807-13.

8. Charnley J (1972) The long term results of low-friction arthroplasty of the hip as a primary intervention. *Journal of Bone and Joint Surgery*, 54B:61.

9. Merle d'Aubigne R (1970) Cotation chiffrée de la fonction de la hanche. *RCO*, 56:481-6.

10. Harris W (1982) Revision surgery for failed, non septic, total hip arthroplasty. *Clin. Orthop.* 170:8-20.

11. Amtutz HC, Ma SN, Jinnah RH, Mai L (1982) Revision of aseptic loose total hip arthroplasty. *Clin. Orthop.* 170:21-3.

12. Kerboull L, Culot Th, Kerboull M (1994) Les reprises d'arthroplasties totales non cimentées par une prothèse cimentée. *RCO*, 80 sup. I-141.

13. Huten D, Bouabdallah N, BassainE M, Wodechi PH (2000) *RCO*, vol. 86 Suppl. I, 72-5.

14. Pierson JL, Harris WH (1994) Cemented revision for femoral osteolysis in cemented arthroplasties. *JBJS (B)*, 76B:40-44.

15. Ling RS, Timperley AJ, Linder L (1993) Histology of cancellous impaction grafting in the femur. A case report. *J. Bone Joint Surg. Br.* 75(5):693-6.

16. Stulberg SD (2002) Impaction grafting: doing it right. *J. Arthroplasty*, 17(4 Suppl 1):147-52.

17. Gie GA, Linder L, Ling RS, Simon JP, Sloof TJ, Timperley AJ (1993) Impacted cancellous allografts and cement for revision total hip arthroplasty. *JBJS*, 75B: 14-21.

18. Kerboull M, Hamadouche M, Kerboull L (2000) The Kerboull acetabular reinforcement device in major acetabular reconstructions. *Clin. Orthop.* (378):155-68.

19. Charrois O, Kerboull L, Vastel L, Courpied JP, Kerboull M (2000) Femoral reconstruction with massive allograft implanted in a split femur. Mid-term results of 18 reconstructions. *Rev. Chir. Orthop. Reparatrice Appar. Mot.* 86(8):801-8.

20. Dujardin F, Mazirt N (2000) Régénération osseuse spontanée. Symposium SOFCOT 1999. *RCO*, Vol. 86, Suppl. I:75-7.

21. Hardy DCR, Frayssinet P, Guilhem A, Lafontaine MA, Delinee PE (1991) Bonding of hydroxyapatite – coated femoral prostheses. *J. Bone joint Surg. RB*, 73B:732-40.

22. Bohm P, Bischel O (2001) Femoral revision with the Wagner SL revision stem : evaluation of one hundred and twenty-nine revisions followed for a mean of 4.8 years. *J. Bone Joint Surg. Am.* 83-A(7):1023-31.

23. Head WC (2001) The Wagner revision prosthesis consistently restores femoral bone structure. *Int. Orthop.* 25(1):63-4.

24. Boisgard S, Moreau PE, Tixier H, Levai JP (2001) Bone reconstruction, leg length discrepancy, and dislocation rate in 52 Wagner revision total hip arthroplasties at 44-month follow-up. Rev. *Chir. Orthop. Reparatrice Appar. Mot.* 87(2):147-54.

CLINICAL EXPERIENCE WITH HYDROXYAPATITE KNEE IMPLANTS AT A MINIMUM OF 10 YEARS

1 Twelve-year Experience with Hydroxyapatite in Primary Knee Arthroplasty

Jean-Alain Epinette, MD and Michael T. Manley, PhD

INTRODUCTION

For years, many questions regarding fixation of prostheses, especially in total knee arthroplasty (TKA) have focused on whether or not there is a need for cementless implants. Perhaps the appropriate question should be, "Is there a need for cement in knees?". Furthermore, the term "cementless" is not appropriate, since the fixation afforded by only metallic porous substrates has often led, in our experience, to poor results, especially on the tibial side. Hydroxyapatite-coated implants must be seen as a distinct means of fixation for prostheses, and as an implant "family" in their own right.

In the long run, lasting, stable implant fixation, without the use of acrylic cement, by means of a bioactive bond between the implant and the host bone, is a goal as important in the knee as it is in the hip. The preservation of bone stock, the elimination of a "third component", and better resistance to bacterial attack are all arguments in favor of a hydroxyapatite (HA) interface. However, looking at the considerable number of large-scale studies of HA-coated hips in the literature, and the paucity of similar studies in the knee, it appears that information on HA knees are lags behind that of HA hips.

HA-coated knee prostheses tend to meet with more skepticism than HA-coated hips. However, for years some papers have reported on promising results with HA-coated knees. Verhaar (1) and Epinette (2) had good clinical reports in two papers published in 1995. More recently, Nilsson et al. (3) published in the *Journal of Arthroplasty* about a prospective randomized comparison of HA-coated and cemented tibial components with 5-years of follow-up using Roentgen Stereophotogrammetric Analysis (RSA). They concluded that the HA knee group could potentially offer longer lasting stability.

Our experience with HA TKA began in 1990 with the Omnifit Knee (Osteonics, Allendale, NJ, USA). Since that first implantation, we have implanted 400 HA-coated primary knees at the Clinique Medico-Chirurgicale of Bruay-Labuissiere, France. We will report on a prospective study detailing our 12-year experience with HA-coated knees. The study was led by CRDA (Center of Orthopaedic Research in Arthroplasty), and OrthoWave outcome study software was used.

MATERIALS AND METHODS

The Series

Beginning in 1990, 400 HA-coated knees were implanted in 342 patients, 74 males and 326 females by one of us (JAE) in the same clinic and using the same operative procedure. Fifty-eight cases involved bilateral implantations. Of the 400 knees, 364 knees remain "on file" (91%), 23 (5.8%) died for reasons unrelated to the hip, 3 (0.75%) were revised for sepsis, 5 (1.25%) were assessed as "out of study" because of major disabling, non knee-related problems, 4 knees (1%) underwent a revision for mechanical failure, and one patient who underwent a unilateral replacement (0.25%) was lost to follow-up. Of the 400 operated knees, 268 had minimum follow-ups greater than five years; 65 had a minimum follow-up greater than 10-years, and 7 had greater than 12-year minimum follow-up.

Type of Implants

In all cases, the type of implant used was a HA-coated knee. Both femoral and tibial components were HA-coated; we excluded from the study the so-called "hybrid" replacements. The first 49 cases (12%) implanted was the partial HA-coated Series 3000 Omnifit knee femoral component. A HA-coated beaded component was used in 25 cases (6%), a fully HA-coated Series 3000 Omnifit component was used in 129 cases (32%), and the Series 7000 OmnifitHA was used in 74 cases (18%). The posterior cruciate ligament was retained in all cases. More recently, we began using posterior cruciate substituting (PS) knees. To date, we have used the HA Scorpio™ PS knee in 104 cases (26%).

In more than 50% of all implanted knee designs (222 knees), the femoral size was 7, followed by size 9 (23%), and size 5 (17%). In the majority of cases (356 knees), the coating was hydroxyapatite plasma-sprayed onto a grit-blasted surface. In 25 cases, the coating was plasma-sprayed hydroxyapatite on microbeads, and the most recent Scorpio™ implants (18 cases) were coated with an electrochemically-deposited hydroxyapatite (referred to as "periapatite"). The underlying substrate was CoCr in all cases.

With regard to the tibial component, 11 trays were coated with HA over beads (3%), 92 tibial components were the regular Series 3000 Omnifit HA cruciate keel (23%), and 272 were the new Series 7000 Omnifit HA fully-coated delta keel (68%), which is currently matched with the Scorpio™ femoral component. The more recently used trays in 25 cases (6%) had a periapatite-coating against the tray itself and were matched with an uncoated keel. The most commonly used thickness for the PE (polyethylene) tibial insert was 8mm (50% of cases). Four screws are routinely used in the tray in order to enhance mechanical fixation.

Patellar replacement using a cemented PE non-metal backed button was performed in 137 cases (34%), mainly in the early procedures. We routinely prefer not to resurface, but perform a double facetectomy of the patella in "upside down ridge roof" shape in order to get a better congruency across the patellar groove. In the past, a systematic release of the lateral parapatellar retinaculum was performed as a routine procedure. However, presently we tend to retain as often as possible the lateral retinaculum in order to preserve an effective blood supply.

Partial weight bearing (WB) is allowed immediately. Patients undergo early mobilization, physiotherapy, and continuous passive motion (CPM). Total weight bearing is generally obtained at 2-3 months.

Methods

All patients are included in this non-selective series. Pre-op status, surgical details, and post-op management are systematically recorded. Post-op clinical and radiological evaluations are performed at the 6th week, at 4-6 months, then yearly. The secretary contacts all patients who did not attend the 5-year visit. Data are entered into the Ortho-Wave™ database, which allows us to easily access clinical and statistical information.

All cases were taken into account for complication rates. No retrievals, clinical, or radiological non re-operated failures were included in the survivorship analysis. Those cases with non knee-related very disabling problems made it difficult to assess their functional abilities; they were classified as "out of study". Of the remaining cases, only reviewed patients who completed clinical and radiological evaluations were included in the clinical study results. Assessment was performed using the International Knee Society Score (IKS) (4) global score, which includes both the 100-point knee score, and the 100-point function score. On the whole, complete post-operative clinical assessments could be achieved for 329 knees according to "knee score", and 278 according to "function score".

With respect to radiographic results, serial films were obtained post operatively, then yearly as possible. Patients were followed routinely at the two- and five-year examinations. Each follow-up included AP and lateral views, weight-bearing films, skyline views, and standing films. In addition, we systematically checked the lines at the HA-bone interface in components with more than two years of follow-up (Figure 1). Attention was given to obtain tangential beams in lateral films of femoral components, as well as AP and lateral views of tibial components, which allowed us to check as precisely as possible the different lines, should they be the so-called "lucent lines" or the "reactive lines" (5) (fig. 2).

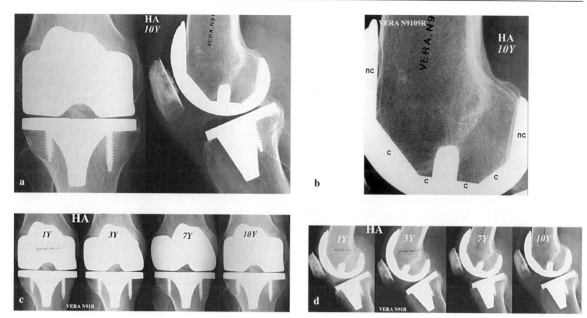

Figure 1a, b, c, d – Excellent clinical (Knee score at 98/ Function score at 100) and radiological result at 10 years post-operatively in a young 43 year-old male operated on in 1991 for osteonecrosis with insertion of a HA Omnifit 3000 knee. AP and lateral films demonstrating excellent bony apposition, and lack of reactive of lucent line onto the HA-coated aspects of the femoral component or beneath the tibial plateau, the keel, and the screws (a). Close view of the femoral component in the same patient showing the distribution of trabecular bone (b), and confirming the intimate bony apposition onto coated zones (c) and conversely the lucent lines and osteolysis onto non HA-coated zones (nc) 1 and 4. Serial films of the same patients at 1 year, 3 years, 7 years, and 10 years on AP (1c) and lateral (1d) views. No modification over time is evident on the X-rays.

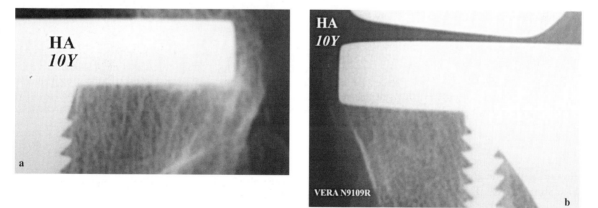

Figure 2a, b – Two close views (2a, 2b) of HA-coated tibial components at 10 years postoperatively demonstrating an intimate metal-bone contact under the tibial tray and absolute lack of gap or any fibrous tissue layer.

RESULTS

Demographics

The average age was 70.3 (34-89) years; 233 cases (58%) were over age 70 and 44 (11%) were over age 80. Conversely, only 34 knees (8.5%) were less than 60 years old. With regard to weight, only 10% were considered "regular". Obesity was "mild" in 39%, "medium" in 44% and "severe" in the remaining 7%. The mean Body Mass Index value was 30.85 (range, 17.3 to 49.8). The Charnley classification (6) placed only 19% of cases in the "A" group (i.e., no other disabling problem except the operated knee), 33% were classified as "B" (other knee affected), and 48% were classified as "C" (significant non knee-related disabling problem). All patients enrolled in the present study were primary cases. Osteoarthritis was the main aetiology (90.8%), followed by rheumatoid arthritis (7.5%), and necrosis (1.7%).

Complications

There were no perioperative adverse effects in the entire series. The post-operative complications included deep venous thrombosis (8.75%), delayed wound healing (6.75%), manipulation under anesthesia (5.25%), deep hematomae (2.5%), and infection (1%). Some of these complications led to reoperation. The 19 reoperations (4.75%) are listed in Table 1, and included 3 deep infections, 10 secondary patellar buttons for patellar pain following a single patelloplasty at the time of replacement, 1 accidental patellar fracture, 1 stiffness of the knee leading to a synoviectomy and articular debridement, and 4 failures, one for pain and stiffness and 3 for osteolysis.

The final failure rate was 1%, including one case of unexpected pain and stiffness in a 68-year old female revised at 2 years, and three cases of severe lysis in three females (age range 73-77) for whom the initial diagnosis was inflammatory (1) (fig. 3) and osteoarthritis (2). These implants underwent revision at 3, 4 and 5 years, respectively.

Reoperations	N	Cases	Comments
Pain-no loosening	1 (0.25%)	Primary case : Retrieval at 2 year Stiffness-inflammatory synovitis (rheumatoid)	
Deep infection	3 (0.75%)	3 primary knees secondary infected due to a distal severe wound infection	The 3 primary implants were retrieved and replaced by 3 stemmed cemented knees
Loosening and osteolysis	3 (0.75%)	• 1 case of severe progressive chondrocalcinosis leading to tremendous lytic femoral and tibial lesions at 5-year • 2 unexpected cases of osteolysis respectively at 3- and 4-year	The three patients are female, over 73 years of age. Prostheses were 2 HA Omnifit 7000 and 1 Scorpio knee (HA-coated)
Patellar traumatic fracture	1 (0.25%)	Only 1 patella had to be reoperated on at 2-year out of a total of 6 traumatic patellar fractures	The reoperated patella had received primarily a cemented button
Synoviectomy	1 (0.25%)	Primary case: severe stiffness due to a very curious phenomenon of "frozen knee" due to a postop retraction of the joint capsule with major non septic inflammatory synovitis	Good result following the Synoviectomy reoperated on at 2-year: no pain and good ROM (flexion over 90°). We had similar cases in shoulders and hips: maybe a sympathetic dystrophy reaction?
Secondary patellar button	10 (2.5%)	Off these 10 cases, 1 had a previous button, whilst 9 had a single patelloplasty	Delays for reoperation were respectively 1-year (6 times), 2-year (2 times), and 3- and 5-year

Table 1 – Numbers and percentages of complications leading to reoperation.

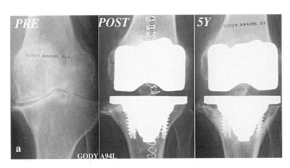

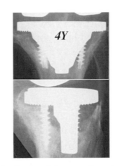

Figure 3 – Severe chondrocalcinosis leading to a tremendous amount of osteolysis at 5 years in a 77 year-old female. She was revised with a long stemmed cemented PS knee. Serial films preoperatively, postoperatively, and at 5 years (a). AP and lateral view of the tibial plateau at 4 years in the same patient (b).

Clinical Results

We first report on clinical status according to post-operative knee-related parameters, such as pain or range of motion, and to functional abilities, such as walking distance or stairs. Secondly, clinical scores based upon the IKS Rating System (4) will be displayed according to the preoperative number of cases (n =400), cases with 2 years of more of follow-up (n =222), and cases with 5 years or more of follow-up (n =87 knees), taking into account both the "Knee Score" and the "Function Score". Finally, survivorship analysis was calculated for the original cohort of 400 knees, of which 34 remain "at risk" at 7-year follow-up.

Descriptive Analysis

Pain within the whole series (n = 328) was post-operatively "none" in 95.4% of cases, "mild" (stairs or walking) in 3.7%, "moderate-occasional" in 1 case (0.3%) and "moderate-continual" in 2 cases (0.6%). No patient experienced "severe" pain post-operatively. Absence of paint remained constant over time in 96.9% of cases (n = 222) at 2 years or more, and in 98.9% (n = 87) at 5 years or more. According to patellar pain, we report "no pain" in 97.3% of cases, "mild" in 2.1% and "moderate" in 0.6%. None of the patient experienced "severe" patellar pain. These patellar results take into account the 10 secondary resurfacing cases for whom at the latest follow-up patellar pain was "none" in 7 knees, and respectively "mild", "moderate", and "severe" in each one of the three remaining knees. When breaking down the patellar results according to the surgical procedure, patellar pain was mild or moderate in 6 cases (5.4%) out of 112 resurfaced patellar replacements *versus* 3 cases (1.4%) out of 207 non-resurfaced patellae. This is highly significant in favor of non-resurfaced patellae (chi square test: p = .001)

Stability was recorded as complete in 97.9% cases in the medial-lateral plane and in 98.5% in the anterior-posterior plane. Interestingly, only 1.5% of the CR knees experienced any anterior-posterior laxity, *ie*, 5 knees out of the 258 CR knees, *versus* no AP laxity in the 63 cases in the Scorpio™ PS group. However, this difference was not significant (Chi square test, p > 0.05), which confirms the good stability obtained in the CR cohort. Observed average values for flexion were 114 ° (35-160°) in the CR group *versus* 120° (40-160) in the PS group. Of the whole population,

only 10 knees had less than 80° of flexion (3.1% of cases) ; 6.1% were recorded as between 80° and 89°, 35.8% between 90 and 119°, and 55% over 120°. No flexion contracture was recorded in 97% of cases, while only 3 knees (0.9%) experienced a flexion contracture over 16°. Observed median value for mechanical axis was ideal at 0° (*ie* femoral-tibial omega angle at 7° valgus) with a SD of 2.157, ranging from 10° valgus to 10° *varus*, while 88.2% of mechanical axis ranged between 3° valgus and 2° *varus*.

Considering *functional abilities*, walking distance was "unlimited" in 74% of cases, limited over 10 blocks in 16%, and under 10 blocks in 10%. Stairs were climbed up and down normally in 52% of the cases, "normal up, rail down" in 33%, "up and down rail" in 13%, and "up rail, unable down" in the remaining 2%. Support was "none" in 80% of the cases, with one cane needed in 19%. Limp was recorded as none in 87% of cases, moderate in 12%. Unipodal stance was normal in 84% of cases, with "slight difficulty" in 14% and "extreme difficulty" in 2%. Activity was recorded as "strenuous" in 2%, "ADL" (normal Activities of Daily Living) in 93%, "independent" in 4%, and "dependent" in the remaining 1%. Nevertheless, when breaking down the results by age this "activity" is significantly different (mean age at 63.6 years for "strenuous", 69.4 for "ADL" and 77.7 for "independent") *ie* p = .05 according to ANOVA and Kruskall & Wallis tests. Similarly, the level of activity was better in males compared to females (chi square and Pearson tests: p =.01). No statistical test was available as far as aetiology is concerned due to an insufficient number of rheumatoid cases.

IKS Results

The mean values of "*Knee Score*" (4) were noted preoperatively as 25.4 of a possible 100 points (0-59 points ; N: 400), up to 95.8 at 2 years post-op. (55-100 ; N: 222), and 96.2 at 5 years post-op. (61-100 ; N:87). Grouping results by categories ("Excellent" 95 points, "Good" 80-94 points, "Fair" 60-79 points, and "Poor" <60 points), IKS Knee results were preoperatively 100% poor. Post-operatively at 2 years or more they were classified as "Excellent"(73.4%), "Good" (22.9%), "Fair" (3.2%), and "Poor" (0.5%). At 5 years or more, cases were classified as "Excellent" (73.6%), "Good" (24.1%), "Fair" (2.3%), and "Poor" (0%) (Table 2).

Knee Score	Pre op	2-year+	5-year+
n	400	222	87
Mean Knee score	25.4 (0-59)	95.8 (55-100)	96.2 (61-100)
Excellent/Good results	0	96.3%	97.7 %

Table 2 – Knee score according to the IKS assessment.

The mean values of *"Function Score"* (4) related to all classes of patients (Charnley A, B, C), were noted preoperatively as 36.8 of a possible 100 points (0-80 points; N: 400), up to 88.4 at 2 years or more postoperatively (40-100; N:184) and 87.1 at 5 years or more postoperatively (45-100; N:69). Grouping results by categories ("Excellent" 95; "Good" 80-94; "Fair" 60-79 and "Poor" <60 points), IKS Function results for all cases were 87.3% "Poor" and 11.0% "Fair" preoperatively, while at 2 years or more postoperatively, cases were classified as "Excellent" (48.4%), "Good" (31.5%), "Fair" (15.2%) and "Poor" (4.9%). At 5 years or more postoperatively, cases were classified as "Excellent" (50.6%), "Good" (27.6%), "Fair" (14.5%) and "Poor" (7.3%) (Table 3).

Function Score	Pre op	2-year+	5-year+
n	400	222	87
Mean Function score	36.8 (0-80)	88.4 (40-100)	87.1 (45-100)
Excellent/Good results	0	79.9%	78.2%

Table 3 – Functional score according to the IKS assessment.

No significant differences were reported when crossing knee and function results with sex, obesity, age and patellar replacement. When crossing Aetiology and Function Scores, there is no significant difference. We found a significant difference (ANOVA: p =.05; Kruskall Wallis: p = .05) when comparing Knee Score and Aetiology. The mean values for Osteoarthritis and Rheumatoid arthritis were, respectively, 96.1 and 96.8 against a mean value of knee score, reaching only 80.5 in the "Necrosis" group.

Radiological Results

Results were recorded in accordance with the IKS radiographic areas, leading to an assessment of the bone bonding areas in 176 HA knees at minimum 2 year follow-up, including 40 partially coated implants on the femoral side, excluding zones 1 and 4 (Omnifit 3000) 19 "HA on Beads" fully-coated (Omnifit "HB"), and 117 fully-coated femoral components (Omnifit7000 and Scorpio™). With respect to the tibial components, 70 uncoated cruciate keels with HA-coated trays are to be compared to both 7 cruciate keels with "HA-on-beads" coated trays, and 99 fully-coated delta keels. Periapatite-coated components did not reach a sufficient follow-up as to be enrolled in the present study (figs 4, 5, 6).

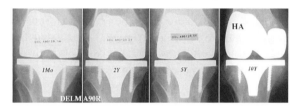

Figure 4 – Serial films of a HA-coated Omnifit 3000 at 1 month, 2 years, 5 years and 10 years: No modification with time, no migration or tilt, and excellent bony apposition under the tibial plateau, the keel and the screws.

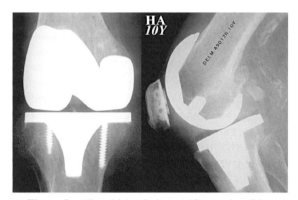

Figure 5 – AP and lateral view at 10 years in a 76 year-old female patient. Excellent radiological result. Clinical result : Knee score at 91 / Function score at 100.

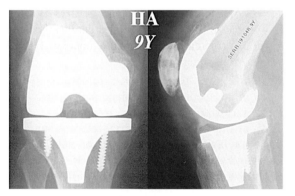

Figure 6 – Excellent radiological result with intimate bony apposition, with no line around the components and the screws at 9 years postoperatively in a 77 year-old rheumatoid patient. (Clinically: Knee score at 92; Function score at 100)

Femoral Components

Lines were more frequent on the smooth non-coated areas (zones 1 and 4 of the partially-coated implants, respectively 23% and 29%, as compared to the HA-coated zones in all groups, where percentages are zero or close to zero in all cases. Despite the "HA on Beads" type of coating, this implant performed better in zones 1 and 4 (5% and 10%) than the uncoated areas of the "partially-coated" components. These beads did not allow better (line free) interfaces compared to the HA-coated grit-blasted substrates (0% in the same zones). The lack of lines around the pegs and surrounding bony structures indicates that hydroxyapatite coating appears to assist in achieving good stability. Our previous experience with HA hips suggested that lines might lead to secondary osteolysis. These findings would have been disastrous regarding our first group of HA components, considering more than 25% of them experienced some lines around uncoated areas. However, we never observed any kind of significant osteolysis in any of these cases.

Osteolysis is not an issue in HA Knees with respect to radiographic changes, as percentages are close to zero in all areas of all types of HA-coated components in this study. Tabulated information on femoral components can be found in Table 4.

Tibial Components

Lines occurred more frequently (from 21% to 42%) in the smooth, uncoated areas of the uncoated cruciate keels (zones 5, 6, and 7 on the A/P view and zone 3 on the lateral view) compared to the HA-coated delta keel, where percentages are zero or close to zero in all cases. However, the coating may only partly be the reason, as the enhanced stability afforded by a better keel design, i.e., the delta keel, may also have a significantly beneficial effect on overall stability. In any case, our experience showed that the fully-coated delta keel design provided the best results with regard to stability.

Lines were commonly found beneath the tibial tray, with no statistical difference between the partially-coated Omnifit HA 3000 series and the fully-coated Omnifit HA 7000 series. Although these percentages are not cause for great concern, they occasionally surpass 10%. Interestingly, we have had an opportunity to compare the type of lines observed in total knees with HA-coated CoCr substrates to the lines found with HA-coated titanium substrate of the HA Unix knees. Percentages of lines and lysis in the long run were close to zero with the HA-coated titanium Unix components (7).

Reactive lines or lucent lines in HA-coated trays were recorded particularly at either the medial aspect of the plateau in AP films (i.e., zone C1) or the anterior aspect in lateral films (i.e., zones L1 and L2). We often defined this as a "scalloping" of the plateau, similar to the way we define limited lysis at the upper part of the femur in hip prostheses. The origin of these lines may be related to some lytic action of the joint fluid under pressure, as documented by Schmalzried and Whiteside (8-10). In any case, neither extensive lysis nor mechanical loosening was demonstrated in the whole series. Osteolytic rates demonstrated throughout the present study were low (under 5%) in all cases with over 2 years of follow-up. In addition, comparison between immediate post-op and later examination confirmed no change, particularly beneath the tibial plateau, around the screws, or around the keel. Tabulated information on tibial components can be found in Table 5.

Finally, the most important finding as regards the HA biological interface was demonstrated by the ability for bone to fill in areas where lucent lines due to a fibrous tissue layer were previously

Femoral component	Partia l coating N: 40		HA on beads N:19		Total coating N: 117	
	Lines	Lysis	Lines	Lysis	Lines	Lysis
Zone 1	23% (NC)	3%	5%	0%	0%	2%
Zone 2	11%	0%	0%	0%	0%	1%
Zone 5/6/7 (pegs)	0%	0%	0%	0%	0%	1%
Zone 3	8%	0%	0%	0%	1%	1%
Zone 4	29% (NC)	0%	10%	0%	0%	1%

Table 4 – (Femoral component): Breakdown of "Lines" (i.e., reactive lines and lucent lines) and osteolytic zones ("Lysis") according to IKS radiographic femoral zones at 2 years + in 176 HA Knees. (Percentages are cumulative for the related zones. NC: Non-coated areas).

Tibial component	HA Partial coating (Cruciate) N: 70		HA on beads partial coating (Cruciate) N:7		HA Total coating (delta HA) N: 99	
	Lines	Lysis	Lines	Lysis	Lines	Lysis
AP Zone 1	9%	1%	28%	0%	6%	3%
AP Zone 2	7%	0%	43%	0%	4%	2%
Zone 5/6/7 (keel)	28% (NC)	0%	42% (NC)	0%	0%	1%
AP Zone 3	6%	0%	43%	0%	5%	2%
AP Zone 4	8%	0%	43%	0%	7%	3%
Lat Zone 1	12%	1%	0%	0%	5%	3%
Lat Zone 3 (keel)	21% (NC)	0%	35% (NC)	0%	1%	1%
Lat Zone 2	5%	0%	14%	0%	1%	2%

Table 5 – (Tibial component): Breakdown of "Lines" (i.e., reactive lines and lucent lines) and Osteolytic zones ("Lysis") according to IKS radiographic tibial zones (respectively AP and lateral films) at 2 years + in 176 HA Knees. (Percentages are cumulative for the related zones – NC: Non-Coated zones).

observed. In some cases, between the first and second year, we observed a lucent line beneath the tibial plateau. In all of these cases, the radiological evaluation over years demonstrated a progressive pattern, i.e., formation of new bony bridges between bone and metal and a progressive new bony structure filling in the gap (fig. 6a, b, c). The explanation can be found in Søballe's works, demonstrating that the fibrous tissue beneath a HA interface contains collagen fibers regularly assembled in a perpendicular axis to the metallic surface and able to guide a secondary bony ongrowth (11). Conversely, the random distribution of collagen fibers in the presences of a porous coating does not cause the bone to fill in the gap. This finding is striking, and this ability to fill in gaps must be seen as a great benefit in favor of HA compared to porous coatings and cemented interfaces.

Survivorship Analysis

Cumulative survival rate, according to Kaplan-Meier analysis, was calculated for primary cases (n = 400) with 34 knees remaining on file at 7 years. (The number of knees examined between 7 and 12 years is not large enough to be statistically significant for cumulative survivorship analysis.) When considering all retrievals (failures + traumatic + deep infection cases), the cumulative survival rate is 0.9461 ± 0.0406. When considering all failures (retrievals for mechanical failures + non-reoperated clinical and radiological failures), the cumulative survival rate is 0.9703 ± 0.0284.

DISCUSSION

The HA results are very encouraging when compared to cemented results

Results in this study may represent an interesting counterweight to both cemented and porous-coated knee series. Our HA-coated knee experience reaches now to 12-year of follow-up. The current series is a consecutive, prospective and non-selective one, the average age was 70 years, and of the 400 operated primary knees at 12-year maximum follow-up, only one patient (0.25%) was lost to follow-up. The mean IKS values at 5 years post-op were 96.2 points and 87.1 points regarding, respectively, "Knee Score" and "Function Score". In such a way, we recorded 96.3% (knee score) and 78.2% (function score) of excellent and good results (>=80 points). Radiographic changes indicated very good HA-bone interface for both the femoral and tibial components. Few lytic lines were observed on HA-coated surfaces and no extensive lysis was demonstrated, especially beneath the tibial plateau and around keel or screws.

The final failure rate was 1%, including one case of unexpected pain and stiffness and three cases of severe lysis. This very low lytic rate suggests that the bigger diameter of debris in knees (compared to the hip) does not lead to a macrophagic reaction and may explain why lysis was not, in our experience, a critical concern. The cumulative survival rate at 7 years, while taking into account all failures, reaches 0.9703 ± 0.0284, which is a very encouraging mid-term result (fig. 7a, b). These results compare favorably with cemented and porous series previously published (12-15).

Over time, prosthetic designs have evolved dramatically

Initially, implants were partially HA-coated (Omnifit 3000) with a non HA-coated cruciate keel. Although these first implants afforded good clinical results, the radiographic changes we observed led us to ask for a fully coated femoral component (Omnifit 7000), which had a fully coated delta keel that seemed to provide significantly better mechanical fixation. Some concerns have been voiced about trying to retrieve a fully coated component during revision surgery without increasing site morbidity. However, retrieval of a tibial tray would mainly occur for two reasons, deep infection or massive osteolysis with loosening. Retrieval would be relatively simple in these cases, since there would be no significant bone bonding around the keel in either instance.

Screws are another controversial concern

Through our experience, these screws never led to any clinical or radiological problem. With the exception of one case, we observed no lysis around the screws in the whole series. In addition, no evidence of PE wear due to the head of screws was ever proved. Therefore, we consider screws a great help in enhancing the mechanical fixation of the tibial component, and we advocate the systematic use of screws in knees.

X-rays have yielded encouraging results

Recent RSA studies by Nilsson *et al.* (3) demonstrated very promising outcomes with HA knees if a sound primary stability is achieved after the operation. Our radiographic findings appear to demonstrate a very good bone-implant interface, as shown by the intimate bony apposition to the HA-coated zones. We had no radiographic loosening and no lucent lines leading to lack of stability. The mechanical fixation afforded by these earlier Omnifit designs and the more current Scorpio™ knee design meets our expectation regarding achievement of primary stability, and allows HA to play its role in a sound biological, long lasting fixation (fig. 7).

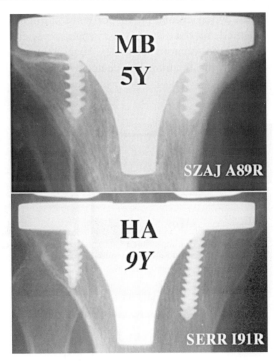

Figure 7 – Typical comparison of a microbeaded porous tibial component (MB) at 5 years and a HA-coated tibial tray (HA) at 9 years in a similar Omnifit 3000 design. The microbeaded device demonstrates lucent line, osteolysis, and bead shedding under the plateau. Conversely, there is no modification at the interface between metal and bone under the HA-coated implant and screws.

Some of our knees experienced a limited lytic area beneath the tibial plateau, mainly medially and anteriorly. We had no clear explanation, since the post-operative films showed very intimate contact, and the short amount of time elapsed makes any polyethylene wear or debris-related problems highly unlikely. However, it seemed to us that in some cases, the lines beneath the tibial plateau and lytic zones, which occurred very shortly after the operation, would be explained by any reaction to kinases caused by the joint fluid. The bone bonding apposing CoCr trays was not excellent at this first stage, and may have provided some pathways for the joint fluid under pressure. We were impressed by the theory proposed by Schmalzried and Whiteside (8-10) about the lytic properties of the joint fluid, and our findings seem to agree with this explanation. Fortunately, in all of these cases, radiological evaluations over time demonstrated the formation of new bony bridges between bone and metal and a progressive new bony structure filling in the gap. This ability to fill in gaps should be seen as a great benefit in favor of HA when compared to porous coatings and cemented interfaces (fig. 8). Further experiences with HA on titanium substrates, such as our findings with the titanium HA-coated Uni Knee (16, 17), would be extremely interesting with respect to this behavior of bone apposing HA under different metallic substrates. Naturally, the ultimate goal is direct and immediate bone bonding.

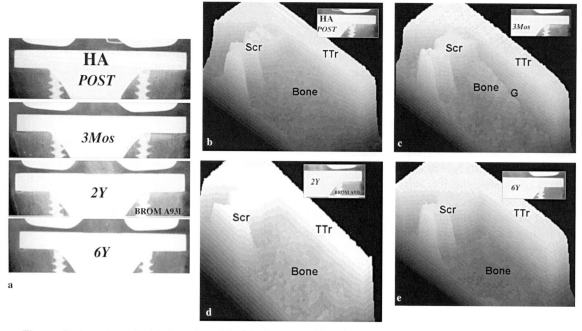

Figures 8a, b, c, d, e – Serial close views (a) of the bone metal interface under a HA-coated tibial component, respectively at post operative period, then at 3 months, 2 years and 6 years. These X-rays have been managed in 3D using Imagika software (b, c, d, e), using bone density as the z axis. Clearly demonstrated is the main advantage afforded by HA coatings, i.e., the ability for HA to fill in fibrous tissue gaps with new bone formation. Figure 8b shows no gap under the plateau; 8c shows typical lysis beneath the plateau at 3 months; 8d shows complete remodeling at 2 years totally filling the previous gap, and 8e shows final intimate bone-metal interface and excellent transmission of loads.

The final issue addresses our behavior regarding the PCL

Should we retain it or substitute it? For the past 17 years, we have retained the PCL, initially using the porous Miller-Galante Knee, and later on the Omnifit HA designs. The results were quite good, as demonstrated in the current study. Almost 75% of our knees were posterior cruciate retaining. Thus, why did we move to the HA Scorpio™ posterior sacrificing knee?

Some studies comparing PR results to PS results have for years reported virtually identical results. Retaining the PCL is a demanding surgical procedure because an effective balance must always be obtained. Additionally, in many cases, the PCL looks a bit loose, and we may anticipate, especially in heavy persons, some instability. Our initial findings seem to demonstrate that in bilateral cases (cruciate retaining on one side, Scorpio™ PS on the other side), patients subjectively spoke about

faster functional recovery, and better subjective stability upon the Scorpio™ PS side. Consequently, we remain satisfied with the Scorpio™ knee (fig. 9). We have to bear in mind that this new

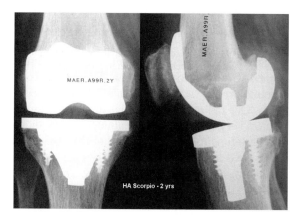

Figure 9 – HA coated postero-cruciate substituting Scorpio Knee at 2 years of follow-up (AP and lateral films in the same patient).

Scorpio™ design incorporates interesting features, including an epicondylar axis that allows a single radius for the femoral curve, and a very well designed patellar groove (fig. 9).

CONCLUSION

HA is not a "magic powder", and HA implants must prove their efficacy when compared to cemented or porous designs. Technical skills and appropriate design are certainly more important than the interface. Nevertheless, the current study demonstrates that we obtained excellent results using HA-coated Omnifit knee implants (fig. 10). These results are as good, and often better, than the best-cemented or porous studies at minimum ten year follow-up. Radiographic findings were encouraging and confirmed the excellent intimate contact between bone and metal, with no appreciable difference between the minimum 2-year and minimum 5-year follow-up examinations. Furthermore, the HA coating appears over time to aid in filling gaps, which should be viewed as an excellent benefit of bioconductive coatings.

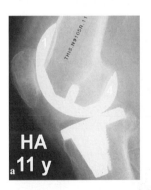 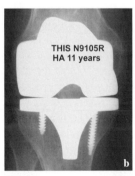

Figures 10a, b – Excellent clinical and radiological results 11 years postoperatively. Lateral (a) and AP (b) films of a 67-year old female who received a HA-coated Omnifit knee for necrosis in 1991. No line or lysis can be observed around HA-coated areas, or around the keel and screws. (The 1 and 4 zones of the lateral femoral component were not HA-coated in these first Omnifit designs; they were smooth areas).

In this way, the current study will serve as a reference for future designs. We must follow-up with these patients in order to get long term results with this "basic HA-coated knee", and each new development or improvement in design or bioconductive coating will have to exhibit a real benefit when compared to the actual findings.

Naturally, the current study must be continued with further examination for at least 15 years in order to confirm actual cumulative survival rates. An appropriate use of survivorship analysis – considering all clinical and radiological failures and revision rates, having a significant number of patients remaining at risk at 10 or 15 year, and ensuring a minimum of patients are lost to follow-up – is an absolute prerequisite if we want to compare different series by as objective a means as possible.

We routinely use HA knees in our daily practice. The very encouraging results reported in the current study make us very confident in the ultimate outcome of bioconductive coatings in knee arthroplasty.

Reference List

1. HA Coating in Knee Arthroplasty. Principles, Importance and Results. Jan Verhaar In Cahiers d'enseignement de la SOFCOT: "Hydroxyapatite Coated Hip and Knee Arthroplasty", 1995, n° 51, pp. 319-22, Paris, Expansion Scientifique Française Ed. (English Volume).

2. Hydroxyapatite and TKR : The HA Omnifit Knee Prosthesis, Jean-Alain Epinette In Cahiers d'enseignement de la SOFCOT: "Hydroxyapatite Coated Hip and Knee Arthroplasty", 1995, n° 51, pp. 323-32. Paris, Expansion Scientifique Française Ed. (English Volume).

3. Kjell G. Nilsson, Johan Kärrholm, Lars Carlsson, and Tore Dalen (1999) Hydroxyapatite Coating *versus* Cemented Fixation of the Tibial Component in Total Knee Arthroplasty. *J. Arthroplasty* 14:9-20.

4. Insall JN, Dorr LD, Scott RD, Scott WN (1989) Rationale of the knee society clinical rating system. *Clin. Orthop.* 248:13-4.

5. Epinette, J.A and Geesink RGT (1996) "Radiographic Assessment in Cementless Arthroplasty, the ARA score" in Cahiers d'enseignement de la SOFCOT: "Hydroxyapatite Coated Hip and Knee Arthroplasty", n° 51, pp. 114-26, Paris, Expansion Scientifique Française Ed. (English Volume).

6. Charnley J (1972) The long term results of Low-Friction arthroplasty of the hip performed as a primary intervention. *J. Bone Joint Surg.* 54-B:61-76.

7. Epinette JA and Edidin AA (1997) Hydroxyapatite coated unicompartmental knee replacement; a report of five to six years' follow-up of the HA Unix Tibial Component, in Cahiers d'Enseignement de la Sofcot, n° 61 (English Volume) "Unicompartmental Knee Arthroplasty", pp. 243-59. Paris, Expansion Scientifique Française.

8. Periprosthetic bone loss in total hip arthroplasty (1992). Polyethylene wear debris and the concept of the effec-

tive joint space. Schmalzried TP, Jasty M, Harris WH in *J. Bone Joint Surg Am.* 74(6):849-63.

9. The role of access of joint fluid to bone in periarticular osteolysis (1997) A report of four cases. Schmalzried TP, Akizuki KH, Fedenko AN, Mirra J in *J. Bone Joint Surg. Am.* 79(3):447-52.

10. Effect of porous-coating configuration on tibial osteolysis after total knee Arthroplasty (1995). Whiteside LA in *Clin. Orthop.* (321):92-7.

11. Søballe K, Hansen ES, Rasmussen HB, Bünger C (1996) Fixation of porous coated *versus* HA coated implants, in Cahiers d'enseignement de la SOFCOT: "Hydroxyapatite Coated Hip and Knee Arthroplasty", n° 51, pp 71-84, Paris, Expansion Scientifique Française Ed. (English volume).

12. Søballe K, Toksvig-Larsen S, Gelineck J, Fruensgaard S, Hansen E-S, Ryd L, Lucht U, Bunger C (1993) Migration of hydroxyapatite coated femoral prostheses. *J. Bone Joint Surg.* 75-B:681.

13. Stern SH, Insall JN (1992) Posterior stabilized prosthesis. Results after follow-up of nine to twelve years. *J. Bone Joint Surg. Am.* (United States), 74(7):980-86.

14. Ranawat CS, Flynn WF, Saddler S *et al.* (1993) Long-term results of the total condylar knee arthroplasty. A 15-year survivorship study. *Clin. Orthop.* (United States), 286:94-102.

15. Schai PA, Thornhill TS, Scott RD (1998) Total knee arthroplasty with the PFC system. Results at a minimum of ten years and survivorship analysis. *J. Bone Joint Surg. Br.* (England), 80(5):850-8.

16. Bauer TW, Jiang M, Epinette JA (1997) Hydroxyapatite-Coated Unicompartimental Knee Arthroplasty: Histologic Analysis of Retrieved Implants in Cahiers d'enseignement de la SOFCOT: "Unicompartment Knee Arthroplasty", n° 61, p. 43-50, Paris, Expansion Scientifique Française Ed. (English Volume).

17. Epinette JA, Edidin AA (1997) 'Hydroxyapatite-Coated Unicompartmental Knee Replacement, A Report of Five to Six Years' Follow-up of the HA Unix Tibial Component" in Cahiers d'enseignement de la SOFCOT: "Unicompartmental Knee Arthroplasty", n° 61, p. 243-59, Paris, Expansion Scientifique Française Ed. (English Volume).

2 Results and Perspectives at Ten-Year Follow-up of a Hydroxyapatite Coated Total Knee Replacement

Oliver Keast-Butler, FRCS, Rami Hussein, FRCS and John Shepperd, FRCS

INTRODUCTION

HA coatings have been shown to be effective in achieving secure bone-prostheses bonding in comparison with simple uncemented implants in total hip arthroplasty. Long term results have proved to be satisfactory (1). Uncemented knee replacements have not been as successful as cemented designs. In a comparison between a cemented and uncemented version of the same knee replacement, the ten year survival of the uncemented group was 72% in comparison with 92% survival in the cemented group (2). Hydroxyapatite coated total knee replacements offer numerous potential advantages in comparison with cement fixation and plain uncemented prostheses.

Cement fixation is associated with high intramedullary pressurisation and high temperatures at the cement interfaces as a result of the exothermic properties of the methylmethacrylate cement. We believe this has harmful local and systemic effects. Damage to the surrounding bone will affect the cement-bone interface, potentially resulting in decreased mechanical stability of the prostheses and creating potential dead spaces. Uncemented techniques avoid these problems and the increased speed of surgery further decreases intraoperative bacterial colonisation decreasing the risk of infection. It also decreases limb ischaemia if a tourniquet is used.

RSA studies have demonstrated that, in comparison with uncemented prostheses, hydroxyapatite coating decreases early subsidence in total knee replacement (3, 4, 5) an important predictor in long term survival (6). RSA studies have also suggested that stability at five years using HA coated tibial components is superior to cement fixation (7). Initial stability provides the optimal

environment for subsequent bonding of the bone and implant, although in experimental models, with the presence of hydroxyapatite, bonding can occur with some motion (8, 9).

Well integrated components, both cemented and uncemented are difficult to revise. Avoidance of cemented techniques will result in an overall preservation of bone stock, an important issue, particularly in younger patients.

While well established in total hip replacements, the introduction of HA as a coating in knee replacements has been slow. Whereas hip replacements are primarily subjected to axial compression, the tibial component of knee replacements is subjected to axial and horizontal shear forces. It is a challenge to provide adequate initial stability in knee replacement to allow bonding to take place.

We have reviewed our first 100 hydroxyapatite coated knee replacements at 8-10 years postoperatively and have subsequently investigated design changes to improve stability of the tibial component.

Patients and Methods

Between March 1990 and November 1992 we performed 100 consecutive primary total knee replacements using a fully hydroxyapatite coated Insall-Burstein II prostheses (Wright Cremascoli). This is a posterior constrained device which sacrifices the posterior cruciate ligament. The components are manufactured from cobalt chrome alloy and the tibial component has a modular polyethylene insert which is fixed into the tibial tray with a cer-clip. The bone interface surfaces of the component are plasma sprayed with hydroxyapatite.

Standard jigs/cutting blocks were used and the tibial component was secured into the tibial metaphysis with 4 cancellous screws. The average age of the patient was 72.5 years (32-92 years). Joint replacement was performed with a medial parapatella incision. Patella replacement was performed if there was excessive wear of the patella surface. Bilateral procedures were performed under the same anaesthetic in 21 people and staged in 1 person. Indications for surgery were osteoarthritis (93 cases), rheumatoid arthritis (5 cases) and PVNS (2 cases). At surgery, 3 knees required cemented tibial components for technical reasons and were excluded from the series. A further 4 knees required cement augmentation of the anterior femur due to the small size of femur and lack of a suitably sized prosthesis. These were included in the series. Antibiotic prophylaxis was used and patients were treated in a compression bandage for 2 days. After this, full weight bearing mobilisation was commenced and patients were discharged when fit.

Patients were seen preoperatively and postoperatively at 6 weeks, 6 months and then annually for assessment. Standard weight bearing AP, lateral, and skyline views were obtained for clinical evaluation. These were evaluated for subsidence and radiolucent areas (10). Patients were scored according to the Hospital for Special Surgery knee score (11), combining function and symptoms, with a maximum score of 100. Perioperative complications were not collected prospectively, and all patients seen for 8-10 year review had this information collected by review of hospital notes.

Survival analysis was calculated using a life table (12, 13). Failures were withdrawn in the year in which they failed. Failure rates were calculated with revision, pain, and knee score as endpoints.

RESULTS

We achieved 100% follow-up of all living patients, including those who moved out of the area, thus ensuring that the survival analysis is reliable (14). At the most recent follow-up, 48 people (60 knees) were alive. All of these patients were assessed by the authors. Forty people (50 knees) attended hospital and had radiographic and clinical examination. Eight people (10 knees) were unable or unwilling to attend the hospital examination and were seen in their homes. Two people (3 knees) unable to attend had radiographs available from within the last 2 years, which were included in the radiographic assessment. Four patients had dementia, and a formal knee score was not possible. We reviewed the notes of people who had died (29). Of these, 3 people had not been seen for 2 years, and 2 people had not been seen for 4 years by an orthopaedic surgeon. None of these had moved away from the region, and other medical notes did not report any problems with regard to their knee replacement. These patients were withdrawn from analysis in their year of death. All other patients had been seen within 1 year of death, and there were no impending failures.

Survival Analysis

Life table analysis has been performed and a survival curve plotted (Table 1). Confidence intervals have been calculated from the effective number at risk using Rothman's formula (13). Using revision as the endpoint for failure, the nine year survival is 92% (CI 0.94-0.84).

Year	Number at start	Revised	With-drawn	Number at risk	Effective number at risk	Failure	Success %	Survival %	95% CI
0-1	97	1	7	92.5	92.5	1.08	98.9	98.9	0.98-0.95
1-2	89		4	87	89.7	0	100	98.9	0.98-0.95
2-3	85	1	4	82.5	87.1	1.21	98.8	97.7	0.98-0.94
3-4	80	1	7	76	84.1	1.32	98.7	96.4	0.97-0.92
4-5	72	1	2	70.5	80.9	1.41	98.6	95	0.96-0.90
5-6	69	1	4	66.5	78.1	1.5	98.5	93.5	0.95-0.88
6-7	64	1	4	62	75.3	1.61	98.4	91.9	0.93-0.8
7-8	59		5	56.5	72.3	0	100	91.9	0.93-0.86
8-9	54		29	39.5	66.2	0	100	91.9	0.93-0.84

Table 1 – Cumulative Survival Rate at 9 Years.

Radiological Evaluation

The Knee Society Radiological Evaluation scoring system was used (fig. 1) (10).

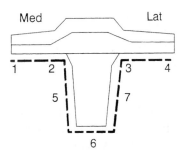

Figure 1 – Knee Society Radiological Evaluation score.

The low incidence of radiolucent lines (0% of knees having a significant score) and the evidence of bone integration demonstrate the long term stability of the bone–prostheses interface (Table 2).

Figures 2a and 2b show 10 year follow up radiographs demonstrating a uniform bone–prostheses interface with trabecular realignment adjacent to

	Tibial Component	Femoral Component
Aseptic Loosening	3	2
Bonded (revised to match other component)	2	2
Infected	1	1
Technical Error	0	1

Table 2 – Distribution of radioculent lines and steolytic lesions adjacent to the proteins according to the various zones.

tibial stem. Table 3 demonstrates the number of knees with radiolucent lines/osteolytic lesions adjacent to the prostheses in 7 zones (47 knees at 8-11 years follow-up). Figures 3a and 3b show 10-year lateral radiographs demonstrating spot welds around the tibial stems.

Pain as Endpoint for Failure

If moderate pain at rest or during exercise at the most recent assessment is used as an endpoint for failure, 5 surviving knees (9.3%) are in this cate-

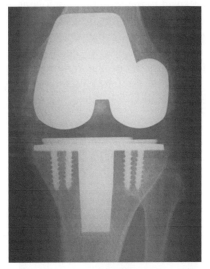
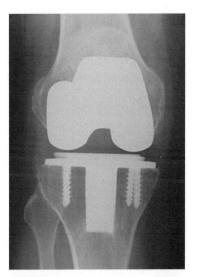

a
b

Figure 2a, b – Ten year follow up radiographs, demonstrating uniform bone – prostheses interface with trabecular realignment adjacent to tibial stem.

	Zone 1	Zone 2	Zone 3	Zone 4	Zone 5	Zone 6	Zone 7	Average score
Tibia AP	3	3	0	1	1	1	2	0,39
Femur Lateral	4	1				2		0,12
Tibia Lateral	3	0	0					0,14

Table 3 – Operative findings with regards to the six revision operations.

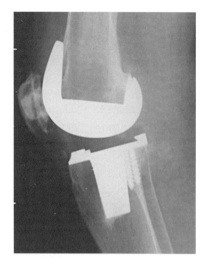 (a)

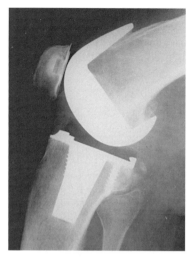 (b)

Figure 3a, b – 10 year lateral radiographs demonstrating spot welds around the tibial stems.

gory. Published results for a series of cemented IB2 TKR's was reported as 17% moderate/severe pain at eight years follow-up (15). This difference may be due to the different methods of symptomatic scoring (direct questioning versus postal questionnaire). There is no suggestion that this uncemented prostheses is more painful than its cemented version. Figures 4a and 4b show retrieved prostheses demonstrating bonding of bone to hydroxyapatite coated prostheses. There have been six revision operations; the operative findings are summarised in Table 2.

Analysis of Failures

Aseptic loosening is caused either by failure of the bone-prostheses interface or delamination of the hydroxyapatite coating from the prostheses.

With respect to the femoral component, accurate cutting of the distal femur is essential to achieve a secure press-fit. Initially, the femoral cutting block design resulted in excessive bone removal with a subsequent loose fit of the femoral component. During the series, the femoral cutting blocks were modified to remove less bone, improving initial

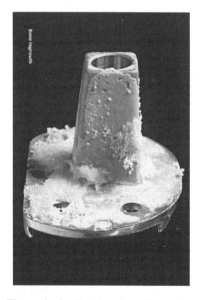 (a)

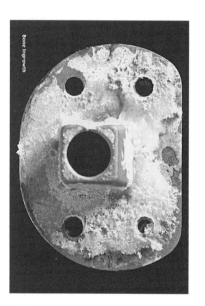 (b)

Figure 4a, b – Retrieved prostheses demonstrating bonding of bone to hydroxyapatite coated prostheses.

stability. The 2 cases of femoral component loosening were from the early part of the series and can be considered as failures of surgical technique, due to lack of initial stability. There have been no further cases of aseptic femoral component loosening.

Uncemented tibial component fixation provides a greater challenge. The IB II knee replacement was designed to be fixed with cement and has a tibial stem to increase stability. To achieve initial fixation with the hydroxyapatite coated prostheses, four screws were used to secure the tibial tray to the metaphysis, augmenting the press-fit nature of the tibial stem. Three tibial components were revised for aseptic subsidence due to failure of bone-prostheses bonding and resulting subsidence. By modifying the design to improve early stability, we believe that the results will be improved.

Design Modification

Work has been carried out on the design of the tibial tray with an aim toward improving initial stability and providing the optimal environment for implant-bone bonding. We have performed loading tests on an IBII tibial tray after attaching various smooth brass tapers to the screw holes (fig. 5). We used two different foams as bone substitute, a phenolic fragile foam, and a harder polymer foam with similar behaviour in compression to bone. The rationale behind this study was to test the effect of the taper on resistance of the prosthesis to subsidence and tilt.

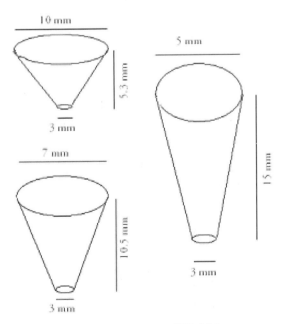

Figure 5 – Loading tests on an IBII tibial tray.

The taper increases the contact area between the prosthesis and foam, thereby allowing a wider distribution of forces at the interface. A mean area of 23mm on the under surface of the tibial tray is converted to a mean of 168.7mm for each peg. The shape of the taper changes the force vectors passing from the prosthesis to the foam, this being affected by the slope. The taper shape changes the force vectors passing from the prosthesis to the bone, and should have a stabilising effect in tension. In the fragile foam, the best improvement in tilt and subsidence resistance of the tibial tray was seen with short pegs, while in the closed cell foam, initial subsidence and tilt resistance improved with the medium pegs. These results support the concept that stability of the tray varies with bone quality, and that instability can be overcome or improved by adding suitable tapered pegs.

While hydroxyapatite delamination has not been a problem in our series, further improvements such increasing the porosity of the component surface and choice of materials (titanium as opposed to cobalt chrome) may further improve results.

Comparison With Cemented Total Knee Replacements

Long term implant success can be analysed with a number of different end points. It has been suggested that, as the initial indication for arthroplasty is for pain relief, that pain and function are the key indicators of success. Other endpoints include revision or need for revision and evidence of component loosening. Good long-term results for various cemented total knee replacements have been published (16, 17, 18). A series of cemented IB II TKR's had a best-case scenario of 92.3% survival at ten years (19).

Radiolucent lines are seen in cemented and uncemented prosthesis and are considered to indicate loosening of the prostheses. The incidence of radiolucent lines in this study was low, and similar findings have been described with hydroxyapatite in total hip replacement.1 In a series of cemented IB II's 19, 10 knees (9.6%) had significant osteolysis (score > 5) around the tibial component. None of the radiographs taken at long-term follow up in our series had a score > 4 around the tibial component, indicating secure fixation at long term follow-up. Furthermore, evidence of bone apposition and ingrowth around the tibial stem was present in 72% of radiographs (spot welding/buttress formation).

CONCLUSION

Uncemented knee replacements have not been popular, and there is a paucity of peer reviewed evidence to suggest that survival matches cemented designs. We feel that the hydroxyapatite coating has enhanced bone fixation in comparison to other uncemented series, resulting in good, long-term results. The consistent findings of serial radiographs taken over the follow-up, as well as evidence of a secure bone-prostheses interface in the majority of cases, suggest that these knees will continue to function well. With improved operative technique and design, we feel these results could be improved, resulting in superior long-term results for HA-coated total knee replacements when compared to cemented total knee replacements.

Reference List

1. McNally SA, Shepperd JAN, Mann CV (2000) The results at nine to twelve years of the use of a hydroxyapatite-coated femoral stem. *J. Bone Joint Surg. Br.* 378-82.

2. Duffy G, Berry DJ, Rand J (1998) *Clinical Orthopaedics and Related Research* 1998 (356):66-72.

3. Toksvig-Larsen S, Jorn LP, Ryd L, Lindstrand A (2000) Hydroxyapatite improves early fixation in comparison to porous coated. RSA study. Hydroxyapatite-Enhanced Tibial Prosthetic Fixation. *Clinical Orthopaedics and Related Research* 370:192-200.

4. Nelissen RG, Valstar ER, Rozing PM (1998) The Effect of Hydroxyapatite on the Micromotion of Total Knee Prostheses. *J. Bone Joint Surg* (A) 80(11):1665-72.

5. Regner L, Carlsson L, Karrholm J, Herberts PJ (2000) Tibial component fixation in pours and hydroxyapatite-coated total knee arthroplasty: A radiostereo metric evaluation of migration and inducible fixation after 5 years. *J. Arthroplasty* 15(6):681-9.

6. Ryd L, Albrektsson BEJ, Carlsson L, Dansgard F, Herberts P, Lindstrand A, Regner L, Toksvig-Larsen S (1995) Roentgen stereophotogrammetric analysis as a predictor of mechanical loosening of knee prostheses. *J. Bone Joint Surg. Br.* 77-B:377-83.

7. Nilsson KG, Karrholm J, Carlsson L, Dalen T (1999) Hydroxyapatite coating *versus* cemented fixation of the tibial component in total knee arthroplasty. *J. Arthroplasty* 14(1):9-63.

8. Søballe K, Hansen ES, Brockstedt-Rasmussen H, Bunger C (1992b) Tissue ingrowth into titanium and hydroxyapatite coated implants during stable and unstable mechanical conditions. *J. Orthop. Research.* 10:285-99.

9. Søballe K, Hansen ES, Rasmussen HB, Bunger C (1993a) Hydroxyapatite coating converts fibrous tissue to bone around loaded Implants. *J Bone Joint Surg. Br.* 75-B:270-78.

10. Ewald FC (1989) The Knee Society Total Knee Arthroplasty Roentgenographic Evaluation and Scoring System. *Clinical Orthopaedics and Related Research* November (248):9-12.

11. Insall JN, Ranawat CS, Aglietti P, Shine J (1976) A comparison of four models of total knee replacement prostheses. *J. Bone Joint Surg. A* 58:754-65.

12. Carr AJ, Morris RW, Murray DW, Pynsent PB (1993) Survival Analysis in Joint Replacement Surgery. *J. Bone Joint Surg. Br.* 75-B:178-82.

13. Murray DW, Carr AJ, Bulstrode C (1993) Survival Analysis of Joint Replacements. *J Bone Joint Surg Br.* 75-B:697-704.

14. Murray DW, Britton AR, Bulstrode CJK (1997) Loss to follow-up matters. *J. Bone Joint Surg. Br.* 79(2): 254-7.

15. Murray DW, Frost SJD (1998) Pain in the Assessment of total knee replacement. *J. Bone Joint Surg. Br.* 80-B: 426-31.

16. Thadani PJ, Vince KG, Ortaaslan SG, Blackburn DC, Cudiamat CV. 10-12 year follow-up of the Insall-Burnstein I total knee prosthesis. *Clinical Orthopaedics and Related Research* 380:17-29.

17. Ritter A, Worland R, Salisiki J, Helphenstine J, Edmondson K, Keating EM, Faris PM, Meding J. Flat-on-Flat, Nonconstrained, Compression Moulded Polyethylene Total Knee Replacement. *Clinical Orthopaedics and Related Research* 321:79-85.

18. Colizza WA, Insall JN, Scuderi GR J (1995) The Posterior Stabilised Total Knee Prosthesis. Assessment of polyethylene damage and osteolysis after a ten-year-minimum follow-up. *J. Bone Joint Surg.* (A) 77(11): 1713-19.

19. Li PLS, Zamora J, Bentley G (1999) The results at ten years of the Insall-Burnstein II total knee replacement. Clinical, Radiological and Survivorship Studies. *J. Bone Joint Surg. Br.* 81-B: 647-53.

3   Hydroxyapatite-Coated Unicompartmental Knee Arthroplasty
A 12-year experience with the HA Unix Prosthesis

Jean-Alain Epinette, MD, David Young, MD and Hayden Morris, MD

INTRODUCTION

Hydroxyapatite (HA) coated Unicompartmental knee arthroplasty (UKA) has for some years been considered a somewhat radical approach to unicompartmental knee arthritis for two fundamental reasons: Firstly, HA coating for joint replacements remains a controversial method for implant fixation. Secondly, unicompartmental knee arthroplasty (UKA) has not yet been universally accepted as a routine method of joint replacement (1). However, studies published in the recent literature (2-7) and results of a fifteen year follow-up presented in this book demonstrate that HA coatings are an effective technique for ensuring implant fixation. This has already been accepted in hip joint replacements. HA is now providing comparable long-term fixation to acrylic cement in both unicompartmental and total knee replacements (4, 5, 8). Furthermore, our experience over the past 20 years suggests that the UKA is able to meet the demands and expec-

tations of all other types of joint replacement. The provisos for this, as with any other joint replacement surgery includes: appropriate selection of patients, adequate surgical technique and correct choice of implant geometry (9).

Following the lead of Philippe Cartier we have since 1982, been keen supporters of the use of the UKA. However, in common with many authors on this subject, we found that the weak link in unicompartmental knee arthroplasty was the tibial component, where loosening, subsidence, wear, implant breakage, and revisions made difficult by bone stock loss were commonplace. These problems prompted us to explore other design approaches (fig. 1). The result of this quest was the creation, in 1986, of the Unix tibial component, featuring a central stabilising fin that is inserted horizontally under the tibial spine. The component has no pegs or vertical keels, and does not require the use of cement. Instead screws are used to augment fixation of the implant. Our experience with HA-coated UKAs dates back to

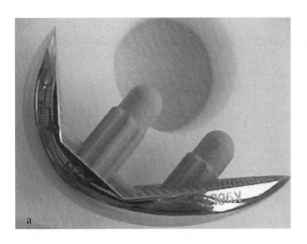
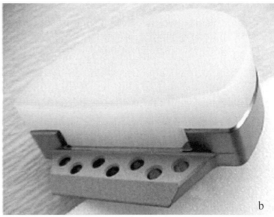

Figure 1a, b – The Unix HA coated knee. The fully HA-coated femoral component (a), and the tibial tray with the up and down HA-coated horizontal fin (b).

September 1990. At the time, the cemented Mod III femoral prosthesis was used in conjunction with HA-coated tibial components. However the Unix HA-coated femoral components were not introduced until 1994. Since then, these HA-coated femoral implants have been routinely used with the HA-coated tibial components in all our patients selected for unicompartmental arthroplasty (fig. 2). The current series is based on a multicenter study comprising 523 consecutive cases of Unix HA Tibial components implanted since 1990, matched with a HA Unix femoral component in 278 cases.

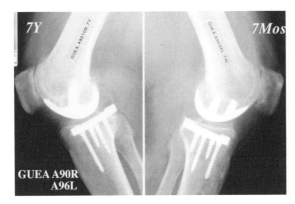

Figure 2 – Bilateral case in a 63 year-old female (osteoarthritis), operated on in 1990 (right) and in 1996 (left). The tibial component is a similar HA-coated Unix, with excellent results both at the 7th month (left) and 7th year (right). The previous cemented Mod III femoral component (right) is not yet used and has been replaced by the HA-coated Unix (left). Note that the external shape of these two components are strictly identical.

The first report on this Unix experience was published in 1997 in the "Unicompartmental Knee Arthroplasty" monograph of the SOFCOT Society (8). With increased experience over the past seven years, two questions remain of interest:

– Do the HA-coated Uni components continue to stand the test of time, i.e., How well are they performing at twelve years' clinical follow-up ?

– What are the real advantages of this "biological" fixation over that of the "tried and tested' cemented components ?

PATIENTS AND METHODS

Patient Selection and Indications

Patient selection is obviously a challenge for the surgeon. To this day, the rightful place of unicompartmental knee arthroplasty versus osteotomy and total knee arthroplasty remains blurred. Taking into account several critical parameters these choices have been described in the previous Unicompartmental monograph (10) leading to important rules we have strictly followed since that time.

Patients managed with unicompartmental replacement were the ones in whom osteotomy would have led to an inadequate outcome, while tricompartmental arthroplasty was considered an "overkill". These patients had a single tibiofemoral compartment affected by a non-inflammatory condition, with a healthy opposite compartment while anterior knee pain was not a dominant feature of the condition and no ligamentous pathology (collateral or cruciate ligaments) had been recorded preoperatively and at the time of the operation.

Whether or not HA-coated components can be used depends only on the quality of the patient's bone stock as seen at surgery and the quality of primary mechanical stabilisation that was achieved.

Principles of Surgical Technique

The principles of the preoperative investigation of the patients, of implant surgery, and of postoperative management have remained largely unchanged since our earliest arthroplasties in 1982. Throughout, we have been following the protocol laid down by Philippe Cartier and Gerard Deschamps (11).

Unicompartmental arthroplasty is a simple procedure that should not be made unnecessarily complicated. The instruments provided must enable the surgeon, at each step in the sequence, to make reproducible cuts and to automatically seat the components. The Unix knee is a "resurfacing device", unlike some unicompartmental prostheses that are really *"half-a-tricompartmental"*. On the femoral side, the bone cuts required for the ideal seating of the component are as sparing as possible. This is, in fact, conservative surgery, which leaves intact the tendons, ligaments, patellofemoral joint and the healthy opposite compartment.

One of the fundamental principles of unicompartmental replacement is under correction of axial alignment. Overcorrection may well overload and sooner or later lead to failure of the opposite compartment. The surgeon should, therefore, deliberately go for a 2-5° under correction. By the same argument, patients who have previously undergone a high tibial osteotomy for the correction of a varus deformity may be unsuitable for "Unix" joint replacement.

Self-stabilization, as defined by Philippe Cartier, is the key design feature of the "Unix". During surgery, a tibial trial is simply laid on the tibial cut surface, underneath the condyle, to carry out full stability testing in flexion and extension. If the tibial trial tends to lift off or shift horizontally in flexion, the bone cuts will need to be redone, and a check should be made to rule out posterior obstacles (meniscal remnants, loose bodies and particularly retained osteophytes), ligament imbalance, or impingement from overhang of the posterior part of the condyle on the tibia in full flexion. Testing must be continued until the two components have "self-stabilized', since it is upon this condition that the longevity of the implant is dependant. Once self-stabilization and self-centering has been obtained, the final position of the tibial trial is marked, to serve as a guide for the implantation of the definitive component. This is a very important step in fixed bearing prostheses.

Our surgical approach was "minimal" in terms of length of skin incision. While "minimal invasive surgery" has recently become fashionable we have always borne in mind that the unicompartmental replacement remains a challenging surgical procedure, and the main goal is to perform adequate surgery, leading to long lasting excellent results. Our surgical protocol does not always dislocate the patella (this practice is reserved for those cases when large osteophytes need to be resected). This point has been crucial over the past 20 years in our experience for faster recovery. This is in accordance with the proposal pointed out recently by the disciples of the "minimally invasive surgery" techniques (12).

Patients are started on a CPM machine immediately after surgery. Protected weight bearing is permitted in the early post operative period, with elbow crutches used for the first 3-5 weeks, as dictated by the patient's age, body weight, and proprioceptive status. Normal walking without a walking aid and return to a full range of activities of daily living usually occurs before the end of the second month.

METHODS

The epidemiological data, findings at surgery, results, and complications were computerised to permit processing of the clinical and radiographic data using the OrthoWave (ARIA, Bruay, France) Knee Data Base (fig. 3). The rating system adopted was the Knee Society Score (IKS) (13), with its dual assessment of the Knee (pain, stability, alignment) and of Function (walking, stairs, walking aids, limp), with a maximum score of 100 points in either section. The cut-off points between the different groups were those commonly adopted, i.e., 95 to 100 points for an excellent rating; 80 to 94 for Good; 60 to 79 for Fair; and 60 or less for Poor.

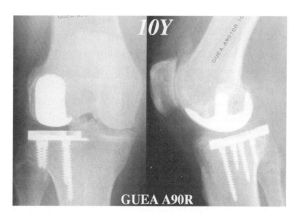

Figure 3 – Typical X-rays at 10 years of follow-up in a 67 year-old female. No radiographic change, especially no osteolysis under the plateau and around screws. Excellent clinical results at 95 points (Knee score) and 100 points (functional score).

This scoring system has been used in many studies of tricompartmental knee replacement. It was therefore important to rate our UKAs using the same system, albeit with a minor modification concerning alignment. For tricompartmental replacements, the corrected mechanical axis should be within 2° of *varus* and 3° of *valgus*. However, UKAs should be under corrected, with a minor "shift" in the penalties for varus or valgus, depending on the deformity to be corrected, and an "ideal" axis of between 0° and 5° of varus for medial compartment replacements and 0° and 5° of *valgus* for lateral compartment replacements.

The survivorship analyses (Kaplan & Meier) (14) were carried out through the "Starwave" statistical module of OrthoWave, providing the cumulative survival rates with respect to different endpoints, i.e., revision due to any cause (irrespective of success or failure of the arthroplasty itself), or aseptic loosening (reporting on the success or failure of the HA fixation). The program allows statistical tests between survival rates comparing two different cohorts. The confidence intervals are computed according to the 0.05 confidence limits. The number of knees remaining "at risk" at the maximum follow-up must stay over 30 cases.

The Series

The present study is based upon a series of 523 UKAs in 457 patients with an HA-coated "Unix" prosthesis (Osteonics, Allendale, NJ-USA), implanted since September 1990: both in France at the Bruay Clinic, and in Melbourne, Australia at three clinics, The Mercy Private The Avenue and Vimy House Private Hospitals. This series is made up of consecutive and homogeneous cases who were operated on by the three authors, using the same protocol. The implanted components were the HA-coated "Unix" tibial component in all cases, while the HA "Unix" femoral component has been used since 1994 in 345 knees (308 patients). Of the total number of UKAs, 140 had a minimum follow-up of ten years in 127 patients who had undergone joint replacement from 1990 to 1992. In all these early patients, the femoral component used was a cemented "Mod III" (Richards, USA), since the "Unix" HA femoral components did not become available until later on in 1994.

In the whole series, 489 knees (93.5%) in 429 patients are still "on file", while 20 patients (22 knees, 4.2%) are deceased. (non knee-related causes) Revisions were 10 (1.9%) in 10 patients, including 9 retrievals of the two components, and 1 isolated tibial revision. Two cases (0.4%) were recorded as "clinical failures". These two patients did not accept offers of reoperation. None of the patients in the whole study were lost to follow-up. Interestingly, in the 10 year+ group of 140 knees, 83.6% of knees remain on file, 11.4% were deceased patients, and failures were recorded in 7 knees (5%), including 6 retrievals of the two components and 1 clinical non reoperated failure.

The distribution regarding right or left and regarding gender, showed the usual pattern observed in studies of this kind. Thus, there was an even distribution between right and left knees (50.8% R, 49.2% L); and a preponderance of female patients, with women accounting for 62.7% of the total patient population. The mean age was 66.65 years (range: 32-99 years; SD 9.14) with 23 patients (4.4%) under 50 years of age and conversely 38 patients (7.2%) over 80. As expected, the medial compartment was affected more often than the lateral one: 87.8% medial *versus* 12.2% lateral. The chief aetiology was osteoarthritis (OA), which accounted for more than 95% of the cases. In the overwhelming majority of cases, the condition was one of primary OA, with only three cases of post-traumatic OA. There were 15 cases (2.9%) of osteonecrosis of the femoral condyle in the weight-bearing zone, as typically seen in elderly subjects; also, there were 2 cases of rheumatoid arthritis (RA) and one of chondrocalcinosis, which would, nowadays, constitute absolute contraindications. Many of the patients had systemic disorders; in particular, cardiopulmonary conditions (including hypertension) were found in over 58% of the cases. This finding was in keeping with the mean age of our patient material. In terms of local conditions, 9 patients had previously undergone *valgus* high tibial osteotomy (19.6%), 8 had had meniscectomies, three had undergone transposition of the anterior tibial tubercle (Elmslie type) and three had been managed with internal fixation for multi-fragment intra-articular fractures of the tibial plateaus. 55.9% of the patients were in Charnley Category A (no other condition interfering with walking); 40.9% were in Category B (both knees involved, but rest of the body normal); and 3.2% were in Category C (general disability, significantly affecting the patient's functional status).

Preoperatively, all the knees had a reasonable range of movement, with an average value of 117° of flexion (range 60°-160°), while only two knees were under 90° of flexion; no, or only low-grade (< 10°) fixed flexion deformities were recorded in 82.9% of knees, while only three knees had presented a preoperatively flexion contracture over 10°. Medio-lateral instability was recorded in only 2% as over 10° laxity. With respect to any preoperative antero-posterior instability, 96.4% of knees had been recorded as anteriorly stable, with no posterior laxity. In all cases, the reason for the patients seeking surgery was pain and the attendant functional impairment; in many of our elderly patients, the knee-related disability was only part of a wider pattern of incapacitating disorders. Body Mass Index averaged 29.14; Weight was considered as regular in 20.9%, while obesity was "mild" in 43.7%, "medium" in 34.2% and "severe" in the remaining 1.2%. Minor ("subsidiary") anterior knee pain was not considered a contraindication to UKA.

At surgery, the ACL was found to be destroyed in four per cent of knees, who were all elderly, with reduced functional demands. In 43% the ACL was noted only to be "stretched", while normal in the remaining 53%. Plica synoviales at the affected femoral condyle were found in almost 5% of the cases. The posterior cruciate ligament (PCL) was always intact. Signs of chondropathology with an inflamed synovial membrane, were seen in about one third of the cases. Minor degrees of chondromalacia patellae were commonplace. The most frequently used tibial insert thicknesses were 8 mm and 10 mm (50.4% and 37% of the cases, respectively), while the 12 mm and 15 mm sizes were less frequently used (11.6% and 1%, respectively). For the past eight years, we have been using the HA-coated Unix femoral components, with mainly size 2 in 48.5% of cases, followed by size 3 (43.7%) and size 1 (7.8%).

The results have been mainly analyzed through the various cumulative survival rates upon the whole series of 523 cases. The clinical assessment is given with respect to both the knee score and functional score following the IKS policy in 350 knees (309 patients) i.e., 303 medial *versus* 47 lateral replacements, who could undergo a complete physical examination and for whom the clinical assessment would not be biased by any other significant non-knee related disabling problem. Conversely, complication rates regarded the whole 523 cases series.

COMPLICATIONS

Intraoperative

Over the past twelve years, we have not experienced any intraoperative complications that might be attributed to the HA Unix design itself. In particular, no screw related problems have occurred.

Conversely, we experienced two vertical fractures of the operated condyle at the time of the insertion of the femoral component: these two components were not HA Unix, but cemented Cartier Mod III femoral components, which were matched with the HA Unix tibial component at the beginning of the study. These fractures may have been due to the aggressive vertical fin of the femoral component inserted into very hard bone. The treatment of these fractures required fixation

with a single cancellous screw. They went on to heal uneventfully.

Post operative

The total postoperative complication rate (from all causes) was 7.1%. 2.2% of patients developed deep vein thromboses. 1.7% of cases in pulmonary embolism without any further adverse events. There was less than 1% local complications observed, with only four patients developing a wound dehiscence. Two of these cases were due to the development of a haematoma which was treated by aspiration and one case was due to a superficial infection. None of these patients required re-operation or plastic surgery and there were no deep articular infections observed.

Five cases of transient inflammation were noted, three of which resolved spontaneously. The remaining two cases developed reflex sympathetic dystrophy, which resolved after three months, with no long-term sequelae. One patient developed a transient incomplete sciatic nerve palsy (complete resolution occurred within sixth months.) Nine patients (1.7%) required subsequent manipulation under anaesthesia.

There were also two cases of fracture from causes not related to the joint replacement. One was a supracondylar fracture in the second postoperative year which was managed with internal fixation. The other was a fracture of the patella following a fall directly onto the knee in an obese patient.

Although the early postoperative complications tended to delay rehabilitation, there were no significant adverse effects impacting on the final result of the arthroplasty.

Late Complications And Adverse Effects

There were few late complications directly related to the joint replacement. The first included three cases of reflex sympathetic dystrophy (without joint stiffness) which resolved within three to five months. There were six cases (1.2%) of patellar-related problems including two subluxations of the patella (one in a medial compartment replacement, the other in a lateral compartment replacement with major under correction), both of which were treated with physiotherapy; three cases of painful chondromalacia patellae, and one patient with an inflammatory reaction secondary to parapatellar osteophytes at 18 months postoperatively. This last patient required a further operation involving synovectomy and excision of osteophytes. The last case involved two patients developed painful knees with inflammatory lesions extended to the non-operated compartments. Both patients were female (age 77 and 90), were operated on in 1991 and 1993 and had chondrocalcinosis noticed at the time of their replacement. Furthermore, both patients have declined further surgery and thus have been recorded as "clinical failures".

Revisions and Failures

Of the entire 523 cases in the series only 10 revisions have led to retrieval of at least one of the major components of the prosthesis (1.9%). These include 1 case with tibial loosening and early osteolysis; 1 case with advanced wear of the prosthesis; 2 cases of ACL tears after subsequent trauma; 2 cases of progression of degenerative change in the non-operated compartment due to overcorrection of alignment; 3 cases of progressive painful inflammatory lesions involving the whole knee secondary to chondrocalcinosis; and 1 unexpected fracture of the tibial plateau.

Failure of fixation of the HA-coated tibial component occurred in one arthritic female aged 72 years. The patient complained of immediate inflammatory-type pain with no clinical features suggestive of infection. Initially, radiographs appeared normal, but by eight months, they revealed an extensive tibial lucent line. At revision, the tibial insert was found to be "floating" in its metal tray, with synovial fluid surrounding the screw holes and the edges. The screws still had a good purchase in the tibia. When the screws had been removed, the resected tibial surface was found to be covered in a layer of fibrous tissue that was soaked in synovial fluid, however the screw holes were not affected. The HA fixation of the femoral component was perfect. Therefore revision involved exchange of the Unix HA tibial component, leaving the femoral component in situ.

One obese (100kg, BMI: 35.4) male patient experienced sudden pain in his knee 4 years after surgery. He initially received a HA Unix tibial component matched with a cemented Mod III femoral component in 1994. The follow-up was excellent at 3 years with a knee score at 99 and a functional score at 100. Revision performed at

another clinic confirmed severe wear and metallosis in the knee.

Two patients required revision procedures to their knees due to secondary ACL deficiencies. The first patient was a 49 year old male with osteoarthritis, who developed anterior laxity and a painful knee 5 years post-operatively. The second patient was an 87year old male, who developed laxity following a fall one year post-operatively. Both patients received a posterior-cruciate retaining HA-coated total knee replacements with satisfactory results.

Two cases of alignment overcorrection occurred. The first patient had previously had a high tibial osteotomy resulting in a post-osteotomy/pre-arthroplasty *valgus* alignment of 8°. In this patient, 5° of *valgus* should have been preserved in order to maintain the balance of the collateral ligaments. As a result of this case we now consider osteotomies resulting in a residual *valgus* to be a contraindication to UKA surgery. The second patient had received a medial compartment replacement for OA of that compartment with correction of a *valgus* deformity. However, the presence of bulky thighs caused the patient to bring her feet closer together for walking and as a result, put excessive varus strain on the knees, despite the axis of the lower limb being anatomically normal. In these two cases, the screws were readily removed and there was no interposed fibrous tissue between the cut bone surface and the underside of the tibial tray. As a result, the removal of the femoral component was straightforward. Both patients were given a cruciate-retaining tricompartmental replacement, with good results.

The three failures from spread of osteoarthritic changes to the other knee compartments occurred in knees noted to have calcific deposits in the joint tissues at the time of surgery. The three patients were elderly and obese, and had a history of inflammatory effusions in the knee. The medial UKAs were not overcorrected, and the radiographic follow-up had not shown anything untoward. Subsequently, at two four and five years (respectively) clinical follow up, the patients had developed severe pain affecting the entire knee joint, and revision was performed. When the UKAs were removed, it was noted that bone was in direct contact with the tibial component, without any interposed fibrous tissue. The patients were given a posterior-stabilized TKR with a satisfactory outcome.

The last case was one of bilateral failure of the tibial bone bed in an arthritic male aged 75 years. We are still at a loss to account for this failure. The patient had initially been operated on by Philippe Cartier, who had inserted a Mod III prosthesis without complication. Subsequently, the patient suffered a vertical fracture of the tibial plateau, against the tibial spine, on the implanted side. There was nothing on history that could have accounted for this event. At time of re-operation he had insertion of an unconstrained tricompartmental knee replacement and the fracture site was treated with internal fixation and a supporting autologous bone graft. By this time, the other knee was showing signs of typical unicompartmental OA, for which the patient was treated with a Unix HA tibial component with supplementary screw fixation. The customary undercorrection of 5° was applied. A few months later the patient suffered a vertical fracture that was a "carbon copy" of the one seen earlier in the contralateral knee. This resulted in the implant tilting into varus. The patient underwent an immediate revision procedure in which a cemented, posterior-stabilized tricompartmental replacement with intramedullary stems was inserted.

The retrieved implants were sent to Dr. Tom Bauer's pathology laboratory in Cleveland, for investigation of the HA-bone interface and examination of what had happened to the original HA coating as well as the state of wear of the tibial component. These studies were the subject of a chapter published in the previous Sofcot Monograph (15).

RESULTS

Clinical Assessment

The main reason for which patients had been seeking arthroplasty was pain. At the latest follow-up, the percentages of pain accounted 85.9% of "no pain", 5.2% of "pain when using stairs", 5.5% of "pain when walking", 2.3% of "moderate and occasional", 0.9% of "moderate and continuous", and finally 0.3% of "severe" pain. Overall, 85.8% of patients with medial replacements and 87 % of patients with lateral replacements were pain-free (not significant; chi square test).

Range of motion is rarely a problem in patients who meet the criteria for unicompartmental knee arthroplasty. The results showed postoperative mean knee flexion values of 127.2° (range: 80°-165°). In fact, less than 1% of knees had a flexion under 90°. Conversely, 27.4% of knees were over 140°, of which 2% exceeded 160°. The flexion averaged 126.8° in medial replacements and 129.9 in lateral, which was not significant at p: .05 according to t-test and Mann-Whitney test.

The patients demonstrated early and usually full recovery of function with 78.5% able to walk unlimited distances (77.3% in medial replacement *versus* 88.6% in lateral), while 16.7% could exceed 10 blocks, 3.5% were limited to 10 blocks, 0.6% to 5 blocks, and the remaining 0.6% of knees compelled patients to rest housebound. The other functional parameters studied showed 71.2% (70.4% in medial *versus* 77.1% in lateral) being able to climb and descend stairs without using a handrail, while 17.6% could climb up normally however using a rail for going down, and 10.9% currently used a rail up and down. Only 0.32% were unable to use stairs, this limitation being mainly due to non-knee related reasons (neurological disease, acute low back pain).

The IKS Knee scores averaged 93.64 /100 points (range: 40-100; SD 9.996) with

90.84% of knees that exceeded 80 points while only 3.72% were under 69 points. There was no significant difference between scores for medial and lateral UKAs, with 93.7 points being scored by medial UKAs (range: 40-100 points), and 93.5 points by lateral UKAs (range: 65-100 points). In terms of qualitative results in this cohort, 65.62% reported excellent results (≥ 95 points); 25.21% good results (80-94 points); 7.74 % fair results (60-79 points); and only 1.43 % reported poor results (< 60 points).

The IKS Function scores averaged 92.84 /100 points (range: 5-100; SD 11.36) with

93.93 % of knees that exceeded 80 points while only 2.88 % were under 69 points. No more than for knee scores, any significant difference could be assessed between medial and lateral UKAs, with 92.5 points being scored by medial UKAs (range: 5-100 points), and 95.4 points by lateral UKAs (range: 75-100 points). In terms of qualitative results on the whole, 61.66 % reported excellent results (≥ 95 points); 32.27 % good results (80-94 points); 4.79 % fair results (60-79 points); and only 1.28 % reported poor results (< 60 points).

Radiographic Results

Mechanical Axis

The mean values of the mechanical axis in our series have been reported separately for medial and lateral replacements.

There were 347 medial Unicompartmental knee replacements performed. The average mechanical axis was 1.8° of *varus* (Range: 14° *varus* to 10° *valgus*; SD: 3.35). 73.2% of knees were within the "ideal" mechanical axis range of 0° to 5° *varus*. Interestingly, 7.5% of knees demonstrated a slight overcorrection of up to 2° of *valgus*, while this overcorrection was over 5° of *valgus* in 5.8% of knees. Conversely, less than 1% were recorded as greatly under corrected with over 10° of *varus*.

For the 53 lateral Unicompartmental knee replacements, the average mechanical axis was 1.7° of *valgus* (Range: 6° *varus* to 9° *valgus*; SD: 3.06). 77.3 % of knees were within the "ideal" limits of 0° to 5° valgus. 9.4% of knees demonstrated a slight overcorrection of up to 2° of varus, while this overcorrection was over 5° of varus in less than 2 % of knees. Conversely, no knee was recorded as greatly under corrected (>10° *valgus*).

There were no statistically significant differences (p<0.05) recorded when comparing overall results with the different groups of the mechanical axis. (Those within the normal range scored 190.0 points, while those under- and over- corrected scored 189.6 points. The overall IKS score was 178.6 points).

Degeneration of The Opposite Compartment

More rapid arthritic degeneration of the compartment opposite to the implant is often used as an argument against unicompartmental arthroplasty. In our series, this occurred in less than 12% of cases. Surprisingly, there was no significant correlation between secondary degenerative changes in the opposite compartment and the mechanical axis of the UKA, in particular whether the joint was over- or under-corrected. However, one of the cases with 8° of *valgus* in a medial UKR, has since required revision as already described in the section on complications.

Interface

With regard to the HA-coated tibial components, the striking finding in the majority of cases was an absolute "mute X-ray", without any adverse bony changes observed over the years. Furthermore, coned views demonstrated intimate bonding at the bone-prosthesis interface (figs. 4 and 5). This supports the earlier work of Tom Bauer (15), who demonstrated on histological views direct osteoapposition (fig. 6).

In just over 10% of cases a non-progressive "scalloping", described as a "droplet of osteolysis", was observed at the anterior border (8.2%) or posterior border (2.5%) of the tibial plateau. In 4.8% of knees, an isolated reactive line was noted in the posterior zone (zone Tib Lat 3), on the lateral films. Less than 1% of patients in this study recorded reactive or lucent lines under the tibial plateau

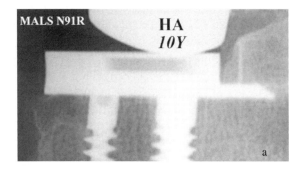

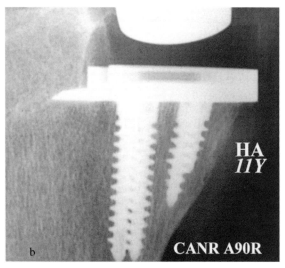

Figure 4a, b – Close view of two HA-coated tibial components respectively at 10 years (a) and 11 years (b). Note the direct bony apposition between metal and bone and the trabeculae directly in contact with the metallic implant, proving an excellent osteointegration.

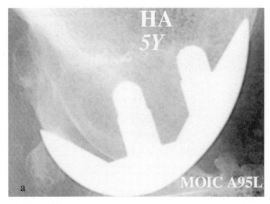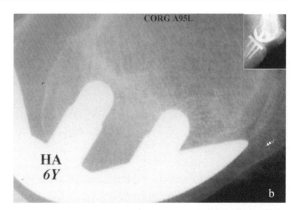

Figure 5a, b – Close view of two typical films demonstrating excellent bone integration of the femoral component respectively at 5 years (a) and 6 years (b). There is intimate contact between metal and bone and harmonious transmission of loads, without any osteolysis of stress shielding.

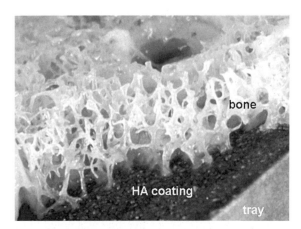

Figure 6 – Photo of a retrieved tibial implant at 5 years postoperatively due to extensive arthritic lesions over the opposite compartment. The retrieval was easily obtained by cutting under the metallic tray. This photo demonstrates an "ideal" bony apposition directly to the metallic surface.

(fig. 7). So far, these radiographic features have not been associated with any symptoms, nor have they spread to involve the screw sites.

The complication of Osteolysis around the screws is frequently cited by the opponents of UKA. In our series of patients it was only observed in six cases and was not associated with clinical symptoms or implant loosening. The radiographic findings in each of these cases, was a limited zone of bone resorption that would not be considered as true osteolysis (fig. 8).

No pattern of pending loosening was ever seen in the group of Mod III cemented femoral components that were matched with the HA tibial tray at the beginning of the series. With respect to the femoral HA-coated component, results were again striking. In all cases, no radiological changes have been observed over 8 years of follow-up.

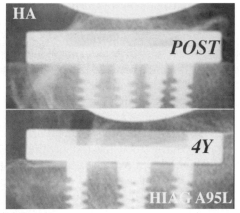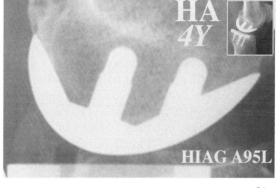

Figure 7a, b – Typical lucent line under a tibial Unix HA-coated plateau at 4 years in a 99 kilograms obese 71 years old patient with excellent clinical result at 100 points for both knee score and functional score (a). Please note the total lack of osteolysis or lines around the screws. Conversely, excellent bony apposition in the same patient onto the HA-coated femur (b).

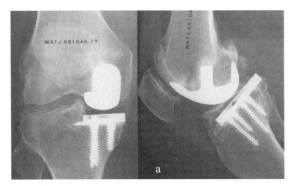
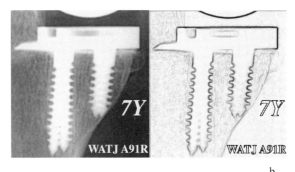

Figure 8a, b – This 7-year radiological evaluation stated a lucent line under the tibial plateau and osteolysis around some of the screws (a). However, an imaging magnification demonstrated around the screws an intimate contact between the threads of the screws and osseous trabeculae (b). No clinical problem in this 92 kilogram obese female patient (osteoarthritis).

Overall, excellent bone ongrowth (without any interposed fibrous tissue) was confirmed in more than 95% of the cases with the HA-coated Unix knee. In the entire study, there was not a single instance of radiographic loosening.

Survivorship

Survivorship analysis in this study was performed under optimum conditions, since the status of all the knees could be checked, with none having been lost to follow-up. Furthermore, all of the knees that had failed on clinical grounds were revised, and placed in the failed group, including additionally the two non revised "clinical failures". No radiographic failure had been observed during the course of the study.

A distinction needs to be made when selecting the endpoint. One must choose between "survival" of the implant (retrieval), "survival" of the replacement itself (failure), and the "survival" of the Hydroxyapatite fixation (aseptic loosening).

With respect to "retrieval for any cause" as endpoint, (i.e., patient selection, surgical technique, and non implant related adverse effects) a total number of 10 revisions had been undertaken, including those due to pathological fracture, extension of the degenerative changes to the opposite compartment and secondary lesions of the ACL.

With respect to "clinical failure", a total of 12 cases were recorded. This includes two non-reoperated clinical failures as well as the ten retrievals previously discussed.

If we were to select "aseptic loosening" as the endpoint, the survivorship analysis would have to take into account failure due to tibial loosening and early osteolysis.

Overall, the arthroplasty survival rate at seven years with 40 knees remaining "at risk" at this follow-up may be estimated to be 93.94 % ± 0.0603 (any retrieval), 92.38 % ± 0.0636 (any failure), and 99.58 % ± 0.0073 (aseptic loosening). No statistically significant differences could be demonstrated between medial and lateral compartment replacements.

DISCUSSION

The clinical results obtained by the HA-coated uni-compartmental knee in this study, may be described as very satisfactory. More than 85 % of operated knees were pain-free at follow-up. The average flexion was recorded as over 125° in all groups. More than 70 % of patients were able to climb up and descend stairs normally. The Knee score is obviously the best yardstick of the success of a knee arthroplasty. In this study, the overall mean score was 93.64 points, with 90.83 % excellent and good results (over 80 points), without any significant difference between the results of medial and lateral UKAs. Regarding the Function score, the overall results obtained in the study were satisfactory, with a mean score of 92.84 points and 93.93 % excellent and good results. Furthermore, these results have stood the test of time as they have been maintained over the years. With respect to "retrieval for any cause" as an endpoint, the arthroplasty survival rate with 40 knees remaining "at risk" at seven years may be estimated to be 93.94 % ± 0.0603 with no significant differences demonstrated between medial and lateral replacements. When selecting "aseptic loosening" as an endpoint, the arthroplasty survival rate was estimated to be 99.58 % ± 0.0073.

With respect to the radiographic analyses, first and foremost it should be noted that there was an absence of any radiographic evidence of pending implant loosening, as well as an absence of any signs of PE insert wear.. Lucent lines were very rarely observed in this study; and reactive lines were seen much less frequently than those reported elsewhere with HA-coated TKRs (5). Scalloping at the anterior border on the lateral views may be a sign of reactive osteolysis brought about by "kinases" in the synovial fluid or by "PE debris", as suggested by Schmalzried (16). Whatever the cause of the phenomenon, the rate observed in this study was low (8.2%) and so far the fixation of the tibial components has not been affected.

The use of supplementary fixation screws is controversial. Opponents of this technique claim that there may be catastrophic osteolysis around the screws. In our series, we had only six cases of osteolysis around the screws and under the anterior border of the tibial tray which would suggest that the lesion may have occurred from the periphery inwards. We feel that screws are a vital means of mechanical implant fixation. They also have the added benefit of neutralising horizontal interface stresses below the metal tray. We have been using screws, both for UKAs and TKRs, over the past 12 years, without any ill effects. It should also be borne in mind that under stable conditions, a titanium screw will become spontaneously covered within about one year, with a layer of physiological bicarbonate hydroxyapatite. This process allows direct bone ongrowth to occur, thereby blocking the route along which any debris may travel.

Our 8-year experience with the HA-coated Unix femoral component has demonstrated absolute osteo-integration of the components and excellent stability afforded over the years, as evidenced by the "mute X-rays" commonly recorded in the patients (fig. 9).

The technique used for the insertion of these devices has also become very specific based on the actual experience of past users of these implants. In this way, unicompartmental joint replacement has become a simple procedure that should not be made unnecessarily complicated. This surgery preserves bone stock and amounts to a true resurfacing, and can avoid any dislocation of the patella. However, if the device is to have a long in-service

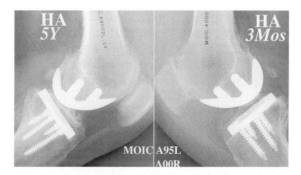

Figure 9 – Bilateral case in a 67 years old female patient respectively at 3 months (right) and 5 years (left). Excellent clinical result for both knees. These films demonstrate the typical evolution of this Unix knee over time, with no radiographic change, leading to speak about "mute x-rays".

life, the implant must be appropriately shaped and fixed; the instruments must be well-designed; and resection must be meticulous, with nothing left to chance. The "minimal invasive surgery" has to be advocated if it does not jeopardize the final outcome of the arthroplasty.

An analysis of the ten cases of UKA failures shows that the problems may be classified under six headings: Failure of the mechanical fixation of the tibial insert, wear and damage of the PE insert, late ACL deficiencies, overcorrection of alignment, spread of degenerative changes to other knee compartments, and unexpected fracture of the bony plateau.

Interestingly, only 2 (0.38%) of the failed cases are related to the implant itself. One of these was a unique case of mechanical aseptic loosening. Thus the failure rate from HA Unix components loosening in our entire arthroplasty population was only 0.2%; all the other failures being attributable to systemic disorders. With hindsight, we have come to recognize that these problems are largely due to poor patient selection or to technical faults. Thus appropriate patients selection and strict observance of surgical principles remain the cornerstones of Unicompartmental knee arthroplasties. Both of these topics are particularly well detailed by Cartier and Deschamps in a previous monograph (10, 11). Interestingly, the various chapters of this monograph (17) provide consistent answers to "some unanswered questions about unicompartmental knee prosthesis" recently asked by Laskin (1).

In cases where revision was required, the procedure could be performed under conditions that were as good as those at primary TKR. All that needs to be done is to undo the screws holding the tibial plateau, and to resect the tibia immediately below the metal tray. The patient's bone stock is left entirely intact. On the femoral side, the guide must be positioned for the distal cut and the cut started before the femoral component is removed. The use of a saw allows the bone to be resected flush against the femoral component, which can then be removed without pulling out a large block of bone. Histological analysis performed by Bauer (8, 15) on retrieved metallic trays confirmed the reality of this "biological fixation".

In the light of the study described in this chapter, we may conclude that HA does indeed produce excellent results on the tibial side, providing that primary self-stabilization has been achieved and that the design of the implant component is such as to optimize implant seating on the host bed and implant fixation in the host bone. The half-moon shape chosen for the Unix tibial tray provides good seating on the cortical rim, while firm seating centrally is ensured by the stabilising fin that is tucked under the tibial spine. This horizontal fin is a vital design feature, since Shinro Takai (18) demonstrated that the central region tends to be the weakest link in conventional systems for the fixation of the tibial component. The fin also allows the patient's bone stock to be preserved, and any revision surgery that may become necessary later on, to be performed under conditions otherwise found at primary surgery. Finally, the use of a titanium alloy could be seen as more beneficial than CoCr in terms of the bone-metal interface, as it provides immediate and long lasting bony apposition in almost all cases (fig. 10).

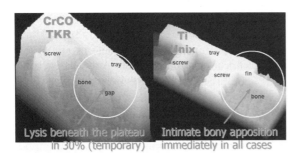

Figure 10 – Comparison of two knee tibial components, the CrCo total knee (left) against the Ti Uni knee (right), focusing on the behavior of the bone, immediately beneath the tibial plateau 6 months postoperatively. These pictures have been enhanced through the Imagika software to produce a 3D-like image, the z axis being the bone density. Obviously, the bony apposition is better with a titanium metallic substrate as compared to CrCo plateau, in which gaps are commonly seen between metal and bone.

Comparing our results to the series published in the literature is a difficult challenge. In a previous paper (19), we reviewed the results of 14 different series of UKAs as a meta analysis. Failure rates varied from 0% up to 21%, Conversely survival rates varied between 67% and 100%. Overall, the newest designs afforded the best results, with no statistically significant differences between different types of fixation or bearings. Recently, a study by Perkins et al (20) reported a 10 year survival rate of 97%, with aseptic loosening as the endpoint. A similar result was obtained by Berger et al (21) who reported a 10-year survival rate of 98% with aseptic loosening as the endpoint. Squire *et al.* (22) examined patients with a minimum of 15 years follow up and found that revision for failure of fixation of the UKAs was comparable with that reported for fixed bearing TKAs. Deshmukh et al (9) reported on two recently published 10-year studies and concluded that results were comparable with those of total knee arthroplasty. Therefore the 99% survival rate of our HA-Unix knees (with aseptic loosening as an endpoint) compares favorably with the best cemented series reported in the current literature.

CONCLUSION

To this day, the use of unicompartmental knee prostheses remains controversial. There is disagreement on the extent of the middle ground between corrective osteotomies and total joint replacement, as well as argument about whether the bearings should be "unconstrained" or "mobile". Notwithstanding these uncertainties, unicompartmentals have matured into an important subgroup of knee arthroplasties. They do however require great clinical skills of patient selection, resection technique, and choice of components (23). Under these conditions, the "enhanced second-decade survivorship and therefore an expansion of the indications for unicompartmental knee arthroplasty are possibilities", according to Deshmukh and Scott (9), while "using stringent selection criteria, UKAs can yield excellent results and represent a superb alternative to TKAs", as stated by Berger, Rosenberg and Galante (19).

In the light of the study presented in this chapter, the HA-coated Unix components have been found to be reliable and effective at 12-years clinical follow-up (fig. 11). The biological fixation was effective and afforded clinical and radiological results at least as good as the best cemented series. Whether the fixation needs to be "bioconductive" or cemented remains an interesting question. Either way, we have been impressed by the excellent fixation – both on radiological and histological findings – as provided by hydroxyapatite for both tibial and femoral components.

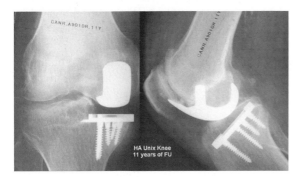

Figure 11 – One of our first HA-coated tibial Unix component implanted in 1990 in a patient who is now 82 years old and who experiences a very good long lasting result at 97 points (knee score) and 100 points (function score). Again no radiographic change with time, no problem onto the opposite compartment, no osteolysis under the plateau and around the screws.

Time and again, experts have warned that hydroxyapatite is not a "magic powder" – and what is true of hip replacement is also applicable to knee joint arthroplasty (24). However, the HA experience in Uni Knees at the current follow-up of twelve years looks encouraging enough to be enthusiastically continued.

Reference List

1. Laskin RS (2001) Unicompartmental knee replacement: some unanswered questions. *Clin. Orthop.* (392):267-71.

2. Capello WN, D'Antonio JA, Feinberg JR, Manley MT. (1997) Hydroxyapatite-coated total hip femoral components in patients less than fifty years old. Clinical and radiographic results after five to eight years of follow-up. *J. Bone Joint Surg. Am.* 79(7):1023-9.

3. D'Antonio JA, Capello WN, Manley MT, and Geesink RGT (2001) Hydroxylapatite femoral stems for total hip arthroplasty: 10-13 year follow-up. *Clin. Orthop.* 393:101-11.

4. Epinette JA (1995) "Hydroxyapatite and TKR: The HA Omnifit Knee Prosthesis" in Cahiers d'Enseignement de la SOFCOT, n° 51 (English Volume), "Hydroxyapatite Coated Hip and Knee Arthroplasty", pp 323-32. Paris, Expansion Scientifique Française.

5. Epinette JA (2001) HA-coated Total Knee Arthroplasty: A 9-year HA Omnifit experience – in "Arthroplasty 2000, recent advances in TJR", Matsui N., Taneda Y. Yoshida Y. eds, pp 189-204. Springer-Verlag Tokyo.

6. Geesink RG (2002) Osteoconductive coatings for total joint arthroplasty. *Clin. Orthop.* (395):53-65. Review.

7. Kirsh G, Roffman M, Kligman M (2001) Hydroxyapatite-coated total hip replacements in patients 65 years of age and over. *Bull. Hosp. Jt. Dis.* 60(1):5-9.

8. Epinette JA and Edidin AA (1997) Hydroxyapatite coated "unicompartmental knee replacement; a report of five to six years" follow-up of the HA Unix Tibial Component, in Cahiers d'Enseignement de la SOFCOT, n° 61 (English Volume) "Unicompartmental Knee Arthroplasty", pp 243-59. Paris, Expansion Scientifique Française.

9. Deshmukh RV, Scott RD (2001) Unicompartmental knee arthroplasty: long-term results. *Clin. Orthop.* (392):272-8.

10. Cartier Ph, Epinette JA, Deschamps G and Hernigou P (1997) Indications and limitations of Unicompartmental Knee Replacement, in Cahiers d'Enseignement de la SOFCOT, n°61 (English Volume) "Unicompartmental Knee Arthroplasty", pp 269-78. Paris, Expansion Scientifique Française.

11. Cartier Ph, and Deschamps G (1997) Surgical Principles of Unicompartmental Knee Replacement, in Cahiers d'Enseignement de la Sofcot, n° 61 (English Volume) "Unicompartmental Knee Arthroplasty", pp 137-43. Paris, Expansion Scientifique Française.

12. Price AJ, Webb J, Topf H, Dodd CA, Goodfellow JW, Murray DW (2001) Oxford Hip and Knee Group. Rapid recovery after oxford unicompartmental arthroplasty through a short incision. *J. Arthroplasty* 16(8):970-6.

13. Insall JN, Dorr LD, Scott RD, Scott WN (1989) Rationale of the knee society clinical rating system. *Clin. Orthop.* 248:13-4.

14. Kaplan EL, Meier P (1958) Nonparametric estimation from incomplete observations. *J. Am. Stat. Assoc.* 457-81.

15. Bauer Th W, Jiang M and Epinette JA (1997) HA-coated Unicompartmental Knee Arthroplasty: Histological analysis of retrieved implants, in Cahiers d'Enseignement de la SOFCOT, n° 61 (English Volume) "Unicompartmental Knee Arthroplasty", pp 43-50, Paris, Expansion Scientifique Française.

16. Schmalzried TP, Jasty M, Harris WH (1992) Periprosthetic Bone Loss in Total Hip Arthroplasty: polyethylene wear debris and the concept of the effective joint space. *J. Bone Joint Surg.* 74A:849-63.

17. Cartier P, Epinette JA, Deschamps G and Hernigou P (1997) Unicompartmental Knee Arthroplasty, in Cahiers d'Enseignement de la SOFCOT, n° 61 (English Volume), Paris, Expansion Scientifique Française.

18. Takai S, Yoshino N, Hirasawa Y and Tsusumi S (1997) Stress analysis of the proximal tibia after unicompartmental knee arthroplasty with finite element method, in

Cahiers d'Enseignement de la SOFCOT, n° 61 (English Volume) "Unicompartmental Knee Arthroplasty", pp 61-7. Paris, Expansion Scientifique Française.

19. Epinette JA (1997) Overview of Clinical Results in Unicompartmental Knee Artrhoplasty Series, in Cahiers d'Enseignement de la SOFCOT, n° 61 (English Volume) "Unicompartmental Knee Arthroplasty", pp 279-86. Paris, Expansion Scientifique Française.

20. Perkins TR, Gunckle W (2002) Unicompartmental knee arthroplasty: 3- to 10-year results in a community hospital setting. *J. Arthroplasty* 17(3):293-7.

21. Berger RA, Nedeff DD, Barden RM, Sheinkop MM, Jacobs JJ, Rosenberg AG, Galante JO (1999) Unicompartmental knee arthroplasty. Clinical experience at 6- to 10-year follow-up. *Clin. Orthop.* (367):50-60.

22. Squire MW, Callaghan JJ, Goetz DD, Sullivan PM, Johnston RC (1999) Unicompartmental knee replacement. A minimum 15 year follow-up study. *Clin. Orthop.* (367):61-72.

23. Lindstrand A, Stenstrom A, Ryd L, Toksvig-Larsen S (2000) The introduction period of unicompartmental knee arthroplasty is critical: a clinical, clinical multi-centered, and radiostereometric study of 251 Duracon unicompartmental knee arthroplasties. *J. Arthroplasty* 15(5):608-16.

24. Epinette JA, Geesink RGT (1995) Hydroxyapatite Coatings: Where do we stand, where do we go ? in Cahiers d'Enseignement de la SOFCOT, n° 51 (English Volume), "Hydroxyapatite Coated Hip and Knee Arthroplasty", p. 345-57. Paris, Expansion Scientifique Française.

4   The Use of Hydroxyapatite in Unicompartmental Arthroplasty

A Brief Note

Philippe Cartier, MD

INTRODUCTION

In light of the excellent, long lasting results we obtained with cemented unicompartmental arthroplasty (UKA) between 1974 and 1991 (1-3), we have broadened the patient selection criteria in favor of this type of replacement in greater numbers of young and active patients.

Due to what is usually a prompt recovery of full functional abilities, as well as a physiological range of motion far better than those obtained by total knee prostheses (TKA), UKA could be seen as better suited than tibial osteotomy for the treatment of osteoarthritic (OA) knees with Ahlbäck Grades III and IV unicompartmental lesions in patients demonstrating a high level of activities in accordance with their young age.

Unicompartmental implants must withstand an overwhelming level of stresses under load compared to TKAs. Because the functional needs of these young patients, mainly males, have become increasingly demanding due to trying physical exercises routinely practiced either during their sport or professional activities, it became obvious that we had to bear in mind the ever increasing risk of implant loosening over time, especially in cemented prostheses.

MATERIALS & METHODS

The quality of the results with hydroxyapatite-coated UKAs reported by Epinette (4) in a previous monograph (5), and the results of the histological evidence provided by Bauer of bone ongrowth in HA implants retrieved at revision (6), were such as to suggest that HA might well be the best choice in properly selected patients. We believe it is possible that this fixation technique may help us overcome the problem of implant loosening in this challenging group of young patients. Hence, in 1991 we designed a novel line of implants belonging to the Unicompartmental Genesis System. They incorporated a 2mm thick metal-backed titanium tibial component, which was hydroxyapatite-coated and permitted complementary fixation by screws.

The first nine patients who received the HA-coated Genesis were included in a larger series of 42 Genesis UKAs presented during the Dallas American Academy (AAOS) in 2002. This reported on 7 years (range, 5 to 9 years) of average follow-up in active middle aged patients averaging 52 years of age (range, 42 to 60 years). Of these nine HA-coated implants, eight patients were male. Aetiology was primary or secondary osteoarthritis, and accounted for six varus and three *valgus* deformities. The postoperative HSS knee score was 99 points *versus* 47 preoperatively. Postoperative HSS function score was 97 *versus* 44.5 preoperatively. All the knees were slightly under-corrected and presented a normally functioning ACL.

RESULTS

No specific implant related complication occurred, as well as no mechanical loosening or lucent lines at the screw fixation adjacent to the tibial plateau. Average polyethylene wear was 0.5mm. Five of the patients with strenuous jobs returned to the same job. Moreover, seven of the nine patients participated regularly in sport activities such as tennis, dance, or gymnastics, before they became disabled by their knee and underwent UKA. Each patient resumed the sport at the same level as before UKA (fig. 1).

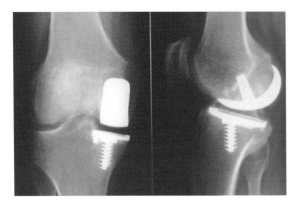

Figure 1 – Postop films at 8 years of follow-up in a 42 years old male who underwent a medial replacement in 1994 with insertion of a Genesis Uni. Excellent bony apposition under the HA-coated tibial component, and no functional limitation in a patient working as a security guard and practicing martial arts.

DISCUSSION

In addition to this very short first experience with the HA-coated genesis UKA reported at the Dallas meeting, we are currently carrying out a prospective study based upon 95 other cases (to date) with a two to five year follow-up period. So far, none of them have encountered any kind of complication except for a single case of limited stable osteolysis around one screw, which did not have any clinical relevance and did not ruin the implant fixation. Thus, it did not led to any reoperation. All 95 cases demonstrated full osteointegration and excellent fixation.

Interestingly, after the tibial cut is made in these young male patients, the bone bed often presents a very dense, sclerotic bone with no real cancellous trabeculae. This is not favorable to a cemented anchorage, even when drilling some holes to enhance this type of fixation. Conversely, this type of underlying surface is well suited for a HA-coated metal-backed tibial tray, although rigorous surgical skills would be needed. For example, the tibial tray would need to lie on a perfectly flat surface to secure an efficient fixation before screwing in any additional screws. There would be no cement to help to fix the irregular surface that results from an inaccurate cut.

Micromotion at the interface after screwing in would be unacceptable. More than ever, the principle of a self-stabilizing tibial component facing the femoral component during the dynamic trials must be achieved as an absolute prerequisite (7).

In order to avoid any theoretical release of HA particles in the knee joint, no part of the metallic rim of the tray should project beyond the bony border of the tibial epiphysis. Naturally, the use of HA-coated tibial components makes any loss of cement debris in the joint space behind the plateau irrelevant.

CONCLUSION

Although UKAs obviously cannot and should not replace tibial osteotomies and total knee replacements in the management of those conditions in which the other treatment modalities are clearly indicated (8), the unicompartmental replacements provide good quality, long-term results and provide for ease of revision if problems are encountered. They should, therefore, keep their legitimate place in the orthopaedic surgeon's armamentarium for the benefit of patients suffering from OA of the knee or from osteonecrosis of the medial condyle. It should also be remembered that the modern resurfacing UKAs will make good functional results even more predictable and more commonplace, because the improvements incorporated into current designs reflect the lessons learned from earlier failures.

This unicompartmental arthroplasty no longer needs to be limited to older patients, since our experience with hydroxyapatite-coated implants during the past ten years has provided evidence that HA performs well for the indications presented by young, active patients. Cementless fixation using a HA coating has produced a satisfying osteointegration in all cases. This permits young, active patients to postoperatively maintain the same preoperative activity level they enjoyed without worrying about implant loosening.

These findings led us to broaden the range of indications for UKA, provided that the bony support width is sufficient to allow the use of a HA-coated Genesis tray of appropriate size (at least medium) and that the underlying subchondral bone is of sufficiently good mechanical quality.

Reference List

1. Cartier Ph, Sanouiller JL, Grelsamer RP (1996) Unicompartmental knee arthroplasty surgery. 10-year minimum follow-up period. *J. Arthroplasty* 11(7):782-8.

2. Grelsamer RP, Cartier Ph (1992) A unicompartmental knee replacement is not "half a total knee": five major differences. *Orthop. Rev.* 21(11):1350-6.

3. Cartier Ph, Cheaib S (1987) Unicondylar knee arthroplasty. 2-10 years of follow-up evaluation. *J. Arthroplasty* 2(2):157-62.

4. Epinette JA, Edidin AA (1997) Hydroxyapatite coated unicompartmental knee replacement; a report of five to six years' follow-up of the HA Unix Tibial Component, in Cahiers d'Enseignement de la SOFCOT, n° 61 (English Volume) "Unicompartmental Knee Arthroplasty", pp 243-59. Paris, Expansion Scientifique Française.

5. Cartier Ph, Epinette JA, Deschamps G, Hernigou Ph (1997) Unicompartmental Knee Arthroplasty in Cahiers d'Enseignement de la Sofcot, n° 61 (English Volume). Paris, Expansion Scientifique Française.

6. Bauer ThW, Jiang M, Epinette JA (1997) HA-coated Unicompartmental Knee Arthroplasty: Histologic analysis of retrieved implants in Cahiers d'Enseignement de la Sofcot, n° 61 (English Volume) "Unicompartmental Knee Arthroplasty", pp 43-50. Paris, Expansion Scientifique Française.

7. Cartier Ph, Deschamps G (1997) Surgical Principles of Unicompartmental Knee Replacement in Cahiers d'Enseignement de la Sofcot, n° 61 (English Volume) "Unicompartmental Knee Arthroplasty", pp 137-43. Paris, Expansion Scientifique Française.

8. Cartier Ph, Epinette JA, Deschamps G, Hernigou Ph (1997) Indications and limitations of Unicompartmental Knee Replacement in Cahiers d'Enseignement de la Sofcot, n° 61 (English Volume) "Unicompartmental Knee Arthroplasty", pp 269-78. Paris, Expansion Scientifique Française.

CLINICAL OVERVIEW, OUTCOMES, AND PERSPECTIVES IN BIOACTIVE COATINGS

1   Global Overview:
Fifteen Years of Clinical Experience
With Hydroxyapatite Coatings

It is our hope – and the hope of the ninety authors who contributed to this work – that this book will provide its readers with current, complete, and detailed information on fifteen years of clinical experience with hydroxyapatite-coated implants. In order to provide the reader with a general overview of the contents, a brief summary of each chapter in each section follows.

The Editors

INTRODUCTION

As pointed out by Rudolph Geesink in the *Preface*, Total Hip Arthroplasty has existed for over 40 years. Since the pioneering days of Sir John Charnley, significant improvements have been achieved through better understanding of the inter-relationship between biomaterials, biomechanics, and biology. With the introduction almost 20 years ago of HA for clinical use, numerous studies have provided an almost exponential increase in knowledge on HA-coatings in orthopaedics. Therefore, the effort was undertaken to provide an update on the current status of calcium-phosphate coatings in orthopaedics.

John Shepperd provides the first chapter in the book, which provides a discussion of *The Early Biological History of Calcium Phosphates,* beginning with the earliest life forms on our planet, including the Precambrian epoch. He includes interesting details about 18th century scientific revelations involving calcium apatite and calcium sulphate, including the 19th century use of plaster of Paris and the use of joint replacements constructed from ivory.

It seemed logical to include in this section a review of HA literature. Michael Manley, Kate Sutton, and John Dumbleton provided this chapter entitled "*Calcium Phosphates: A Survey of the Orthopaedic Literature*". Interestingly, during their review of the literature on HA and calcium phosphates, they observed inconsistencies in the way authors use the terms osteogenic, osteoconductive, and osteoinductive to describe different bone healing and forming processes. Additionally, they note that some investigators use the term "hydroxyapatite" loosely, referring to a material with a calcium-phosphorous (Ca/P) ratio ranging anywhere from 1.3 to 2.0. It can be difficult – and potentially misleading – to compare studies using various or undefined ratios to those using the generally accepted Ca/P ratio for hydroxyapatite of 1.67. *In vitro, in vivo*, and clinical studies using different forms of HA, such as blocks, granules, pastes, and coatings, are discussed as well as combinations of HA and TCP.

BASIC SCIENCE: HISTOLOGY & EXPERIMENTAL WORKS

Many of the HA coatings used in earlier clinical studies involving plasma-sprayed HA-coated products were not as consistent in chemistry and mechanical properties as those now found on contemporary prostheses. As demonstrated by Paul Serekian in "*Hydroxyapatite: From Plasma Spray to Electrochemical Deposition*", alternate processing advancements are currently available. This chapter discusses the advent of three-dimensional interstitial porous and textured surfaces and the considerable level of interest and focus directed toward exploring non-line-of-site coating techniques. Topics of discussion include HA solution deposition, electrophoretic technique, electrophoretic nanotechnology, and ion beam assisted deposited coatings (IBAD).

Ole Rahbek, Søren Overgaard, and Kjeld Søballe provided very detailed analyses about *"Calcium Phosphate Coatings for Implant Fixation"*. This chapter describes a series of experimental and human studies performed in order to evaluate systematically potential improvements of bone implant fixation using hydroxyapatite (HA) and fluorapatite (FA) coating when subjected to pathological and mechanical conditions mimicking the clinical situation. The authors also studied factors influencing resorption of the coatings *in vivo*, and they report on the effect of hydroxyapatite on peri-implant migration of wear debris.

Florence Barrere, Pamela Habibovic, and Klaas de Groot report on *"Biological Activities of Biomimetic Calcium Phosphate Coatings"*. The deposition of Ca-P coatings on and in porous material has been incomplete because of the line-of-sight application required by the current plasma-spraying coating technique. However, it is currently possible to evenly coat porous implants with Ca-P by using a biomimetic coating method. The aim of this paper is to study the biological activity of these novel biomimetic coatings, which includes *in vitro* and *in vivo* degradation, the osteogenecity in osseous sites, and the osteoinductivity.

The goal of the chapter by Thomas W. Bauer and Satoshi Takikawa entitled, *"Histology and Fate of Bioactive Coatings"* is to describe the basic histology of the interface between HA-coated devices and bone, as well as the fate of coatings and the potential consequences of coating loss. Although the biocompatibility and osteoconductive properties of calcium phosphate coatings have been well established, some controversial concerns remain, such as the mechanisms of coating loss, the optimum physiochemical properties of the coating, the long term consequences of coating loss, and the optimum substrate texture beneath the coating. The authors hypothesize about four mechanisms whereby HA can be lost from the surface of implants: osteoclastic resorption of the coating as part of normal bone remodeling, delamination, dissolution at neutral pH and, finally, abrasion. These mechanisms are discussed in detail within the chapter.

Another histological analysis regarding the outcome of the HA coating is provided by Alfons Tonino, Cees Oosterbos, Ali Rahmy, and M. Thèrin in their chapter, *"What is the Function and Fate of the HA Coating in Cementless HA-coated Hip Prostheses?"*, which is based upon the histology and histomorphometry of eight hip prostheses retrieved at post mortem. When radiographic and clinical findings are unreliable in predicting exact ingrowth or ongrowth of bone, only histology and histomorphometry in human autopsy retrievals after a long period of successful implantation can provide answers about the relationship between hydroxyapatite resorption and persistence of implant osseointegration, or about the morphology and exact location of polyethylene induced osteolysis. The purpose of this study of eight clinically successful hydroxyapatite-coated hip prostheses retrieved at post mortem (between 3 and 9 years after insertion) was to document the extent and pattern of bone apposition in relation to the hydroxyapatite coating and implantation time. The tissue reactions on detected particles (titanium, polyethylene, and hydroxyapatite) were also studied.

In a previous paper within this "experimental" section, Pamela Habibovic, Florence Barrère, and Klaas de Groot described the biological activities of biomimetic calcium phosphate coatings. This chapter provides complementary information about these *"Biomimetic Hydroxyapatite Coatings"*, and discusses a variety of different methods that can be used to coat implants with HA. According to the authors, the formation of thick, homogeneous calcium phosphate coatings on Ti6Al4V implants and porous tantalum substrates can be consistently achieved using a two-step biomimetic method.

The peri-implant osteolysis that can follow total joint arthroplasty is responsible for the majority of orthopedic implant loosening and can be caused either by stress shielding or by a wear particle induced inflammatory reaction. Recently, a new therapy using a systemic treatment with drugs that specifically target osteolysis has been considered. However, the systemic use of drugs presents drawbacks, including serious side effects such as throat or stomach ulcers. Additionally, determining the appropriate dosage can be difficult. In order to resolve those issues, Dominique P. Pioletti, Bastian Peter, Lalao R. Rakotomanana, Pascal Rubin, and Pierre-François Leyvraz in their chapter entitled, *"Combination of HA and Bisphosphonate Coating to Control the Bone Remodeling Around an Orthopedic Implant"*, suggest a new way to use implants. The implants would provide not only structural support, but would also serve as a local drug delivery system. This innovative concept, among others, is expanded upon within this chapter.

Numerous procedures for the coating of metallic implants with hydroxyapatite exist. At present, the most current industrial application is plasma spraying. However, laser surface treatments are quickly becoming an attractive alternative to that technology. Pascal Deprez and Philippe Hivart in the chapter, entitled *"Coating Of Titanium With Hydroxyapatite By Laser Surface Powder Cladding : Exploratory Results"*, expound on a novel technology called laser powder cladding. This pre-study suggests that laser processes are worth being studied in detail and developed. Though the two methodologies are similar in principle, the authors explain why the advantages of laser over plasma spraying are important.

In the chapter *"Comparative Experimental Study of The Behavior of Polyethylene Particulates around Hydroxyapatite-Coated Implants versus Cemented Ones"*, Ph. Massin, E. Viguier, B. Flautre, P. Hardouin, and B. Duponchel performed an experimental study in sheep to examine the migration of polyethylene wear debris at the bone-metal interface of a hydroxyapatite-coated implant. They tested a proximally HA-coated implant with a smooth distal portion and compared it to an entirely smooth cemented control implant of the same shape. It is believed that an intimate bond at the fixation interface, such as the microinterlocking of bone into the porous coating, or of the cement into the cancellous bone, may prevent excessive particle migration. This may explain why the use of circumferential porous coating as well as an optimal cement technique may prevent distal osteolysis. The effect of particles migrating through the cancellous bone and the role of implant stiffness on particle migration are some of the issues examined in this chapter.

The stability of the components is vital for successful, long-term results of total knee arthroplasty (TKA). Loosening of the tibial component is more common than that of the femoral component. The objective of, *"Finite Element Analysis in Bioactive-coated Tibial Components"*, by Nobuyuki Yoshino, Shinro Takai, and Sadami Tsutsumi, is to assess the effectiveness of bioactive coating with tibial components. For this objective, the two-dimensional finite element method (FEM) was employed for four different modalities of fixation with the same stem-type design. The modalities

examined were rigid interface, rigid interface only at the tibial tray, early stage of bioactive coating, and fibrous fixation. The findings indicate that the advantage of the bioactive coating should be evaluated by long-term clinical results.

BIOACTIVE COATINGS: CLINICAL WORKS

Shunsuke Fujibayashi and Takashi Nakamura begin this section with a report on *"Current Status of Bioactive Coatings in Japan"*. In order to establish a mechanical anchor, a bioactive ceramic coating is one way of enhancing bone tissue formation around and into the surface of a prosthesis. In this chapter, the authors focus on bioactive glass coating and bioactive titanium. They discuss their attempt to combine AW glass ceramic with titanium alloy implants to further accelerate the bone-bonding process of the implants, and to improve the bone-bonding strength. Also discussed are reports on other research involving the surface modification of titanium metal.

The chapter entitled *"Radiological Assessment and Predictive Meaning of Bone Remodeling in Cementless Implant"*, by Philippe Massin and Jean-Alain Epinette, deals with several kinds of radiographic changes that are currently observed following insertion of a cementless femoral component in total hip arthroplasty, including bone modeling and particle-induced osteolysis. The purpose of this chapter is to assess the predictive value of these radiographic changes on implant fixation.

"The Extent of Hydroxyapatite Coating : Proximal versus Full Coating with Custom Stems Using Compacted Bone Preparation", is addressed by Jean-Noël A. Argenson, Pierre-Paul Ettore, and Jean-Manuel Aubaniac. Numerous experimental and clinical studies have shown the effectiveness of hydroxyapatite coating in providing rigid biological fixation of femoral components. However, the clinical and radiographic effects of varying the extent of hydroxyapatite on a femoral component of one design has not been evaluated. This chapter focuses on a study that compares the clinical and radiographic findings of one cementless femoral stem design that is coated with hydroxyapatite in two different ways, fully-coated, and proximally-coated. All patients received a cementless custom femoral component designed using computed

tomography and made using computer-aided manufacturing techniques. This chapter details the results of this study, and suggests that further study is required to extend this comparison to traditional stem systems implanted into a reamed femoral preparation.

In *"The Effect of the Metal Substrate on Biologic Fixation with Hydroxyapatite"*, William L. Jaffe and Harlan Levine review the effect of the metal substrate on the biologic fixation of hydroxyapatite and evaluate the influence of the metal substrate, surface texture, and HA on biologic fixation. In this chapter, they discuss the results obtained from an implantable bone chamber model used to assess the effects of different metal substrates, varying surface textures, and hydroxyapatite in a canine model of bone-to-prosthesis apposition. The chapter concludes with a brief review of the results of using HA-coated metal substrates in different mechanical environments; the femoral and acetabular components of a total hip arthroplasty are used as a paradigm.

The design of the implant is interesting with respect to the primary stability as well as the long term fate of the prosthesis. In *"Proximal Modularity in a Cementless HA-Coated Hip Replacement: Assessment of Utility"*, Michel P. Philippe, Gérard Gacon, André Ray, and Alain Dambreville report on preliminary experience with a modular system. According to the authors, some questions regarding the different modes of fixation for uncemented stems remain unanswered. Therefore, they set out to design an implant that would obtain both primary and secondary fixation in the metaphysis alone, since there was evidence that stress transfer to the rest of the femur takes place in that part of the bone. The Esop stem is presented by the authors as an original design with three features that may be of fundamental importance: fixation confined to the metaphysis, HA coating, and modularity. This study cannot be considered a consecutive one and, therefore, serves simply as a trial clinical series to achieve a better understanding of the proposed design, focusing mainly on the intraoperative selection of implants and technical tips, as well as demographics, complications and radiological findings.

On the acetabular side, Scott W. Siverhus and Dawanna R. Bryant report on *"Early Clinical Results of an Arc-Deposited Hydroxyapatite-Coated Acetabular Component in Total Hip Arthroplasty"*. There is conflicting literature support for the use of HA coating on acetabular components. Implant design has been implicated in the variable failure rates reported at early follow up in HA-coated shells. Specifically, the ability of the acetabular shell to provide adequate bone interlock to resist shear forces is considered critical to long term stability. Given the biocompatibility and osteoconductive properties of HA, combining it with a macrostructured biocompatible metal surface theoretically presents an appealing combination for an acetabular design. In this chapter, the authors review their early clinical and radiographic results of a consecutive series of 78 patients (93 hips) that have been prospectively evaluated and followed annually after primary total hip arthroplasty using an arc-deposited HA-coated titanium acetabular component. To date, no patients have required revision of any of the components for septic loosening, aseptic loosening, mechanical failure, osteolysis, or pain.

As stated by J.M. Oosterbos, H. Ch. Vogely, W.J.A. Dhert, and A.J. Tonino in their paper *"Hydroxyapatite-coated Ti6Al4V Implants and Peri-implant Infection – Microbiological, histological and histomorphometrical studies in a rabbit tibial model and a human hip"*, the relationship between implant bioactivity and infection susceptibility has not yet been clarified. Therefore, they formulated several questions such as: "Will the use of noncemented HA-coated titanium implants influence the rate of postoperative infection?", and "Will the use of noncemented HA-coated titanium implants also influence the way in which an infection develops if it does occur?" Female New Zealand White rabbits were used for this study, which was designed to investigate the infection susceptibility and osseointegration related to peri-implant infection of two commonly used surfaces for noncemented fixation of orthopaedic implants, grit blasted Ti6Al4V as a biocompatible surface, and hydroxyapatite plasma-sprayed Ti6Al4V as a bioactive surface. Additionally, the authors also report on a postmortem study they conducted on a patient who sustained a postoperative infection after total hip replacement and recovered without removal of the prosthesis.

A clinical report on the critical relationship between HA and infection has been provided by Jean-Pierre Vidalain and the ARTRO Group: *"Hydroxyapatite and Infection – Results of a consecutive series of 49 infected total hip replacements"*. The biological properties of hydroxyapatite

(HA) in the promotion of osseointegration and the achievement of early stabilization have been extensively documented. The authors believe it is also possible that the biological fixation provided by HA may also improve the behavior of implant components exposed to infection. There are, however, very few clinical studies in the literature to show in what way the presence of an HA coating could affect the resistance to infection of the implant components. Interestingly, the authors present herein the experience of the ARTRO Group with regard to infective complications which, although rare, may cause a poor functional outcome or worse. Although this study was not performed to show that the risk of infection is less with HA-coated prostheses than with conventional prostheses, HA could be seen as an effective means of controlling infection.

The last chapter belonging to this section has been authored by Hironobu Oonishi and Hiroshi Fujita and describes long term results with an original use of HA combined with bone cement, detailed in, *"The 13 Year Experience of a Novel Cementing Technique Using HA Granules Interface Bioactive Bone Cement (IBBC)"*. With respect to cemented hip arthroplasty, even with contemporary cementing techniques, cement pressurization is often imperfect, especially in the fixation of acetabular components. This contributes to the high failure rate and aseptic loosening observed with cemented acetabular components. Despite the use of the best surgical techniques, there is a limit to what can be achieved with pressurized cement. The use of bioactive materials interposed at the bone-cement interface, with the hope of achieving further interdigitation, may be an attractive option. In this chapter, the pros and cons of IBBC and HA coatings are compared and examined in great detail.

CLINICAL EXPERIENCES IN PRIMARY HIPS AT A MINIMUM OF 10 YEARS

In, *"Two Decades Of Hydroxyapatite Coatings In Total Hip Replacement"*, M. George, M. Mueller, and J. Shepperd report on extensive experience with HA hips. During a sixteen year period beginning in 1986, the authors evaluated five different

stem designs and six different cup designs. Between 1986 and 1991, 346 HA-coated total hip replacements were performed in 301 patients. With results now at up to 16 years, the only case of femoral loosening followed major trauma. The authors placed no lifestyle limitations on their patients, and their long-term clinical results are excellent.

The French ARTRO Group has the longest experience in France with the HA-coated CORAIL stem. Jean-Pierre Vidalain elaborates on this experience in, *"Corail Stem Long Term Results – 15-Year ARTRO Group Experience"*. It has been 15 years since the Corail prostheses were first implanted. From September 1986 to December 2000, the ARTRO Group performed 2,956 CORAIL prostheses surgeries in 2,580 patients. Excluding patients deceased or lost to follow-up, over 2,775 cases remain available for analysis. Two hundred forty-three cases have more than 10 years follow-up. On the femoral side, the HA fully-coated standard Corail stem has been used in all cases. If one takes as an end point any failure of the biological fixation, the survival probability of the Corail prosthesis is 100%. Although no revision has been performed on the femoral side for aseptic loosening, polyethylene wear is a reality, and any subsequent osteolysis may pose a potential risk of destabilization in the future.

Survivorship analysis has become one of the most reliable tools when determining the long term outcome of implants. With reference to the works of the Scandinavian registers, the main goals of this method of analysis are to first report an updated epidemiological analysis of hip replacement, then to identify risk factors for failures leading to revision procedures, and finally, to describe the importance of continual improvement of surgical technique by independent risk factor analysis. As a contribution to the evaluation of the long-term outcome of hydroxyapatite (HA)-coated hips, the study by Jean-Alain Epinette and Michael T. Manley report on *"Long-Term Survivorship Analysis of Hydroxyapatite-Coated Hips, based upon a 15-Year Clinical Experience with Three Different Models of HA-Coated Omnifit Stems"*. This study reports on a series of 2,199 cases where HA stems used in primary surgery were followed up from 1987 to 2002. Of the 2,199 primary hips in the current study, 1,892 hips (86.04%) in 1,570 patients remain "on file". Interestingly, when selecting only hip related failures as an end point, revised or not, the cumulative survival rates were 98.98% ±0.0043 at 5 years, then 98.47% ±0.0080 at 10 years, and finally, 98.15 ±0.0080 at 12 years. In addition, comparative survivorship analyses were also carried out. These included patient-related factors, such as age, gender, weight, or aetiology, which would likely affect changes in the outcome of the arthroplasty.

The chapter entitled *"Hydroxyapatite Femoral Stems for Total Hip Arthroplasty: 10-14 Year Follow-up"* by James A. D'Antonio, William N. Capello, Michael T. Manley, Rudolph G. T. Geesink, and William L. Jaffe, discusses the results of hip replacement surgeries performed from 1987 to 1990 by five surgeons in four centers. From 1987 to 1990, fifteen surgeons implanted 380 Omnifit-HA stems in eight centers. Five surgeons in four centers continue to follow 267 of these hips beyond ten years. Their primary objectives were to evaluate long-term stem fixation, functional results, and radiographic bony response to the implant. Of the cups implanted with the 267 hip stems still followed, 143 were hydroxyapatite threaded, 74 were hydroxyapatite press-fit, 47 were porous press-fit, and three patients (three hips) received a bipolar prosthesis. A complete evaluation (a calculable Total Harris Hip Score) was available at latest follow-up for 186 hips evaluated between 10 and 14 years. No stems were radiographically loose. However, it is noted that the overall success rate with the acetabular components has not matched that of the hydroxyapatite-coated femoral stem.

Ch. Nourissat, J. Adrey, D. Berteaux, and C. Goalard report on their *"Clinical Experience with the ABG Total Hip Arthroplasty"*. Between February 1989 and March 1990, 294 ABG total hip prostheses, with cementless cups and cementless stems, were implanted by the authors in a continuous series. At present, 96% of the hips are pain-free. This retrospective analysis of the clinical results demonstrated very high stability and the absence of the early thigh pain often observed with cementless implants without bioactive coating. Osteointegration was observed at the third month postoperatively and remained constant due to the initial stability of the implant. Taking all 294 primary interventions into consideration, results showed that the ABG-HA prosthesis has a 92.18% survival rate at 10 years post implantation, if the change of the implant or only a part of the implant is a criteria of failure. The analysis of explants originating from revisions on account of wear or

osteolysis revealed no third body wear associated with the resorption of HA coating.

Another chapter devoted to study of the ABG stem is presented by A. J. Tonino, C. J. M. Oosterbos, A. I. A. Rahmy, and W. D. Witpeerd in *"The ABG Hydroxyapatite-coated Hip Prosthesis Followed-up for 9-11 Years"*. The hip prosthesis described in this article is designed for proximal osseointegration only and, therefore, only proximal off loading. To enhance further proximal offloading and to inhibit distal off loading, the stem has an anatomic shape, which permits distal over-reaming. The HA coating was applied with a vacuum plasma-spray torch on a sublayer of pure titanium in order to improve the tensile adhesion of the HA of the implant. The first goal was to evaluate, through clinical and radiographic assessment, whether or not the prosthesis did fulfill the design criteria. The second goal of the study was to confirm that proximal circumferential osseointegration reduces or eliminates femoral diaphyseal osteolysis. The poor performance of press-fit cups in these studies has been the success limiting factor of the procedure. Therefore, there is reason for concern about the relatively high percentage of polyethylene induced acetabular osteolysis in these kind of press-fit metal-backed cups with open screw holes. In contrast to the noted acetabular osteolysis, no distal or linear osteolysis around the stem was observed in any case after 9 to 11 years of follow up. Also, in the cases that augmented acetabular osteolysis, where the extended joint space surely had also extended to the femoral side, only very moderate local cystic osteolysis was noted in 8 cases. This can only be explained by a complete proximal sealing of the medullary cavity by circumferential bone ongrowth. Histology of retrieved autopsy specimens have acknowledged this circumferential sealing through circumferential osseointegration.

The Italian experience with HA-coated implants comes from Bologna and is presented in *"10 Years Follow Up Experience With A Hydroxyapatite-Coated Hip Arthroplasty"*, by Aldo Toni, Francesco Traina, Susanna Stea, Barbara Bordini, Enrico Guerra, Alessandra Sudanese, and Armando Giunti. The authors report the ten year results of 151 An.C.A hip systems, the design of which includes a collarless hydroxyapatite-coated femoral stem and a ceramic-on-ceramic coupling. The AnCA hip arthroplasty uses a cobalt-chrome alloy stem, 13cm long, anatomically shaped, proximally porous-coated in the medial, anterior, and posterior faces, and fully-coated with plasma-sprayed hydroxyapatite (HA). Six cups required revision surgery for aseptic loosening, and 6 stems were revised for thigh pain. At revision surgery, the stems were firmly fixed to the bone. A whitish powder mould surrounded the stems retrieved; the HA coating loss was macroscopically evident, since the metallic stem surface was largely exposed. The authors found a 92.5% survival rate of the AnCA prosthesis at 10 years follow up, which does not differ significantly from the 93% rates of other prostheses followed by The Swedish National Total Hip Arthroplasty Register.

Apart from standard stems, the HA-coated customized systems are of great interest, mainly because the bioactive coating must deal with the particularly challenging geometry of the femoral shapes. Thus, the contribution to this book of *"The Symbios HA Custom Stem At Ten Years"*, by Jean-Noël Argenson and Jean-Manuel Aubaniac is notable. The custom made hip prosthesis is now integrated into the whole concept of computer assisted hip arthroplasty, which includes computer assisted preoperative planning, computer assisted designing of custom hip prostheses, and computer assisted hip surgery. The extramedullary custom neck has been able to solve many of the surgical difficulties faced in the cases of excessively anteverted upper femurs, often found in dysmorphic or dysplastic hips. Between January 1990 and January 2000, 1,156 cementless custom stems were implanted. Focusing only on patients 65 years old or less, and excluding revisions of another prostheses, the initial series consisting of 726 hips left 680 hips to study at an average of 5.6 years of follow-up. The authors report clinical results at 10 years that are at least as good as or better than previously reported clinical reports results in young age groups where modern cementing techniques were used with conventional cemented implants, or where standard cementless prostheses were used.

An interesting contribution from Spain and the USA has been afforded by Joaquín Sánchez-Sotelo and Miguel E. Cabanela regarding the *"Clinical Results with the Omniflex HA Femoral Stem"*. Periprosthetic osteolysis caused by the effects of wear particles on bone is noted to be one of the most common failure modes of hip arthroplasty. It is theorized that wear-related bone loss might be prevented by decreasing the amount of debris produced by hip arthroplasty components, or by limiting the access of particles to the bone-implant interface. To the authors' knowledge, no study has focused solely on the role of HA coating in generating femoral osteolysis. The authors conducted a retrospective study of patients who underwent primary hip replacement with insertion of an Omniflex HA-coated femoral component. None of the 68 hips in this study developed osteolysis in Gruen zones two to six. Although HA particulate material found at the periprosthetic tissue of retrieved implants has been implicated in third body wear, the authors did not find any increase in polyethylene wear.

Whether or not an implant is being successfully integrated into the host bone can be judged from X-ray films only. Radiographic evidence can often be obtained well before there are clinical manifestations and is of paramount importance for predicting the eventual outcome of the arthroplasty. J. A. Epinette, M. T. Manley, and Ph. Massin carried out a detailed study on the *"Radiographic Analysis of HA-coated Hip Femoral Components at 10-15 Years of Follow-up"*. In this chapter, the authors report on radiographic results of a prospective continuous series of 500 HA-coated Omnifit and Omniflex stems with a minimum of 10 years radiological follow-up.

Designed in 1987, the PRA stem was intended to reflect the lessons learned from the frequent failures of cementless implants and the hopes raised by the introduction of HA coatings. The results of this device, which has been in clinical use since 1988, encouraged Roland Petit to present *"Ten-Year Results of the PRA Stem"*. The PRA stem is characterized by its pronounced proximal flare and distal taper. It is collarless and its HA coating involves only the proximal one-third of the stem, while the rest of the stem has a mat surface. The device is made of grit-blasted anodized titanium alloy. The series was composed of 87 hips in 83 consecutive patients operated on between January 1988 and June 1991. On the acetabular side, a variety of implants were used. Survivorship analysis using only implant-related failures as the endpoint accounted for two cases (2.3%) out of a total of 87 hips, including one operative error (inappropriate choice of stem size) and one failure of implant fixation. Therefore, the failure rate at ten years of the HA fixation of the PRA stem was 1 case in 87 (1.15%).

On the acetabular side, HA threaded cups remain controversial. J.A. Epinette, M.T. Manley and E. Duthoit report on *"Long-term Results with the HA-coated Arc2f in Primary Hip Surgery"*. Acetabular replacement is a challenging procedure in hip arthroplasty. The implanted cup and its fixation interfaces must cope with the stresses imposed by patient activity as well as stresses imposed by neck impingement at the extremes of motion. For many years, a stable fixation alone was considered to be the ultimate goal in acetabular arthroplasty, but currently, complex problems such as wear, migration of particles, and osteolytic lesions tend to be the major concern. The authors enter the debate about threaded cups by reporting on a continuous series of 602 primary HA-coated screw cups (Arc2f) implanted from 1989 to 1991. These cups have a minimum follow-up of 10 years and a maximum of 13 years. Clinical and radiological results reported in this chapter cover only those patients reviewed both clinically and radiologically at 10 year minimum follow-up. The success achieved with this Arc2f implant suggests that early threaded designs that performed poorly did so because no provision for long-term stability in the form of secondary fixation was provided.

The so-called "expansion cups" are another option in acetabular components. Alain Dambreville reports on the *"Minimum Ten-Year Follow-Up Of The HA-Coated Atlas Cup"*. The Atlas cup is a press-fit acetabular component. It consists of a hemispherical shell made of a titanium alloy (Ti6Al4V) with a split in the lower part to provide elasticity. The titanium shell is very thin (2.5 mm), so as to allow a maximal thickness of polyethylene (PE) to be inserted. This study was a prospective study of a consecutive series of 151 primary hip replacements performed between 1990 and 1991. In this study, 109 cups were reviewed, 61 at a follow-up of eleven years, and 48 at a follow-up of ten years. This study suggests that HA-coated metal-backed cups are reliable, provided the PE insert has been firmly seated in the shell and is of sufficient thickness. The HA coating was found to be effective in terms of providing secondary stabilization of the implant and in limiting the migration of PE wear particles.

HA IN REVISION HIP SURGERY

The first paper in this section, written by N. Passuti, J. Delécrin, and G. Daculsi, focuses on *"Experimental Data Regarding Macroporous*

Biphasic-Calcium Phosphate Ceramics: Can they replace bone grafting ?". Calcium phosphate ceramics are bioactive products and the closest relatives to the mineral phases of calcified tissues. Calcium phosphates and their composites with a calcium phosphate ceramic base, such as autogenous bone, collagen, and fibrin glue, show considerable potential and value for bone reconstruction. In comparison with the other biocompatible biomaterials, calcium phosphates are bioactive ceramics. They take part in exchanges between the cells and neighboring tissues, which is in contrast to the bioinert ceramics, such as alumina. This chapter examines in detail the unique bioactive properties of hydroxyapatites, tricalcium phosphates, and bicalcium phosphates.

Another interesting means of reconstructing acetabular defects is presented by Hironobu Oonishi and Hiroshi Fujita, each of whom have extensive experience using *"HA Granules in Acetabular Reconstruction"*. In 1986, the authors began using sintered HA granules clinically. During the "first generation" of use (1986-1992), HA granules were used to fill cavitary deficiencies, after which the entire surface of the exposed HA granules at the peripheral deficiencies were covered with bone cement. However, spaces were subsequently observed between HA granules and nearby bone and, in cases of large acetabular wall deficiencies, the prostheses migrated. Consequently, in the second generation (1993 to present), peripheral segmental deficiencies were covered with bulk allografts to gain stable filling of HA granules. This chapter reports on the results of this innovative reconstructive approach.

The use of allograft material to restore bone stock and promote bone healing and implant stabilization is a crucial part of total joint arthroplasty, especially in the revision situation. Allograft bone is an attractive alternative to autograft bone because it supports bone formation, its supply is less limited than autograft, and large structural restorations are possible. However, allograft bone has only a fraction of the osteoinductive capacity of autograft bone and a lower capacity to incorporate with host bone. Stephen D. Cook and Robert L. Barrack report on an osteogenic protein-1 device in their paper entitled *"The Use of the OP-1 Implant in Reconstructive Surgery of the Hip and Knee"*. The use of an OP-1 Implant alone or in conjunction with autograft or allograft bone offers many potential advantages. In addition to better defect healing, bone ingrowth to a porous surface may be enhanced with the use of the OP-1 Implant. Theoretically, this speeds the rehabilitation process and shortens the time of protected weight bearing and the attendant functional disability for the patient. The results of the effectiveness of OP-1 for healing bone defects are presented.

Bruno Balaï and the ARTRO Group authored a chapter about their experience with *"Management of Severe Acetabular Defects Using A Hydroxyapatite-Coated Reconstruction Ring"*. According to the authors, when there has been acetabular component loosening with severe segmental or cavitary bone defects, a threaded or screw-fixed cup cannot be adequately stabilized. There is agreement in the literature that such cases should be managed with reconstruction grafting (to restore the deficient bone stock) and a reinforcement ring (to enhance the strength of the construct and improve graft compression). The authors report herein on their experience with the Octopus cementless ring in the management of some cases of cup loosening with extensive loss of bone stock.

Another paper devoted to cementless HA-coated cups in revision cases is by J. A. Epinette, M. T. Manley, and B. Tillie on *"The Use of the Hydroxyapatite-Coated Arc2f Cup in Acetabular Revision Surgery"*. As an alternative to cement, porous and hydroxyapatite-coated implants have shown positive results in achieving direct bone-implant bonding and preservation of bone stock in the revised acetabulum. The authors present up to 13 years of follow-up experience with a hydroxyapatite-coated threaded hemispherical acetabular component used routinely in the revision setting, and indicate that the Arc2f results compare favorably with the more successful revision hip series in the literature.

The third option in acetabular revision surgery, after reconstruction rings and threaded cups, is addressed by Alfons J. Tonino, Mathijs van der Linde, Will Meijers, and Jelle Schaafsma, in *"Acetabular Revision Using Cementless Hydroxyapatite-Coated Components"*. Although the best method for revising the deficient acetabulum is not known, it has become increasingly obvious that, to achieve long-term cup fixation in the structurally-deficient revision acetabulum, the primary goal is to achieve a sufficient amount of stability on host bone. As new bone bonding surfaces like hydroxyapatite (HA) have been repeatedly shown to promote bone ongrowth, it was tempting to perform

acetabular revision with a HA-coated component under the hypothesis that the HA coating could theoretically compensate for the reduced amount and vitality of the host bone bed. The authors report on the intermediate results of 81 consecutive hip revisions, in which 59 cups were revised for aseptic loosening with a cementless HA-coated ABG acetabular component.

The chapter, by J. C. Chatelet and L. Setiey from the Artro Group, entitled *"Femoral Component Revision With HA-Coated Revision Stems"*, is the only chapter dedicated to femoral revision surgery with an HA-coated femoral stem. Revision following major femoral component loosening can be difficult, both in terms of finding a means of stable fixation of the revision implant and in terms of finding viable bone stock. Adequate primary stability must be obtained, in order to allow the restoration of the badly damaged bone around the new implant, and to ensure the sound and lasting integration of the new device. This means that specially designed implants will be required to obtain the necessary primary stability and to find a solution to the individual patient's needs. The results of two HA-coated femoral implant designs are presented.

HA KNEE IMPLANTS AT OVER 10 YEARS

The first TKA chapter in this section, *"12-year Experience with HA in Primary Knee Arthroplasty"*, was authored by Jean-Alain Epinette and Michael T. Manley. Beginning in 1990, 400 HA-coated knees were implanted in 342 patients. Of the 400 knees, 364 knees remain "on file" (91%). Although the authors argue that technical skills and appropriate design are more important than the interface, this study shows that excellent results were obtained using HA-coated Omnifit knee implants. At minimum ten year follow-up, these results are as good as, and often better than, the best-cemented or porous studies. Radiographic findings were encouraging and confirmed the excellent intimate contact between bone and metal, with no appreciable difference between the minimum 2-year and minimum 5-year follow-up examinations. Furthermore, the HA coating appears over time to aid in filling gaps, a benefit of bioconductive coatings. The encouraging results reported in this study encourage confidence in the ultimate outcome of bioconductive coatings in knee arthroplasty.

The second chapter relays long term HA TKA experience by Oliver Keast-Butler, Rami Hussein, and John Shepperd, the results of which are reported in the chapter, "*Results and Perspectives at Ten Year Follow-Up of a Hydroxyapatite-Coated Total Knee Replacement*". Between March 1990 and November 1992, the authors performed 100 consecutive primary total knee replacements using a fully hydroxyapatite-coated Insall-Burnstein II prostheses, a posterior constrained device that sacrifices the posterior cruciate ligament. The bone interface surfaces of the component are plasma sprayed with hydroxyapatite. If moderate pain at rest or during exercise at the most recent assessment is used as an endpoint for failure, 5 surviving knees (9.3%) are in this category. However, there is no suggestion that this uncemented prostheses is more painful than its cemented version. Uncemented knee replacements have not been popular, and there is a paucity of peer reviewed evidence to suggest that survival matches cemented designs. According to this series, the hydroxyapatite coating has enhanced bone fixation in comparison to other uncemented series, resulting in good, long term results.

The third chapter involves a French and Australian multicenter study on UKAs. Jean-Alain Epinette, David Young, and Hayden Morris present their experiences in, "*Hydroxyapatite-coated Unicompartmental Knee Arthroplasty - A 12-year Experience with the HA Unix Prosthesis*". For some years, hydroxyapatite-coated UKA has been considered a somewhat radical approach to unicompartmental knee arthritis. The present study is based upon a series of 523 UKAs in 457 patients beginning in September of 1990. All patients received HA-coated uni-knee prostheses. This series is made up of consecutive cases who were operated on by the three authors at three clinics using the same protocol. The implanted components were the HA-coated uni-tibial components in all cases. Of the total number of UKAs, 140 (127 patients) had a minimum follow-up of ten years. In all these patients, the femoral component used was a cemented "Mod III"(Richards, USA), since the Unix HA (Osteonics, USA) components did not become available until 1994. Of the entire 523 cases in the series 10 revisions led to retrieval of at least one of the components of the prosthesis (1.9%). Overall, 85.8% of patients with medial replacements and 87% of patients with lateral replacements were pain-free. Less than 1% of knees had a flexion under 90 degrees, 27.4% could flex 140 degrees, and 2% exceeded 160 degrees flexion. Overall, excellent bone ongrowth (without any interposed fibrous tissue) was confirmed in more than 95% of the cases with the HA-coated Unix knee.

The last chapter is a brief note by Philippe Cartier about his own experience with "*The Use of Hydroxyapatite in Unicompartmental Arthroplasty*". In light of the excellent, long lasting results obtained with cemented UKA between 1974 and 1991, the author has broadened the patient selection criteria in favor of this type of replacement in greater numbers of young and active patients. However, unicompartmental implants must withstand an overwhelming level of stresses under load compared to TKAs. Because the functional needs of these young patients, mainly males, have become increasingly demanding due to trying physical exercises routinely practiced either during their sport or professional activities, it became obvious that the ever increasing risk of implant loosening over time had to be borne in mind, especially in cemented prostheses.

2 The "Frequently Asked Questions" About Hydroxyapatite Coatings

Thomas W. Bauer, MD, PhD, James A. D'Antonio, MD, Hironobu Oonishi, MD, PhD, Aldo Toni, MD, Alfons J. Tonino, MD, PhD, William K. Walter, FRCS, William N. Capello, MD and P. Serekian, MS

For the past fifteen years, similar questions have been asked about HA-coated implants. We asked our advisory board to respond to five common questions about the use of hydroxyapatite in orthopaedics.

Q1 - Why would you choose to use HA-coated implants in your practice instead of cemented implants or porous metallic coated implants? In what cases would you choose not to use an HA-coated implant?

The ultimate goal of any joint arthroplasty is intimate bone contact and stabilization by bone. As demonstrated by the chapters in this book, the gold standard for such stabilization is hydroxyapatite coating fixation.

Avoid cement when possible in young active patients would be of interest. It is known that when the design of a stem and its surface roughness are improperly matched, the result can be early failure of the cement-stem interface. Also, over-reaming of cancellous bone or the absence of robust cancellous structures at surgery can lead to early loosening of the cement-bone interface. During surgery, modern cemented procedures need complex devices to mix and inject the cement, the bone bed must be dried, the cement must cure leading to longer surgery times. When cemented implants are done poorly, cement particulates may participate in a third body wear process and jeopardize the longevity of the bearing. Cementless HA coated stems require simply the attainment of a stable implant at surgery. The HA/bone interfaces have proven to be durable and excellent results are achieved routinely in young active patients as well as in the elderly.

Porous metallic coatings may allow bone ingrowth and stabilization of the implant. However, surgery must be more precise than with HA coated devices as the gaps that can be filled in between metal and bone must be less than 50 microns. In the presence of gaps or lack of proper implant stability, fibrous tissue ingrowth is common. Even when an excellent fit is achieved at the time of the insertion, micromotion may occur later on. Such micromotion may lead to unstable and painful implants, especially in hip stems and knee tibial plateaus. If fibrous tissue fixation is achieved, the fibrous layer does not seal the implant interface to debris penetration and osteolytic lesions may occur in supporting structures. Experimental evidence suggests strongly that HA coated implants are always stabilized more quickly by bone ongrowth than the porous implants stabilized by bone ingrowth.

It is now accepted that when properly applied, hydroxylapatite coatings enhance the speed, strength and quantity of bony attachment. Histological analyses reflecting clinical studies carried out for more than 15 years, show that a direct and intimate bonding between implant and bone is obtained. In some instances, gaps of over 300 microns were observed to be filled with bone. As long as the implant design is appropriate for the stresses applied during daily activity, osseointegration is obtained within a few weeks, the implant interfaces are sealed and appear to stand the test of time (15 years) in clinical applications.

In summary, the use of HA-coated implants can be supported in most patients as long as primary mechanical stability of the device can be achieved at surgery. The literature suggests no limitation because of patient age, weight, or aetiology is necessary. If primary mechanical fixation cannot be achieved at surgery, the use of cement fixation is recommended.

Q2 – Do you use HA-coated hip implants in the femur, acetabulum, or both ? Do you use HA-coated knee implants in the femur, tibia, patella, or all three ? What is your experience using HA-coated implants for primary surgery compared to revision surgery ?

With primary hips, there is generally no limitation to the use of HA-coated implants. However, the requirements for fixation in acetabulum are different from the requirements for fixation in the femur. Each site is subjected to different stresses and strains. For the acetabulum, we know now that interlock of bone into the implant shell is crucial to the longevity of fixation. Interlock is especially important in zone 3, below the implant, so that tensile loading of the interface can be resisted. The design of the implant is important also in the femur. Here a grit-blasted surface for the femoral component is not only adequate for fixation, but allows the implant to be extracted if this is required later during the life of the patient. The stem design must provide initial stability. Later ongrowth onto the HA surface provides long-term fixation and seals the fixation interface to debris penetration.

In total knee arthroplasty, the use of hydroxyapatite fixation has been adopted more slowly than in hips. HA-coated knees became available only in 1990, when technical obstacles related to coating of complex internal shapes of the implants were overcome. Adoption of HA knees has been slow, perhaps because of good results with cemented knees or because of a less forgiving surgical environment for cementless designs. Again fixation with the femoral component was resolved more readily than for the opposing side of the joint. The femoral component is inherently stable and only requires the HA coating for interface maintenance and interface sealing. In the tibia, the tibial tray is subjected to in plane and to tilting stresses, especially if the knee is not balanced correctly or if the cuts are not precise. Thus, similarly to the acetabulum, loosening may occur in tibial components not designed properly for the stress environment encountered during daily living. In the patella, the reality of thin polyethylene and a metal backing required by application of the HA coating has meant adoption of knees without patella replacement or simple cementing of a patella button. We know now that HA-coated TKR, and HA-coated UKR provide extremely encouraging results at follow-up of more than 10 years. These knees are performing as well as the best cemented and porous series in the literature.

With regard to using HA-coated implants for primary versus revision surgery, the same benefits that the HA coating brings to the primary situation are desirable for the revision scenario. In the revision situation all the problems of primary surgery regarding implant stabilization are magnified. Any implant surface that will help the host to recover bone quality and bone quantity is an asset. We know that for bone ongrowth, there must be direct contact between the hydroxyapatite coating and living bone. Thus the two prerequisites for using HA in revision are first a secured primary mechanical fixation, and second at least 50% of direct contact between bone and coating. This principle works for both stem and cup. To quote Tonino, "especially in revision, where bone stock can be very compromised, the use of HA-coated implants is even more compelling, not only for faster osseointegration, but also to compensate for the less vital host bone". The fate of bone grafts in apposition to an HA coating is controversial. Generally speaking, HA cannot induce new bone formation if the coating is in contact with dead bone. Bone conduction along the HA coating from the nearest viable bone is the best result that may be expected in this situation.

Q3 – Are you confident in the stability of the HA-bone interface over the long term, even though the HA coating will eventually be resorbed ?

This probably is the most frequently asked question regarding HA-coatings. The coating may be resorbed or may be remodeled. As the coating is resorbed after implantation, the release of calcium and phosphate ions provides a calcium rich region around the implant enhances new bone formation. In this way, the HA coating works as a starter for new bone formation. The hydroxyapatite surface acts as a substrate for the new bone and void filling around the implant occurs both from the bone bed and from the implant surface. Once the implant is embedded in bone, the primary goal of the coating has been achieved. As time goes by, the HA coating participates in the physiological turn over of bone around the implant. Osteoclastic resorbtion of bone close to the coating will remove regions of the coating also. Osteoblasts lay down new bone, and in areas where the coating has been removed, this new bone may be in contact with the implant substrate. Coating resorbtion differs according to the location and the amount of stresses that is applied (Wolfe's Law) in a particular area. Where the stress is high, new bone formation replaces the former coating. When the area is a bit "quiet", the coating can be found intact, even after many years implantation.

Within this natural life of the HA coating, the coating must withstand the mechanical stresses applied to the implant surfaces. For interfaces subjected to bending and moderate shear stresses (e.g., hip stems) a microstructured or grit-blasted surface provides good stability of the coating on metal, and allows simple extraction of the implant from the bone bed. For implants subjected to high shear and tensile stresses (e.g., hip cups, tibial implants), protection of the coating by surface features of the implant is required. Macroporous HA-coated substrates can enhance biological fixation while insuring an augmented interlocking mechanism.

Clinical experience has suggested that long term stability of HA-coated implants is a multifactorial process, dependent upon the physiochemical nature of the interface between bone and implant, the microtexture of the implant surface, the shape and flexibility of the device, local physiologic Ph, and other factors that can be attributed to device, surgeon, and patient. HA coatings of many different formulations induce nearly complete bone apposition within several weeks after the device is implanted into a suitable host site. Experience has shown us that bone will remain in close contact with the implant. In areas of high stress where the HA coating has been remodeled away, direct attachment of bone to the implant substrate has been demonstrated in evaluation of retrieved human specimens. Toni's conclusion would be, summing up the consensus from the panel: HA may resorb but this does not mean that this resorbtion jeopardizes the quality of osseintegration.

Q4 – Have you experienced any complications or adverse reactions, such as third body wear, that you believe are directly related to the HA coating ?

Some 10 years ago a number of investigators suggested that particles released from HA coatings could be involved in "third body wear" in the hip. A few years ago, Frayssinet and the ARTRO group reported an interesting case of calcium phosphate particulates embedded into the polyethylene insert of an acetabular component...however, the prosthesis was a cemented one. Other reports of hydroxyapatite particulates detected in the joint space were dismissed by Doyle, who demonstrated that the tests used could not determine the origin of these hydroxyapatite particles, and the particle type is found in numerous locations within the body. According to Bauer: " Calcium phosphates have been detected on the articular surface of retrieved implants, but have not been proven to have originated from HA coatings. Although delamination and third body wear will remain a theoretical concern, clinical results and the results of animal studies and human retrievals suggest that for contemporary designs, it is not a clinically important problem."

Q5 – In general, are you satisfied with plasma-sprayed hydroxyapatite in its current state, or do you think it could be improved upon by combining it with bioglasses, improved substrates, or biologic factors ?

It is difficult to be unsatisfied with HA-coated implants applied by plasma spray technology, especially when the superb clinical results described in this book are compared to other fixation technologies. Most of the implants described in this volume were grit-blasted plasma-sprayed titanium and despite this 20 years old technology, they have stood the test of time, without the need of major changes in the technical process. Nevertheless, some problems have occurred giving the way to some novel developments. In acetabular replacement, the unexpected rate of failures in HA-coated grit blasted cups led to development of a rough HA coated fixation surface. In tibial trays, an HA-coating applied onto rough titanium or titanium foam offer advantages in resistance to implant lift-off. Despite proven longevity of these plasma sprayed coatings, the plasma-spray techniques now begins to look dated.

As stated by the members of the panel, some tracks should be explored. The first idea is to enhance the quality of the actual coating. The choice of coating chemistry remains a balance between a higher resorption coating, that increases the bioactivity, and a higher durability coating, that decreases the bioactivity. Thus, Tri Calcium Phosphates (TCP) coatings are bioactive but resorbable. High crystallinity HA is very stable but less bioactive. Perhaps a multiphase coating, with a high activity layer over a stable substrate will be the next coating of choice.

Another possibility is to use electrochemical deposition of hydroxyapatite rather than plasma spray. This is currently achieved with the solution deposited Peri-Apatite™ process. The thin periapatite coating, active because of its high surface to volume ratio, is applied onto a porous metal substrate. This coating develops enhanced "bone ingrowth" instead of ongrowth, and allows development of a new generation of three-dimensional coatings for bone interlock.

The new coating technologies, such as laser surface powder cladding, electrophoretic nanotechnology or ion-beam-assisted-deposition (IBAD), are exciting, but will have to be proven clinically. The coating of porous implants with Ca-P by using the biomimetic route, based on the nucleation and growth of Ca-P from supersaturated calcifying solutions called Simulated Body Fluids (SBF); will allow the coating of complex shaped non metallic materials. If they could be validated clinically, such coatings will be less fragile than the plasma sprayed or electrochemically deposited coatings. Conversely, the use of bioglasses holds little future as a real competitor for calcium phosphates. According to Bauer: "The replacement of a hydroxyapatite coating with a bioactive glass defies logic."

With regard to bone growth factors, the panel showed little support for their use in the primary total joint. There is a need for less expensive versions of growth factors for new developments in difficult or revision cases with major bony defects: "The incorporation of osteoinductive or other bioactive factors may have a role in revision arthroplasty, but is unlikely to improve the results of primary arthroplasty...". All members of the panel showed interest in combining HA coatings with bioactive coatings, osteoinductive proteins or any other drug delivery products. As stated by Tonino: "Combining these coatings with bioglasses to fill cavities, or with biological factors like OP-1 for faster bone in- or ongrowth or with alendronate to prevent periprosthetic bone loss from stress shielding may give even better clinical performance", or Walter: "Combining hydroxyapatite with other materials and biological factors promises to become an important tool in joint replacement surgery, particularly in revision surgery in the future..."

While "current hydroxyapatite or periapatite are working well with no adverse reaction", Toni confirmed, further developments are needed. If validated, these might afford new possibilities in joint replacement. As stated by D'Antonio: "With regard to improving its (HA coating) biologic activity by combining it with other biologic factors or improved substrates, the search is essential and certainly should be carried out. However, any improvement over what is known today with regard to HA advantages must be measured against any increased cost versus increased benefit..." The final word from Bauer regarding the future of HA coatings is "The search for improved substrate texture, optimum geometry and flexibility appears to be unending..."

3 Afterword
"Hydroxyapatite Coatings: The First Fifteen Years"

In this book we have attempted to describe the "state of the art" in hydroxyapatite coatings in orthopaedics as this stands at the close of 2002. The book attempts to present an up-to-date summary of studies with hydroxyapatite coatings, from fundamental research to the clinical results obtained with HA-coated hip and knee replacements in patient populations. From around the world, some ninety scientists – surgeons, biophysicists, histologists, and bioengineers – have contributed their results to this volume. The book exists only because of their efforts, and we are grateful to them.

From conception, our interest was to provide a forum to allow some of the most prominent researchers in this subject to express their views, however contradictory these views might be. We received manuscripts from Europe, the United States, Australia, and Japan and simply assembled these into our volume, although allowing ourselves some latitude to edit for language or layout. We trust we have not changed the sense of an author's work and have assembled a coherent document. We hope also that the comprehensive bibliographies presented with each chapter will be a useful tool and source of further reading for those interested in studying the field further.

Review of the manuscripts collected show that, in much of the world, HA coatings are an accepted fixation technology and are an integral part of the orthopaedic scene. Together with hip and knee prostheses fixed with polymethylmethacrylate cement or by ingrowth into porous metal surfaces, HA-coated joint replacements are now considered mainstream orthopaedic products, and HA coatings are a distinct fixation technology in their own right. Proponents claim that HA coatings provide a unique fixation surface that is more forgiving of errors in implant placement and is less dependent on initial implant stabilization to bone than either cement or porous fixation. Further, claims of more rapid patient rehabilitation than with the more traditional fixation methods are frequently made. Unfortunately, standard clinical scoring systems are incapable of determining this potential improvement in patient recovery in an objective manner, and doubters remain unconvinced of what they perceive to be simple anecdotal evidence of the superiority of HA fixation over other methods.

In spite of the limitation of patient scoring systems to assess nuances of implant and patient performance, even skeptics should now be impressed by the long term implant survivorship and the favorable radiographic results achieved by HA-coated implants when compared to older fixation technologies. The manuscripts contained in this volume alone detail a number of studies with survivorship of better than 98% at more than ten years follow-up together with radiographic evidence of bone remodeling that suggests a stable fixation interface. Case reports show that, in spite of concerns of coating dissolution or digestion leading to a loose implant, as suggested by some authors, bone remodeling around the implant now includes remodeling of the coating. Studies described both here and in the literature suggest that the remodeling bone adapts itself to the base material of the implant, and that the implant remains stable *in situ*. Surgeons removing an HA-coated implant for reasons other than loosening often report that the bone bed is a mirror image of the topography of the fixation interface of the implant. This finding is rarely reported for other cementless devices removed for reasons unrelated to fixation.

In Europe, HA-coated implants are often referred to as "HA: The Third Track" and form a major part of the cementless implant market. In Asia, Australasia, and Canada, too, hydroxyapatite-coated hip and knee devices enjoy widespread use. In the United States, although there are fierce proponents of the technology, many surgeons see little advantage with HA-coated hip stems compared to ingrowth or ongrowth metal designs. This skepticism remains, even though peer reviewed publications in the North American literature show compelling clinical results with HA-coated hips at thirteen or more years follow-up. With respect to TKA, in spite of twelve years clinical experience in Europe, Asia, and the Antipodes with HA-coated unicompartmental and total knee implants associated with the type of excellent results published in this text, HA-coated knees of any type are not yet commonly used in the United States. Whether this lack of adoption is due to a perception that results with cemented knees cannot be beaten, or to a more onerous regulatory environment in the US than elsewhere, or to a lack of commitment from an orthopedic manufacturer is unclear. We trust that the data contained in this volume will help to convince the more skeptical surgeons and the manufacturers of orthopaedic implants in the United States that hydroxyapatite fixation technology is worth a second look.

Finally, as editors of this volume, we feel we should acknowledge those individuals who have collaborated with us over the years and who were responsible for the beginning of the use of hydroxyapatite coatings in orthopaedics. In the United Kingdom, Ronald Furlong and his group; in the Netherlands, Rudolf Geesink, Klaas deGroot and his group, and Gied Hermsen; in France, Jean-Pierre Vidalain and the Artro Group; in Scandinavia, Kjeld Søballe and his group; and in the United States, John Kay, Paul Serekian, and Thomas Bauer. We remain enthusiastic about the use of hydroxyapatite fixation. In the Preface to *Hydroxyapatite Coatings in Orthopaedic Surgery (1993)*, it was noted that HA-coated implants were remarkably stable and pain free at four to six years follow-up. The hope was expressed that "only time is required to see whether this favorable trend continues into long-term ten year results". Now that these same implants are successful out to fifteen years follow-up, we must trust that, at twenty years post implantation, clinical performance and clinical survivorship of HA implants will be as compelling as it is now.

Jean-Alain Epinette, MD
Bruay La Buissiere, France
Michael T. Manley, PhD
Franklin Lakes, New Jersey, USA
Août 2003

Achevé d'imprimer sur les presses de l'Imprimerie BARNÉOUD
BP 44 - 53960 BONCHAMP-LÈS-LAVAL
Dépôt légal : septembre 2004 - N° d'imprimeur : 13781
Imprimé en France